ATLAS OF
Radiologic
Measurement

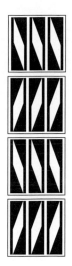

ATLAS OF
Radiologic
Measurement

SEVENTH EDITION

Theodore E. Keats, M.D.
Professor of Radiology
University of Virginia
Charlottesville, Virginia

Christopher Sistrom, M.D.
Department of Radiology
University of Florida
Gainesville, Florida

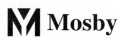 **Mosby**
A Harcourt Health Sciences Company
St. Louis   London   Philadelphia   Sydney   Toronto

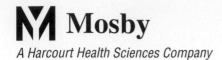

Mosby
A Harcourt Health Sciences Company

Acquisitions Editor: Janice Gaillard
Project Manager: Evelyn Adler
Production Manager: Natalie Ware
Illustration Specialist: Rita Martello
Book Designer: Marie Gardocky-Clifton

SEVENTH EDITION
Copyright © 2001, 1990, 1985, 1978, 1972, 1967, 1959 by Mosby, Inc.

Mosby, Inc.
A Harcourt Health Sciences Company
11830 Westline Industrial Drive
St. Louis, Missouri 63146

Printed in the United States of America.

Library of Congress Cataloging-in-Publication Data

Keats, Theodore E. (Theodore Eliot)
Atlas of radiologic measurement / Theodore E. Keats, Christopher Sistrom.—7th ed.

p.; cm.

Rev. ed. of: Atlas of roentgenographic measurement / Theodore E. Keats, 6th ed.
© 1990.
Includes bibliographical references and index.

ISBN 0–323–00161–0

1. Radiography, Medical—Measurement—Tables. 2. Radiography,
Medical—Atlases. I. Sistrom, Christopher. II. Keats, Theodore E. (Theodore
Eliot), Atlas of roentgenographic measurement. III. Title.

[DNLM: 1. Radiography—Atlases. 2. Reference Values—Atlases. 3. Tomography,
X-Ray Computed—Atlases. 4. Ultrasonography—Atlases. WN 17 K25ab 2001] RC78.K315
2001

616.07′572—dc21   00–060938

01 02 03 04 05 9 8 7 6 5 4 3 2 1

This book is dedicated to Howard L. Steinbach,
the originator of the concept of this work.

Preface

When you can measure what you are speaking about, and express it in numbers you know something about it; but when you cannot measure it, when you cannot express it in numbers, your knowledge is of a meager and unsatisfactory kind; it may be the beginning of knowledge, but you have scarcely in your thoughts, advanced to the stage of science.

WILLIAM THOMSON, LORD KELVIN
Popular Lectures and Addresses
(1891–1894)

This seventh edition serves to introduce a new author, Dr. Chris Sistrom, who will carry on this work in subsequent editions. In this current edition we have introduced changes in format, organization, and scope that we believe will improve the usefulness of the work. In accordance with the many changes that have taken place in diagnostic imaging in recent years, we have again attempted to select those new entities that have practical utility and to avoid esoterica. The work is now called *Atlas of Radiologic Measurement* to reflect the fact that many of the measurements that we commonly deal with now come from modalities other than radiography. We have also eliminated or replaced those measurements that have not been found to have great usefulness in clinical practice. This work is not intended to be encyclopedic, yet we hope that our readers will find it a useful aid in their everyday work.

In addition to the normative data that has formed the core content of past editions, we have added sections dealing with quantitative and semiquantitative methods for diagnosis and prediction. Examples of techniques using direct measurement include ultrasound examination of the pylorus for hypertrophic stenosis, Doppler ultrasound of native renal arteries for stenosis, and magnetic resonance imaging to detect hepatic iron overload. Newly added semiquantitative methods include a scoring system for ovarian masses, grading of avascular necrosis of the hip, and bayesian analysis for predicting malignancy in pulmonary nodules.

We have not included material about nuclear medicine because by its very nature the discipline is quantitative, and standard texts address the subject well. Obstetric ultrasound has matured in the past two decades so as to virtually have become a separate specialty. We have included updated material about pelvimetry, standard biometry, amniotic fluid quantification, and umbilical artery velocimetry. However, we did not attempt to cover fetal measurement in its entirety, as it would fill a whole book and the subject is well covered in comprehensive texts. Cardiac magnetic resonance, echocardiography, and coronary artery calcification scoring were not included because of the huge volume and dynamic nature of research in these fields. Functional brain imaging, magnetic resonance spectroscopy, and perfusion/diffusion brain imaging are rapidly being brought to the point of general utility, and like quantitative cardiac imaging, would merit inclusion in the next revision.

To address these issues, we may change the title of subsequent editions to *Quantitative Imaging*, seek additional editorial help in specialty areas, and split the book into several volumes. We hope that this text will continue the fine tradition established by Drs. Lusted and Keats in producing a practical, useful, and authoritative reference for practitioners and researchers. Readers are encouraged to contact Dr. Sistrom with criticism, suggestions, and important new references to help plan the scope and format of later editions.

THEODORE E. KEATS, M.D.
CHRIS L. SISTROM, M.D.

Acknowledgments

We gratefully acknowledge the generosity of the many imaging scientists throughout the world who graciously allowed us to adapt material from their works for use in this forum. The American College of Radiology was very helpful in allowing us to use their coding system to provide a familiar and useful ordering of the material. We wish to express our appreciation to our secretary, Pat Steele, for her great help and for her unfailing equanimity in the face of author-engendered stress. We also thank Janice Gaillard and the rest of the staff at Harcourt Health Sciences for helping to bring this book to fruition. Most importantly, we express our deep gratitude to our spouses, Patt and Brenda. Throughout this process, they freely gave us their unflagging devotion, invaluable help, and constant encouragement.

THEODORE E. KEATS, M.D.
CHRIS L. SISTROM, M.D.

Contents

CHAPTER 1

Intracranial Contents

▪▪
▪

▪: VOLUMES OF INTRACRANIAL STRUCTURES
▪ ACR Code: 1 (Skull and Contents)

Technique ▪

MR images were performed on a 1.5-T scanner (GE Signa). Sagittal T1-weighted (500/11), axial proton density (3000/31), and axial T2 (3000/90) sequences were obtained on all subjects.

Measurements ▪

The axial image data were transferred to a SPARC workstation (SUN Microsystems) running the ANALYZE software (Biomedical Imaging Resource, Mayo Foundation). A combination of multispectral tissue segmentation, interactive

Table 1 ▪ Volumes of the Ventricles, Subarachnoid CSF, and Total CSF in 194 Subjects by Gender and Age

AGE (Yr)	NUMBER	LATERAL VENTRICLES	THIRD VENTRICLE	FOURTH VENTRICLE	VENTRICULAR CSF	SUBARACHNOID CSF	TOTAL CSF	VBR
Women								
16–25	20	14.7 ± 6.8	0.7 ± 0.2	1.5 ± 0.6	17.4 ± 7.2	72.0 ± 30.9	89.4 ± 36.7	1.32 ± 0.53
26–35	24	14.3 ± 6.9	0.7 ± 0.2	1.5 ± 0.4	16.9 ± 7.2	79.0 ± 29.6	95.9 ± 32.7	1.36 ± 0.56
36–45	22	12.8 ± 4.7	0.7 ± 0.3	1.5 ± 0.4	15.4 ± 5.0	95.8 ± 29.9	111.2 ± 31.7	1.24 ± 0.37
46–55	24	13.2 ± 3.7	0.8 ± 0.2	1.3 ± 0.5	15.5 ± 3.8	100.8 ± 28.9	116.3 ± 30.3	1.27 ± 0.28
56–65	15	21.1 ± 11.3	1.2 ± 0.6	1.4 ± 0.5	24.2 ± 12.2	123.1 ± 30.9	147.4 ± 34.9	2.08 ± 1.11
Men								
16–25	24	15.3 ± 6.2	0.7 ± 0.2	1.7 ± 0.6	18.1 ± 6.6	67.7 ± 29.2	85.8 ± 29.8	1.20 ± 0.42
26–35	19	15.2 ± 4.5	0.7 ± 0.2	1.9 ± 0.7	18.3 ± 4.5	94.5 ± 35.7	112.8 ± 37.8	1.27 ± 0.31
36–45	16	16.1 ± 6.3	1.0 ± 0.4	2.1 ± 0.6	19.7 ± 6.5	118.9 ± 35.0	138.6 ± 38.0	1.40 ± 0.45
46–55	15	17.0 ± 4.8	1.1 ± 0.4	1.5 ± 0.5	21.0 ± 5.1	115.5 ± 36.5	136.4 ± 38.8	1.52 ± 0.43
56–65	15	24.8 ± 12.1	1.3 ± 0.4	1.5 ± 0.4	28.1 ± 12.3	163.0 ± 62.3	191.4 ± 65.5	2.07 ± 0.88

Measurements are in cubic centimeters (mean ± standard deviation). The ventricle/brain ratio (VBR) is also shown and is equal to ventricular CSF volume/total brain volume.
From Blatter DD, Bigler ED, Gale SD, et al: AJNR Am J Neuroradiol 1995; 16(2):241–251. Used by permission.

Table 2 ▪ Volumes of Gray Matter, White Matter, Total Brain Volume, and Total Intracranial Volume (TICV) of 194 Subjects by Gender and Age

AGE (Yr)	NUMBER	GRAY MATTER	WHITE MATTER	TOTAL BRAIN	TICV
Women					
16–25	20	694.78 ± 112.71	616.21 ± 109.00	1310.99 ± 79.74	1400.33 ± 93.09
26–35	24	647.54 ± 98.61	586.26 ± 79.34	1233.79 ± 102.43	1329.67 ± 112.37
36–45	22	611.71 ± 105.79	628.68 ± 108.83	1240.39 ± 102.96	1351.62 ± 110.79
46–55	24	580.94 ± 81.68	645.95 ± 103.27	1226.89 ± 138.06	1343.19 ± 146.41
56–65	15	597.59 ± 60.71	590.55 ± 106.22	1188.14 ± 95.75	1335.49 ± 82.98
Men					
16–25	24	761.84 ± 106.99	746.45 ± 89.25	1508.29 ± 106.90	1594.10 ± 101.39
26–35	19	749.09 ± 83.62	687.56 ± 106.49	1436.66 ± 79.85	1549.43 ± 81.98
36–45	16	740.70 ± 112.63	666.61 ± 120.34	1407.31 ± 99.34	1545.91 ± 130.94
46–55	15	712.74 ± 73.27	683.77 ± 108.43	1396.51 ± 108.58	1532.89 ± 89.29
56–65	15	691.47 ± 130.51	666.37 ± 137.92	1357.84 ± 100.59	1548.91 ± 106.09

Measurements are in cubic centimeters (mean ± standard deviation).
From Blatter DD, Bigler ED, Gale SD, et al: AJNR Am J Neuroradiol 1995; 16(2):241–251. Used by permission.

image editing, and region of interest pixel counting was used to define outlines of structures to be measured on all pertinent slices. These areas were summed and corrected for slice thickness and interval to obtain volumes. Table 1 gives volumes of CSF compartments and the ventricle/brain ratio (VBR) for all subjects, segregated by age and gender. Table 2 shows volumes of gray matter, white matter, total brain, and total intracranial volume (TICV) grouped by gender and age of the subjects.

Source ▪

Healthy volunteers whose age ranged from 16 years to 65 years, consisting of 105 women and 89 men.

REFERENCE

1. Blatter DD, Bigler ED, Gale SD, et al: Quantitative volumetric analysis of brain MR: Normative database spanning 5 decades of life. AJNR Am J Neuroradiol 1995; 16(2):241–251.

▪▪ VOLUMES OF YOUNG ADULT BRAIN STRUCTURES
▪ ACR Code: 1 (Skull and Contents)

Technique ▪

Coronal spoiled gradient echo T1-weighted images were done on two scanners. Ten scans (4 men, 6 women) were done on a 1.5-T Magnetom machine (Siemens Medical Systems, Iselin, NJ), using FLASH sequences (TR = 40 msec, TE = 8 msec, flip angle = 50 deg). Ten scans (6 men, 4 women) were imaged on a 1.5-T Signa system (General Electric Corporation, Milwaukee, WI) using 3D-CAPRY sequences (TR = 50 msec, TE = 9 msec, flip angle = 50 deg).

Measurements ▪

Image data were transferred to computer workstations (Sun Microsystems, Mountainview, CA). A 3-D Cartesian coordinate system was used, referenced to the commissures and bisecting the interhemispheric fissure. Anatomic segmentation was done using intensity contour mapping and differential intensity contour algorithms on coronal images. Pri-

mary borders were automatically registered where possible and were defined as signal intensity transitions (e.g., CSF/brain interfaces or gray-white matter borders). Secondary borders were defined by hand to define structures, using knowledge-based anatomic subdivisions where needed. To obtain volumes, the total number of voxels for each structure was multiplied by the absolute volume of each voxel. Table 1 gives combined volumes of all structures studied for men and women and the sum of both sides where bilateral. Table 2 shows the volumes of all structures with men and women combined and divided by left and right. Table 3 gives the volumes of all structures with both sides summed and divided by gender.

Source ▪

Healthy female volunteers (n = 10) with an average age of 26.9 years, and male volunteers (n = 10) whose average age was 27.4 years.

Table 1 ▪ Volumes of Normal Brain Structures

STRUCTURE	MEAN ± SD	MINIMUM	MAXIMUM	% TOTAL VOLUME
Whole brain	1380.1 ± 113.9	1173.3	1625.6	100.0
Total cerebrum	1192.1 ± 102.5	1007.5	1403.5	86.4
Neocortex	688.8 ± 65.0	573.7	828.5	57.8
White matter	443.8 ± 42.4	376.2	515.8	37.2
Caudate	9.5 ± 1.3	7.3	11.7	0.8
Lenticulate	14.1 ± 1.1	11.9	16.6	1.2
Putamen	10.1 ± 0.9	8.7	1.4	0.9
Pallidum	3.9 ± 0.5	3.1	5.2	0.3
Hippocampus	9.9 ± 1.2	7.2	11.5	0.8
Amygdala	5.5 ± 0.8	4.0	7.0	0.5
Central gray nuclei	20.5 ± 1.7	18.1	24.1	1.7
Total cerebellum	143.4 ± 12.5	123.8	175.1	10.4
Cortex	119.7 ± 10.6	102.9	146.3	83.5
Central mass	23.7 ± 2.9	19.1	29.6	16.5
Ventricular system	21.3 ± 7.4	10.3	36.4	1.5
Lateral	18.1 ± 7.3	7.3	33.7	85.0
Third	1.3 ± 0.5	0.3	2.2	6.1
Fourth	1.9 ± 0.6	1.0	36	8.9
Brain stem	23.4 ± 3.1	19.5	32.3	1.7

All measurements (except percent of total) are in cubic centimeters (mean ± standard deviation).
From Filipek PA, Richelme C, Kennedy DN, Caviness VS Jr: Cerebral Cortex 1994; 4(4):344–360. Used by permission.

Table 2 ▪ Volumes of Normal Brain Structures by Side

STRUCTURE	RIGHT	LEFT
Total cerebrum	606.3 ± 53.5	603.9 ± 54.1
Neocortex	346.2 ± 33.0	342.6 ± 32.2
White matter	221.8 ± 20.7	221.1 ± 22.2
Caudate	4.7 ± 0.7	4.8 ± 0.7
Putamen	5.1 ± 0.4	5.0 ± 0.5
Pallidum	1.9 ± 0.3	1.9 ± 0.3
Central gray nuclei	10.2 ± 0.9	10.3 ± 0.9
Amygdala	2.9 ± 0.4	2.6 ± 0.4
Hippocampus	4.9 ± 0.7	5.1 ± 0.7
Lateral ventricle	8.1 ± 3.1	9.9 ± 4.6
Cerebellum	71.5 ± 6.4	71.9 ± 6.1

All measurements are in cubic centimeters (mean ± standard deviation).
From Filipek PA, Richelme C, Kennedy DN, Caviness VS Jr: Cerebral Cortex 1994; 4(4):344–360. Used by permission.

Table 3 ▪ Volumes of Normal Brain Structures by Gender

STRUCTURE	MEN	WOMEN
Whole brain	1434.8 ± 116.2	1325.4 ± 85.4
Total cerebrum	1235.6 ± 109.6	1148.5 ± 77.2
Neocortex	714.4 ± 69.4	663.2 ± 51.5
White matter	462.4 ± 46.2	425.3 ± 30.0
Caudate	8.8 ± 1.2	10.1 ± 1.1
Lenticulate	14.4 ± 1.2	13.7 ± 1.1
Hippocampus	9.6 ± 1.4	10.4 ± 1.1
Amygdala	5.5 ± 0.7	5.6 ± 0.9
Central gray nuclei	20.7 + 1.7	20.3 ± 1.8
Total cerebellum	152.2 ± 10.5	134.6 ± 6.8
Cerebellar cortex	127.2 ± 8.9	112.3 ± 5.9
Central mass	24.9 ± 3.3	22.4 ± 2.0
Ventricular system	22.6 ± 7.6	20.0 ± 7.3
Lateral ventricle	18.9 ± 7.6	17.3 ± 7.2
III ventricle	1.5 ± 0.5	1.1 ± 0.4
IV ventricle	2.1 ± 0.7	1.7 ± 0.5
Brain stem	24.5 ± 3.4	22.3 ± 2.3

All measurements are in cubic centimeters (mean ± standard deviation).
From Filipek PA, Richelme C, Kennedy DN, Caviness VS Jr: Cerebral Cortex 1994; 4(4):344–360. Used by permission.

Comments ▪

Male cerebellar volumes were larger than female volumes. Also, male cerebral white matter volume and caudate volume were larger than in the women. The neocortex and amygdala were larger on the right, whereas the lateral ventricle was larger on the left.

REFERENCE

1. Filipek PA, Richelme C, Kennedy DN, Caviness VS Jr: The young adult human brain: An MRI-based morphometric analysis. Cerebral Cortex 1994; 4(4):344–360.

▪: SULCAL, VENTRICULAR, AND WHITE MATTER CHANGES IN THE AGING BRAIN
▪ ACR Code: 1 (Skull and Contents)

Technique ▪

MRI scans of the brain in the axial projection were performed with T1 weighting (500/15–25), PD weighting (3000/20–35), and T2 weighting (3000/70–100). Intravenous contrast was not employed.

Measurements ▪

A visual grading system for sulcal size (Fig. 1), ventricular size (Fig. 2), and white matter hyperintensities (Fig. 3) was developed, with 8 steps in each of the three parameters.

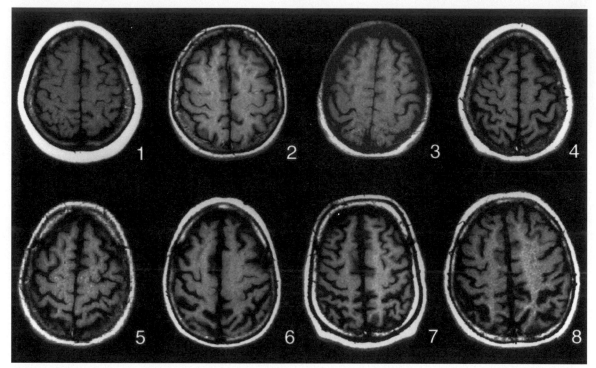

Figure 1 ▪ MR images of sulcal grades 1 through 8. (From Yue NC, Arnold AM, Longstreth WT, et al: Radiology 1997; 202:33–39. Used by permission.)

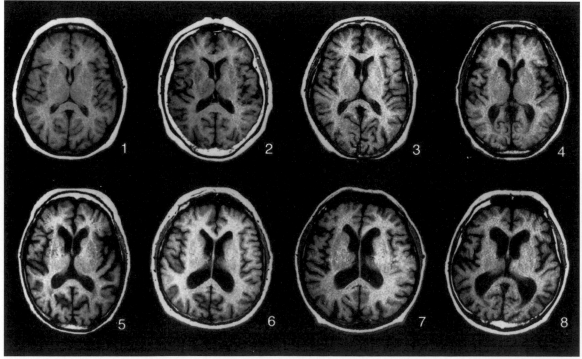

Figure 2 ▪ MR images demonstrating ventricular grades 1 through 8. (From Yue NC, Arnold AM, Longstreth WT, et al: Radiology 1997; 202:33–39. Used by permission.)

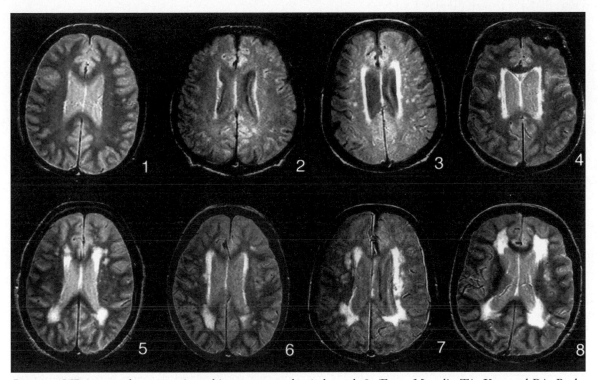

Figure 3 ▪ MR images demonstrating white matter grades 1 through 8. (From Manolio TA, Kronmal RA, Burke GL, et al: Stroke 1994; 25:318–327. Used by permission.)

Table 1 ▪ MR Findings for Different Age Groups in the Entire Cohort

AGE GROUP (Yr)	SULCAL	VENTRICULAR	WHITE MATTER
65–69	2.9 ± 1.0	3.0 ± 1.2	1.7 ± 1.2
70–74	3.2 ± 1.1	3.4 ± 1.2	2.0 ± 1.3
75–79	3.5 ± 1.2	3.7 ± 1.2	2.4 ± 1.4
80+	3.9 ± 1.3	4.2 ± 1.3	2.9 ± 1.7
All	3.4 ± 1.2	3.6 ± 1.3	2.3 ± 1.5

The mean ± standard deviations of assigned scores are given.
From Yue NC, Arnold AM, Longstreth WT, et al: Radiology 1997; 202:33–39. Used by permission.

Table 2 ▪ MR Findings in the Healthier Subgroup by Gender and Age

AGE GROUP (Yr)	SULCAL		VENTRICULAR		WHITE MATTER	
	Men	Women	Men	Women	Men	Women
65–69	5	4	5	4	3	3
70–74	5	5	6	5	4	4
75–79	5	5	6	5	4	5
80+	6	5	6	6	6	5

Numbers are the grade category containing the 95th percentile for each group (95% of patients will have a score less than or equal to the grade shown).
From Yue NC, Arnold AM, Longstreth WT, et al: Radiology 1997; 202:33–39. Used by permission.

MRI scans of the patients were graded according to this system and correlated with age (Tables 1 and 2).

Source ▪

The study population consisted of 3660 adults from the cohort of the Cardiovascular Health Study (CHS). A subgroup of 1488 healthier adults was identified. These had no history of CNS disease or cardiac problems and no focal abnormalities on the MRI scans.

Comments ▪

Sulcal size, ventricular size, and white matter hyperintensity grades all increased with age (p = <.0001).

REFERENCES

1. Yue NC, Arnold AM, Longstreth WT, et al: Sulcal, ventricular, and white matter changes at MR imaging in the aging brain: Data from the Cardiovascular Health Study. Radiology 1997; 202:33–39.
2. Manolio TA, Kronmal RA, Burke GL, et al: Magnetic resonance abnormalities and cardiovascular disease in older adults. Stroke 1994; 25:318–327.

▪▪ T1 VALUES IN NORMAL BRAIN TISSUES
- ▪ ACR Code: 13 (Brain and Meninges, Supratentorial)

Technique ▪

Seven studies of T1 values in normal brain structures are included.[1-7] The machines used ranged in field strength from .02 T to 4 T. All imaging was done in the axial plane for both localizing scans and signal strength determinations. Typically, a scan at the level of the lateral ventricles, including the head of the caudate and thalamus, was chosen from a standard T1 sequence. After that, a second set of sequences was performed in that plane only, mostly using inversion recovery technique with a long TR (1500–2500) and 3 or 4 more different T1 values (range, 50–2400). In one study at .28 T,[5] a triple spin echo sequence was used with 3 different TR values (320, 640, 1920). At 4 T, 3 different techniques were used to obtain T1 information.[1] These included the fast low-angle shot (FLASH) with progressive saturation, the Look-Locker method,[8] and inversion recovery with interleaved echo-planar imaging.

Measurements ▪

The images obtained in the single-level multi-acquisition sequences were analyzed by placing region of interest (ROI) cursors over structures to be analyzed and recording signal intensity values. The series of values from each structure was applied to a curve-fitting algorithm (usually nonlinear regression), using various simplifications and modifications of the Bloch equations[9] so as to obtain T1 relaxation time values. Table 1 lists T1 values in various brain tissues as reported.[1-7]

Source ▪

In one study at .28 T, scans were done on patients with various abnormalities, including tumors, hematoma, and edema.[5] The normal values were obtained from areas of brain well away from any pathology. In the rest of the series, normal volunteers or patients with scans judged to be normal were used as subjects. The number of subjects ranged from 23 to 164.

Comments ▪

Note that the T1 values in brain strongly depend on field strength.

Table 1 ▪ T1 Relaxation Times Obtained from Normal Brain Tissues at Various Field Strengths (.02 T to 4 T)

Reference	Jezzard[1]	Steen[2]	Steen[3]	Breger[4]	Just[5]	Wahlund[6]	Agartz[7]
No. Subjects	23	26	55	164	160	24	79
Age Range	24–65	18–60	18–72	5–90	5–80	75–85	19–85
Average Age	not given	35	41	38	not given	79	50
Field Strength	4	1.5	1.5	1.5	.28	.02	.02
Technique	3 methods (see technique)	IR	IR	IR	TRIPLE SE	IR	IR
No. Measurements	multiple	4	4	4	3	3	3
Cortical White Matter	1043 ± 27	570 ± 18	572 ± 21	752	401 ± 38	220 ± 16	208 ± 18
Cortical Gray Matter	1724 ± 51	1013 ± 62	999 ± 54		625 ± 50		
Caudate	1458 ± 38	928 ± 26	928 ± 24	1220		248 ± 12	239 ± 16
Thalamus		758 ± 24	764 ± 31	996		245 ± 19	224 ± 19
CSF	4550 ± 800	4282 ± 1552					

Relaxation times given as mean ± standard deviation. IR = inversion recovery, SE = spin echo.

REFERENCES

1. Jezzard P, Duewell S, Balaban RS: MR relaxation times in human brian: Measurement at 4 T. Radiology 1996; 199:773–779.
2. Steen RG, Gronemeyer SA, Kingsley PB, et al: Precise and accurate measurement of proton T1 in human brian in vivo: Validation and preliminary clinical application. J Magn Reson Imaging 1994; 4(5):681–691.
3. Steen RG, Gronemeyer SA, Taylor JS: Age-related changes in proton T1 values of normal human brain. J Magn Reson Imaging 1995; 5(1):43–48.
4. Breger RK, Yetkin FZ, Fischer ME, et al: T1 and T2 in the cerebrum: Correlation with age, gender, and demographic factors. Radiology 1991; 181:545–547.
5. Just M, Thelen M: Tissue characterization with T1, T2, and proton density values: Results in 160 patients with brain tumors. Radiology 1988; 169:779–785.
6. Wahlund LO, Agartz I, Almqvist O, et al: The brain in healthy aged individuals: MR imaging. Radiology 1990; 174:675–679.
7. Agartz I, Saaf J, Wahlund LO, Wetterberg L: T1 and T2 relaxation time estimates in the normal human brain. Radiology 1991; 181:537–543.
8. Look DC, Locker DR: Time saving in measurement of NMR and EPR relaxation times. Rev Sci Instrum 1970; 41:250–251.
9. Bloch F: Nuclear induction. Phys Rev 1946; 70:460–473.

▪: T2 VALUES IN NORMAL BRAIN TISSUES
▪ ACR Code: 13 (Brain and Meninges, Supratentorial)

Technique ▪

Five studies of T2 values in normal brain structures are included.[1–5] The machines used ranged in field strength from .02 T to 4 T. All imaging was done in the axial plane for both localizing scans and signal strength determinations. Typically, a scan at the level of the lateral ventricles, including the head of the caudate and thalamus, was chosen from a standard T2 sequence. After that, measurements were performed in the chosen plane using either a multiple echo spin echo (1920–2000/20–272) sequence[2, 3] or three separate single echo SE (2000/100,150,200) sequences.[4, 5] In the study done at 4 T, an interleaved echo-planar SE (10,000/25–700) sequence as well as a multiecho SE (2500/25–700) sequence was done at the selected level.[1]

Measurements ▪

The images obtained in the single level multiecho or separate single echo sequences were analyzed by placing region of interest (ROI) cursors over structures to be analyzed and recording signal intensity values. The series of values from each structure was applied to a curve-fitting algorithm (usually non-linear regression) using various simplifications and modifications of the Bloch equations[6] so as to obtain T2 relaxation time values. Table 1 lists T2 values in normal brain tissues as reported.[1–5]

Source ▪

In one study at .28 T, scans were done on patients with various abnormalities, including tumors, hematoma, and edema.[3] The normal values were obtained from areas of brain well away from any pathology. In the rest of the series, normal volunteers or patients with scans judged to be normal were used as subjects. The number of subjects ranged from 23 to 164.

Table 1 ▪ T2 Relaxation Times Obtained from Normal Brain Tissues at Various Field Strengths (.02 T to 4 T)

Reference	Jezzard[1]	Breger[2]	Just[3]	Wahlund[4]	Agartz[5]
No. Subjects	23	164	160	24	79
Age Range	24–65	5–90	5–80	75–85	19–85
Average Age	not given	38	not given	79	50
Field Strength	4	1.5	.28	.02	.02
Technique	2 methods (see technique)	SE MULTI-ECHO	SE MULTI-ECHO	SE SINGLE ECHO ± X3	SE SINGLE ECHO ± X3
No. Measurements	multiple	4	8	3	3
Cortical White Matter	50 ± 2	75	122 ± 3	95 ± 10	95 ± 15
Cortical Gray Matter	63 ± 6		143 ± 17		
Caudate	46 ± 11	77		98 ± 14	99 ± 21
Thalamus		76		100 ± 14	98 ± 21
CSF	704 ± 245				

Relaxation times given as mean ± standard deviation. SE = spin echo.

REFERENCES

1. Jezzard P, Duewell S, Balaban RS: MR relaxation times in human brain: Measurement at 4 T. Radiology 1996; 199:773–779.
2. Breger RK, Yetkin FZ, Fischer ME, et al: T1 and T2 in the cerebrum: Correlation with age, gender, and demographic factors. Radiology 1991; 181:545–547.
3. Just M, Thelen M: Tissue characterization with T1, T2, and proton density values: Results in 160 patients with brain tumors. Radiology 1988; 169:779–785.
4. Wahlund LO, Agartz I, Almqvist O, et al: The brain in healthy aged individuals: MR imaging. Radiology 1990; 174:675–679.
5. Agartz I, Saaf J, Wahlund LO, Wetterberg L: T1 and T2 relaxation time estimates in the normal human brain. Radiology 1991; 181:537–543.
6. Bloch F: Nuclear induction. Phys Rev 1946; 70:460–473.

▪: TEMPORAL LOBE AND HIPPOCAMPAL VOLUMES RELATED TO AGE
▪ ACR Code: 134 (Temporal Lobe)

Technique ▪

A 1.5 T Signa (General Electric, Milwaukee, WI) MRI machine was used for the study by Sullivan.[1] Oblique coronal images were made using a multiecho, flow-compensated, cardiac-gated sequence (2800/40,80). The imaging plane was defined from a parasagittal scout image to be perpendicular to the sylvian fissure. A 1.5 T machine (manufacturer not given) was used in Bigler's study.[2] Fast spin echo (3800/21, 105), intermediate, and T2-weighted oblique coronal images were made through the temporal lobes.

Measurements ▪

Image data were transferred to a computer graphics workstation in both studies.[1, 2] The hippocampal formations (HF), temporal lobe white and gray matter, and temporal cerebral sulci were outlined manually from each slice, aided by automated tissue segmentation algorithms. The areas were summed and corrected for slice interval to obtain volumes in cubic centimeters.[1] Similar techniques were used to measure bilateral HF volumes and the volume of the temporal horn of the lateral ventricle.[2] Figure 1 shows the HF volumes for each side plotted against age.[1] Figures 2 and 3 depict the volumes of temporal white and gray matter plotted against age.[1] Tables 1 and 2 give the HF and temporal horn volumes for 5 age groups, by gender and for the population as a whole.[2]

Source ▪

Sullivan's group recruited 77 healthy male volunteers, aged 21 to 70 years. There was an average of 14 subjects within each decade. There were 53 right-handed, 8 left-handed, and 10 undefined dominance subjects as judged by answers to a questionnaire.[1] Subjects for Bigler's study included 96 healthy volunteers (37 male and 59 female) ranging in age from 16 to 65 years old.[2] Candidates who reported drinking more than 53 grams (4 drinks) of ethanol per day were excluded, as were any with dementia or any significant medical or psychologic condition.[1, 2]

Comments ▪

Sullivan found no significant differences in HF volumes based on age or handedness, whereas the temporal lobe gray matter decreased in volume with age and the temporal sulcal CSF volume increased with age.[1] Bigler found a modest correlation of HF volume with age (r = −0.33, p = 0.001). However, analysis of variance (ANOVA) across decades showed no significant effect. Men had slightly larger raw HF volumes, and this difference reversed with correction for overall brain size. Temporal horn volume did not change with age.[2] Right to left differences are detailed in another section of this chapter.

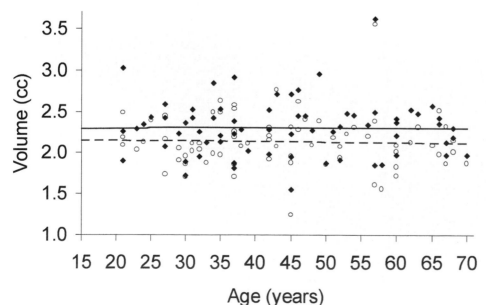

Figure 1 ▪ Scatterplot of left (*open circles*) and right (*solid diamonds*) HF volumes related to age (20–70 years). Linear regressions for both sides (*left = dashed line, right = solid line*) are shown. (From Sullivan EV, Marsh L, Mathalon DH, et al: Neurobiol Aging 1995; 16(4):591–606. Used by permission.)

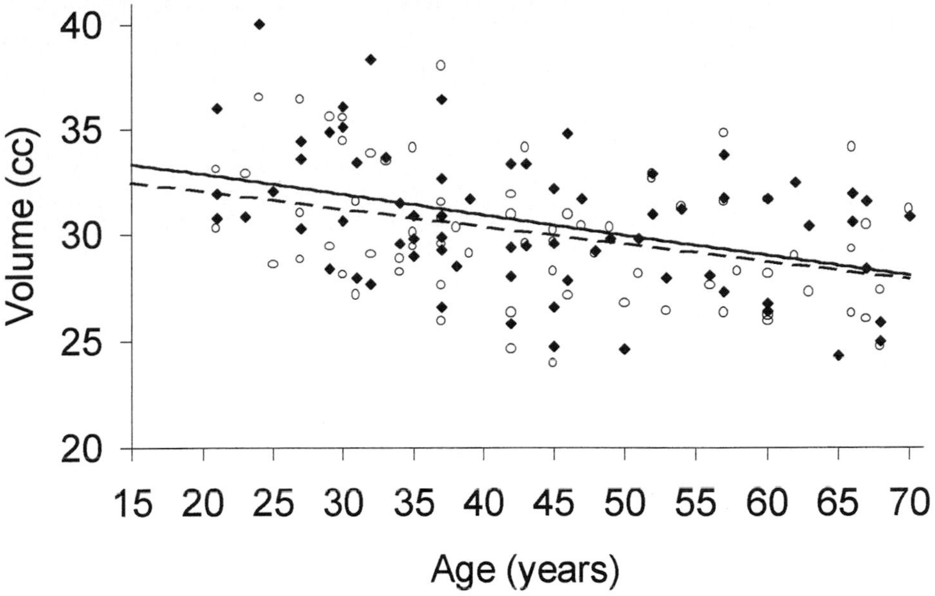

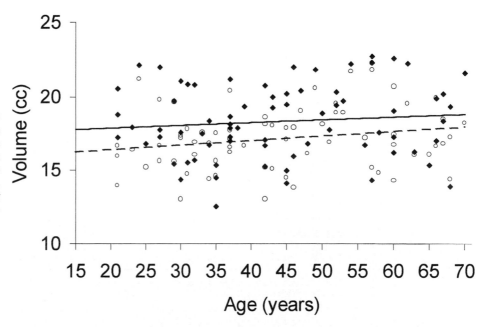

Figure 2 ▪ Scatterplot of left (*open circles*) and right (*solid diamonds*) temporal lobe gray matter volumes related to age (20–70 years). Linear regressions for both sides (*left = dashed line, right = solid line*) are shown. (From Sullivan EV, Marsh L, Mathalon DII, et al: Neurobiol Aging 1995; 16(4):591–606. Used by permission.)

Table 1 ▪ **Volumes of the Hippocampal Formations Related to Age and Gender**

AGE RANGE (Yr)	GENDER	NUMBER	R HIPPOCAMPUS	L HIPPOCAMPUS	TOTAL HIPPOCAMPUS
16–25	Both	16	2.73 ± 0.3	2.68 ± 0.33	5.41 ± 0.58
26–35	Both	15	2.58 ± 0.3	2.47 ± 0.31	5.05 ± 0.56
36–45	Both	18	2.56 ± 0.3	2.51 ± 0.19	5.07 ± 0.43
46–55	Both	23	2.41 ± 0.2	2.38 ± 0.27	4.80 ± 0.47
56–65	Both	24	2.45 ± 0.3	2.36 ± 0.30	4.81 ± 0.56
16–65	Male	59	2.65 ± 0.29	2.58 ± 0.32	5.23 ± 0.59
16–55	Female	37	2.45 ± 0.24	2.39 ± 0.26	4.85 ± 0.48
16–55	Both	96	2.53 ± 0.26	2.46 ± 0.29	4.99 ± 0.54

Measurements are in cubic centimeters (mean ± standard deviation).
From Bigler ED, Blatter DD, Anderson CV, et al: AJNR Am J Neuroradiol 1997; 18:11–23. Used by permission.

Figure 3 ▪ Scatterplot of left (*open circles*) and right (*solid diamonds*) temporal lobe white matter volumes related to age (20–70 years). Linear regressions for both sides (*left = dashed line, right = solid line*) are shown. (From Sullivan EV, Marsh L, Mathalon DH, et al: Neurobiol Aging 1995; 16(4):591–606. Used by permission.)

Table 2 • Volumes of the Temporal Horns of the Lateral Ventricles Related to Age and Gender

AGE RANGE (Yr)	GENDER	NUMBER	R TEMPORAL HORN	L TEMPORAL HORN	BOTH TEMPORAL HORNS
16–25	Both	16	0.34 ± 0.11	0.37 ± 0.22	0.70 ± 0.27
26–35	Both	15	0.30 ± 0.15	0.23 ± 0.09	0.53 ± 0.19
36–45	Both	18	0.31 ± 0.14	0.43 ± 0.26	0.57 ± 0.23
46–55	Both	23	0.28 ± 0.13	0.47 ± 0.24	0.52 ± 0.21
56–65	Both	24	0.36 ± 0.19	0.56 ± 0.30	0.66 ± 0.30
16–65	Male	59	0.36 ± 0.16	0.31 ± 0.15	0.67 ± 0.28
16–55	Female	37	0.29 ± 0.14	0.26 ± 0.13	0.55 ± 0.23
16–55	Both	96	0.31 ± 0.15	0.28 ± 0.14	0.6 ± 0.25

Measurements are in cubic centimeters (mean ± standard deviation).
From Bigler ED, Blatter DD, Anderson CV, et al: AJNR Am J Neuroradiol 1997; 18:11–23. Used by permission.

REFERENCES

1. Sullivan EV, Marsh L, Mathalon DH, et al: Age-related decline in MRI volumes of temporal lobe gray matter but not hippocampus. Neurobiol Aging 1995; 16(4):591–606.

2. Bigler ED, Blatter DD, Anderson CV, et al: Hippocampal volume in normal aging and traumatic brain injury. AJNR Am J Neuroradiol 1997; 18:11–23.

BILATERAL HIPPOCAMPAL VOLUMES IN ADULTS
- ACR Code: 1341 (Hippocampus, Inferior Temporal Gyri)

Technique •

Sixteen studies in which the normal right and left adult hippocampal formations (HF) were measured are included in this analysis.[1-16] MRI field strength varied from 1.0 T to 1.5 T, and various high resolution 2D coronal or 3D sequences were employed (Table 1). Most of the 2D coronal sequences were angled to be perpendicular to the long axis of the Sylvan fissure as determined from sagittal scans. When 3D sequences were used, a similar oblique coronal plane was selected to mark and measure the HF.

Table 1 • Hippocampal Volumetrics in Normal Adults from 16 Published Studies

STUDY	FIELD STRENGTH	SEQUENCE	NUMBER	NORMALIZED	RIGHT VOLUME	LEFT VOLUME	R − L VOLUME	SUGGESTED THRESHOLDS
Jack[1]	1.5	SE (600/20)	52	TICV	2.8 ± 0.1	2.5 ± 0.1	0.3	
Jack[2]	1.5	SE (500/20)	35	—	2.5 ± 0.3	2.3 ± 0.3	0.2 ± 0.2	− 0.2, 0.6
Ashtari[4]	1.0	FLASH (40/15/50°)	28	—	2.62	2.70	− 0.08	
Cook[5]	1.5	SPGR (35/5/35°)	10	—	3.19 ± 0.39	3.23 ± 0.39	− 0.04 ± 0.07	
Lencz[6]	1.5	SE (400/20)	14	—	—	—	0.08	
Cendes[7]	1.5	3D (75/16/60°)	13	TBV	4.71 ± 0.24	4.59 ± 0.24	0.12 ± 0.09	
Tien[8]	1.5	FSE (4000/100)	33	—	—	—	0.13 ± 0.09	− 0.05, 0.31
Bhatia[9]	1.5	SPGR (24/5/45°)	29	TBV	3.59 ± 0.51	3.59 ± 0.48	0.005	
Kim[10]	1.5	FSE (4000/100)	30	—	—	—	0.08 ± 0.18	
Honeycutt[11]	1.5	SE ± 500/10	24	—	2.90 ± 0.35	2.78 ± 0.26	0.12	
Honeycutt[11]	1.5	MPRAGE (11/4/10/15°)	24	—	3.04 ± 0.33	2.82 ± 0.34	0.22	
Lehtovirta[12]	1.5	MPRAGE (10/4/250/12°)	16	TBA	3.71 ± 0.11	3.35 ± 0.11	0.36	
Gilmore[13]	1.0	MPRAGE (10/4/300/10°)	22	—	—	—	0.085 ± 0.25	− 0.67, 0.84
Sheline[14]	1.5	MPRAGE (10/4/300/8°)	10	—	2.58 ± 0.33	2.54 ± 0.26	0.04	
Parnetti[15]	1.5	T1IR (2200/20/80°)	6	TICV	1.81 ± 0.18	1.76 ± 0.24	0.05 ± 0.33	
Bigler[16]	1.5	FSE (3800/21,105)	96	—	2.53 ± 0.26	2.46 ± 0.29	0.07	

All mean volumes and R-L differences are in cubic centimeters, with error terms listed where available.
TICV = total intracranial volume, TBV = total brain volume, TBA = total brain area.

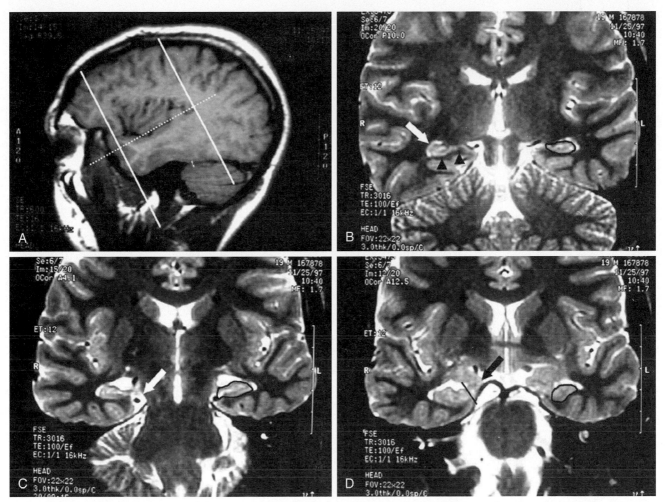

Figure 1 ▪ Scan geometry and hippocampal outlining. *A*, Parasagittal T1 MRI scan showing the selection of oblique coronal slice angle and limits (*solid lines*) perpendicular to the sylvian fissure (*dotted line*). *B–D*, Oblique coronal T2 MRI scans through the temporal lobes from posterior to anterior, with the left HF outlined in black. *B*, The right temporal horn (*arrow*), and subiculum (*arrowheads*). *C*, Ambient cistern (*arrow*). *D*, Uncinate gyrus (*arrow*) and separation from HF (*line*).

Measurements ▪

Typically, MRI data were transferred to an imaging workstation, and the outlines of the HF were drawn by hand. Sometimes boundary-finding software was used to aid in this task. The posterior limit of the HF was most often taken to lie at the level of the posterior commissure. The medial border of the HF was often defined as the uncal or ambient cistern. It was often reported that separation of the HF from the amygdala was a difficult task that was aided by using the alveolar covering of the HF as a boundary. Figure 1 shows selection of coronal angle from a parasagittal image and outlines of the HF on three images. The volumes of the right and left HF were calculated by summation of the outlined volumes and correction for slice interval. In 5 of the papers, these volumes were corrected for total intracranial volume (TICV) or total brain volume or area (TBV, TBA) to normalize them. Table 1 gives the mean values of the right and left HF from each study (when provided), as well as the right minus left hippocampal volume difference (HVD). Figure 2 shows the distribution of the HVD obtained from each study, with 6 additional data points from Honeycutt,[11] in which a meta-analysis was done in addition to studying 24 normal adults.

Source ▪

Subjects were either normal adult populations[1, 9, 11] or control patients with no MRI abnormalities and no disease process expected to affect the temporal lobe or hippocampal morphology. Table 1 lists the number of subjects in each study. All but two of the case-control studies were done with patients who had temporal lobe seizures in an attempt to identify hippocampal sclerosis/atrophy on the smaller side.[2–8, 10, 13] The remaining case-control studies were done with patients with Alzheimer dementia[12, 15] or major depression.[14]

Comments ▪

The reported volumes of the right and left HF vary considerably owing to differences in definition of the structure, normalization of data, and biologic variation. Perhaps more reproducible and useful is the HVD, which tends to favor the right side slightly (positive numbers). Suggested cut-

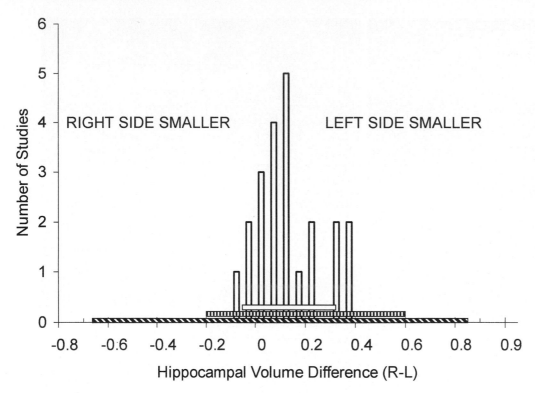

Figure 2 • Hippocampal volume differences (right-left) from the 16 papers cited, with 6 additional points from Honeycutt.[11] Each vertical bar indicates the number of series falling within each range of values. The horizontal bars depict the suggested normal ranges cited in three of the papers.[2, 8, 13]

off values (when cited by the authors) are noted on Table 1 and Figure 2. From these data, we suggest − 0.3 cc for a cut-off, indicating that the right HF is smaller, and 0.6 cc as the cut-off for an abnormally small left HF.

REFERENCES

1. Jack CR, Twomey CK, Zinsmeister AR, et al: Anterior temporal lobes and hippocampal formations: Normative volumetric measurements from MR images in young adults. Radiology 1989; 172:549–554.
2. Jack CR, Sharbrough FW, Twomey CK, et al: Temporal lobe seizures: Lateralization with MR volume measurements of the hippocampal formation. Radiology 1990; 175:423–429.
3. Jack CR, Sharbrough FW, Cascino GD, et al: Magnetic resonance image–based hippocampal volumetry: Correlation with outcome after temporal lobectomy. Ann Neurol 1992; 31:138–146.
4. Ashtari M, Barr WB, Schaul N, Bogerts B: Three-dimensional fast low-angle shot imaging and computerized volume measurement of the hippocampus in patients with chronic epilepsy of the temporal lobe. AJNR Am J Neuroradiol 1991; 12:941–947.
5. Cook MJ, Fish DR, Shorvon SD, et al: Hippocampal volumetric and morphometric studies in frontal and temporal lobe epilepsy. Brain 1992; 115 (Pt 4):1001–1015.
6. Lencz T, McCarthy G, Bronen RA, et al: Quantitative magnetic resonance imaging in temporal lobe epilepsy: Relationship to neuropathology and neuropsychological function. Ann Neurol 1992; 31(6):629–637.
7. Cendes F, Leproux F, Melanson D, et al: MRI of amygdala and hippocampus in temporal lobe epilepsy. J Comput Assist Tomogr 1993; 17:206–210.
8. Tien RD, Felsberg GJ, deCastro CC, et al: Complex partial seizures and mesial temporal sclerosis: Evaluation with fast spin-echo MR imaging. Radiology 1997; 189:835–842.
9. Bhatia S, Bookheimer SY, Gaillard WD, Theodore WH: Measurement of whole temporal lobe and hippocampus for MR volumetry: Normative data. Neurology 1993; 43:2006–2010.
10. Kim JH, Tien RD, Felsberg GJ, et al: MR measurements of the hippocampus for lateralization of temporal lobe epilepsy: Value of measurements of the body vs. the whole structure. AJR Am J Roentgenol 1994; 163(6):1453–1457.
11. Honeycutt NA, Smith CD: Hippocampal volume measurements using magnetic resonance imaging in normal young adults. J Neuroimaging 1995; 5(2):95–100.
12. Lehtovirta M, Laakso MP, Soininen H, et al: Volumes of hippocampus, amygdala and frontal lobe in Alzheimer patients with different apolipoprotein E genotypes. Neuroscience 1995; 67(1):65–72.
13. Gilmore RL, Childress MD, Leonard C, et al: Hippocampal volumetrics differentiate patients with temporal lobe epilepsy and extratemporal lobe epilepsy. Arch Neurol 1995; 52(8):819–824.
14. Sheline YI, Wang PW, Gado MH, et al: Hippocampal atrophy in recurrent major depression. Proc Natl Acad Sci USA 1996; 93(9):3908–3913.
15. Parnetti L, Lowenthal DT, Presciutti O, et al: 1H-MRS, MRI-based hippocampal volumetry, and 99mTc-HMPAO-SPECT in normal aging, age-associated memory impairment, and probable Alzheimer's disease [see comments]. J Am Geriatr Soc 1996; 44(2):133–138.
16. Bigler ED, Blatter DD, Anderson CV, et al: Hippocampal volume in normal aging and traumatic brain injury. AJNR Am J Neuroradiol 1997; 18:11–23.

▪: THE INTERUNCAL DISTANCE
▪ ACR Code: 134 (Temporal Lobe)

Technique ▪

All studies included herein were done on commercially available MRI units using standard sequences (detailed in Table 1) and a head coil. Field strength was 1.5 T in all series.[1-6]

Measurements ▪

The minimum interuncal distance (IUD) was measured on the axial slice through the suprasellar cistern with electronic calipers.[1, 2, 4, 6] For coronal measurement, the anteriormost slice showing the temporal horn was employed. The minimum distance between the unci of the temporal lobe was measured with electronic calipers.[3, 5] The intracranial width (IW) at the same level was measured by two investigators and used to express the interuncal distance as a fraction (IUD/IW) to correct for interindividual variation.[2, 4] Figure 1 shows the technique for measurement of the IUD on axial and coronal MRI images, and Table 1 lists the results from each study (in chronologic order).

Source ▪

Doraiswamy and associates examined 75 healthy volunteers to establish normative values for the interuncal distance.[3]

The remaining papers employed case-control design, with cases being patients with Alzheimer dementia (AD) by clinical criteria and controls being age-matched volunteers or patients seen for reasons other than dementia who had normal MRI scans.[1, 2, 4, 5] Numbers of patients and age distributions are included in Table 1.

Comments ▪

Interuncal distance variation is largely due to differences in hippocampal volume. The IUD might provide a simple indirect measurement of relative hippocampal volume, which is known to be significantly decreased in patients with AD. Dahlbeck and associates suggested that patients with an IUD of more than 30 mm are likely to have AD.[1] However, because of significant overlap of the measurements for controls and AD patients in their series, Howieson and Laakso and their colleagues felt that the method was not useful as a screen for AD.[2, 4] Frisoni and associates found the IUD to be useful in combination with 3 other linear measures of hippocampal atrophy to separate AD from controls.[5, 6]

Table 1 ▪ Interuncal Distances in Normal Subjects and Those with Alzheimer Dementia

AUTHOR/CATEGORY	TECHNIQUE	AGE (Yr)	NUMBER	IUD (mm)	IUD/IW
Dahlbeck					
Control	Axial, PD	>60	10	22.2 ± 4.4	—
AD	"	>60	10	37.3 ± 3.0	—
Howieson					
Control	Axial, T1	mean = 75	10	28.4 ± 5.6	0.21 ± 0.05
AD	"	mean = 74	10	29.6 ± 2.7	0.21 ± 0.02
Howieson					
Control	Coronal, T2	mean = 75	10	24.1 ± 3.7	0.18 ± 0.03
AD	"	mean = 74	10	30.5 ± 2.8	0.22 ± 0.03
Doraiswamy					
Normals	Axial, T1	20–30	15	18.3 ± 3.0	—
"	"	31–40	11	19.9 ± 3.0	—
"	"	41–50	8	17.4 ± 3.0	—
"	"	51–60	9	22.2 ± 3.0	—
"	"	61–70	17	23.5 ± 4.0	—
"	"	>70	15	25.0 ± 3.0	—
Laakso (Coronal)					
Controls	Coronal, GRE	mean = 29	20	22.8 ± 3.7	0.17 ± 0.03
Controls	"	mean = 71	27	27.4 ± 2.8	0.21 ± 0.02
AD	"	mean = 70	54	29.4 ± 4.8	0.22 ± 0.03
Frisoni (Axial)					
Controls	Axial, GRE	mean = 69	31	26.8 ± 4.0	—
Mild AD	"	mean = 75	33	30.2 ± 3.8	—
Moderate AD	"	mean = 70	13	30.1 ± 4.9	—

Measurements are given as mean ± standard deviation.
IUD = interuncal distance, IW = intracranial width, AD = Alzheimer dementia, GRE = gradient echo, PD = proton density.

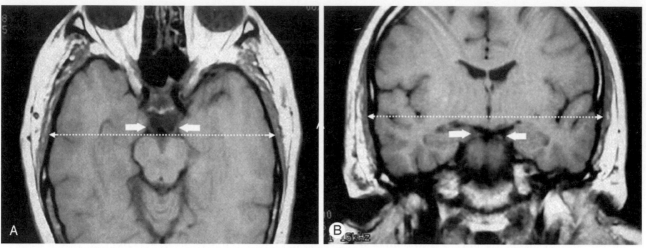

Figure 1 ▪ Measurement of the interuncal distance *(arrows)* and intracranial width *(dotted lines)* from T1-weighted images of the brain. The axial image *(A)* chosen is the one through the suprasellar cistern, and the coronal image *(B)* used is the most anterior that still contains the temporal horns of the lateral ventricles.

REFERENCES

1. Dahlbeck JW, McCluney KW, Yeakley JW, et al: The interuncal distance: A new MR measurement for the hippocampal atrophy of Alzheimer disease AJNR Am J Neuroradiol 1991; 12(5):931–932.
2. Howieson J, Daye JA, Holm L, Howieson D: Interuncal distance: Marker of aging and Alzheimer disease. AJNR Am J Neuroradiol 1993; 14:647–650.
3. Doraiswamy PM, McDonald WM, Patterson L, et al: Interuncal distance as a measure of hippocampal atrophy: Normative data on axial MR imaging. AJNR Am J Neuroradiol 1993; 14(1):141–143.
4. Laakso M, Soininen H, Partanen K, et al: The interuncal distance in Alzheimer disease and age-associated memory impairment. AJNR Am J Neuroradiol 1995; 16(4):727–734.
5. Frisoni GB, Beltramello A, Weiss C, et al: Linear measures of atrophy in mild Alzheimer disease. AJNR Am J Neuroradiol 1996; 17(5):913–923.
6. Frisoni GB, Beltramello A, Weiss C, et al: Usefulnes of simple measures of temporal lobe atrophy in probable Alzheimer's disease. Dementia 1996; 7(1):15–22.

⁚ LINEAR MEASUREMENTS OF THE CORPUS CALLOSUM IN INFANTS
▪ ACR Code: 135 (Corpus Callosum)

Technique ▪

Two groups of infants were studied by Fujii and colleagues.[1] The babies were scanned with a 1.5-T Signa (General Electric Corporation, Milwaukee, WI) unit to produce sagittal images with T1 weighting (300/20). Barkovich and associates also used a 1.5-T Signa unit to perform T1 (400–600/20) sagittal images.[2]

Measurements ▪

Fujii measured the thickness (cephalocaudal) of the corpus callosum from the midsagittal image one third of the dis-

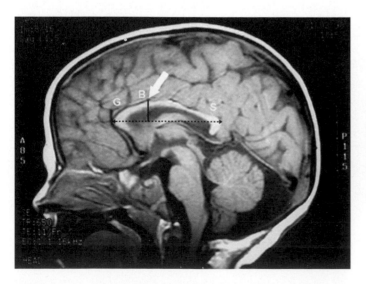

Figure 1 ▪ Measurement of the corpus callosum in infants from a midsagittal T1-weighted MR image. A line is drawn from the anteriormost part of the genu to the posteriormost part of the splenium. This delineates the length *(dotted line)*. The thicknesses of the genu and splenium are measured where this line crosses the structures *(G and S)*. The thickness of the body *(B)* of the corpus callosum is measured at a point one third of the way between the genu and splenium perpendicular to the long axis *(arrow)*.

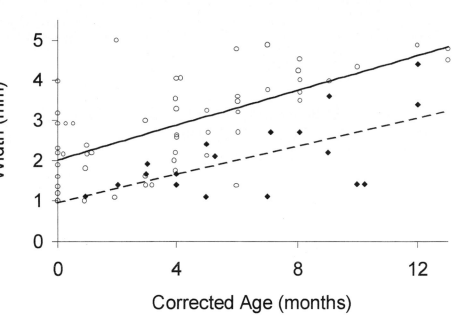

Figure 2 ▪ Scatterplot of thickness of the corpus callosum (body) in normal *(open circles)* and developmentally delayed *(solid diamonds)* infants. The age is corrected to adjust for preterm infants by subtracting the difference between the gestational age at birth and 40 weeks from the given age from birth. The least squares linear regression line is shown for normal *(solid line)* and developmentally delayed *(dotted line)* infants. (From Fujii Y, Konishi Y, Kuriyama M, et al: Pediatr Neurol 1994; 11:219–223. Used by permission.)

tance from the genu to the splenium, with electronic calipers.[1] Barkovich and Kjos also measured the thickness of the genu and splenium (anteroposterior) as well as the length of the whole structure.[2] These measurements are shown in Figure 1. Figure 2 is a scatterplot of thickness of the body in developmentally normal and delayed infants by age.[1] Table 1 shows the three thicknesses and the overall length by two-month age intervals in tabular form.[2] The predicted normal thickness of the body of the corpus callosum may be calculated as follows:

$$\text{Thickness in millimeters} = 0.217 \\ \times \text{ age in months} + 2.039$$

Source ▪

The study by Fujii included 54 scans of 38 developmentally normal infants whose gestational age ranged from 30 to 42 weeks at birth.[1] The second cohort (18 scans of 18 subjects) was composed of developmentally retarded infants (Enjoji developmental scale < 70 at 2 years of age). There was no evidence of aneuploidy, intracranial hemorrhage, leukomalacia, CNS infection, or structural abnormality. The subjects in both cohorts were of gestational ages ranging from 30 to 42 weeks at birth, had normal body weights and head circumferences for age, and were within 1 to 13 months of age when studied. Barkovich examined 63 infants from 3 days old to 12 months of age for various reasons. All the scans were judged to be normal, and the babies had achieved appropriate developmental milestones.[2]

Comments ▪

The thickness of the corpus callosum was significantly less in developmentally delayed infants when compared with normals. There was a significant positive correlation between age and corpus callosum thickness in both groups (p < 0.01).

Table 1 ▪ Linear Corpus Callosum Measurements During the First Year of Life in Normal Infants

AGE (Mon)	NUMBER	THICKNESS			LENGTH
		Genu	Body	Splenium	
0–2	12	5.1 ± 1.0	2.3 ± 0.5	3.7 ± 0.6	47.7 ± 2.8
2–4	18	5.0 ± 1.3	2.5 ± 0.5	4.5 ± 0.9	51.2 ± 4.5
4–6	7	7.0 ± 1.3	3.0 ± 0.8	5.8 ± 1.3	50.8 ± 3.4
6–8	7	6.3 ± 1.0	2.8 ± 0.4	6.6 ± 0.6	54.0 ± 0.8
8–10	8	7.7 ± 1.3	4.2 ± 1.0	7.6 ± 1.6	59.0 ± 8.2
10–12	11	7.8 ± 1.1	4.2 ± 0.8	8.3 ± 1.2	57.6 ± 4.9

All measurements are given in millimeters (mean ± standard deviation).
From Barkovich AJ, Kjos BO: AJNR Am J Neuroradiol 1988; 9:487–491. Used by permission.

REFERENCES

1. Fujii Y, Konishi Y, Kuriyama M, et al: Corpus callosum in developmentally retarded infants. Pediatr Neurol 1994; 11:219–223.

2. Barkovich AJ, Kjos BO: Normal postnatal development of the corpus callosum as demostrated by MR imaging. AJNR Am J Neuroradiol 1988; 9:487–491.

⁚ AREA MEASUREMENTS OF THE CORPUS CALLOSUM IN ADULTS RELATED TO AGE AND GENDER
- ACR Code: 135 (Corpus Callosum)

Technique ▪

Three studies of adults are included here. Johnson and associates used a 1.5-T Signa (General Electric Corporation, Milwaukee, WI) scanner to make T1 (500/11)-weighted sagittal scans.[1] Pozzilli and associates performed T1 (400/30)-weighted sagittal images on a 0.2-T machine (ESATOM 2000, Ansaldo).[2] Biegon and associates used a 0.5-T magnet (unspecified manufacturer) to make T1 (33/0.4)-weighted sagittal scans.[3]

Table 1 ▪ Area of the Corpus Callosum in the Midsagittal Plane in Five Age Groups by Gender

AGE RANGE	BOTH SEXES		MEN		WOMEN	
	Number	Area	Number	Area	Number	Area
16–25	49	6.71 ± 1.0	30	6.80 ± 0.96	19	6.58 ± 1.07
26–35	42	6.64 ± 0.9	20	6.94 ± 1.02	22	6.36 ± 0.76
36–45	34	6.74 ± 1.1	14	6.78 ± 1.16	20	6.72 ± 1.03
46–55	42	6.51 ± 1.0	18	6.76 ± 1.08	24	6.32 ± 0.93
56–65	33	6.17 ± 0.9	18	6.16 ± 0.83	15	6.18 ± 0.93
16–65	200	6.57 ± 1.0	100	6.70 ± 1.02	100	6.44 ± 0.94

Measurements are in square centimeters (mean ± standard deviation).[1]

Table 2 ▪ Midsagittal Area Measurements of the Corpus Callosum in Adults in Two Age Groups

REFERENCE (Age)	NUMBER	TOTAL	GENU	BODY	SPLENIUM
Pozzilli					
13–49	85	6.91 ± 1.1	1.75 ± 0.4	3.16 ± 0.3	1.91 ± 0.4
50–80	45	6.88 ± 1.0	1.67 ± 0.4	3.13 ± 0.3	1.98 ± 0.3
Biegon					
26–41	16	5.70 ± 1.07	1.76 ± 0.34	2.24 ± 0.45	1.71 ± 0.36
54–78	13	5.62 ± .98	1.66 ± 0.40	1.92 ± 0.45	2.04 ± 0.39

Measurements are in square centimeters (mean ± standard deviation).[2, 3]

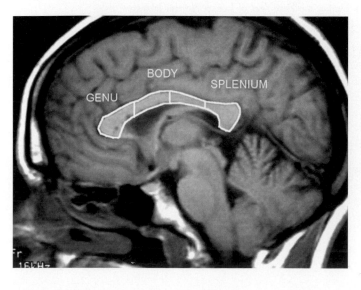

Figure 1 ▪ Area measurements of the corpus callosum from a T1-weighted midsagittal MRI image. The length from genu to splenium is divided into fourths. The area of the genu is the anterior fourth, the body the middle half, and the splenium the posterior fourth. The overall area is the sum of all subregions or the area subtended by the outline of the whole structure.

Measurements •

The cross-sectional area of the corpus callosum on the midsagittal scan was measured by hand tracing its perimeter and recording the resulting area.[1-3] The midsagittal area of several subregions was measured in the same way.[2, 3] Figure 1 shows the measurements, and Tables 1 and 2 list the results.

Source •

Johnson and associates used 200 normal adult volunteers.[1] Pozzilli and associates studied 46 normal volunteers and 84 patients in whom neurologic findings and MRI scans were normal.[2] Biegon and associates included 31 normal volunteer control subjects in a study of Alzheimer dementia.[3]

REFERENCES

1. Johnson SC, Farnworth T, Pinkston JB, et al: Corpus callosum surface area across the human adult life span: Effect of age and gender. Brain Res Bull 1994; 35(4): 373–377.
2. Pozzilli C, Bastianello S, Bozzao A, et al: No differences in corpus callosum size by sex and aging. A quantitative study using magnetic resonance imaging. J Neuroimaging 1994; 4(4): 218–221.
3. Biegon A, Eberling JL, Richardson BC, et al: Human corpus callosum in aging and Alzheimer's disease: A magnetic resonance imaging study. Neurobiol Aging 1994; 15(4): 393–397.

•: MEASUREMENTS OF THE CORPUS CALLOSUM IN NORMAL ADULTS AND THOSE WITH SCHIZOPHRENIA OR HYDROCEPHALUS
• ACR Code: 135 (Corpus Callosum)

Technique •

Three studies are included herein. Laissy and associates used a 0.5-T MR Max system (GE Medical Systems, Milwaukee, WI) to obtain gradient echo T1 (400/20)-weighted sagittal images that were 7 mm thick.[1] Steinmetz and associates performed fast low-angle-shot sagittal images (machine and parameters not specified).[2] Hofmann used a 1.5-T machine (manufacturer not given) to perform T2* (~80/35/10 deg flip angle), ECG-gated, multiphase fast-field-echo sequences.[3] Woodruff and associate performed a meta-analysis of corpus callosum size in schizophrenia, which included measurements of 281 control subjects from 17 MRI studies.[4]

Measurements •

Measurements of the corpus callosum area, length, thickness, and height (Fig. 1) were made from midsagittal images, using electronic calipers and tracing functions available on the MRI scanners.[1-3] Measurements from midsagittal MR images, as reported in the source papers (area: 11 papers, length: 8 papers), were compiled in the meta-analysis.[4] Table 1 lists the reported measurements.

Source •

Laissy and associates included 124 healthy subjects (63 men and 61 women) ranging in age from 12 to 85 years (mean, 37.5 years).[1] Steinmetz and associates recruited 120 volunteers (71 men with a mean age of 25 years and 49 women with a mean age of 26 years).[2] Hofmann and associates studied 22 healthy individuals (8 men and 14 women, aged 22 to 92 years; mean, 45 years) and 163 patients with hydrocephalus (75 men and 88 women, aged 2 to 81 years; mean, 49 years).[3] The meta-analysis by Woodruff included 281 control subjects (mean age, 33.3 years; men, 68%, women, 32%) and 313 with schizophrenia (mean age, 32.1 years; men, 68%, women, 32%).[4]

Comments •

Women had slightly smaller area, length, and thickness measurements (p = 0.01), and these differences disappeared with correction for brain area.[7] The height of the corpus callosum was significantly greater in patients with hydrocephalus (communicating and noncommunicating) than in normal subjects (p = 0.001). The length of the

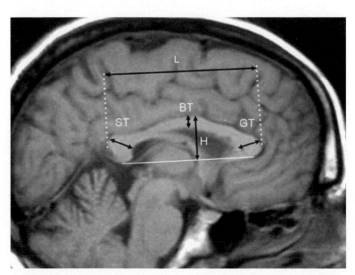

Figure 1 • Measurements of the corpus callosum from midsagittal T1-weighted MRI images. Length *(L)* is measured from anterior genu to posterior splenium, and thicknesses of the genu *(GT)*, body *(BT)*, and splenium *(ST)* as shown. Height *(H)* is midway between a baseline drawn between the genu and septum *(white line)*. Area was measured by use of a freehand tracing function (not shown).

Table 1 ▪ Composite Table of Corpus Callosum Measurements in Normal Adults and Those with Schizophrenia or Hydrocephalus

REFERENCE/CATEGORY	NUMBER	AREA	LENGTH	HEIGHT	THICKNESS		
					Genu	Body	Splenium
Laissy normals							
Men	63	6.54 ± 1.26	7.15 ± 0.33		0.98 ± 0.19	0.62 ± 0.13	1.1 ± 0.17
Women	61	6.17 ± 1.07	7.01 ± 0.54		0.94 ± 0.19	0.58 ± 0.1	1.06 ± 0.14
All subjects	124	6.36 ± 1.19	7.06 ± 0.48		0.96 ± 0.19	0.6 ± 0.11	1.08 ± 0.15
Steinmetz normals							
Men	71	6.63 ± 0.82					
Women	49	6.64 ± 0.81					
All subjects	120	6.63 ± 0.9					
Hoffmann							
Controls	22	7.0 ± 1.2	7.1 ± 0.5	2.5 ± 0.4			
Communicating hydrocephalus	74	6.7 ± 1.2	7.7 ± 0.7	3.6 ± 0.7			
Obstructive hydrocephalus	27	7.4 ± 1.1	8.1 ± 1.3	4.2 ± 1.1			
Woodruff							
Controls	281	6.31 ± 1.84	6.83 ± 1.51				
Schizophrenia	313	6.06 ± 1.69	6.90 ± 1.43				

All measurements are in centimeters (mean ± standard deviation).[1–3]

corpus callosum was greater in both forms of hydrocephalus (p = 0.002).[3] Schizophrenic patients had significantly smaller corpus callosum areas than did controls (p = 0.019).[4]

REFERENCES

1. Laissy JP, Patrux B, Dachateau C, et al: Midsagittal measurements of the corpus callosum in healthy subjects and diseased patients: A prospective study. AJNR Am J Neuroradiol 1993; 14: 145–154.
2. Steinmetz H, Staiger JF, Schlaug G, et al: Corpus callosum and brain volume in women and men. Neuroreport 1995; 6(7): 1002–1004.
3. Hofmann E, Becker T, Jackel M, et al: The corpus callosum in communicating and noncommunicating hydrocephalus. Neuroradiology 1995; 37(3): 212–218.
4. Woodruff PW, McManus IC, David AS: Meta-analysis of corpus callosum size in schizophrenia. J Neurol Neurosurg Psychiatry 1995; 58(4): 457–461.

▪ᛁ MEASUREMENT OF THE NORMAL PITUITARY STALK BY CT IN CHILDREN
- ACR Code: 145 (Pituitary Gland, Stalk)

Technique ▪

1. Scans were obtained on a GE 8800 scanner; 10-mm slice thickness was used.
2. Scans were begun during a bolus injection of 2 ml/kg of Hypaque meglumine 60%

Measurements ▪

The ideal stalk diameter is made through the midstalk in the suprasellar cisterns. Measurement of the basilar artery is made on the same slice, shown in Figure 1.

Table 1 ▪ Pituitary Measurements in "Pure" Population of Normal Boys Aged 0–19 Years

AGE (Mon)	MINIMUM NO. (n = 659)	MEAN DIAMETER IN mm (SD)		MEAN STALK/BASILAR RATIO (SD)
		Pituitary Stalk	Basilar Artery	
0–6	11	1.9 (0.34)	2.7 (0.74)	0.73 (0.20)
7–12	12	1.9 (0.35)	3.4 (0.54)	0.57 (0.10)
13–24	37	2.0 (0.31)	3.6 (0.43)	0.55 (0.10)
25–36	22	1.9 (0.37)	3.9 (0.57)	0.50 (0.11)
37–48	23	2.1 (0.47)	3.8 (0.40)	0.57 (0.12)
49–60	23	2.1 (0.36)	3.9 (0.53)	0.52 (0.09)
61–72	23	2.1 (0.36)	3.9 (0.46)	0.56 (0.12)
73–84	29	2.2 (0.31)	3.7 (0.46)	0.60 (0.12)
85–96	27	2.1 (0.31)	3.8 (0.46)	0.56 (0.11)
97–108	35	2.2 (0.37)	3.9 (0.56)	0.57 (0.12)
109–120	25	2.4 (0.42)	3.9 (0.40)	0.62 (0.11)
121–132	22	2.4 (0.47)	3.9 (0.51)	0.62 (0.16)
133–144	14	2.6 (0.46)	4.1 (0.56)	0.64 (0.15)
145–156	20	2.3 (0.38)	3.7 (0.65)	0.62 (0.12)
157–168	9	2.4 (0.55)	3.8 (0.54)	0.62 (0.10)
169–180	11	2.4 (0.34)	3.5 (0.51)	0.68 (0.10)
181–192	4	2.8 (0.74)	3.8 (0.46)	0.72 (0.20)
193–204	5	2.3 (0.49)	3.8 (0.46)	0.61 (0.13)
205–216	3	2.3 (0.50)	3.6 (0.05)	0.64 (0.13)
217–228	1	1.8	3.2 (0.23)	0.54

From Seidel FG, Towbin R, Kaufman RA: AJR Am J Roentgenol 1985; 145:1297–1302. Used by permission.

Table 2 ▪ Pituitary Measurements in "Pure" Population of Normal Girls Aged 0–19 Years

AGE (Mon)	MINIMUM NO. (n = 659)	MEAN DIAMETER IN mm (SD)		MEAN STALK/BASILAR RATIO (SD)
		Pituitary Stalk	Basilar Artery	
0–6	8	1.9 (0.41)	2.5 (0.47)	0.74 (0.09)
7–12	9	1.8 (0.34)	3.3 (0.47)	0.57 (0.13)
13–24	37	2.1 (0.42)	3.5 (0.56)	0.59 (0.11)
25–36	30	2.0 (0.31)	3.6 (0.66)	0.57 (0.15)
37–48	28	2.0 (0.40)	3.5 (0.44)	0.58 (0.11)
49–60	17	2.0 (0.31)	3.6 (0.63)	0.60 (0.16)
61–72	22	2.2 (0.48)	3.7 (0.47)	0.60 (0.18)
73–84	24	2.2 (0.33)	3.5 (0.52)	0.62 (0.09)
85–96	19	2.2 (0.52)	3.7 (0.51)	0.61 (0.10)
97–108	20	2.2 (0.45)	3.9 (0.53)	0.57 (0.15)
109–120	9	2.4 (0.57)	3.5 (0.53)	0.69 (0.13)
121–132	11	2.2 (0.28)	3.6 (0.50)	0.60 (0.09)
133–144	15	2.5 (0.39)	3.7 (0.51)	0.68 (0.08)
145–156	13	2.8 (0.50)	3.5 (0.30)	0.80 (0.17)
157–168	10	2.6 (0.49)	3.7 (0.49)	0.70 (0.10)
169–180	5	2.5 (0.63)	3.2 (0.69)	0.73 (0.10)
181–192	10	2.7 (0.68)	3.6 (0.71)	0.74 (0.21)
193–204	1	2.7	3.4 (0.54)	0.64
205–216	4	3.0 (0.82)	3.8 (0.59)	0.79 (0.21)
217–228	3	2.4 (0.32)	3.1 (0.47)	0.79 (0.18)

From Seidel FG, Towbin R, Kaufman RA: AJR Am J Roentgenol 1985; 145:1297–1302. Used by permission.

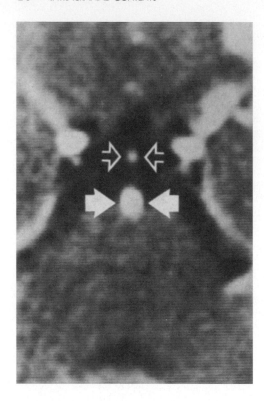

Figure 1 ▪ Normal pituitary stalk with pituitary stalk/basilar artery ratio less than 1.0. Pituitary stalk diameter *(open arrows)*; basilar artery diameter *(closed arrows)*. (From Seidel FG, Towbin R, Kaufman RA: AJR Am J Roentgenol 1985; 145:1297–1302. Used by permission.)

The absolute pituitary stalk and basilar artery diameters are shown in Tables 1 and 2.

The pituitary stalk to basilar artery ratio is easily estimated visually. Ratios greater than or equal to 1 are unusual in normal children. A ratio greater than or equal to 1 should prompt direct measurement of the stalk and comparison with age-matched normal values. A stalk measurement greater than 2 SD above the age-matched mean is presumably abnormal.

Source ▪

Data are based on a study of 1005 normal CT scans in 990 patients aged newborn to 18 years. Fifty-three percent were boys and 47% were girls.

REFERENCE

1. Seidel FG, Towbin R, Kaufman RA: Normal pituitary stalk size in children: CT study. AJR Am J Roentgenol 1985; 145:1297–1302.

▪▪ MEASUREMENT OF THE NORMAL PITUITARY STALK BY CT IN ADULTS
▪ ACR Code: 145 (Pituitary Gland, Stalk)

Technique ▪

1. Scans were performed on a GE 8800 immediately after drip infusion of 150 ml Conray 60.
2. Scan plane was parallel to the orbitomeatal line. Five- or 10-mm slices were obtained.

Measurement ▪

Measurements were taken to the nearest half millimeter of the smallest diameter of the stalk and basilar artery when both were visualized at the level of the dorsum sellae and at the suprasellar levels, shown in Figure 1.

Table 1 ▪ Measurements of Normal Pituitary Stalk and Basilar Artery on High-Resolution Axial CT with Contrast Enhancement

STRUCTURE AND LEVEL	NO. VISUALIZED	DIMENSIONS		CONFIDENCE INTERVALS (mm)	
		Mean ± SD	Range	95%	99%
Pituitary stalk					
At dorsum sellae	137	2.1 ± 0.7	0.5–4.0	0.5–3.5	0.0–4.0
Above dorsum sellae	32	2.8 ± 0.6	1.5–4.0	1.5–4.0	1.0–4.5
Basilar artery					
At dorsum sellae	152	3.2 ± 0.8	1.5–7.5	1.5–4.5	1.5–5.5
Above dorsum sellae	29	3.6 ± 0.9	2.5–6.0	2.0–5.5	1.0–6.0

Subjects were 184 normal patients.
From Peyster RG, Hoover ED, Adler LP: AJNR Am J Neuroradiol 1984; 5:45–47. Used by permission.

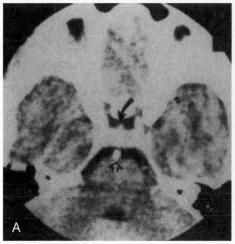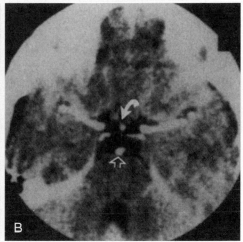

Figure 1 ▪ Two contiguous axial CT sections. Normal pituitary stalk *(solid arrow)* and basilar artery *(open arrow)*. *A,* Stalk is seen at level of dorsum. *B,* Stalk is slightly above level of dorsum and just posterior to optic chiasm. (From Peyster RG, Hoover ED, Adler LP: AJNR Am J Neuroradiol 1984; 5:45–47. Used by permission.)

Table 1 shows the normal measurements of normal pituitary stalk and basilar artery.

The upper size limit of the normal pituitary stalk is 4 mm at the level of the dorsum sellae and 4.5 mm above the dorsum. Stalks longer than this should be viewed with suspicion. Comparison with the size of the basilar artery is a quick and reliable visual check of stalk size with a 1:1 ratio.

Source ▪

Data are based on a CT study of 98 male and 86 female subjects 9 to 84 years of age.

REFERENCE

1. Peyster RG, Hoover ED, Adler LP: CT of the normal pituitary stalk. AJNR Am J Neuroradiol 1984; 5:45–47.

▪▪ SIZE, SHAPE, AND ENHANCEMENT OF THE PITUITARY STALK
▪ ACR Code: 145 (Pituitary Gland, Stalk)

Technique ▪

Examinations were performed on a Siemens 1.5-T machine. Spin echo T1-weighted (400/12) sagittal and coronal sequences with 3.0-mm slices were done. Spin echo T1-weighted (600/20) and T2-weighted (2500/30,80) axial images were obtained. The sagittal and coronal sequences were done before and after injection of Gd-DTPA intravenously.

Measurements ▪

The transverse diameter of the stalk was measured at the optic chiasm and at the pituitary. The signal intensities before and after enhancement were noted by comparison with the neurohypophysis and optic chiasm. The stalk was smoothly tapered with no abrupt changes in caliber in all cases. The transverse dimension at the chiasm was 1.56 to 4.58 mm (mean +/− SD, 3.25 +/− 0.56). The transverse dimension at the insertion on the gland was 1.04 to 2.93 mm (mean +/− SD, 1.91 +/− 0.40). Unenhanced signal intensity was uniform and hypointense relative to the neurohypophysis in all cases. It was hypointense compared with the optic chiasm in 84% and isointense in 16%. After enhancement, the signal intensity of the stalk increased uniformly in all cases to be hyperintense with respect to the optic chiasm. The enhanced stalk was hypointense compared with the neurohypophysis in all cases but one.

Source ▪

Fifty-eight patients with no pituitary or juxtasellar abnormalities were included. There were 17 men and 41 women, aged 19 to 71 years (mean, 40 years).

REFERENCE

1. Simmons GE, Suchnicki JE, Rak KM, Damiano TR: MR imaging of the pituitary stalk: Size, shape, and enhancement pattern [see comments]. AJR Am J Roentgenol 1992; 159(2):375–377.

⁘ INFUNDIBULAR TILT OF THE PITUITARY GLAND
- ACR Code: 145 (Pituitary Gland, Stalk)

Technique •

Coronal images were made on a 1.5-T Signa machine (GE Medical Systems) using T1-weighted spin echo sequences (500–600/20–30) and a 3- to 5-mm section thickness. Gadolinium was given intravenously prior to all scans.

Measurements •

The midpoint of the gland was defined as being between the signal voids of the internal carotid arteries in the cavernous sinuses. Assessment of infundibular tilt and insertion point was made by consensus of three reviewers. Fig-

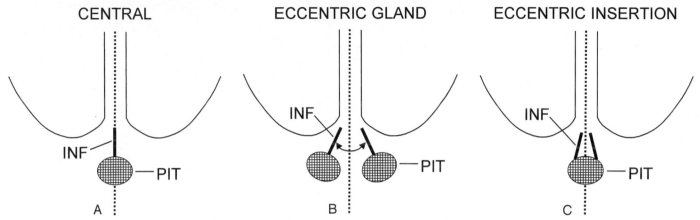

Figure 1 • Relationships of the infundibulum (*INF*) to the pituitary gland (*PIT*) on coronal MR images. *A*, Midline insertion with no tilt. *B*, Lateral tilt caused by eccentric position of the gland in the sella. *C*, Lateral tilt caused by eccentric insertion of the stalk into the gland. (From Ahmadi H, Larsson EM, Jinkins JR: Radiology 1990; 177:389–392. Used by permission.)

Table 1 • Relationships of the Infundibulum to the Pituitary Gland on Coronal MRI Images in 50 Normal Subjects

TYPE	NUMBER		
	Male (%)	Female (%)	Both (%)
Central, no tilt	8 (42)	19 (61)	27 (54)
Lateral tilt, eccentric gland	8 (42)	9 (29)	17 (34)
Lateral tilt, eccentric insertion	3 (16)	3 (10)	6 (12)
TOTAL	19	31	50

From Ahmadi H, Larsson EM, Jinkins JR: Radiology 1990; 177:389–392. Used by permission.

ure 1 shows the categories of infundibular tilt, and Table 1 shows their frequency.

Source •

Random patients (n = 50) scanned for diseases not related to the pituitary, who ranged in age from 9 to 73 years (mean, 39 years).

REFERENCE

1. Ahmadi H, Larsson EM, Jinkins JR: Normal pituitary gland: Coronal MR imaging of infundibular tilt. Radiology 1990; 177:389–392.

▪ː MEASUREMENT OF NORMAL PITUITARY GLAND BY CT

▪ ACR Code: 145 (Pituitary Gland, Stalk)

Technique ▪

1. GE 8800 CT/T scanner with 5-mm thick sections in the coronal plane.
2. Localization with lateral scout image, with the head hyperextended in the auxiliary head holder. Coronal sections set perpendicular to the sellar floor.
3. One hundred fifty milliliters of 30% iodinated contrast was infused in 3 to 4 minutes. The infusion was then slowed during coronal imaging.
4. Axial images with and without enhancement were compared but not measured.

Measurement ▪

Figure 1 shows that the pituitary was homogeneously isodense or slightly hyperdense with respect to brain tissue. The top of the gland was outlined with cerebrospinal fluid and was flat or concave.

The lateral margin of the gland was difficult to distinguish from the cavernous sinus on routine and enhanced views.

Height of the pituitary gland:

Females: 4.8 + 1.3 mm plus 1 SD (range, 2.7–6.7 mm)
Males: 3.5 + 1.5 mm plus 1 SD (range, 1.4–5.9 mm)

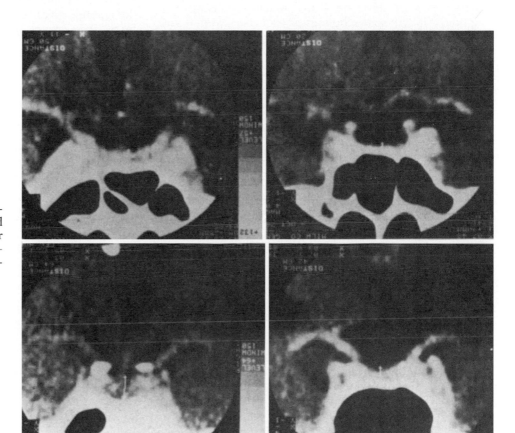

Figure 1 ▪ The pituitary gland on coronal CT images. Measurement of gland height is illustrated with cursor in four patients. (From Syvertsen A, et al: Radiology 1979; 133:385. Used by permission.)

The infundibulum could be identified between the top of the gland and the infundibular recess of the third ventricle, often slightly off midline.

Source ▪

Twenty patients (14 females and 6 males) between the ages of 6 and 74 years. These subjects had no clinical suspicion of pituitary adenoma.

REFERENCE

1. Syvertsen A, et al: The computed tomographic appearance of the normal pituitary gland and pituitary microadenomas. Radiology 1979; 133:385.

▪: SIZE OF THE PITUITARY RELATED TO AGE AND SEX
▪ ACR Code: 145 (Pituitary Gland, Stalk)

Technique ▪

MRI scans were done on 1.5-T machines, using T1-weighted (500/20) spin echo sagittal sequences with 4- and 5-mm section thickness. Intravenous contrast was not given in either study.

Measurements ▪

The maximum gland height was measured from the midsagittal image with electronic calipers in both studies.[1, 2] The maximum gland length was measured with electronic calipers parallel to the floor of the sella, and an ROI function was used to measure gland area in the second work.[2] Table 1 shows combined measurements of pituitary height from both studies broken down by decade and gender. Table 2 gives the height, length, and area of the gland in two age groups by gender and for all subjects in two age groups.[2]

Source ▪

The first study included 213 patients with no clinical symptoms relating to the pituitary gland and scans judged to be normal in the sellar region.[1] The second included 71 normal volunteers.[2] The age distributions are detailed in Tables 1 and 2.

Table 1 ▪ Pituitary Gland Height (mm) on Midsagittal Thin-Section MRI Segregated by Age and Gender

	MALE		FEMALE		BOTH	
DECADE	Number	Mean	Number	Mean	Number	Mean
1	5	3.8 ± 1.4	2	3.1 ± 0	7	3.6 ± 1.3
2	9	5.7 ± 1.2	7	6.1 ± 0.9	16	6.0 ± 1.1
3	18	5.8 ± 0.9	12	6.6 ± 1.2	30	6.1 ± 1.1
4	12	5.0 ± 0.7	19	5.9 ± 1.3	31	5.5 ± 1.1
5	24	4.8 ± 1.4	15	5.3 ± 1.4	39	5.0 ± 1.4
6	28	4.4 ± 1.6	34	4.5 ± 1.6	62	4.4 ± 1.6
7	30	4.3 ± 1.2	26	5.1 ± 1.6	56	4.7 ± 1.4
8	22	4.6 ± 1.3	21	4.1 ± 1.6	43	4.4 ± 1.5

Data for the first and second decades from Suzuki.[1] Measurements from the third through eighth decades are combined data from both studies.[1, 2]

Table 2 ▪ Midsagittal Pituitary Gland Height (mm), Length (mm), and Area (mm²)

	MALE		FEMALE		BOTH		ALL
Age range	20–49	50–90	20–49	50–90	20–49	50–90	20–90
Number	16	15	17	23	33	38	71
Height	5.2 ± 0.9	4.4 ± 1.2	6.1 ± 1.7	4.7 ± 1.5	5.7 ± 1.4	4.6 ± 1.4	5.1 ± 1.4
Length	10.8 ± 1.4	10.7 ± 1.7	10.8 ± 1.1	10.4 ± 1.7	10.8 ± 1.2	10.5 ± 1.7	10.6 ± 1.5
Area	38.3 ± 9.3	32.5 ± 8.5	45.8 ± 13.7	36.5 ± 13.3	42.2 ± 11.8	34.9 ± 11.7	38.3 ± 11.7

Arranged by gender and two age groups, with 50 years as the cut-off. The last column on the right contains data for all 71 subjects.[2]

REFERENCES

1. Suzuki M, Takashima T, Kadoya M, et al: Height of normal pituitary gland on MR imaging: Age and sex differentiation. J Comput Assist Tomogr 1990; 14(1): 36–39.

2. Doraiswamy PM, Potts JM, Axelson DA, et al: MR assessment of pituitary gland morphology in healthy volunteers: Age- and gender-related differences. AJNR Am J Neuroradiol 1992; 13(5): 1295–1299.

∴ LOCALIZATION OF THE PINEAL GLAND: LATERAL PROJECTION
▪ ACR Code: 147 (Pineal Gland)

Vastine-Kinney Method ▪

Technique

Central ray: Perpendicular to film centered over midportion of skull.
Position: True lateral.
Target-film distance: Immaterial.

Measurements (Figures 1 and 2)

A = The greatest distance from the pineal body to the inner table of the frontal bone.
B = The greatest distance from the pineal body to the inner table of the occiput.
C = The greatest distance from the pineal body to the inner table of the vault.
D = The greatest distance from the pineal body to the occipital bone in the vertical direction.

Source

This material is based on the roentgen examination of 200 skull films that were essentially negative for intracranial lesions.

Pawl-Walter Method ▪

Technique

Central ray: Perpendicular to film centered over midportion of skull.

Position: True lateral.
Target-film distance: Immaterial.

Measurements (Figure 3)

Line A is drawn from nasion to the lowest point of the basiocciput just posterior to the opisthion.

Line B is drawn perpendicular to line A and passes through the center of the calcified pineal body (P).

Point P_1 is one half the distance from the baseline A to the inner table of the cranial vault.

Line C is drawn through the pineal body (P) perpendicular to line B.

Point P_2 is one half the distance from the inner table of the frontal bone to the outer table of the occipital bone.

The pineal body (P) should lie 1 cm below point P_1 and 1 cm posterior to point P_2.

The range of normal is 5 mm superior, inferior, anterior, or posterior to this calculated point.

The accuracy in Pawl and Walter's series was 100% in the superoinferior dimension and 98.5% in the anteroposterior dimension.

Note: Pawl and Walter reviewed the various methods for localization of the calcified pineal body. The Vastine-Kinney method has been included because it is familiar to many radiologists. However, the Pawl-Walter method, which does not require use of overlays and tables, has much to recommend it.

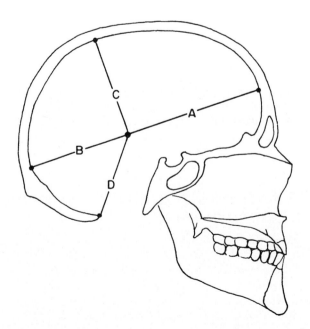

Figure 1 ▪ Vastine-Kinney chart for pineal position measurements.

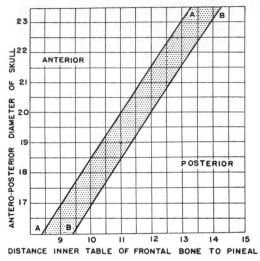
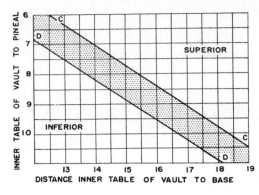

Figure 2 ▪ Dyke modification of Vastine-Kinney chart for pineal position measurements. **A**, normal anteroposterior variation. The measurement of *A* is plotted against the sum of *A* + *B*. This sum is approximately equal to the greatest anteroposterior diameter of the skull. The pineal glands of normal skulls lie between *A-A* and *B-B*. **B**, normal vertical variation. The measurement of C is plotted against the sum of *C* + *D*. This sum is approximately equal to the vertical diameter of the skull. The pineal glands of normal skulls lie between *C-C* and *D-D*. Note: Dyke advocates moving forward 4 mm the normal zone of Vastine and Kinney. (From Dyke CG: AJR Am J Roentgenol 1930; 23:598. Used by permission.)

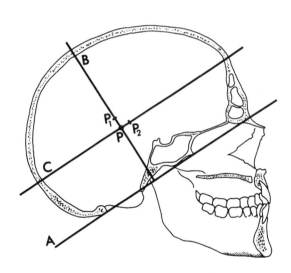

Figure 3 ▪ The Pawl-Walter method of pineal gland measurement. (Adapted from Pawl RP, Walter AK: AJR Am J Roentgenol 1969; 105:287.)

Source

One hundred twenty skull examinations at Tripler Army Medical Center.

Note: A calcified pineal may normally be shifted 2 to 3 mm from the midline on a good PA skull. This is considered a normal variation.

REFERENCES

1. Vastine JH, Kinney KK: AJR Am J Roentgenol 1927; 17:320.
2. Dyke CG: AJR Am J Roentgenol 1930; 23:598.
3. Pawl RP, Walter AK: Localization of the calcified pineal body on lateral roentgenograms. AJR Am J Roentgenol 1969; 105:287.

▪▪ SIZE AND ENHANCEMENT OF THE PINEAL GLAND
▪ ACR Code: 147 (Pineal Gland)

Technique ▪

Inoue and associates performed examinations of the brain on a Siemens 1.5-T-machine, using gradient echo T1-weighted sagittal sequences (400–600/15–22) with 3.0-mm slices. These were done before (39 subjects) and 10 minutes after (all subjects) the intravenous administration of 0.1 mmol/kg of Gd-DTPA.[1] Rajarethinam and associates used a General Electric 1.5-T Signa machine and Spoiled GRASS coronal sequences (24/5 flip angle of 40 degrees) with 1.5-mm slices. Images were resampled in the axial plane normalized to a line between the commissures.[2]

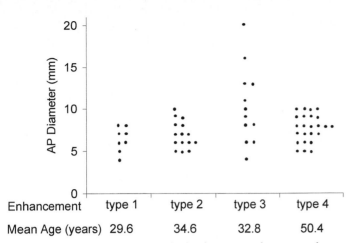

Enhancement	type 1	type 2	type 3	type 4
Mean Age (years)	29.6	34.6	32.8	50.4

Figure 1 ▪ Distribution of pineal gland patterns by age and sex. The diameter of the gland is indicated by the position of the dots against the y axis in millimeters. The four types of enhancement are

type 1 = solid gland, homogeneous enhancement
type 2 = solid gland, partial enhancement
type 3 = cystic gland, ring enhancement
type 4 = cystic gland, partial enhancement of cyst wall

(From Inoue Y, Saiwai S, Miyamoto T, Katsuyama J: J Comput Assist Tomogr 1994; 18(2):182–186. Used by permission.)

Measurements ▪

The largest diameter of the gland was measured by Inoue and associates; the signal intensity of the central portion was noted, and the enhancement pattern was classified. Four patterns of gland morphology and enhancement pat-

tern were noted, and their distribution is shown in Figure 1. The gland was considered to be solid in 40% of cases and cystic (fluid intensity center) in 60%. The gland diameter ranged from 4 to 10 mm in 55 subjects, and in five cases it was larger, ranging from 11 to 20 mm.[1] Rajarethinam and associates manually traced the pineal gland from the resampled images and a volume calculated with locally developed software. The mean volume of the normal pineal gland was 0.213 ml with a standard deviation of 0.097 ml. Assuming a perfect sphere, this would give a mean diameter of 7.4 mm, which is in nice agreement with Inoue and associates' direct measurements.[2]

Source ▪

In Inoue and associates' study, the population consisted of 55 adults who had brain MRI for reasons unrelated to pineal pathology and 5 normal volunteers, for a total of 60 subjects. The mean age was 34 years.[1] Rajarethinam and associates' subjects consisted of 86 normal control adults with a mean age of 27 years. Forty-five patients with schizophrenia were also evaluated.[2]

Comments ▪

There was no significant difference in volume of the pineal between normal controls and schizophrenics. [2]

REFERENCES

1. Inoue Y, Saiwai S, Miyamoto T, Katsuyama J: Enhanced high-resolution sagittal MRI of normal pineal glands. J Comput Assist Tomogr 1994; 18(2):182–186.
2. Rajarethinam R, Gupta S, Andreasen NC: Volume of the pineal gland in schizophrenia; an MRI study. Schizophrenia Res 1995; 14(3):253–255.

▪▪ LINEAR MEASUREMENTS OF THE BRAIN STEM RELATED TO AGE
- ▪ ACR Code: 15 (Brain and Meninges, Infratentorial)

Technique ▪

MRI of the brain was done with a 1.0 T machine (manufacturer not given) on all subjects. Axial sequences were done with T2-weighted (2500/22–90) SE technique. With children under 4 years of age, a longer TR (3500) was used. Sagittal sections were obtained with one of two techniques: T1 (250–500/15) SE or gradient echo (FLASH-3D, TR = 30, TE = 6, flip angle = 40).

Measurements ▪

All measurements were made with the electronic calipers from the console of the MRI unit. The midsagittal scan was used to measure the mesencephalon (upper border of the pons to midway between colliculi), pons (anterior surface to floor of V4), medulla (anterior to posterior just above the cervicomedullary junction). Figure 1 shows these measurements. Axial scans at the appropriate levels were used to measure the maximum peduncular diameter at the mesencephalon, the transverse pons (at the level of the trigeminal or acoustic nerves), and the transverse medulla

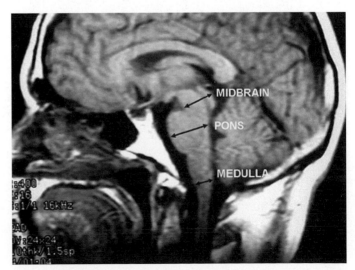

Figure 1 ▪ Midsagittal T1-weighted MRI scan through the posterior fossa, showing measurement of the anteroposterior diameter of the midbrain, pons, and medulla.[1]

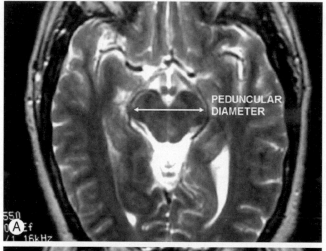

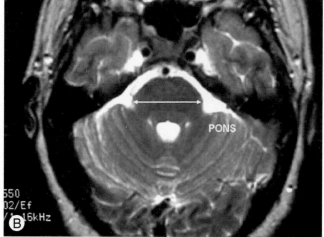

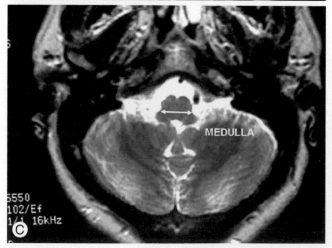

Figure 2 ▪ Axial T2-weighted MRI scans showing transverse measurements of the midbrain (*A*) (peduncular diameter), pons (*B*), and medulla (*C*).[1]

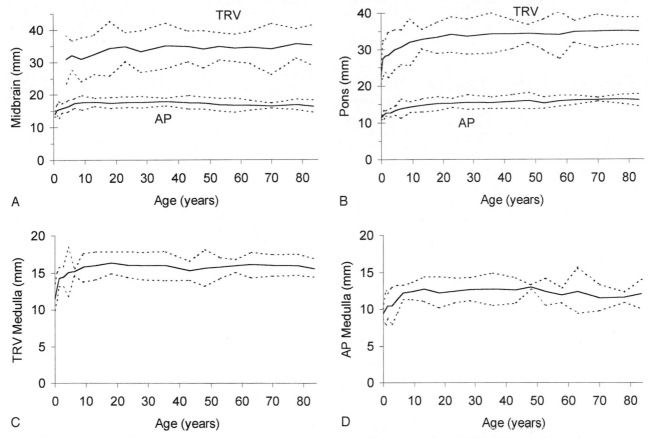

Figure 3 ▪ Plots of linear brain stem measurements versus age. The mean values (*solid lines*) and plus and minus 2 standard deviations (*dotted lines*) are shown. *A*, Midbrain, *B*, pons, *C*, transverse medulla. *D*, anteroposterior medulla. AP = anteroposterior, TRV = transverse. (From Raininko R, Autti T, Vanhanen SL, et al: Neuroradiology 1994; 36(5):364–368. Used by permission.)

Table 1 ▪ **Normal Ranges of Dimensions of Brain Stem Structures Versus Age**

AGE GROUP	NUMBER (Male/Female)	MIDBRAIN AP	PONS AP	PONS TRV	MEDULLA AP	MEDULLA TRV
Months						
4	6 (3/3)	13–15	16–18	21–25	8–10	10–14
12–14	15 (8/7)	13–17	17–20	23–32	8–13	11–15
15–23	8 (7/1)	13–17	17–20	24–33	8–13	13–16
Years						
2–3	7 (2/5)	14–17	17–21	25–35	8–13	13–16
4–5	8 (5/3)	15–18	18–22	25–35	10–13	13–18
6–7	6 (2/4)	16–19	18–24	26–36	11–14	13–18
8–10	11 (4/7)	16–19	18–24	26–38	11–14	14–18
11–15	14 (4/10)	16–19	19–25	29–38	11–14	14–18
16–20	11 (4/7)	16–19	20–25	29–38	11–14	14–18
21–40	31 (17/14)	16–19	21–25	30–38	11–14	14–18
41–50	16 (4/12)	16–19	21–25	30–38	11–14	14–17
51–65	21 (10/11)	15–18	21–25	30–38	10–14	14–17
66–86	20 (11/9)	15–18	21–25	30–38	10–12	14–17

AP = anteroposterior, TRV = transverse.
From Raininko R, Autti T, Vanhanen SL, et al: Neuroradiology 1994; 36(5):364–368. Used by permission.

(most caudal section visible). Figure 2 shows these measurements. Table 1 gives the normal ranges for all these dimensions for various age groups. Figure 3 (A–D) graphically depicts these same measurements.

Source ▪

Patients with no known brain disease (other than single seizures in some of the children) with scans interpreted as normal (n = 37) and healthy volunteers (n = 137) were included in the study. The age of all subjects (n = 174) ranged from 4 months to 86 years. There were 81 males and 93 females. The age distribution is given in Table 1.

REFERENCE

1. Raininko R, Autti T, Vanhanen SL, et al: The normal brain stem from infancy to old age. A morphometric MRI study. Neuroradiology 1994; 36(5):364–368.

▪: MEASUREMENT OF NORMAL BRAIN STEM IN ADULTS AND CHILDREN BY CT CISTERNOGRAPHY
▪ ACR Code: 15 (Brain and Meninges, Infratentorial)

Technique ▪

1. GE 8800 CT/T scanner with 10-mm slices (occasional 5 mm).
2. Patient lies supine with transverse slices, parallel to the canthomeatal line. Coronal scanning is used in some, depending on individual circumstances.
3. Six milliliters of metrizamide (190 mg iodine/ml) are injected in the lumbar subarachnoid space (proportionately smaller volume in younger patients). The prone patient is tilted into a 45°-angle Trendelenburg position, with head flexed for 2 minutes to fill the intracranial cisterns. The patient remains in the prone hanging-head position during transport to the CT suite.

Measurements ▪ (Figure 1 and Table 1)

Measurements were done on hard copy images, corrected for minification.

Transverse measurements of the medulla, pons, and cerebral peduncles were made when possible. These are easily made, except at the level of the brachium pontis, where lateral margins are not readily defined; at that level, the transverse measurement is 5 mm posterior to the anterior pontine margin.

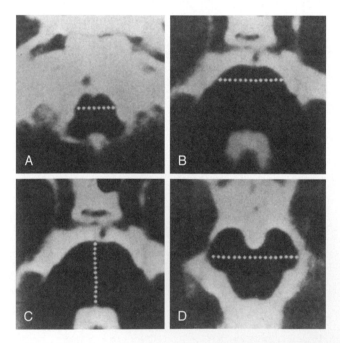

Figure 1 ▪ Locations at which transverse medullary (A), transverse pontine (B), pons—fourth ventricle (C), and transverse peduncular (D) dimensions were obtained. (From Steele JR, Hoffman JC: AJR Am J Roentgenol 1981; 136:287. Used by permission.)

Table 1 ▪ Normal Brain Stem Measurements

LOCATION	NO. CASES	MEAN (mm)	SD (σ)	RANGE (± 2σ) (mm)
Transverse peduncular	41	25.4	3.1	19.5–31.5
Transverse pontine	43	24.8	2.2	20.4–29.2
Transverse medullary	29	13.8	1.9	10.0–17.6
Pons—fourth ventricle	39	22.8	2.3	18.1–27.4

From Steele JR, Hoffman JC: AJR Am J Roentgenol 1981; 136:287. Used by permission.

Distance from the anterior pons to the floor of the fourth ventricle is sometimes not possible because of incomplete mixing of contrast with cerebrospinal fluid in the fourth ventricle.

Measurements on young and elderly patients tend to be in the lower end of the normal range.

Minor asymmetry was noted in about 10% of normal patients, particularly in the cerebral peduncles. Causes include positioning and ectatic arteries.

Sources ▪

Seventy-eight CT cisternograms were reviewed. About half had satisfactory images of the basal cisterns. All such patients examined for reasons unrelated to brain stem or posterior fossa were considered "normal."

REFERENCE

1. Steele JR, Hoffman JC: Brainstem evaluation with CT cisternography. AJR Am J Roentgenol 1981; 136:287.

▪: LINEAR MEASUREMENTS OF VENTRICLES AND POSTERIOR FOSSA STRUCTURES
▪ ACR Code: 15 (Brain and Meninges, Infratentorial)

Technique ▪

All scans were done on a 0.5-T Toshiba machine. T1-weighted (500/30) sagittal and axial images were done. Intravenous contrast was not administered.

Measurements ▪

Measurements were made with sliding calipers from hard copies. All ventricular measurements (except V4 height), as well as the transverse cerebellar diameter, were made from the T1-weighted axial images. V4 height measurement, as well as all the anteroposterior and height measurements, was made from T1-weighted sagittal scans at midplane. Table 1 gives these values for two subgroups of age (cutoff = 50 years) and for all subjects.

Source ▪

The subjects were 40 normal controls included in a study of chronic alcoholic patients. They were scanned for headache, head trauma, and cervical syndrome. All examinations were interpreted as normal, and none of the patients had neurologic symptoms or signs. All but 3 of the subjects were men.

Comments ▪

The ventricular sizes were significantly greater in the alcoholic patients (p < 0.05 to p < 0.001).

REFERENCE

1. Hayakawa K, Kumagai H, Suzuki Y, et al: MR imaging of chronic alcoholism. Acta Radiol 1992; 33(3):201 206.

Table 1 ▪ Composite of Linear Ventricular and Posterior Fossa Structure Measurements from T1-Weighted MRI Scans in 40 Adults

Age range	31–50	51–70	All
Number	20	20	40
Frontal horn TRV	3.5 ± 0.3	3.7 ± 0.3	3.6 ± 0.3
Cellae media TRV	1.6 ± 0.2	1.9 ± 0.3	1.7 ± 0.3
V3 TRV	0.61 ± 0.13	0.81 ± 0.21	0.71 ± 0.2
Evan's ratio	0.25 ± 0.017	0.27 ± 0.02	0.26 ± 0.02
Midbrain AP	1.27 ± 0.11	1.26 ± 0.08	1.27 ± 0.09
Pons AP	2.45 ± 0.13	2.5 ± 0.12	2.48 ± 0.13
Medulla AP	1.56 ± 0.12	1.56 ± 0.07	1.56 ± 0.1
V4 height	1.02 ± 0.13	1.03 ± 0.11	1.03 ± 0.12
V4 TRV	1.62 ± 0.3	1.64 ± 0.25	1.63 ± 0.27
CBL TRV	3.6 ± 0.24	3.55 ± 0.19	3.57 ± 0.21
CBL height	4.87 ± 0.23	4.82 ± 0.3	4.84 ± 0.27
CBL vermis height	2.74 ± 0.18	2.62 ± 0.15	2.68 ± 0.18

All measurements are in centimeters (mean ± standard deviation) except the Evan's ratio (dimensionless).
TRV = transverse (from axial scans), AP = anteroposterior (from midplane sagittal scan), height = cephalo-caudal dimension (from midplane sagittal scans), CBL = cerebellum.
From Hayakawa K, Kumagai H, Suzuki Y, et al: Acta Radiol 1992; 33(3):201–206. Used by permission.

⫶ CEREBELLAR VERMIS AREA IN NEONATES
- ACR Code: 153 (Cerebellum)

Technique ▪

Neonatal neurosonograms were performed with a 7702A unit (Hewlett Packard) using 3.5 MHz real-time sector transducers. Scans were done through the anterior fontanel in the segittal plane.[1]

Measurements ▪

The cerebellar vermis was identified on a frozen midsagittal scan in each case, and an ellipse was superimposed over it

and adjusted to cover the structure. The cerebellar vermian area (CVA) in square centimeters was calculated by multiplying the axes together with pi.[1] Figure 1 shows this measurement, Table 1 lists the data in tabular form, Figure 2 is a scatterplot of CVA versus gestational age, and Figure 3 is a scatterplot of CVA versus birth weight.[1]

Source ▪

A total of 51 neonates were studied, consisting of 38 appropriate for gestational age (GA) infants, 10 small for GA

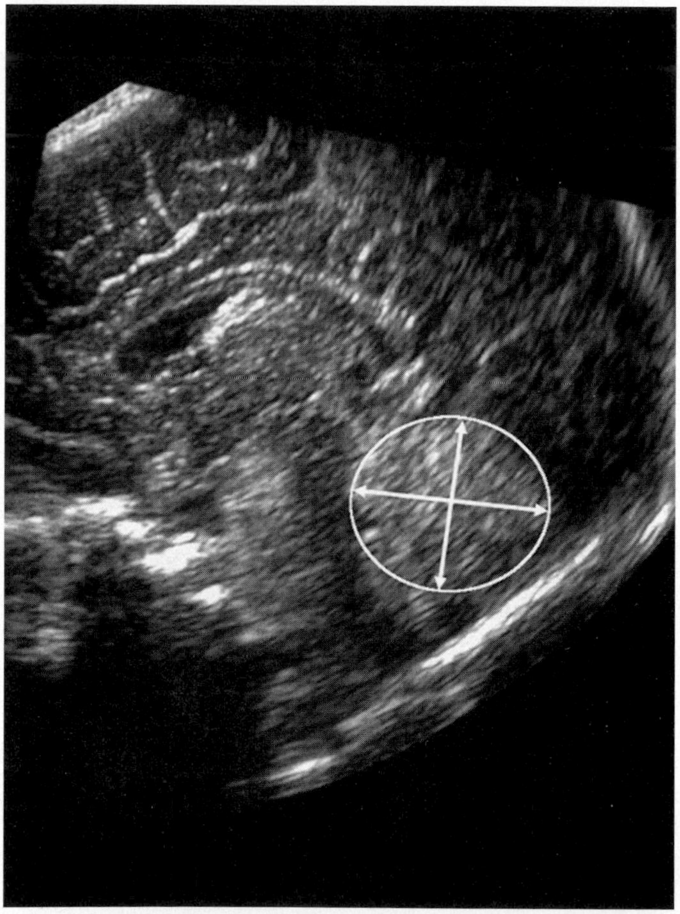

Figure 1 ▪ Midsagittal sector ultrasound scan of a neonatal brain showing measurement of cerebellar vermis area. An ellipse is superimposed over the structure (*white*), and the area was derived by multiplying the two axes (*white lines*) and pi.[1]

Table 1 ▪ Cerebellar Vermis Area, Gestational Age, and Birth Weight of 51 Neonates

	GESTATIONAL AGE (wk)	BIRTH WEIGHT (gm)	VERMIS AREA (cm)
AGA (n = 35)			
Mean ± SD	34.0 ± 4.6	2028 ± 902	2.72 ± 1.02
Range	26–42	600–3680	0.75–4.74
SGA (n = 10)			
Mean ± SD	35.7 ± 2.6	1735 ± 349	2.54 ± 0.36
Range	32–41	1220–2180	1.92–3.14
LGA (n = 6)			
Mean ± SD	34.2 ± 3.5	2435 ± 754	2.68 ± 0.68
Range	28–38	1240–3320	1.52–3.41

AGA, SGA, LGA = appropriate, small, and large for gestational age; SD = standard deviation.

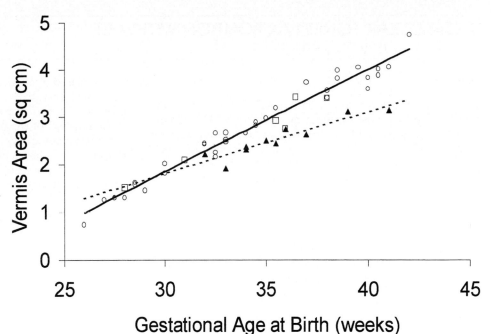

Figure 2 • Scatterplot of cerebellar vermis area versus gestational age (GA) of 51 neonates. Circles represent appropriate for GA, triangles small for GA, and squares large for GA. Linear regression lines are shown for appropriate for GA (*solid*) and small for GA (*dotted*). (From Birnholz JC: Pediatrics 1982; 70:284–287. Used by permission.)

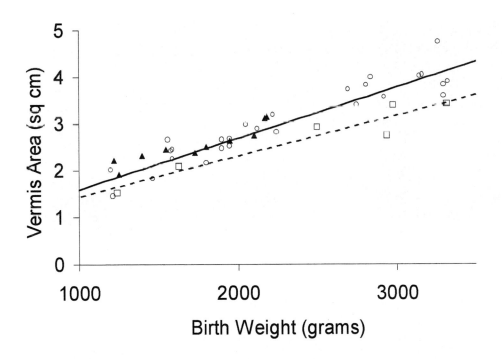

Figure 3 • Scatterplot of cerebellar vermis area versus birth weight of 51 newborns. Circles represent appropriate for GA, triangles small for GA, and squares large for GA. Linear regression lines are shown for appropriate for GA (*solid*) and large for GA (*dotted*). (From Birnholz JC: Pediatrics 1982; 70:284–287. Used by permission.)

infants, and 6 large for GA babies. Gestational age and birth weight demographics are shown in Table 1. The large for GA infants were all born of diabetic mothers. The brains were morphologically normal (inclusion criteria), and all studies were performed within 24 hours of birth.[1]

Comments •

Linear regressions of CVA to gestational age (r squared = .96) and CVA to birth weight (r squared = .93) were both good for appropriate-for-GA infants. Using the parameter estimates, one may calculate expected CVA from gestational age or birth weight as follows:

$$\text{CVA (cm}^2) = 0.213 \times \text{GA (wk)} - 4.56$$
$$\text{CVA (cm}^2) = 0.0011 \times \text{birth weight (gm)} + 0.507$$

REFERENCE

1. Birnholz JC: Newborn cerebellar size. Pediatrics 1982; 70:284–287.

∴ CEREBELLAR TONSILLAR POSITION WITH AGE
- ACR Code: 1532 (Cerebellar Tonsil)

Technique •

MRI of the brain was done with a 1.5-T Signa machine (General Electric Medical Systems, Milwaukee, WI). Sagittal T1-weighted (600/20) sequences at 5-mm, section thickness were done on all subjects. The midsagittal and adjacent images on either side (left and right parasagittal) were chosen in each case for measurements.

Measurements •

All measurements were done on the MRI console using electronic calipers, line-drawing functions, and the measure distance function. The basion and opisthion were identified by the most inferior cortical bone of the clivus and occiput, respectively. These points were connected by a reference line on the midsagittal image. The recorded coordinates of these reference points were used to draw a reference line on the parasagittal images. The perpendicular distance between the reference lines and the inferiormost tonsillar tissue was measured on the midsagittal and each parasagittal slice. Figure 1 illustrates these measurements. The measured position of the lowest tonsil (in millimeters) was used for subsequent analysis and was assigned a positive number if above the reference and a negative number if below the reference (0 mm). Subjects were grouped by decade (about 25 per group) and descriptive statistics of tonsillar position tabulated (Table 1). These same data are depicted graphically in Figure 2.

Source •

Randomly selected outpatients (male = 106, female = 115, n = 221), ranging in age from 8 months to 89 years, were enrolled in the study. None had any known disease or abnormality on the scans affecting the position of the cerebellar tonsils.

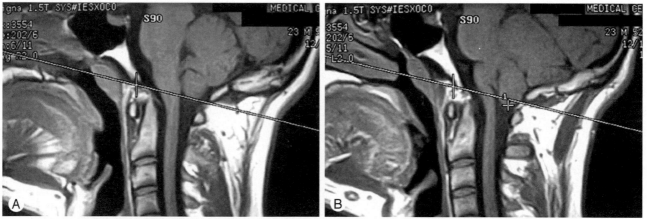

Figure 1 • Midsagittal T1-weighted MRI of the brain showing measurement of cerebellar tonsil position with respect to the foramen magnum. *A*, The reference line is drawn on the midsagittal image connecting the basion and opisthion. *B*, The distance between this line and the bottom of each tonsil is measured. Often the lowest part of the tonsil is on a parasagittal image, as is the case here. Most MRI measurement packages allow the user to change images while leaving the reference line in its previous position.[1]

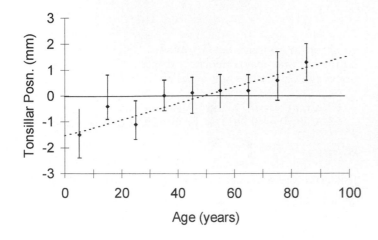

Figure 2 • Plot of mean cerebellar position (*diamonds*) and 95% confidence limits (*error bars*) for decades 1–9. The zero line on the y axis indicates the position of the foramen magnum. The published regression of position on age is also included (*dotted line*). (From Mikulis DJ, Diaz O, Egglin TK, Sanchez R: Radiology 1992; 183(3):725–728. Used by permission.)

Table 2 ▪ Position of the Cerebellar Tonsils on Sagittal MRI Scans Grouped by Decade of Life

DECADE	NUMBER	TONSIL POSITION Mean ± SD	95% CL Lower	95% CL Upper	SUGGESTED CUT-OFF VALUE
1	24	−1.5 ± 2.2	−2.4	−0.5	−6
2	18	−0.4 ± 1.0	−0.9	0.8	−5
3	26	−1.1 ± 1.9	−1.7	−0.2	−5
4	30	0.0 ± 1.7	−0.6	0.6	−4
5	27	0.1 ± 1.7	−0.7	0.7	−4
6	23	0.2 ± 1.6	−0.5	0.8	−4
7	26	0.2 ± 1.6	−0.5	0.8	−4
8	21	0.6 ± 2.1	−0.2	1.7	−4
9	26	1.3 ± 1.8	0.6	2.0	−3

Measurements are in millimeters. Negative numbers indicate that the tonsils are below the foramen magnum. CL = confidence limits.
From Mikulis DJ, Diaz O, Egglin TK, Sanchez R: Radiology 1992; 183(3):725–728. Used by permission.

Comments ▪

There was a significant difference in tonsillar position between different age groups by analysis of variance (ANOVA) testing (p < .001). There was no significant side-to-side difference. Based on this study and a review of the literature, the authors suggest criteria for definition of tonsillar ectopia for different age groups (see Fig. 1).

REFERENCE

1. Mikulis DJ, Diaz O, Egglin TK, Sanchez R: Variance of the position of the cerebellar tonsils with age: Preliminary report. Radiology 1992; 183(3):725–728.

▪: FRONTAL VENTRICLE WIDTH IN NEONATES
▪ ACR Code: 16 (Cerebral Ventricles)

Technique ▪

Neonatal neurosonography was done through the anterior fontanel with a 7.0-MHz linear transducer and a real time scanner (ADR, Tempe, AZ). An oblique coronal section through the level of the foramina of Monro was recorded for measurements.[1]

Measurements ▪

The ventricular width was measured from the medial wall to the floor of the ventricle at the widest point. The measurement was recorded as 0 mm, when the ventricle appeared as a thin line less than 0.5 mm in width. Otherwise, measurements were recorded to the nearest millimeter. Figure 1 shows a representative coronal scan with measurement sites indicated. Table 1 lists the percentages of widths from 0 to 5 mm versus gestational age.

Source ▪

A total of 533 neurologically normal infants was examined. All examinations were done between 48 and 96 hours after delivery. Gestational age was determined from the last menstrual period (LMP) and a pediatric assessment using the Ballard score.[2] When the two methods differed by

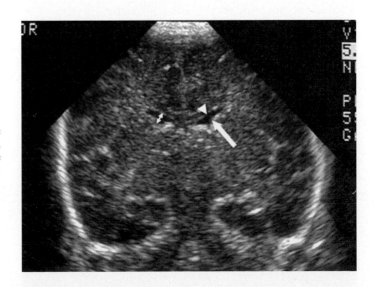

Figure 1 ▪ Oblique coronal ultrasound of the frontal horns of the lateral ventricles, showing measurement of ventricular width on the right (*line with arrowheads*), the roof of the left lateral ventricle (*arrowhead*), and the floor of the left lateral ventricle (*arrow*).

Table 1 ▪ Frontal Ventricular Widths in Neonates of Various Gestational Ages

GESTATIONAL AGE RANGE (Wk)	NUMBER	FRONTAL HORN SIZE (mm) Percent Having Each Width						MEAN WIDTH (Calculated)
		0.0	1.0	2.0	3.0	4.0	5.0	
26–27	10	30	50	20	0	—	—	0.9
28–29	18	35	33	28	4	—	—	1.01
30–31	28	13	55	21	9	2	—	1.32
32–33	82	23	57	14	4	2	—	1.05
34–35	102	47	34	12	4	3	—	0.82
36–37	71	51	35	7	4	2	1	0.74
38–39	92	28	51	14	5	2	—	1.02
40–41	123	43	38	11	3	3	2	0.91
42	7	14	63	23	—	—	0	1.09

From Perry RNW, Bowman ED, Roy RND, et al: J Ultrasound Med 1985; 4:475–477. Used by permission.

more than 2 weeks (in 3 patients), the Ballard score was used. The gestational ages at time of delivery ranged from 26 to 42 weeks.[1]

Comments ▪

There was no significant difference in frontal ventricular width among different gestational age groups. A large majority (97 to 100%) of ventricles were smaller than 3 mm. Of all 533 infants scanned, 15 (2.8%) had ventricular widths greater than 3 mm. Of these 15 infants, 13 were examined in follow-up between 3 and 12 months of age and were found to be developmentally and neurologically normal.

REFERENCES

1. Perry RNW, Bowman ED, Roy RND, et al: Ventricular size in newborn infants. J Ultrasound Med 1985; 4:475–477.
2. Ballard JL, Novak KK, Driver M: A simplified score of the assessment of fetal maturation of newly born infants. J Pediatr 1979; 95:769.

▪: VENTRICULAR SIZE IN NEONATES
- ▪ ACR Code: 16 (Cerebral Ventricles)

Technique ▪

Neonatal neurosonograms were performed using a Sono III EP (Unirad, Denver, CO) B-mode unit. Transducers used included 3.5- and 5-MHz short or medium focus. Scans were done in sagittal and coronal planes through the anterior fontanel and in transverse plane through the squamous portion of the temporal bone.[1]

Measurements ▪

Measurements were made in the transverse plane at the level of the midbody on the side contralateral to the transducer, using electronic calipers, of the ventricular width (VW) from the midline echo complex to the lateral ventricular wall, as well as the hemispheric width (HW) from the midline to the inner skull margin. A ventricular ratio (VR) was calculated as follows: VR = VW/HW. Figure 1 shows these measurements, and Table 1 lists the results.

Source ▪

Twenty-five full-term infants from a well-baby nursery were examined. The mean gestational age was 39.3 wks

Figure 1 ▪ Measurement of the lateral ventricular ratio in the neonate. Transverse image through the squamous temporal bone at the level of the bodies of the lateral ventricles. The distance from the midline echo to the wall of the lateral ventricle at its midportion is divided by the distance from the midline to the inner table of the skull (short and long arrows respectively).

Table 1 ▪ Ultrasound Measurements of the Lateral Ventricle and Hemisphere Widths and Their Ratios[1]

| | TERM NEONATES (n = 25) | | PREMATURE NEONATES (n = 25) | |
	Mean	Range	Mean	Range
Width of lateral ventricle (cm)	1.1	0.9–1.3	1.0	0.5–1.3
Width of hemisphere (cm)	3.9	3.1–4.7	3.1	2.1–4.3
Ventricle/hemisphere ratio × 100 (%)	28	24–30	31	24–34

(range = 38–42 wk), and the mean birth weight was 3128 gm (range = 2610–4040 gm). Twenty-five premature infants thought to be normal by clinical examination were also studied. The mean gestational age was 31.6 wk (range = 26–37 wk), and the mean birth weight was 1333 gm (range = 690–2820 gm). All ultrasound examinations were morphologically normal.[1]

Comments ▪

The ventricular ratio (VR) is rather easy to measure and calculate and is useful in identifying and following hydrocephalus in neonates.

REFERENCE

1. Johnson ML, Rumack CM: B-mode echoencephalography in the normal and high risk infant. AJR Am J Roentgenol 1979; 133:375–381.

▪: THE VENTRICULAR AND CISTERNAL SPACES IN CHILDREN AND ADOLESCENTS
▪ ACR Code: 16 (Cerebral Ventricles)

Technique ▪

CT scans of the head were done using an LX scanner (Phillips Medical Systems, Irvine, CA). Slice orientation was not specified. Scanning was done at 5-mm intervals through the posterior fossa in all subjects and continued

through the vertex at 5 mm for infants and at 10 mm in older children.[1, 2]

Measurements ▪

Using electronic calipers on the CT console, the transverse (TRV) widths of the lateral ventricles (three sites), third

Table 1 ▪ Normal Values of Ventricular/Cisternal Ratios and Sum of Maximal Skull Diameters in Children

AGE	NUMBER	LATERAL VENTRICLE RATIO	ANTERIOR HORN RATIO	BICAUDATE RATIO	V3 RATIO	V4 RATIO	CHIASMATIC CISTERN RATIO*	PONTINE CISTERN RATIO	SUM OF CRANIAL DIAMETERS (cm)	
Months									Boys and Girls	
3–6	12	104 ± 5	102 ± 6	32 ± 1	7 ± 1	78 ± 5	151 ± 8	50 ± 2	23.9 ± 1.1	
6–9	12	108 ± 4	108 ± 6	34 ± 1	8 ± 1	80 ± 4	148 ± 7	47 ± 2	25.2 ± 1.0	
9–12	12	112 ± 4	114 ± 6	36 ± 1	8 ± 1	81 ± 4	145 ± 7	44 ± 2	26.0 ± 1.3	
12–15	12	113 ± 4	115 ± 5	36 ± 1	9 ± 1	78 ± 4	142 ± 6	42 ± 2	26.2 ± 1.3	
15–18	12	115 ± 5	117 ± 5	37 ± 1	8 ± 1	77 ± 4	140 ± 4	42 ± 1	26.7 ± 1.0	
18–21	12	116 ± 4	119 ± 4	39 ± 1	9 ± 2	79 ± 4	138 ± 4	38 ± 2	26.8 ± 1.0	
21–24	12	113 ± 5	116 ± 5	37 ± 1	9 ± 1	80 ± 4	136 ± 4	38 ± 2	27.2 ± 1.0	
24–27	12	110 ± 4	114 ± 5	36 ± 1	8 ± 1	79 ± 4	135 ± 4	37 ± 2	27.6 ± 0.9	
Years									Boys	Girls
0–1	15	106 ± 12	108 ± 12	34 ± 5	8 ± 2	78 ± 9	148 ± 12	47 ± 8	25.8 ± 1.3	23.4 ± 1.1
1–2	26	115 ± 11	118 ± 13	38 ± 5	9 ± 3	76 ± 11	139 ± 11	40 ± 10	27.3 ± 1.4	26.1 ± 1.5
2–3	21	102 ± 14	112 ± 11	34 ± 6	8 ± 3	79 ± 8	131 ± 14	38 ± 11	27.6 ± 0.8	26.8 ± 1.9
3–4	20	103 ± 12	104 ± 11	29 ± 6	8 ± 2	74 ± 8	128 ± 7	38 ± 10	28.2 ± 1.1	27.2 ± 0.8
4–5	29	99 ± 13	106 ± 7	28 ± 4	7 ± 2	72 ± 9	130 ± 8	42 ± 12	28.4 ± 1.4	27.2 ± 1.1
5–6	22	103 ± 12	108 ± 8	30 ± 6	7 ± 3	75 ± 7	124 ± 11	40 ± 11	28.4 ± 1.9	27.4 ± 2.1
6–7	15	104 ± 13	109 ± 12	29 ± 5	7 ± 1	76 ± 7	126 ± 9	38 ± 9	28.4 ± 2.3	27.5 ± 1.7
7–8	13	105 ± 11	108 ± 11	28 ± 5	8 ± 2	75 ± 9	122 ± 8	35 ± 8	28.2 ± 3.1	27.4 ± 2.6
8–9	14	98 ± 14	105 ± 9	31 ± 5	9 ± 3	72 ± 11	130 ± 9	31 ± 9	28.3 ± 1.1	27.8 ± 1.3
9–10	12	98 ± 13	107 ± 9	28 ± 5	8 ± 2	76 ± 8	125 ± 9	37 ± 10	28.7 ± 1.2	27.8 ± 1.2
10–11	13	103 ± 13	107 ± 11	29 ± 5	7 ± 1	75 ± 8	125 ± 10	35 ± 9	29.0 ± 1.7	27.6 ± 1.6
11–12	11	105 ± 13	105 ± 8	31 ± 7	8 ± 1	75 ± 9	130 ± 10	33 ± 8	29.1 ± 0.8	28.0 ± 1.9
12–13	10	101 ± 15	103 ± 7	32 ± 6	7 ± 2	77 ± 12	134 ± 9	39 ± 9	29.7 ± 1.8	28.3 ± 1.4
13–14	14	102 ± 14	105 ± 7	28 ± 5	7 ± 1	78 ± 6	134 ± 7	32 ± 7	29.8 ± 2.1	28.4 ± 1.8
14–15	12	101 ± 15	106 ± 8	31 ± 6	7 ± 2	73 ± 9	130 ± 11	36 ± 7	29.5 ± 2.2	28.3 ± 1.6

*The chiasmatic cistern ratio was formed by dividing the sum of the AP and TRV dimensions by the sum of posterior fossa inner skull diameters.
All ratios are unitless and have been multiplied by 1000 (mean ± standard deviation). V3 = third ventricle, V4 = fourth ventricle.
From Prassopoulos P, Cavouras D: Eur J Radiol 1994; 18:22–25. Used by permission.

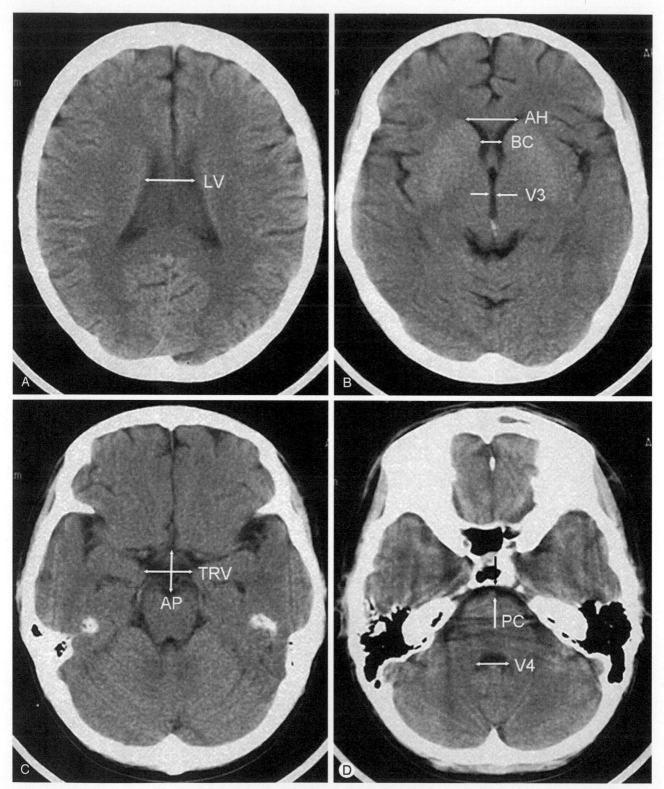

Figure 1 ▪ Measurements of ventricles and cisterns. *A,* Lateral ventricles *(LV)* at the level of the cella media. *B,* Anterior horns *(AH)*, bicaudate distance *(BC)*, and third ventricle *(V3)*. *C,* Chiasmatic cistern *(AP* and *TRV)*. *D,* Prepontine cistern *(PC)*, fourth ventricle *(V4)*. The inner skull measurements are not shown but were made between the inner tables (midsagittal and maximum transverse) at the level of measurement. The anterior landmark for the posterior fossa was the posterior clinoids or the clivus.[1, 2]

ventricle, fourth ventricle, and chiasmatic cistern were measured. The anteroposterior (AP) dimensions of the chiasmatic and prepontine cisterns were also measured. Ratios were formed by dividing the various measures made of these structures (summed AP and TRV of the chiasmatic cistern) by the sum of the AP and TRV inner skull dimensions of the cranium or posterior fossa at the measurement level.[1, 2]

Examples of these measurements are shown in Figure 1. Table 1 lists the ratios grouped by age in months from 3 to 27,[1] and by year from 0 to 15.[2] The sums of maximum AP and TRV cranial diameters are included for each age group and are divided by gender for the older children. Posterior fossa dimensions are not given.

Source ■

Ninety-six infants and young children ranging in age from 3 to 27 months (gender not specified), with normal head CT scans, were included in one study.[1] In a second series, 145 boys and 102 girls ranging in age from 3 months to 14 years, with normal CT findings, were evaluated.[2] In both studies, children with evidence of increased intracranial pressure, abnormal head circumference, CNS infection, or any other condition or therapy that would potentially alter brain or skull morphology, was excluded.[1, 2]

Comments ■

Note that the ratios of the ventricular measurements are quite stable with age, whereas the cisternal spaces grow at a slower rate than the skull, as reflected by decreasing ratios.[1, 2]

REFERENCES

1. Prassopoulos P, Cavouras D, Golfinopoulos S, Nezi M: The size of the intra- and extraventricular cerebrospinal fluid compartments in children with idiopathic benign widening of the frontal subarachnoid space. Neuroradiology 1995; 37:418–421.
2. Prassopoulos P, Cavouras D: CT evaluation of normal CSF spaces in children: Relationship to age, gender, and cranial size. Eur J Radiol 1994; 18:22–25.

▪▪ LINEAR MEASUREMENTS OF THE VENTRICULAR SYSTEM RELATED TO AGE
- ACR Code: 16 (Cerebral Ventricles)

Technique ■

Unenhanced CT scans of the brain were done with EMI[1, 2] and Siretom[3] scanners. Measurements were made from hard copies, using a transparent ruler and calibration scale.[1–3] In another study, brain CT scans (unspecified model) were printed on 35-mm film and projected on the screen of a Vanguard Motion Analyzer for measurement.[4] MRI scans were done on a Signa 1.5-T system (General Electric Corp, Milwaukee, WI). T2 (2800/30 or 80) axial images were done at 5-mm-slice thickness.[5] A computer-generated transparent scale calibrated to 0.5 mm was placed over the MRI images, and measurements were made with the aid of a head-mounted magnifying glass.[5] In all studies, the physicians performing measurements were blinded to the age of the subjects.[1–5]

Measurements ■

Figure 1 shows the various linear measurements that have been reported. These are commonly given in the form of ratios to correct for overall head size and are listed below. The ER, BFI, and BCI are often multiplied by 100 to yield percents.

Evan's ratio (ER) = A/F
Bifrontal index (BFI) = A/D
Bicaudate index (BCI) = B/E
Cella media index (CMI) = H/I
Frontal horn index (FHI) = G/A
Ventricular index (VI) = B/A
Huckman number (HN) = A + B
3rd ventricle width (V3) = C
4th ventricle width (V4, not shown) is the greatest transverse diameter of the structure.

Tables 1 and 2 show CMI, ER, and V3 related to age in tabular form.[1, 3] Table 3 gives proposed normal cut-off values of CMI, FHI, HN, VI, V3, and V4 for young children, adults, and aged individuals based on the study results.[2] Figure 2 shows ER based on age.[1, 3] Figure 3 shows

	Table 1 ▪ Ventricular Size Related to Age, from Newborn to 15 Years								
Age (yr)		0–3			4–15			0–15	
Number		46			109			155	
Mean ± SD									
CMI		4.4 ± 0.87			5.2 ± 1.12			5.0 ± 1.12	
ER		0.28 ± 0.036			0.26 ± 0.026			0.27 ± 0.026	
V3		3.7 ± 1.48			3.3 ± 0.87			3.3 ± 1.68	
Percentiles	5th	50th	95th	5th	50th	95th	5th	50th	95th
CMI	3.7	4.4	6.1	4.2	5.2	7.4	3.9	5.0	7.2
ER	0.22	0.28	0.35	0.21	0.26	0.31	0.21	0.27	0.32
V3	1.9	3.7	6.6	1.7	3.3	5.0	1.7	3.3	6.6

ER = Evan's ratio, CMI = cella media index, V3 = 3rd ventricle.[1]

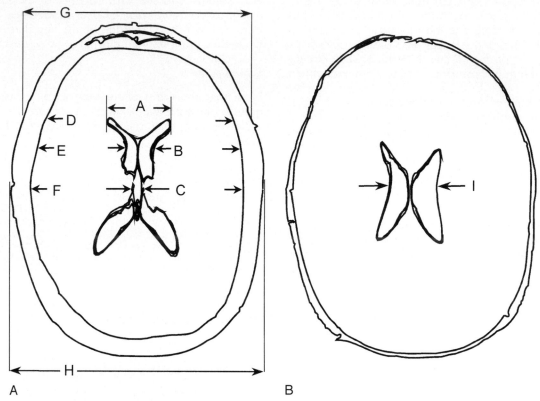

Figure 1 ▪ Measurements of ventricular size on axial CT or MRI scans. *A*, Axial scan at the level of the lateral and 3rd ventricles. *B*, Axial scan at the level of the bodies of the lateral ventricles. Standard linear measurements are depicted on appropriate levels.

A = maximum frontal horn diameter
B = minimum width of the lateral ventricles at the heads of the caudate nuclei
C = maximum width of the 3rd ventricle
D = inner skull diameter at the level of the frontal horns
E = inner skull diameter at the heads of the caudate nuclei
F = maximum inner skull diameter (may be at a different level)
G = outer skull diameter at the frontal horns
H = maximum outer skull diameter (may be at a different level)
I = minimum width of the lateral ventricles separated by the septum (cella media)

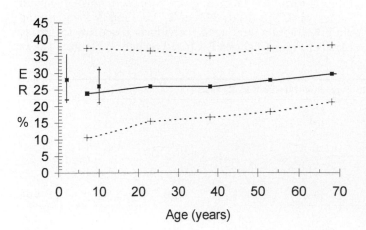

Figure 2 ▪ Evan's ratio (ER) related to age from neonate to 75 years. The mean values (*squares/solid line*) as well as 5th and 95th percentile values (*crosses/dotted lines*) are shown.[1, 3]

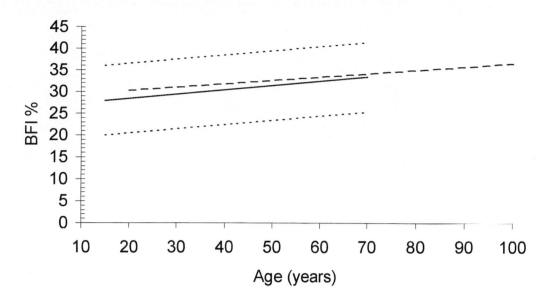

Figure 3 ▪ Bifrontal index (BFI) expressed as percent (× 100) related to age. The linear regressions of the mean (*solid*) as well as plus and minus 2 standard deviations (*dotted*) on age (10–70 years) are from Hahn.[4] The dashed line is the regression of mean BFI on age (20–100 years) from Doraiswamy.[5]

Table 2 ▪ Ventricular Size Related to Age, from Newborn to 75 Years														
Age	0–15			16–30			31–45			46–60			61–75		
Number	15			40			62			40			14		
Mean ± SD															
CMI	6.7 ± 1.7			5.6 ± 1.5			5.4 ± 1.3			5.0 ± 1.0			4.4 ± 1.0		
ER	0.24 ± 0.067			0.26 ± 0.053			0.26 ± 0.046			0.28 ± 0.048			0.30 ± 0.043		
V3	2.4			3.0			3.6			4.5			5.4		
Percentiles	5th	50th	95th	5th	50th	95th	5th	50th	95th	5th	50th	95th	5th	50th	95th
CMI	3.3	6.7	10	2.7	5.6	8.5	2.8	5.4	7.9	3.0	5.0	7.0	2.4	4.4	6.4
ER	0.11	0.24	0.37	0.16	0.26	0.36	0.17	0.26	0.35	0.19	0.28	0.37	0.22	0.30	0.38

ER = Evan's ratio, CMI = cella media index, V3 = 3rd ventricle.[3]

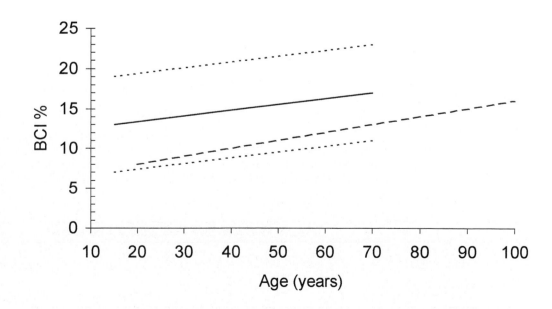

Figure 4 ▪ Bicaudate index (BCI) expressed as percent (× 100) related to age. The linear regressions of the mean (*solid*) as well as plus and minus 2 standard deviations (*dotted*) on age (10–70 years) are from Hahn.[4] The dashed line is the regression of mean BFI on age (20–100 years) from Doraiswamy.[5]

Table 3 ▪ Proposed Normal Values for Various Linear Measurements of the Ventricular System

	AGE RANGE		
	Through 2 Years	Through 60 Years	Above 60 Years
Upper limit of normal			
V3 width (mm)	5	7	9
V4 width (mm)	9	11	13
Huckman number (mm)	35	45	55
Lower limit of normal			
Frontal horn index	3.5	3.7	3.5
Cella media index	3.8	4.0	3.8
Ventricular index	1.6	1.6	1.4

Upper limits of normal are given for 3rd ventricle width (V3), 4th ventricle width (V4), and Huckman number. Lower limits are given for frontal horn index, cella media index, and ventricular index.[2]

linear regressions of BFI on age, and Figure 4 depicts linear regressions of BCI on age.[4, 5]

Source ▪

The populations studied with CT included 155 children, ranging in age from newborn to 15 years, with normal scans,[1] 170 neurologically normal subjects ranging in age from newborn to 75 years,[2] 160 healthy subjects ranging in age from newborn to 80 years,[3] and 200 normal individuals ranging in age from 10 to 81 years.[4] MRI of the brain was done on 49 healthy volunteers aged 22 to 82 years.[5]

REFERENCES

1. Pedersen H, Gyldensted M, Gyldensted C: Measurement of the normal ventricular system and supratentorial subarachnoid space in children with computed tomography. Neuroradiology 1979; 17(5):231–237.
2. Meese W, Kluge W, Grumme T, Hopfenmuller W: CT evaluation of the CSF spaces of healthy persons. Neuroradiology 1980; 19:131–136.
3. Haug G: Age and sex dependence of the size of normal ventricles on computed tomography. Neuroradiology 1977; 14:201–204.
4. Hahn FJY, Rim K: Frontal ventricular dimensions on normal computed tomography. AJR Am J Roentgenol 1976; 126:593–596.
5. Doraiswamy PM, Patterson L, Na C, et al: Bicaudate index on magnetic resonance imaging: Effects of normal aging. J Geriatr Psychiatry Neurol 1994; 7(1):13–17.

▪: AREA MEASUREMENTS OF THE LATERAL VENTRICLES
▪ ACR Code: 16 (Cerebral Ventricles)

Technique ▪

CT scans (unspecified model) through the bodies of the lateral ventricles were printed on Polaroid film and traced with a planimeter.[1] A meta-analysis of 29 studies (23 using CT scans and 6 with MRI scans) of ventricular size and mood disorders was undertaken.[2]

Measurements ▪

The area of the ventricles traced by hand was divided by the area of the whole brain (also traced by hand) at the level of the body of the lateral ventricles, to derive the

ventricle-brain ratio (VBR) both in the cited study and in all the articles included in the meta-analysis.[1, 2] The average VBR in normal adult control subjects calculated by meta-analysis[1] was 5.46 (SD = 2.39; range, 2.9 to 9.1). Figure 1 shows the measurement, Table 1 lists results in tabular form, and Figures 2 and 3 show results in graphic format.

Source ▪

Normal subjects (n = 135), ranging in age from 9 months to 90 years.[1] In the meta-analysis, 932 control subjects with an average age of 45 years (range, 28 to 74 years) were pooled.[2]

Table 1 ▪ Ventricle to Brain Ratio (VBR) Related to Age[1]

Decade	1	2	3	4	5
VBR ± SD	1.8 ± 0.4	3.3 ± 0.7	3.1 ± 0.6	4.2 ± 0.8	4.4 ± 0.8
Decade	6	7	8	9	
VBR ± SD	5.2 ± 0.6	6.4 ± 0.8	11.5 ± 1.2	14.1 ± 1.4	

VBR expressed as percent: (ventricle area/brain area) ×100.

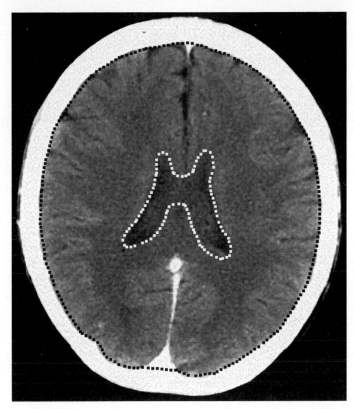

Figure 1 ▪ Measurement of the ventricle to brain ratio (VBR). The slice at the foramen of Monro or the next one caudal (whichever showed the lateral ventricles to be larger) is used. The outline of the ventricles is traced *(white dotted line)* and the area measured. The outline of the inner table of the skull is outlined *(black dotted line)* and the area measured. Most scanners have software for outlining regions of interest and calculating areas at the operator's console.

Figure 2 ▪ Ventricle to brain ratio (VBR) plotted against age.[1] The circles are mean values for each decade, and the error bars are plus and minus 2 standard deviations. The horizontal solid line is the mean value of VBR from the meta-analysis.[2] The horizontal dotted lines are plus and minus 2 standard deviations from the same analysis.

Figure 3 ▪ Ventricle to brain ratio (VBR) plotted against age. The solid line is a 3rd degree polynomial regression on the mean values against age. The dotted lines are similar regressions on plus and minus 2 standard deviations.[1]

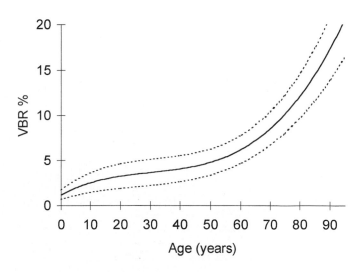

REFERENCES

1. Barron SA, Jacobs L, Kinkel WR: Changes in size of normal lateral ventricles during aging determined by computerized tomography. Neurology 1976; 26:1011–1013.

2. Elkis H, Friedman L, Wise A, Meltzer HY: Meta-analyses of studies of ventricular enlargement and cortical sulcal prominence in mood disorders. Comparisons with controls or patients with schizophrenia. Arch Gen Psychiatry 1995; 52(9):735–746.

⠂ AQUEDUCTAL CSF FLOW VOID IN NORMAL AND HYDROCEPHALIC STATES
- ACR Code: 163 (Aqueduct of Sylvius)

Technique ▪

Standard axial MRI images were obtained with a 0.35T MT/S machine (Diasonics, Milpitas, CA). Double-spin echo T2-weighted (2000/28,56) sequences were done, with slice thickness being 5 or 7 mm. Optimal images through the aqueduct and the lateral ventricles were chosen for study.

Measurements ▪

A ten-pixel region of interest was placed in the lateral ventricle on the appropriate slice, and signal intensity (SI) was recorded for both first and second echo images. A one-pixel region of interest was placed in the center of the cerebral aqueduct on both first and second echo images for SI measurement of all patients. The SI readings from ventricles and aqueduct obtained by these measurements were subtracted to obtain mean differences (lateral ventricle SI − aqueduct SI) in all cases and the standard error of the mean for each group. The absolute SI values in each individual were submitted for one-tailed Student's t-testing. Table 1 lists these results. There was a 95% chance of finding lower aqueductal intensity in normal subjects and a 99.9% chance in normal pressure hydrocephalus (NPH),

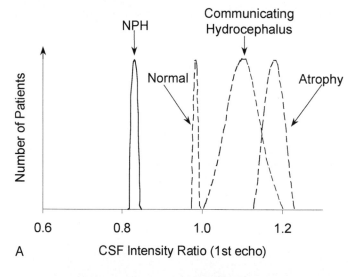

A

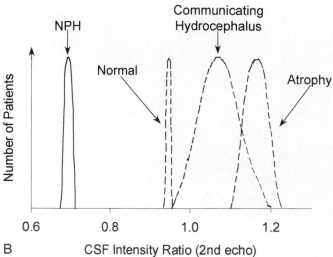

B

Figure 1 ▪ T2 signal intensity (SI) ratios (aqueduct SI/lateral ventricle SI) in healthy subjects and patients with various hydrocephalic states. Ratios are plotted against number of patients (no units) in normalized curves for the first echo (28 msec) (A) and the second echo (56 msec) (B). (From Bradley WG, Kortman KE, Burgoyne B: Radiology 1986; 159:611–615. Used by permission.)

Table 1 ▪ T2 Signal Intensity (SI) Differences Between the Cerebral Aqueduct
and Lateral Ventricle in Healthy Subjects and Patients with Various Hydrocephalic States

CLINICAL STATE	NO. OF PATIENTS	MEAN DIFFERENCE (VENTRICLE-AQUEDUCT)	STANDARD ERROR	SIGNIFICANCE
Normal	16	116	66	$p < 0.05$
NPH	20	481	106	$p < 0.0005$
Acute communicating hydrocephalus	7	−83	99	NS
Atrophy (hydrocephalus ex vacuo)	5	−290	129	NS

NPH = normal pressure hydrocephalus. NS = not significant.
From Bradley WG, Kortman KE, Burgoyne B: Radology 1986; 159:611–615. Used by permission.

with considerable overlap in communicating hydrocephalus and atrophy. The SI ratios (aqueduct SI/ventricular SI) were plotted to show these distributions (Fig. 1).

Source ▪

A total of 48 adult patients were studied (age distribution not given). Of these, 16 were clinically normal with negative scans, 20 had clinical NPH, 7 had acute communicating hydrocephalus, and 5 had atrophy.

Comments ▪

This method should be applicable to other scanners since T2 values are not particularly affected by field strength.

Even though the absolute SI values and differences may vary, SI ratio measurement would obviate these. The SI ratio on less heavily T2-weighted images (first echo) may be the most useful since there is a greater difference among populations. Numbers less than 1 indicate a flow void caused by pulsatile CSF motion in the aqueduct. This is most marked in NPH, whereas the SI is greater in the aqueduct with communicating hydrocephalus and atrophy, reflecting relatively decreased pulsation.

REFERENCE

1. Bradley WG, Kortman KE, Burgoyne B: Flowing cerebrospinal fluid in normal and hydrocephalic states: Appearance on MR images. Radiology 1986; 159:611–615.

▪▪ SIZE OF THE INTERNAL CAROTID, MIDDLE CEREBRAL, AND ANTERIOR CEREBRAL ARTERIES
▪ ACR Code: 17 (Cerebral Vessel)

Technique ▪

Central ray: Anteroposterior: Directed to superior forehead with the beam angulated 20° cranially.
Lateral: Perpendicular to the film, centered 1 inch anterior and 1 inch superior to the external auditory meatus.
Position: Anteroposterior and lateral.

Target-film distance: 85 cm, using a 10-by-12-inch Elema-Schönander film changer.

Measurements ▪ (Figure 1; Tables 1 and 2)

1. Anteroposterior view:
   C = Diameter of the internal carotid artery 5 mm proximal to its bifurcation into the anterior and middle cerebral arteries.

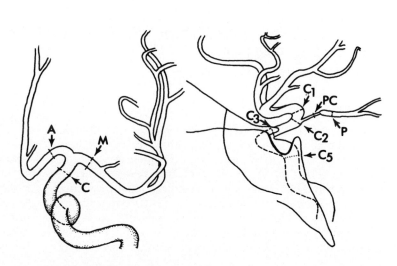

Figure 1 ▪ (From Gabrielsen TO, Greitz T: Normal size of the internal carotid, middle cerebral and anterior cerebral arteries. Acta Radiol Diagn 1970; 10:1.)

Table 1 ▪ Mean Values for Various Diameters of Normal Cerebral Arteries

MEASUREMENT	MEAN DIAMETER (mm)	SD (mm)
M	3.82	0.43
A	3.02	0.50
C	4.57	0.46
C_1	3.78	0.43
C_2	4.08	0.47
C_3	5.12	0.63
C_5	5.80	0.76
C_6	5.90	0.73
Siphon length	15.1	2.45

Based on 156 normal carotid angiographies. No correction for gender and skull size.
From Gabrielsen TO, Greitz T: Acta Radiol Diagn 1970; 10:1. Used by permission.

Table 2 ▪ Influence of Gender and External Biparietal Diameter (W in cm) on Size of Internal Carotid and Middle Cerebral Arteries (in mm)

MEASUREMENT	MALE	FEMALE
M	$1.97 + 0.118\ W$	$1.78 + 0.118\ W$
C	$2.99 + 0.100\ W$	$2.81 + 0.100\ W$
C_5	$4.56 + 0.112\ W$	$3.91 + 0.112\ W$
$M + C + C_5$	$9.52 + 0.330\ W$	$8.50 + 0.330\ W$

From Gabrielsen TO, Greitz T: Acta Radiol Diagn 1970; 10:1. Used by permission.

A = Diameter of the anterior cerebral artery 5 mm distal to origin.

M = Diameter of the middle cerebral artery 5 mm distal to origin.

2. Lateral view:

C_1 = Diameter of the internal carotid artery 5 mm distal to its junction with the posterior communicating artery.

C_2 = Diameter of the internal carotid artery just proximal to the junction with the posterior communicating artery.

C_3 = Diameter of the internal carotid artery at the level of the tuberculum sellae.

C_5 = Diameter of the internal carotid artery just proximal to its bend at the posterior aspect of the cavernous sinus.

C_6 = Diameter of the internal carotid artery at the level of the atlas (not depicted in Fig. 1).

PC = Diameter of the posterior communicating artery 5 mm distal to its junction with the internal carotid artery.

P = Diameter of the posterior cerebral artery 5 mm distal to its junction with the posterior communicating artery.

Source ▪

One hundred fifty-six angiograms from 72 males and 84 females, ranging in age from 13 to 69 years. Mean age was 33 years. Great care was taken to select normal cases. Excluded from the study were cases with even minimal atherosclerosis or cerebral spasm.

REFERENCE

1. Gabrielsen TO, Greitz T: normal size of the internal carotid, middle cerebral, and anterior cerebral arteries. Acta Radiol Diagn 1970; 10:10.

▪▪ TRANSCRANIAL DOPPLER VESSEL LOCATIONS AND NORMAL VALUES
▪ ACR Code: 17 (Cerebral Vessel)

Technique ▪

Pulsed Doppler devices dedicated to transcranial Doppler ultrasound (TCDU) are required. They typically operate at 2 MHz rather than the higher frequencies used for duplex examination of the extracerebral vessels. The devices are handheld, range gated, and directionally sensitive, and they operate at a depth of 2.5 to 10 cm from the transducer face. The sample volume is typically 3 to 6 mm. The signals are computer processed to extract spectral information and displayed on a video monitor as well as on hard copy. Figures 1, 2, and 3 show the orbital, temporal, and suboccipital windows.

Measurements ▪

Peak systolic velocity (PSV) is the maximum velocity at systole. End-diastolic velocity (EDV) is the velocity just prior to the systolic acceleration. Mean velocity (MV) is obtained from one typical cycle and may be approximated by $MV = (PSV + [EDV \times 2])/3$. Many dedicated TCDU

Text continued on page 51

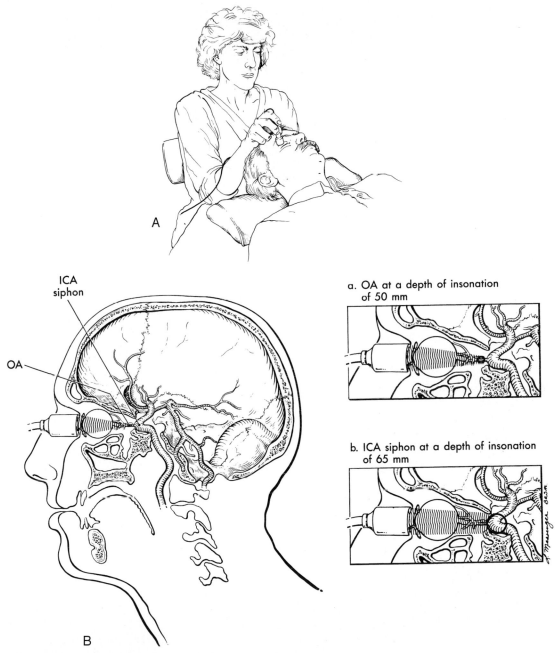

a. OA at a depth of insonation
of 50 mm

b. ICA siphon at a depth of insonation
of 65 mm

ICA
siphon

OA

A

B

Figure 1 ▪ Orbital window for TCDU. *A*, Patient and transducer position. *B*, Diagram of vessels reached by this approach. OA = ophthalmic artery; ICA = internal carotid artery siphon. (From Saver JL, Feldman E: Mosby–Year Book, St. Louis, 1993, pp. 11–28. Used by permission.)

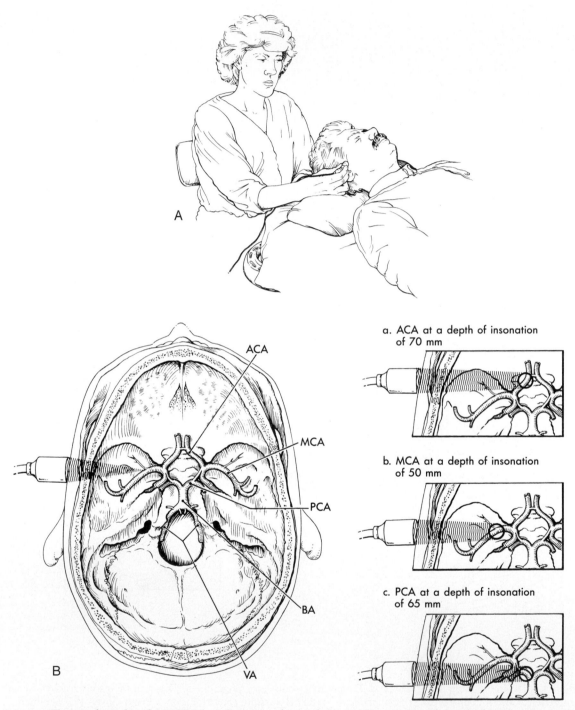

Figure 2 ▪ Temporal window for TCDU. *A*, Patient and transducer position. *B*, Vessels reached by this approach. ACA = anterior communicating artery; MCA = middle cerebral artery; PCA = posterior cerebral artery; BA = basilar artery; VA = vertebral artery. (From Saver JL, Feldman E: Mosby-Year Book, St. Louis, 1993, pp. 11–28. Used by permission.)

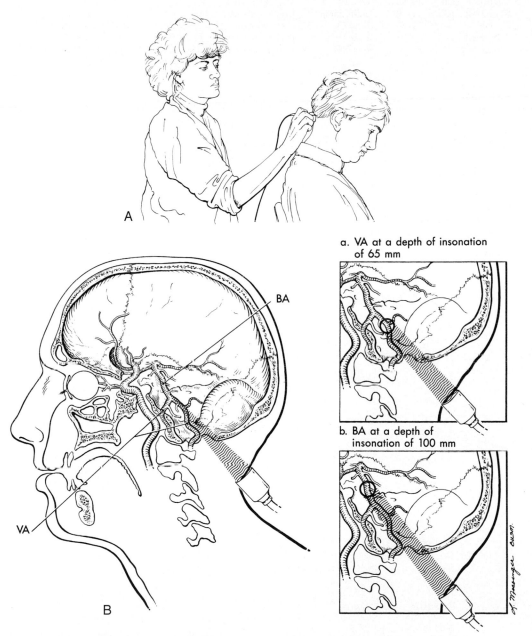

a. VA at a depth of insonation of 65 mm

b. BA at a depth of insonation of 100 mm

Figure 3 ▪ Suboccipital window for TCDU. *A*, Patient and transducer position. *B*, Vessels reached by this approach. VA = vertebral artery; BA = basilar artery. (From Saver JL, Feldman E: Mosby–Year Book, St. Louis, 1993, pp. 11–28. Used by permission.)

Table 1 ▪ Criteria for Identification of Intracranial Arteries with Transcranial Doppler Ultrasound

VESSEL	WINDOW	TRANSDUCER ORIENTATION	DEPTH (mm)	FLOW DIRECTION FROM TRANSDUCER	WAVEFORM CONTOUR	RESPONSE TO CAROTID VIBRATION	RESPONSE TO IPSILATERAL CAROTID COMPRESSION	RESPONSE TO CONTRALATERAL CAROTID COMPRESSION
OA	Orbital	Slightly medial	40–50	Toward	High resistance	—	—	—
ICS	Orbital	Slightly medial	55–70	Bidirectional	Low resistance	—	—	—
MCA	Temporal	En face	35–60	Toward	Low resistance	Responds	Reduced velocities	No change
ACA	Temporal	Anteriorly	60–75	Away	Low resistance	Responds	Flow reversal*	Increased velocities
PCA	Temporal	Posteriorly	55–70	Toward	Low resistance	Does not respond*	Increased velocities or no change*	No change
VA	Suboccipital	Superiorly and obliquely	45–75	Away	Low resistance	—	—	—
BA	Suboccipital	Superiorly	70–120	Away	Low resistance	—	—	—

OA = ophthalmic artery, ICS = internal carotid siphon, MCA/ACA/PCA = middle/anterior/posterior cerebral arteries, VA = vertebral artery, BA = basilar artery.
*Isolated findings will vary in nonstandard patients.
From Saver JL, Feldman E: Mosby–Year Book, St. Louis, 1993, pp 11–28. Used by permission.

Table 2 ▪ Normal Intracerebral Arterial Flow Velocities in Children at Transcranial Doppler Ultrasound

ARTERY	AGE	MEAN	PEAK SYSTOLIC	END-DIASTOLIC
ICA	0–10 days	25 ± 6	47 ± 9	12 ± 6
	11–90 days	43 ± 12	77 ± 19	24 ± 8
	3–11.9 mon	67 ± 10	104 ± 12	40 ± 8
	1–2.9 yr	81 ± 8	118 ± 24	58 ± 5
	3–5.9 yr	93 ± 9	144 ± 19	66 ± 8
	6–9.9 yr	93 ± 9	140 ± 14	68 ± 10
	10–18 yr	79 ± 12	125 ± 18	59 ± 9
MCA	0–10 days	24 ± 7	46 ± 10	12 ± 7
	11–90 days	42 ± 10	75 ± 15	24 ± 8
	3–11.9 mon	74 ± 14	114 ± 20	46 ± 9
	1–2.9 yr	85 ± 10	124 ± 10	65 ± 11
	3–5.9 yr	94 ± 10	147 ± 17	65 ± 9
	6–9.9 yr	97 ± 9	143 ± 13	72 ± 9
	10–18 yr	81 ± 11	129 ± 17	60 ± 8
ACA	0–10 days	19 ± 5	35 ± 8	10 ± 6
	11–90 days	33 ± 11	58 ± 15	19 ± 9
	3–11.9 mon	50 ± 11	77 ± 15	33 ± 7
	1–2.9 yr	55 ± 13	81 ± 19	40 ± 11
	3–5.9 yr	71 ± 15	104 ± 22	48 ± 9
	6–9.9 yr	65 ± 13	100 ± 20	51 ± 10
	10–18 yr	56 ± 14	92 ± 19	46 ± 11
PCA1	0–10 days			
	11–90 days			
	3–11.9 mon			
	1–2.9 yr	50 ± 17	67 ± 18	36 ± 13
	3–5.9 yr	56 ± 13	84 ± 20	40 ± 12
	6–9.9 yr	57 ± 9	82 ± 11	42 ± 7
	10–18 yr	50 ± 10	75 ± 16	39 ± 8
PCA2	0–10 days			
	11–90 days			
	3–11.9 mon			
	1–2.9 yr	50 ± 12	69 ± 9	35 ± 7
	3–5.9 yr	48 ± 11	81 ± 16	35 ± 9
	6–9.9 yr	51 ± 9	75 ± 10	38 ± 7
	10–18 yr	45 ± 9	66 ± 10	33 ± 7
BA	0–10 days			
	11–90 days			
	3–11.9 mon			
	1–2.9 yr	51 ± 6	71 ± 6	35 ± 6
	3–5.9 yr	58 ± 6	88 ± 9	41 ± 5
	6–9.9 yr	58 ± 9	85 ± 17	44 ± 8
	10–18 yr	46 ± 8	68 ± 11	36 ± 7

Velocities are in centimeters/second (mean ± standard deviation). Vessel abbreviations are standard (see Table 1).
From DeWitt LD, Rosengart A, Teal PA: Mosby–Year Book, St. Louis, 1993, pp 29–38. Used by permission.

Table 3 ▪ Normal Intracerebral Arterial Flow Velocities in Adults at Transcranial Doppler Ultrasound

ARTERY	AGE (Yr)	DEPTH (mm)	MEAN	PEAK SYSTOLIC	END-DIASTOLIC
MCA	20–65	—	62 ± 12		
	20–35	—	67 ± 7		
	49–63	—	58 ± 10		
	12–81	50	—	90 ± 16	45 ± 10
	<40	50	—	94 ± 18	48 ± 10
	>60	50	—	80 ± 18	36 ± 9
	20–70	35–45	56 ± 13	82 ± 21	40 ± 9
	<40	50	58 ± 8	95 ± 14	46 ± 7
	40–60	50	58 ± 12	91 ± 17	44 ± 10
	>60	50	45 ± 11	78 ± 15	32 ± 9
	<40	45–55	—	104 ± 14	51 ± 9
	40–59	45–55		87 ± 18	43 ± 9
	>60	45–55	—	81 ± 20	34 ± 9
	20–66	—	79 ± 16		
ACA	20–65	—	51 ± 12		
	<40	55–80	—	72 ± 14	34 ± 7
	>60	55–80	—	66 ± 11	23 ± 9
	20–70	65	50 ± 13	71 ± 18	35 ± 10
	<40	70	47 ± 14	76 ± 17	36 ± 9
	40–60	70	53 ± 11	86 ± 20	41 ± 7
	>60	70	45 ± 14	73 ± 20	34 ± 9
	20–66		63 ± 12		
PCA	20–65	—	44 ± 11	—	
	<40	50–80		60 ± 13	30 ± 7
	>60	50–80	—	51 ± 8	24 ± 5
	20–70	60	41 ± 9	57 ± 12	28 ± 8
	<40	60	34 ± 8	53 ± 11	26 ± 7
	40–60	60	37 ± 10	60 ± 21	29 ± 8
	>60	60	30 ± 9	51 ± 12	22 ± 7
	—	—	40 ± 9	56 ± 12	27 ± 7
	20–66	—	47 ± 13		
VA	<40	75	—	64 ± 13	32 ± 6
	>60	75	—	51 ± 9	23 ± 6
	20–70	75	39 ± 9	56 ± 13	27 ± 7
	<40	75	35 ± 8	56 ± 8	27 ± 5
	40–60	75	36 ± 12	60 ± 17	29 ± 8
	>60	75	30 ± 12	51 ± 19	21 ± 9
BA	<40	85	—	64 ± 13	32 ± 6
	>60	85	—	52 ± 9	23 ± 6
	20–70	75	39 ± 9	56 ± 13	27 ± 7
	22–79	100	—	59 ± 17	31 ± 9
	22–79	110	—	60 ± 14	33 ± 10

Velocities are in centimeters/second (mean ± standard deviation). Vessel abbreviations are standard (see Table 1).
From DeWitt LD, Rosengart A, Teal PA: Mosby–Year Book, St. Louis, 1993, pp 29–38. Used by permission.

machines will calculate this value by averaging instantaneous velocities over a user-defined time interval.

Source ▪

This material is contained in an excellent textbook of TCDU.[1,2] Criteria for artery identification (Table 1) were compiled based on the author's clinical experience and review of the literature. Flow velocities in children (Table 2) were compiled from a study of 25 neonates and 112 healthy children and from a text by Bode.[3,4] Flow velocities in adults (Table 3) were compiled from several studies of normal values as well as other texts.[5–12]

REFERENCES

1. Saver JL, Feldman E: Basic transcranial Doppler examination: Technique and anatomy. In Babikian VL, Wechsler LR (eds): Transcranial Doppler Ultrasonography. Mosby–Year Book, St. Louis, 1993, Chapter 2, pp 11–28.

2. DeWitt LD, Rosengart A, Teal PA: Transcranial doppler ultrasonography: Normal values. In Babikian VL, Wechsler LR (eds): Transcranial Doppler Ultrasonography. Mosby–Year Book, St Louis, 1993, Chapter 3, pp 29–38.

3. Bode H, Wais U: Age dependence of flow velocities in basal cerebral arteries. Arch Dis Child 1988; 63:606–611.

4. Bode H: Pediatric Applications of Transcranial Doppler Sonography. Springer-Verlag, Vienna, 1988.

5. Aaslid R, Markwalder TH, Nornes H: Noninvasive transcranial Doppler ultrasound recording flow velocity in basal cerebral arteries. J Neurosurg 1982; 57:769–774.

6. Lindegaard KF, et al: Assessment of intracranial hemodynamics in carotid artery disease by transcranial Doppler ultrasound. J Neurosurg 1985; 63:890–898.

7. Arnolds BJ, von Reutern GM: Transcranial Doppler sonography: Examination technique and normal reference values. Ultrasound Med Biol 1986; 12:115–123.

8. Harders A: Neurosurgical Applications of Transcranial Doppler Sonography. Springer-Verlag, Vienna, 1986.

9. Hennerici M, Rautenberg W, Sitzer G, Schwartz A: Transcranial Doppler ultrasound for the assessment of intracranial arterial flow velocity; Part I: Examination technique and normal values. Surg Neurol 1987; 27:439–448.

10. Von Reutern GM, Budingen HJ: Ultraschalldiagnostik der Hirversor-genden Arterien. Theime-Verlag, Stuttgart, 1989.
11. Harders A, Gilsbach J: Transcranial Doppler sonography and its application in extra-intracranial bypass surgery. Neurol Res 1985; 7:129–144.
12. Sorteberg W, Langmoen IA, Lindegaard K, Nornes H: Side-to-side differences and day-to-day variations of transcranial Doppler parameters in normal subjects. J Ultrasound Med 1990; 9:403–409.

▪: CEREBRAL BLOOD FLOW CHANGES WITH AGE
▪ ACR Code: 17 (Cerebral Vessel)

Technique ▪

All studies were performed with a Gyroscan-NT (Philips, Best, The Netherlands) 1.5-T MRI unit, using ungated 2D phase-contrast (TR/TE/flip angle: 16.4/9.3/7.50) MR angiography in a transverse plane at the skull base perpendicular to the precavernous portions of the internal carotid arteries (ICA) and the middle or distal part of the basilar artery (BA). Section thickness was 5 mm, 8 signals were acquired, and 100-cm/sec velocity encoding was used, by subtracting two images obtained with opposed, bipolar, velocity-encoding gradients.[1]

Measurements ▪

Flow velocities were calculated from phase-difference images by drawing regions of interest (ROI) over the entire lumen of each carotid and the basilar artery. The resultant value of mean signal intensity within the ROI represented the space- and time-averaged flow velocity (AFV). The volume flow rate (VFR) was obtained by multiplying the AFV by the cross-sectional area of the vessel. Total cerebral blood flow (CBF) was calculated by summing the VFRs from both carotid arteries and the basilar artery. Table 1 lists the results. Table 2 lists linear regression equations for volume flow in

Table 1 ▪ Volume Flows of the Internal Carotid and Basilar Arteries and Total Cerebral Blood Flow Versus Age in 250 Subjects

AGE RANGE (Yr)	NUMBER MEN/WOMEN	VOLUME FLOW RATE (ml/min)			TOTAL CEREBRAL BLOOD FLOW (ml/min)		
		Right ICA (% of CBF)	Left ICA (% of CBF)	BA (% of CBF)	Men	Women	All
19–29	23/20	294 ± 63 (39 ± 7)	303 ± 74 (40 ± 6)	152 ± 47 (20 ± 6)	757 ± 122	739 ± 122	748 ± 121
30–39	21/19	291 ± 70 (41 ± 7)	275 ± 79 (38 ± 8)	145 ± 43 (21 ± 5)	723 ± 140	699 ± 107	712 ± 125
40–49	23/18	258 ± 65 (41 ± 6)	250 ± 60 (40 ± 6)	115 ± 41 (18 ± 6)	612 ± 109	637 ± 127	623 ± 116
50–59	13/13	235 ± 58 (39 ± 6)	249 ± 48 (42 ± 7)	111 ± 40 (18 ± 5)	607 ± 95	583 ± 111	595 ± 102
60–69	22/37	221 ± 57 (41 ± 6)	209 ± 55 (39 ± 6)	107 ± 36 (20 ± 7)	551 ± 90	527 ± 105	536 ± 99
70–79	15/17	213 ± 60 (41 ± 7)	217 ± 64 (42 ± 8)	86 ± 46 (17 ± 8)	527 ± 131	508 ± 92	517 ± 110
80–89	5/4	201 ± 51 (43 ± 6)	188 ± 74 (39 ± 10)	86 ± 40 (19 ± 8)	443 ± 96	514 ± 116	474 ± 105
All	122/128	250 ± 69 (41 ± 6)	247 ± 72 (40 ± 7)	120 ± 47 (19 ± 6)	630 ± 146	604 ± 139	616 ± 143

All measurements are given as mean ± standard deviation. ICA = internal carotid artery, BA = basilar artery, % of CBF = percent of cerebral blood flow.
From Buijs PC, Krabbe-Hartkamp MJ, Bakker CJG: Radiology 1998; 209:667–674. Used by permission.

Table 2 ▪ Regression Equations for Cerebral Flow Versus Age from 20–90 Years

ARTERY	PERCENTILE	FORMULA
Internal carotid flow (ml/min)	90th	= −2.3994 (age) + 411.15
	50th	= −1.655 (age) + 293.03
	10th	= −1.5501 (age) + 231.38
Basilar flow (ml/min)	90th	= −1.0607 (age) + 202.83
	50th	= −1.2851 (age) + 161.31
	10th	= −1.2095 (age) + 107.06
Total cerebral flow (ml/min)	90th	= −5.2664 (age) + 935.14
	50th	= −4.6945 (age) + 744.64
	10th	= −4.2117 (age) + 623.76

From Buijs PC: Personal communication, 1999. Used by permission.

the internal carotid and basilar arteries, as well as total CBF versus age (20 to 90 years). With age, there was a gradual and continuous decrease in CBF of 4.8 ml/min/yr (p < .001). Gender had no significant influence on CBF.[1]

Source ▪

A total of 250 adult subjects was drawn from healthy volunteers (n = 20), relatives of patients with subarachnoid hemorrhage (n = 142), and individuals screened in a study on cerebrovascular risk factors in elderly people (n = 88).

Some individuals in the latter two groups had histories of hypertension, diabetes, coronary artery disease, or cerebrovascular disease; these were noted but not excluded, as exclusion did not substantially alter the results.[1]

REFERENCES

1. Buijs PC, Krabbe-Hartkamp MJ, Bakker CJG, et al: Effect of age on cerebral blood flow: Measurement with ungated two-dimensional phase contrast MR angiography in 250 adults. Radiology 1998; 209:667–674.
2. Buijs PC: Personal communication, 1999.

▪: ULTRASOUND OF THE TEMPORAL ARTERIES FOR ARTERITIS
▪ ACR Code: 171 (External Carotid Artery; Include: Meningeal Branch)

Technique ▪

Color Doppler and duplex ultrasound of the temporal arteries was done with an Ultramark 9 HDI unit (Advanced Technology Laboratories, Bothell, WA), with 5- or 10-MHz linear transducers.[1]

Measurements ▪

The common superficial temporal artery (proximal), frontal ramus (proximal and middle), and parietal ramus (middle)

were imaged in all subjects bilaterally in longitudinal and transverse planes (Fig. 1). Measurements included systolic luminal diameter, arterial wall diameter, and maximal velocity (duplex angle-corrected Doppler). The entire arterial distribution was scanned with B-mode gray scale, color Doppler, and duplex Doppler to look for stenosis, occlusion, and a hypoechoic halo around the artery. Occlusion was defined by lack of flow in an arterial segment, stenosis by focally increased velocities with distal decreased velocities, and a halo by a hypoechoic rim around the arterial

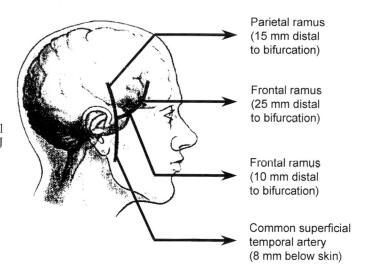

Parietal ramus
(15 mm distal
to bifurcation)

Frontal ramus
(25 mm distal
to bifurcation)

Frontal ramus
(10 mm distal
to bifurcation)

Common superficial
temporal artery
(8 mm below skin)

Figure 1 ▪ Locations of measurements of the superficial temporal artery. (From Schmidt WA, Kraft HE, Vorpahl K, et al: N Engl J Med 1997; 337:1336–1342. Used by permission.)

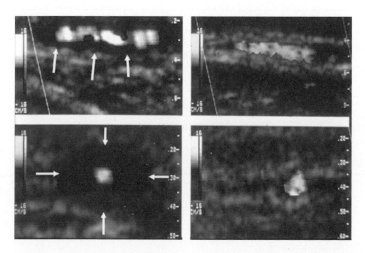

Figure 2 ▪ Superficial temporal artery (parietal ramus) in a patient with temporal arteritis (*left side*) and in a normal subject (*right side*). Longitudinal images are on the top and transverse images are on the bottom. Note the hypoechoic halo (*arrows*) around the artery in the patient with temporal arteritis. (From Schmidt WA, Kraft HE, Vorpahl K, et al: N Engl J Med 1997; 337:1336–1342. Used by permission.)

Table 1 ▪ Measurements of the Superficial Temporal Arteries in Normal Subjects and Three Patient Groups

SITE	PATIENTS WITH TEMPORAL ARTERITIS (n = 301)	PATIENTS WITH POLYMYALGIA RHEUMATICA (n = 37)	CONTROL SUBJECTS (n = 30)	PATIENTS WITH NEGATIVE HISTOLOGIC FINDINGS AND OTHER DIAGNOSES (n = 15)
Parietal Ramus				
Systolic lumen (mm)	0.79 ± 0.29	0.76 ± 0.20	0.89 ± 0.24	0.81 ± 0.30
Wall (mm)	0.94 ± 0.28	0.70 ± 0.08	0.72 ± 0.13	0.79 ± 0.11
Maximal velocity (cm/sec)	52 ± 18	59 ± 14	54 ± 14	57 ± 18
Frontal Ramus (25 mm distal to bifurcation)				
Systolic lumen (mm)	0.67 ± 0.20	0.66 ± 0.22	0.74 ± 0.24	0.68 ± 0.23
Wall (mm)	0.95 ± 0.20	0.66 ± 0.07	0.65 ± 0.13	0.72 ± 0.09
Maximal velocity (cm/sec)	48 ± 13	53 ± 16	47 ± 15	55 ± 19
Frontal Ramus (10 mm distal to bifurcation)				
Systolic lumen (mm)	0.74 ± 0.24	0.71 ± 0.17	0.86 ± 0.26	0.78 ± 0.30
Wall (mm)	0.95 ± 0.22	0.69 ± 0.09	0.71 ± 0.13	0.76 ± 0.10
Maximal velocity (cm/sec)	50 ± 14	56 ± 15	48 ± 13	59 ± 20
Common Superficial Temporal Artery				
Systolic lumen (mm)	1.51 ± 0.44	1.54 ± 0.41	1.70 ± 0.35	1.85 ± 0.54
Maximal velocity (cm/sec)	62 ± 22	61 ± 16	55 ± 13	64 ± 16

Values are given as mean ± standard deviation.
From Schmidt WA, Kraft HE, Vorpahl K, et al: N Engl J Med 1997; 337:1336–1342. Used by permission.

Table 2 ▪ Sensitivity and Specificity of Ultrasound Findings for Diagnosis of Temporal Arteritis

FINDING	CLINICAL DIAGNOSIS		HISTOLOGIC DIAGNOSIS	
	Sensitivity-Positive Tests/Total (%)	Specificity-Negative Tests/Total (%)	Sensitivity-Positive Tests/Total (%)	Specificity-Negative Tests/Total (%)
Halo	22/30 (73)	82/82 (100)	16/21 (76)	24/26 (92)
Stenosis or occlusion	24/30 (80)	76/82 (93)	18/21 (86)	23/26 (88)
Halo, stenosis, or occlusion	28/30 (93)	76/82 (93)	20/21 (95)	22/26 (85)

From Schmidt WA, Kraft HE, Vorpahl K, et al: N Engl J Med 1997; 337:1336–1342. Used by permission.

Table 3 ▪ Patient Demographics

	NORMAL SUBJECTS	TEMPORAL ARTERITIS	POLYMYALGIA RHEUMATICA	OTHER DIAGNOSES
Number	30	30	37	15
Mean age	matched→	73	70	70
Age range	matched→	52–86	51–86	49–90
Male/female	matched→	9/21	9/28	9/6
Steroids < 24 hours	—	10	7	0
Steroids 1–10 days	—	11	16	4
Biopsies done	—	27	7	0
Positive biopsies (for temporal arteritis)	—	21	0	0

wall measuring 0.3 to 1.2 mm.[1] Figure 2 is an example of a normal artery and one with a halo.

Table 1 lists the measurements in each group of subjects. Table 2 details the sensitivity and specificity of the findings of periarterial halo, stenosis, and occlusion with respect to temporal arteritis (disease-positive).

Source ▪

Patients with clinical temporal arteritis (n = 30), polymyalgia rheumatica (n = 37), other diagnoses (n = 15), and normal controls (n = 30) age- and gender-matched to the temporal arteritis patients were studied.[1] Table 3 shows the demographics of the subjects, as well as the steroid treatment history.

Comments ▪

There was no significant difference among groups with respect to systolic luminal diameter and velocity, whereas the wall thickness was greater in temporal arteritis patients. The morphology of the Doppler curve did not differ significantly among groups.[1]

REFERENCE

1. Schmidt WA, Kraft HE, Vorpahl K, et al: Color duplex ultrasonography in the diagnosis of temporal arteritis. N Engl J Med 1997; 337:1336–1342.

▪: DIAMETERS AND FLOW PARAMETERS OF THE COMMON CAROTID ARTERY
  ▪ ACR Code: 172 (Common Carotid Artery)

Technique ▪

Examinations were performed with a vascular color Doppler ultrasound device (Phillips Medical Systems, Irvine, CA) and a 7.5-MHz transducer. The unit employs time-domain processing (color velocity imaging, CVI, and color velocity imaging-quantification, CVI-Q) for velocity determination and flow estimation. The common carotid artery (CCA) was examined from the lateral aspect of the neck and the measurement tracings taken from the midportion, with an insonation angle between 40 and 70 degrees.[1]

Measurements ▪

The systolic (greatest width) and diastolic (smallest width) luminal diameters were measured from color M-mode trac-

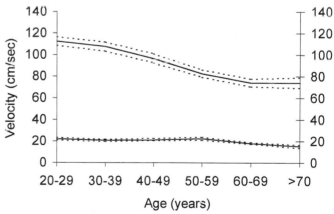

Figure 1 ▪ Graph of peak systolic velocity and end-diastolic velocities in the common carotid artery related to age (both sexes). Mean (solid line) values and 95% confidence intervals (dotted lines) are shown. Peak systolic velocities are plotted in the upper part and end-diastolic velocities in the lower portion. (From Weskott HP, Holsing K: Radiology 1997; 205:353–359. Used by permission.)

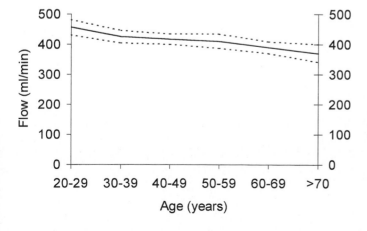

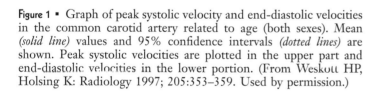

Figure 2 ▪ Graph of volume flow rates in the common carotid artery related to age (both sexes). Mean (solid line) and 95% confidence intervals (dotted lines) are shown. (From Weskott HP, Holsing K: Radiology 1997; 205:353–359. Used by permission.)

Table 1 • Common Carotid Artery Flow Parameters in 164 Adults by Age and Gender

DECADE	NUMBER (Male/Female)	PSV (cm/sec) Male	PSV (cm/sec) Female	EDV (cm/sec) Both	VOLUME FLOW (ml/min) Male	VOLUME FLOW (ml/min) Female
2	17/15	119.8 ± 17.4	106.0 ± 11.6	21.9 ± 4.2	487.6 ± 116.7	429.3 ± 69.2
3	16/15	114.5 ± 14.7	100.8 ± 11.6	20.7 ± 4.0	466.6 ± 84.2	492.3 ± 69.2
4	17/15	105.8 ± 16.0	88.4 ± 12.1	21.3 ± 4.0	434.6 ± 67.4	384.1 ± 57.2
5	15/15	84.7 ± 13.2	80.5 ± 13.4	22.2 ± 5.0	445.1 ± 90.7	401.6 ± 66.0
6	16/16	81.3 ± 15.7	67.0 ± 9.0	18.0 ± 3.0	408.2 ± 86.1	375.8 ± 77.6
7	9/8	74.6 ± 17.7	73.3 ± 10.9	15.0 ± 4.0	375.5 ± 94.7	371.2 ± 62.2
All	90/84	98.5 ± 22.8	87.4 ± 19.0	20.2 ± 4.6	440.1 ± 96. 3	390.2 ± 70.6

All measurements given as mean ± standard deviation. There were no gender differences for EDV.
PSV = peak systolic velocity, EDV = end-diastolic velocity.
From Weskott HP, Holsing K: Radiology 1997; 205:353–359. Used by permission.

Table 2 • Common Carotid Artery Functional Luminal Diameters in 164 Adults by Age and Gender

DECADE	NUMBER (Male/Female)	SYSTOLIC LUMEN (mm) Male	SYSTOLIC LUMEN (mm) Female	DIASTOLIC LUMEN (mm) Male	DIASTOLIC LUMEN (mm) Female
2	17/15	7.00 ± 0.49	6.58 ± 0.52	5.52 ± 0.48	5.30 ± 0.43
3	16/15	7.15 ± 0.54	6.24 ± 0.28	5.50 ± 0.46	4.87 ± 0.32
4	17/15	6.85 ± 0.46	6.43 ± 0.32	5.31 ± 0.52	5.09 ± 0.39
5	15/15	6.85 ± 0.34	6.35 ± 0.39	5.53 ± 0.45	5.23 ± 0.43
6	16/16	7.03 ± 0.74	6.69 ± 0.53	5.47 ± 0.66	5.34 ± 0.54
7	9/8	7.17 ± 0.69	6.65 ± 0.41	5.13 ± 1.11	5.03 ± 0.54
All	90/84	6.99 ± 0.55	6.48 ± 0.45	5.43 ± 0.61	5.15 ± 0.46

Measurements are given as mean ± standard deviation.
From Weskott HP, Holsing K: Radiology 1997; 205:353–359. Used by permission.

ings. Measurement of the CCA flow parameters was done from 3-second Doppler samples, and each was repeated 5 times. Using the flow velocity display mode, the peak systolic velocity and end-diastolic velocities were measured. Volume flow was calculated from all displayed cardiac cycles within the 3-second sweep time. Tables 1 and 2 list these parameters by age (decade) and gender. Figure 1 is a graphic depiction of peak systolic and end-diastolic velocity versus age, and Figure 2 shows volume flow rate related to age in graphic form.[1]

Source •

Of 205 adult volunteers, 15 were excluded because of hypertension (> 140/70 mm/Hg), and 12 were excluded because of CCA or internal carotid artery stenosis (> 50%). The remaining 174 subjects were included in the study. The age distribution is given in Table 1.[1]

Comments •

In a validation study using the same color Doppler machine, Westra and colleagues compared measurements of blood flow in swine CCAs with the time domain (CVI-CVI-Q) technique, a transit time ultrasound flowmeter, and timed collection (true volume flow). They found good correlation up to flow rates of 500 ml/min among the three methods. True flow was underestimated by 10% with time domain processing and by 21% with the ultrasound flowmeter. They concluded that at least three measurements with time-domain technique were required for accurate flow estimation because of inter- and intraobserver variability.[2]

REFERENCES

1. Weskott HP, Holsing K: US-based evaluation of hemodynamic parameters in the common carotid artery: A nomogram trial. Radiology 1997; 205:353–359.
2. Westra SJ, Levy DJ, Chaloupka JC, et al: Carotid artery volume flow: In vivo measurement with time-domain processing US. Radiology 1997; 202:725–729.

▪: MULTICENTER RECOMMENDATION FOR CAROTID DOPPLER CRITERIA
▪ ACR Code: 1721 (Common Carotid Artery Bifurcation)

Technique ▪

A multicenter task force met to establish reproducible criteria for carotid ultrasound and Doppler criteria to facilitate standardized reporting of atherosclerotic disease.

Measurements ▪

Duplex Doppler angle-corrected sampling of flow velocity profiles in the common carotid artery (CCA) and the internal carotid artery (ICA) is used to classify stenoses. Peak systolic and end-diastolic velocities are obtained at the point of maximal stenosis (usually in the bulb or ICA). The velocity ratios are calculated by dividing the maximum systolic and end-diastolic velocities by those obtained in a non-stenotic portion of the CCA. Figure 1 shows the relationship between diameter reduction and area reduction in a circular vessel. Figure 2 shows associated peak velocities plotted against the severity of stenosis. Figure 3 shows velocity ratios plotted against severity of stenosis. Table 1 is a summary of the criteria recommended by the task force

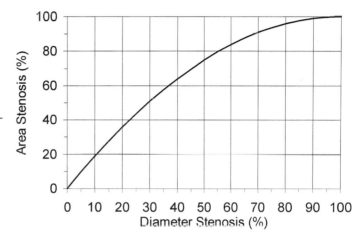

Figure 1 ▪ Relationship between area reduction and diameter reduction of stenosis in a circular vessel.[1]

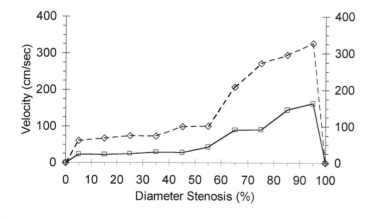

Figure 3 ▪ Velocity ratios (*systolic—diamonds, dashed line; diastolic—squares, solid line*) of the stenotic area over a normal portion of the common carotid artery plotted against severity of stenosis (diameter reduction). (From Bluth EI, Stavros AT, Marich KW, et al: Radiographics 1988; 8:487–506. Used by permission.)

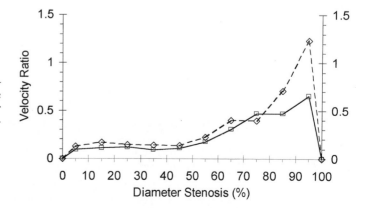

Figure 2 ▪ Peak systolic (*diamonds, dashed line*) and diastolic (*squares, solid line*) velocities in the stenotic area plotted against stenosis severity in the carotid arteries (diameter reduction). (From Bluth EI, Stavros AT, Marich KW, et al: Radiographics 1988; 8:487–506. Used by permission.)

Table 1 ▪ Doppler Criteria for Carotid Artery Stenosis

CATEGORY	DIAMETER STENOSIS (%)	AREA STENOSIS (%)	PEAK SYSTOLIC VELOCITY (cm/sec)	PEAK DIASTOLIC VELOCITY (cm/sec)	SYSTOLIC VELOCITY RATIO (ICA/CCA)	DIASTOLIC VELOCITY RATIO (ICA/CCA)	SPECTRAL BROADENING (BANDWIDTH cm/sec)
Normal	0	0	<110	<40	<1.8	<2.4	<30
Mild	1–39	1–63	<110	<40	<1.8	<2.4	<40
Moderate	40–59	64–83	<130	40	<1.8	<2.4	<40
Severe	60–79	84–95	>130	>40	>1.8	>2.4	>40
Critical	80–99	96–99	>250	>100	>3.7	>5.5	>80

ICA = internal carotid artery; CCA = common carotid artery.
From Bluth EI, Stavros AT, Marich KW, et al: Radiographics 1988; 8:487–506. Used by permission.

for grading carotid stenosis. The systolic velocity ratio and spectral broadening criteria are included for reference but were not shown to be as accurate as peak systolic velocity and end-diastolic velocity at the point of maximum stenosis.[1]

Source ▪

Sonographers from six different institutions met, reviewed the current literature, and decided on a common protocol and standards for stenosis grading. The centers represented included the Oschner Clinic, New Orleans; Swedish Medical Center, Englewood, CO; UCSF Medical Center, San Francisco; Whidden Memorial Hospital, Everett, MA; and UCI School of Medicine, Irvine, CA.

Comments ▪

The slopes of the peak velocity and velocity ratio versus percent stenosis curves are too shallow below 60% diameter stenosis to permit accurate grading of low-grade lesions. The authors recommend using gray scale images in the transverse plane to quantify stenoses in this range.

REFERENCE

1. Bluth EI, Stavros AT, Marich KW, et al: Carotid duplex sonography: A multicenter recommendation for standardized imaging and Doppler criteria. Radiographics 1988; 8:487–506.

▪: ULTRASOUND CAROTID STENOSIS CRITERIA MATCHING THOSE USED IN NORTH AMERICAN ENDARTERECTOMY TRIALS
▪ ACR Code: 1721 (Common Carotid Artery Bifurcation)

Technique ▪

Ultrasound examinations of the carotid arteries were performed with QUAD I or Quantum 2000 machines. (Quantum Medical Systems, Isaquah, WA). Gray scale images, color Doppler velocity maps, and duplex Doppler waveforms were obtained from the common (CCA), internal (ICA), and external (ECA) carotid arteries. Peak systolic (PSV) and end-diastolic velocities (EDV) were recorded with duplex technique from these vessels. Digital subtraction or cut film arteriograms in at least two planes were used to measure "gold standard" ICA stenosis.

Measurements ▪

Arteriographic ICA stenosis was calculated as follows: % ICA stenosis = (1 – ICA stenosis diameter/normal distal ICA diameter) × 100. Receiver operator curves (ROC) were generated to find optimal values of ICA, PSV, and EDV to detect stenoses at thresholds of 30%, 50%, and 70%. Sensitivity, specificity, and predictive values were generated for various absolute velocities and velocity ratios. Table 1 shows these criteria.

Source ▪

Arteriograms of 770 internal carotid arteries from 405 patients were compared with ultrasound scans of the carotid bifurcations done contemporaneously.

Comments ▪

A combination of maximum PSV > 130 and EDV > 100 proved to be the most accurate at predicting 70% or

Table 1 ▪ Carotid Duplex Criteria for Grading Stenoses of the Internal Carotid Arteries

CATEGORY	DIAMETER STENOSIS (%)	AREA STENOSIS (%)	PEAK SYSTOLIC VELOCITY (cm/sec)	END-DIASTOLIC VELOCITY (cm/sec)	SYSTOLIC VELOCITY RATIO (ICA/CCA)	SPECTRAL BROADENING
Mild	0–29	0–50	≤110	—	<1.7	None
Moderate	30–49	51–74	111–130	—	1.7–2.0	Mild
Severe	50–69	75–90	>130	≤100	2.1–3.2	Moderate
Critical	70–99	91–99	>130	>100	>3.3	Severe

greater stenosis (sensitivity = 81%, specificity = 98%, accuracy = 95%). Velocity criteria alone were not felt to be sufficiently accurate in distinguishing between the 30% and 50% stenosis thresholds. Gray scale findings and spectral broadening are suggested to supplement velocity criteria. For example, with little or no visible plaque and minimal spectral broadening, the vessel would be classified as having < 30% stenosis even with a PSV between 111 and 130 cm/sec. If the PSV is below 111 and there is significant visible plaque and spectral broadening, the vessel would be classified as having 30 to 49% stenosis. The ratio of ICA/CCA PSV did not add to the accuracy of predicting higher-grade lesions but may be helpful for the 30% and 50% thresholds.

REFERENCE

1. Faught WE, Mattos MA, van Bemmelen PS, et al: Color-flow duplex scanning of carotid arteries: New velocity criteria based on receiver operator characteristic analysis for threshold stenoses used in the symptomatic and asymptomatic carotid trials. J Vasc Surg 1994; 19:818–827.

CHAPTER. 2

Skull, Bony Orbit, and Sinuses

": TRANSVERSE CRANIAL AREA
- ACR Code: 11 (Calvaria)

Technique

CT scans through the head were made with an 8800-JC scanner (General Electric, Milwaukee, WI). Scans were done at 5 to 10 degrees from the canthomeatal line, with a scan time of 9.6 seconds. The slice thickness was not given.[1]

Measurements

The slice showing the most prominent frontal horns was used for measurement. Using built-in software on the scanner, the outer diameter of the skull was traced, yielding an area. The greatest anteroposterior (AP) and transverse (TRV) dimensions were measured from outer table to outer table. Figure 1 shows these measurements. Tables 1 and 2 list the cranial area by age (0–24 months and 3–18 years). Figures 2 and 3 graphically depict the cranial area and the product of AP and TRV dimensions. Regression formulas for cranial area and the AP×TRV product against age were calculated for 2 years or less (in months) and above 2 years (in years). These are listed below along with the r values:

Area (cm²) = 75.55 + 26.5 × ln (age in months), r = 0.96
Area (cm²) = 140.11 + 21.44 × ln (age in years), r = 0.86
Product (cm²) = 96.18 + 34.51 × ln (age in months), r = 0.96
Product (cm²) = 181.64 + 28.06 × ln (age in years), r = 0.83

		Table 1 • Cranial Area in Infants and Children from Birth to 24 Months	
AGE (Mon)	NUMBER	CRANIAL AREA MEAN (cm²)	CRANIAL AREA RANGE (cm²)
1	17	75.5	(63.0–88.0)
2	6	93.9	(81.4–106.4)
3	4	104.7	(92.2–117.2)
4	6	112.3	(99.8–124.8)
5	8	118.2	(105.7–130.7)
6	6	123.0	(110.5–135.5)
7	3	127.1	(114.6–139.6)
8	7	130.7	(118.2–143.2)
9	7	133.8	(121.3–146.3)
10	1	136.6	(124.1–149.1)
11	3	139.1	(126.6–151.6)
12	9	141.4	(128.9–153.9)
13	1	143.5	(131.0–156.0)
14	1	145.5	(133.0–158.0)
15	1	147.3	(134.8–159.8)
16	3	149.0	(136.5–161.5)
17	3	150.6	(138.1–163.1)
18	3	152.1	(139.6–164.6)
19	1	153.6	(141.1–166.1)
20	1	154.9	(142.4–167.4)
21	2	156.2	(143.7–168.7)
22	1	157.5	(145.0–170.0)
23	2	158.7	(146.2–171.2)
24	14	159.8	(147.3–172.3)

Mean values are derived from the regression formulas in the text. The range reflects the 90% of the population closest to the mean.
From Hahn FJ, Chu WK, Cheung JY: AJR Am J Roentgenol 1984; 142:1253–1255. Used by permission.

Table 2 ▪ Cranial Area in Infants and Children from 3 to 18 Years

AGE (Yr)	NUMBER	CRANIAL AREA MEAN (cm²)	CRANIAL AREA RANGE (cm²)
3	13	163.0	(146.4–179.4)
4	14	169.4	(152.9–185.9)
5	5	174.4	(157.9–190.9)
6	8	178.6	(162.1–195.1)
7	7	182.0	(165.5–198.5)
8	8	185.0	(168.5–201.6)
9	6	187.7	(171.2–204.2)
10	8	190.1	(173.6–206.6)
11	7	192.2	(195.7–208.7)
12	1	194.2	(177.7–210.7)
13	11	196.0	(179.6–212.6)
14	5	197.7	(180.7–213.7)
15	6	199.2	(182.7–215.7)
16	6	200.7	(184.2–217.2)
17	7	202.1	(185.6–218.6)
18	3	204.4	(187.9–220.9)

Mean values are derived from the regression formulas in the text. The range reflects the 90% of the population closest to the mean.
From Hahn FJ, Chu WK, Cheung JY: AJR Am J Roentgenol 1984; 142:1253–1255. Used by permission.

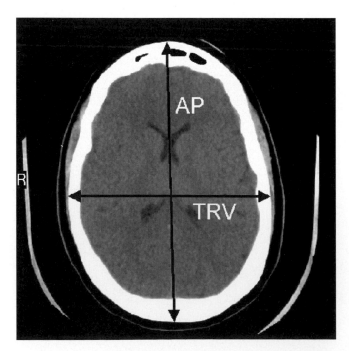

Figure 1 ▪ Measurement of maximal anteroposterior (*AP*) and transverse (TRV) outer dimensions of the skull on the midventricular slice.

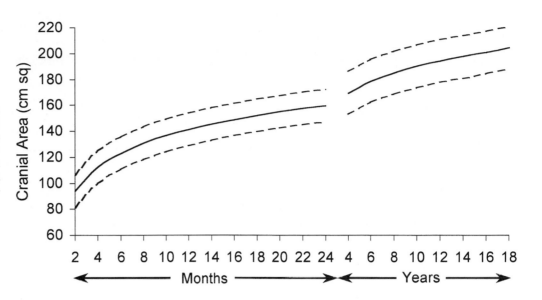

Figure 2 ▪ Cranial area of infants and children. The mean (*solid line*) values and 90% confidence limits (*dotted lines*) are shown. Cm sq = centimeters squared. (From Hahn FJ, Chu WK, Cheung JY: AJR Am J Roentgenol 1984; 142:1253–1255. Used by permission.)

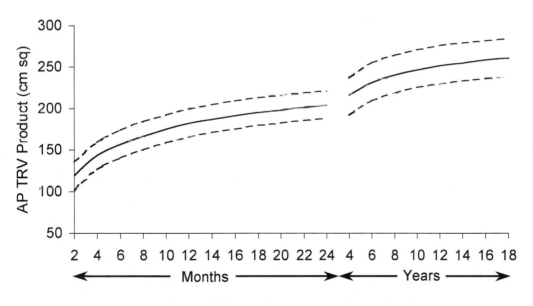

Figure 3 ▪ Product of AP and TRV cranial diameter in infants and children. The mean (*solid line*) values and 90% confidence limits (*dotted lines*) are shown. Cm sq = centimeters squared. (From Hahn FJ, Chu WK, Cheung JY: AJR Am J Roentgenol 1984; 142:1253–1255. Used by permission.)

Source ▪

Two hundred and five pediatric neurology patients were scanned; those with possible microcephaly or hydrocephalus were excluded. There were 125 boys and 90 girls, with ages ranging from newborn to 18 years.[1]

REFERENCE

1. Hahn FJ, Chu WK, Cheung JY: CT measurements of cranial growth: Normal subjects. AJR Am J Roentgenol 1984; 142:1253–1255.

▪: POSTERIOR FOSSA AND SUPRATENTORIAL VOLUMES IN CHILDREN
▪ ACR Code: 11 (Calvaria)

Technique ▪

Computed tomographic scans (machine details not given) of the head were done in the axial plane parallel to the supraorbital meatal line, with 5-mm slices through the posterior fossa (PF) and 10-mm slices through the supratentorial cranial cavity (SC). All scans were done after intravenous contrast was administered.[1]

Measurements ▪

Measurements were made on the CT console, using vendor-supplied software on images displayed with a window of 2000 HU and a level of 500 HU. Area measurements of the PF and SC were done by hand, tracing the inner table of the skull on each image. The areas were then summed and corrected for slice interval to yield volumes. The maximal anteroposterior (AP) and transverse (TRV) dimensions were also measured for the PF and SC. The cephalocaudal (CC) dimension was calculated by multiplying the number of slices containing the PF and SC cavities and multiplying by the slice interval. Figure 1 shows the linear measurements.

Table 1 gives the 95% limits of tolerance for the PF and SC volumes (area summing method) by age and gender of the subjects. The PF volume by the area method was strongly correlated with the linear measurements (r = 0.945, p < 0.001), and the SC volume was also strongly correlated with corresponding linear measurements (r = 0.953, p < 0.001). The authors give simple formulas for calculated PF and SC volume from linear measurements (in centimeters) as follows:

PF volume (ml) = 0.34 × (AP × TRV × CC) + 51.17
SC volume (ml) = 0.46 × (AP × TRV × CC) + 89.10

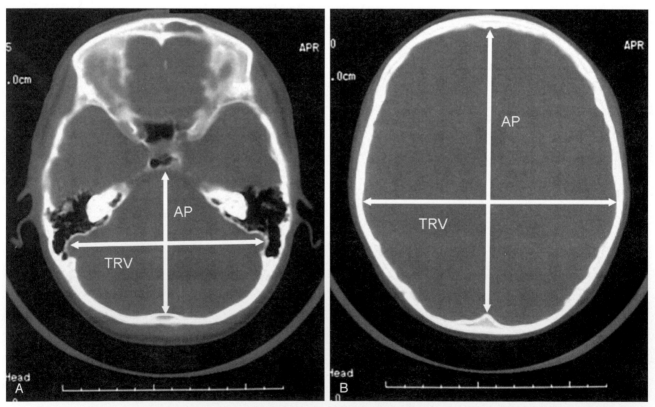

Figure 1 ▪ Measurements of the posterior fossa (*A*) and supratentorial (*B*) intracranial compartments. Maximum AP and TRV dimensions are shown. The authors also traced the inner table of the skull to obtain the area of each section, and these were summed to obtain volumes.

Table 1 ▪ Posterior Fossa and Supratentorial Cranial Cavity Volumes in Children

AGE (Mon)	BOYS	GIRLS	POSTERIOR FOSSA VOLUME (cc)		SUPRATENTORIAL CRANIAL VOLUME (cc)	
			Boys	Girls	Boys	Girls
Months						
3–5	3	3	95–143	90–135	616–924	574–862
6–8	3	2	102–154	96–145	661–992	619–929
9–11	5	4	108–162	101–153	695–1043	653–980
12–14	6	1	112–168	106–159	723–1085	680–1021
15–17	4	4	116–174	109–164	746–1120	704–1056
18–20	5	9	119–179	112–169	767–1150	724–1087
21–23	8	4	122–183	115–173	785–1177	742–1114
24–26	7	4	125–187	117–177	801–1202	759–1138
27–29	5	4	127–191	120–180	816–1224	774–1161
30–32	6	4	129–194	122–183	830–1245	787–1181
33–35	5	2	132–198	124–187	842–1264	800–1201
Years						
4	9	3	139–208	130–195	884–1327	843–1264
5	5	2	144–216	136–204	919–1378	878–1317
6	3	5	149–224	140–211	950–1425	909–1364
7	2	2	153–230	144–217	977–1466	936–1405
8	3	2	157–236	148–223	1002–1503	962–1443
9	5	4	161–242	152–228	1024–1537	985–1478
10	2	4	164–247	155–232	1046–1569	1007–1510
11	9	2	168–252	158–237	1065–1598	1027–1540
12	2	2	171–256	161–242	1084–1626	1045–1568
13	2	6	174–261	164–246	1101–1652	1063–1594
14	2	2	176–265	166–249	1117–1676	1080–1620
15	2	3	179–268	168–253	1132–1699	1096–1644

Measurements given as upper-lower 95% tolerance intervals.
From Prassopoulos P, Cavouras D, Golfinopoulos S: Neuroradiology 1996; 38:80–83. Used with permission.

Source ▪

Subjects included 103 boys and 78 girls (age distribution given in Figure 1) who were scanned for headache, seizure, or abnormal EEG and were otherwise normal. All scans were interpreted as normal.[1]

REFERENCE

1. Prassopoulos P, Cavouras D, Golfinopoulos S: Developmental changes in the posterior cranial fossa of children studied by CT. Neuroradiology 1996; 38:80–83.

▪: MEASUREMENT OF THE THICKNESS OF THE SKULL[1, 2]
▪ ACR Code: 11 (Calvaria)

Technique ▪

Central ray: To a point 1 inch anterior and 1 inch superior to the external auditory meatus.
Position: Lateral.
Target-film distance: 70 cm (Orley[1]); 7 feet (Hansman[2]).

Measurements ▪

Outer table: Average thickness, 1.5 mm.[1]
Inner table: Average thickness, 0.5 mm.[1]

Cranial wall: Frontal region, average thickness, 5.0 mm.[1] Parietal region (measured on anteroposterior skull film) also has an average thickness of 5.0 mm except in the region of parietal thinning.[1]
Floor of skull: Average thickness, 2.0 to 3.0 mm.[1]
Occipital (lambda[2]): See Figures 1 and 2.

Source ▪

These dimensions are from Dr. Orley's extensive experience in skull measurement. No statistics were available.

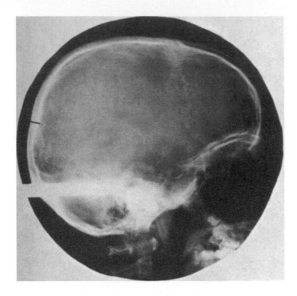

Figure 1 ▪ Straight line at lambda indicates site of measurement of skull thickness. (From Hansman CF: Radiology 1966; 86:87. Used by permission.)

Figure 2 ▪ Percentile standards for measurements of skull thickness for both sexes. The ranges for the two dimensions are indicated. (From Hansman CF: Radiology 1966; 86:87. Used by permission.)

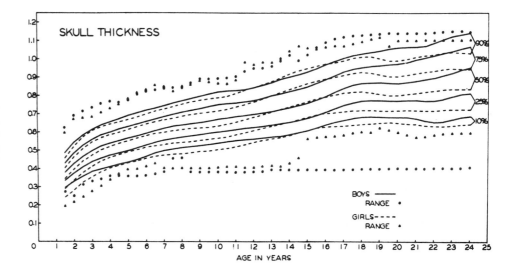

Hansman used several hundred normal individuals who have been studied by the Child Research Council of the University of Colorado.

REFERENCES

1. Orley A: Neuroradiology. Springfield, IL, Charles C Thomas, Publisher, 1949, p. 3.
2. Hansman CF: Growth of interorbital distance and skull thickness as observed in roentgenographic measurements. Radiology 1966; 86:87.

▪: NORMAL DEVELOPMENT OF MARROW IN THE SKULL
▪ ACR Code: 11 (Skull Marrow)

Technique ▪

In one study,[1] sagittal T1-weighted images of the brain (TR and TE not given) were made with a 5-T machine (Picker International, Highland Heights, OH) or 1.5-T machine (General Electric, Milwaukee, WI). A second study[2] used a 1.5-T Signa machine (General Electric, Milwaukee, WI), and sagittal T1 sequences (400–600/20) of the brain were analyzed.

Measurements ▪

In both studies, marrow signal was subjectively assessed, comparing marrow intensity in various locations with muscle and fat. A four-step scale was used in the first study,[1] and a three-step scale was used in the other.[2] In both scales, low numbers were associated with lower signal (nearer to muscle) and larger numbers with higher signal (nearer to fat). Pneumatization of the sphenoid sinus was graded by percentage in one series.[1]

Figure 1 is a tracing of a midline image of the skull in the sagittal plane showing various marrow regions and the progression of conversion to fatty marrow. Figure 2 is a graphic depiction of changes in marrow intensity with age.[1] Table 1 shows changes in signal intensity in skull marrow with age in tabular form.[2]

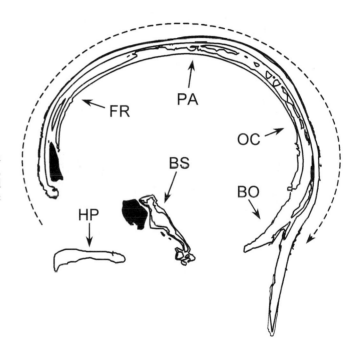

Figure 1 ▪ Tracing of a midsagittal section through the skull, with defined regions of marrow development indicated. The frontal (*FR*), parietal (*PA*), occipital (*OC*), basiocciput (*BO*), basisphenoid (*BS*), and hard palate (*HP*) are shown. The dashed line with arrow indicates the general progression of marrow conversion with maturation.

Table 1 ▪ Distribution of Marrow Signal Intensity by Age in Four Regions of the Skull on Sagittal MRI Images

AGE (Yr)	NUMBER	BASIOCCIPUT			BASISPHENOID			OCCIPITAL			PARIETAL			FRONTAL		
		1	2	3	1	2	3	1	2	3	1	2	3	1	2	3
0	28	89	11	0	89	11	0	96	4	0	96	4	0	89	7	4
1–2	35	46	51	3	48	46	6	60	31	9	68	23	9	52	31	17
3–4	37	5	68	27	8	70	22	16	43	41	22	43	35	19	43	38
5–6	32	9	47	44	6	56	38	13	31	56	19	31	50	16	31	53
7–9	25	0	32	68	0	44	56	0	32	68	0	36	64	0	16	84
10–14	41	0	17	83	0	29	71	0	12	88	2	10	88	2	12	86
15–19	27	0	8	92	0	8	92	4	15	81	4	15	81	4	11	85
20–24	21	0	5	95	0	5	95	0	14	86	0	24	76	0	19	81

Percentages of three intensities are given: low = 1 (hematopoietic), intermediate = 2, high = 3 (fat).
From Okada Y, Aoki S, Barkovich AJ, et al: Radiology 1989; 171:161–164. Used by permission.

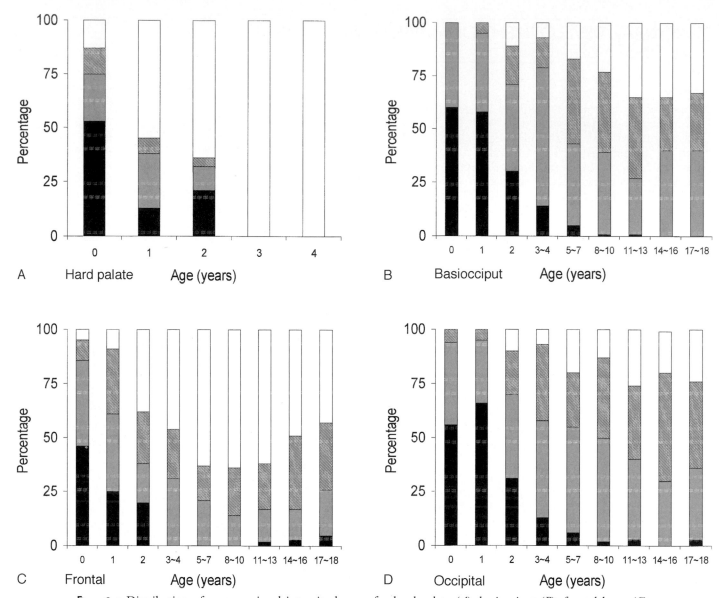

Figure 2 ▪ Distribution of marrow signal intensity by age for hard palate (*A*), basiocciput (*B*), frontal bone (*C*), and occipital (*D*) regions. Black = grade 1 (similar to muscle), gray = grade 2, hatched = grade 3, white = grade 4 (similar to fat). (From Simonson TM, Kao SC: Pediatr Radiol 1992; 22[8]:556–559. Used by permission.)

Source ▪

A total of 324 examinations of children and adolescents (171 boys, 153 girls, aged newborn to 18 years), with no diseases or treatments known to affect bone marrow, was analyzed in the first series.[1] The subjects were divided into 9 age groups (range of n = 21 to 59, mean of n = 36). The second study included 246 examinations of 238 patients (127 male, 119 female, aged newborn to 24 years), who also had no known condition affecting the marrow.[2]

These subjects were divided into 8 age groups (range of n = 21–41, mean of n = 39).

REFERENCES

1. Simonson TM, Kao SC: Normal childhood developmental patterns in skull bone marrow by MR imaging. Pediatr Radiol 1992; 22(8):556–559.
2. Okada Y, Aoki S, Barkovich AJ, et al: Cranial bone marrow in children: Assessment of normal development with MR imaging. Radiology 1989; 171:161–164.

·: MEASUREMENT OF THE BASE OF THE SKULL FOR BASILAR INVAGINATION
- ACR Code: 12 (Base of Skull)

Technique ·

1. McGregor's, McRae's, and Chamberlain's lines:
   Central ray: Perpendicular to lateral skull.
   McGregor's: Centered to C2.
   McRae's and Chamberlain's: Over midportion of skull.
   Position: McGregor's: True lateral of cervical spine and skull. Patient sitting with head in neutral position.
   McRae's and Chamberlain's: True lateral of skull. Include upper portion of cervical spine.
   Target-film distance:
   72 inches for McGregor's measurements.
   36 inches for Chamberlain's measurements.
2. Method of Bull:
   As above, except that the roentgenograms must be made with the patient in the prone position and the chin in neutral position, neither flexed nor extended. Criteria do not apply in the erect position.
3. Digastric line:
   Central ray: To line connecting outer canthus of eye and external auditory meatus.

Position: Patient supine and skull so positioned that the line connecting the outer canthus of the eye and external auditory meatus is perpendicular to the table top. Anteroposterior tomograms are used.
Target-film distance: 40 inches.

Measurements ·

Chamberlain's line (Fig. 1): Line from the posterior margin of the hard palate to the posterior margin of the foramen magnum.
   McRae's line (Fig. 2): Foramen magnum line. Line from the anterior margin of the foramen magnum (basion) to the posterior border (opisthion).
   Method of Bull (Fig. 3):

C = Line drawn along plane of hard palate.
D = Line drawn along plane of atlas.

   McGregor's line (Fig. 4; Tables 1 and 2): Line from the posterosuperior margin of the hard palate to the lowest point on the midline occipital curve.

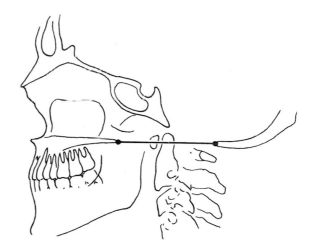

Figure 1 · Chamberlain's line.[1] The odontoid process should not project above Chamberlain's line in the normal case (SD ± 3.3 mm).[2] In any individual case, an odontoid process 6.6 mm (2 SD) or more above this line should be considered strongly indicative of basilar impression.

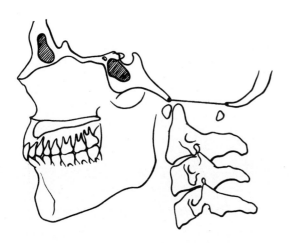

Figure 2 · McRae's line.[3] If the line of the occipital squama is convex upward or if it lies above the line of the foramen magnum, basilar impression is present. In addition, a perpendicular line drawn from the apex of the odontoid to the reference line should intersect it in its ventral quarter. (From Hinck V, et al: Radiology 1961; 76:572. Used by permission.)

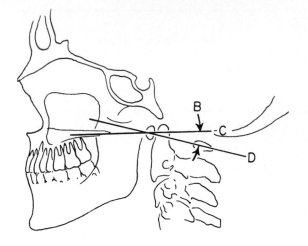

Figure 3 ▪ Method of Bull.[4] If angle B is more than 13°, the position of the odontoid process is abnormal.

Figure 4 ▪ McGregor's line.[5] See Tables 1 and 2 for values.

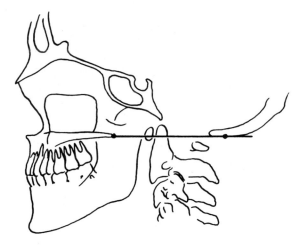

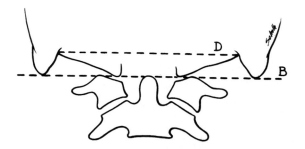

Figure 5 ▪ D = digastric line; B = bimastoid line. (From Hinck VC, Hopkins CE: AJR Am J Roentgenol 1960; 84:945. Used by permission.)

Table 1 ▪ McGregor's Line to Odontoid Tip: Children, Both Sexes (mm)[5]		
AGE (Yr)	MEAN BASE LINE	90% TOLERANCE RANGE
3	1.94	− 0.8 + 4.7
4	2.07	− 0.7 + 4.8
5	2.17	− 0.6 + 4.9
6	2.24	− 0.5 + 5.0
7	2.29	− 0.4 + 5.1
8	2.31	− 0.4 + 5.1
9	2.30	− 0.4 + 5.1
10	2.27	− 0.5 + 5.0
11	2.21	− 0.5 + 5.0
12	2.13	− 0.6 + 4.9
13	2.01	− 0.7 + 4.8
14	1.88	− 0.9 + 4.6
15	1.71	− 1.0 + 4.5
16	1.52	− 1.2 + 4.3
17	1.31	− 1.4 + 4.1
18	1.07	− 1.7 + 3.8

Table 2 ▪ McGregor's Line to Odontoid Tip: Adults (mm)[5]

	MEAN	SD	90% TOLERANCE RANGE FOR NORMALS
Male subjects	0.33	3.81	−7.4 to + 8.0
Female subjects	3.67	1.69	−2.4 to + 9.7
Male-female average difference	−3.06	—	—

Table 3 ▪ Digastric to Bimastoid Line: Adults: Measured on Laminagrams to Atlanto-occipital Joint (mm)[3]

	MEAN	SD	90% TOLERANCE RANGE FOR NORMALS
Either sex	11.66	4.04	3.8–19.5

Table 4 ▪ Digastric to Bimastoid Line: Adults: Measured on Laminagrams to Apex of Dens (mm)[3]

	MEAN	SD	90% TOLERANCE RANGE FOR NORMALS
Either sex	10.70	5.06	1.0–20.4

Digastric line (Fig. 5; Tables 3 and 4): Line between the two digastric grooves that lie just medial to the bases of the mastoid processes.

Source ▪

The measurements of the normal position of the odontoid process in relation to Chamberlain's line were based on a series of roentgenograms of 102 normal skulls (Poppel).

McRae's measurements were based on roentgenograms of 26 skulls.

Bull's measurements were based on roentgenograms of 120 normal skulls.

Hinck's measurements of McGregor's line were based on roentgenograms of 66 normal adult skulls and a series of 258 films taken at yearly intervals on 43 normal children, aged 3 to 18 years.

Hinck's measurements of the digastric line were based on skull laminagrams of 68 normal adults.

Note: Studies by Hinck show that, of the various diagnostic systems to determine basilar invagination, McRae's line and the digastric line appear to be the best. McGregor's line seems to be the best measurement for use on the lateral skull film.

REFERENCES

1. Chamberlain WE: Yale J Biol Med 1939; 11:487.
2. Poppel MH; et al: Radiology 1953; 61:639.
3. McRae DL, Barnum AS: AJR Am J Roentgenol 1953; 70:23.
4. Bull JW, et al: Brain 1955; 78:229.
5. Hinck VC, Hopkins CE: AJR Am J Roentgenol 1960; 84:945.

▪: MEASUREMENT OF THE BASE OF THE SKULL FOR PLATYBASIA
▪ ACR Code: 12 (Base of Skull)

The Basal Angle[1] ▪

Technique

Central ray: Perpendicular to film centered over midportion of skull.
Position: True lateral. Midline tomogram may be used.
Target-film distance: Immaterial.

Measurements (Figure 1 and Table 1)

1 = Line drawn from the nasion to the center of the sella turcica.
2 = Line drawn from the center of the sella turcica to the anterior margin of the foramen magnum.

The basal angle is not a measurement of degree of impression of the base but is an index of the position of one part of the base relative to another. The base may be impressed with or without disturbance of this relationship.

Table 1 ▪ Normal Range of the Basal Angle

Maximum	152°
Minimum	123°
Mean	137°

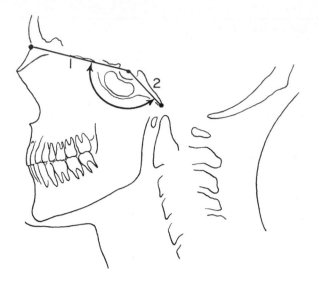

Figure 1 ▪ The basal angle.[1] See Table 1 for values.

Source

These measurements were based on roentgen examination in 102 normal cases.

REFERENCE

1. Poppel MH, et al: Radiology 1953; 61:639.

▪▪ MEASUREMENT OF INTERORBITAL DISTANCE
 ▪ ACR Code: 221 (Bony Orbit)

Technique ▪

Central ray: To anterior nasal spine.
Position: Sinus film, using an angle board with nose and forehead touching the cassette and the tube in a vertical position.
Target-film distance: 28 inches.

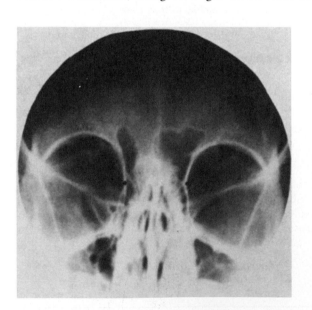

Figure 1 ▪ Black dots indicate the points at which the interorbital distance is measured. (From Hansman CF: Radiology 1966; 86:87. Used by permission.)

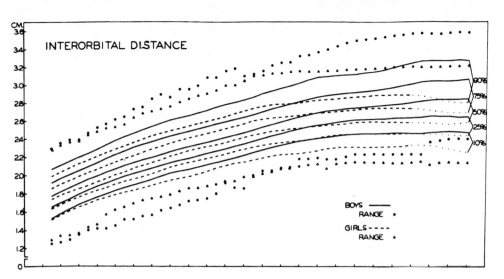

Figure 2 • Percentile standards for measurement of interorbital distance for both sexes. Distance (*cm*) on the left and percentile scale on the right. (From Hansman CF: Radiology 1966; 86:87. Used by permission.)

Measurements (Figures 1 and 2) •

Source •

Hansman used several hundred normal individuals who have been studied by the Child Research Council, University of Colorado.

REFERENCE

1. Hansman CF: Growth of interorbital distance and skull thickness as observed in roentgenographic measurements. Radiology 1966; 86:87.

⠶ MEASUREMENT OF THE HEIGHT OF THE ORBIT[1]
- ACR Code: 221 (Bony Orbit)

Technique •

Central ray: Perpendicular to the plane of the film centered over the midportion of the skull.
Position: Posteroanterior with the head in nose-chin position.
Target-film distance: Immaterial.

Measurements (Figure 1) •

The measurement is taken from the highest point of the orbit to the lowest part of the floor, ignoring the intraorbi-

tal margin or supraorbital ridge. A difference of 2 mm in height of the orbits is likely to be of significance in a patient with unilateral exophthalmos. Dysthyroid patients do not show any variation from normal. Over 25% of proven intraorbital space-occupying lesions show a significant increase in vertical diameter of the affected orbit.

Source •

Measurements were made on a control series of 200 consecutive nonproptosed patients, 61 patients with unilateral

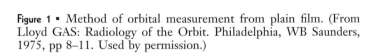

Figure 1 • Method of orbital measurement from plain film. (From Lloyd GAS: Radiology of the Orbit. Philadelphia, WB Saunders, 1975, pp 8–11. Used by permission.)

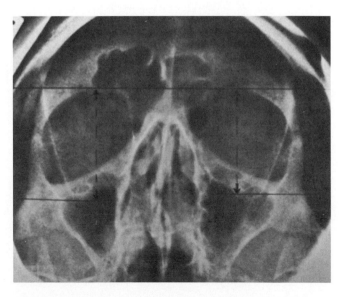

proptosis caused by dysthyroid disease, and 78 patients with proven intraorbital space-occupying lesions of the orbit.

REFERENCE

1. Lloyd GAS: Radiology of the Orbit. Philadelphia, WB Saunders, 1975, pp. 8–11.

▪: NORMAL MEASUREMENTS OF THE SUPERIOR ORBITAL FISSURE[1]
▪ ACR Code: 221 (Bony Orbit)

Technique ▪

Central ray: Directed toward the external occipital protuberance and angulated 15° toward the feet.
Position: Posteroanterior. Head placed with forehead and nose touching the table top.
Target-film distance: 40 inches.

Measurements (Figure 1 and Table 1) ▪

A = Greatest length.
B = Maximum width.
    Normal sphenoid fissures showed asymmetric development, compared with the opposite side, in 9% of cases measured.

Table 1 ▪ Superior Orbital Fissure Dimensions	
A (length)	15 mm (av)
B (maximum width)	5 mm (av)

av = average.

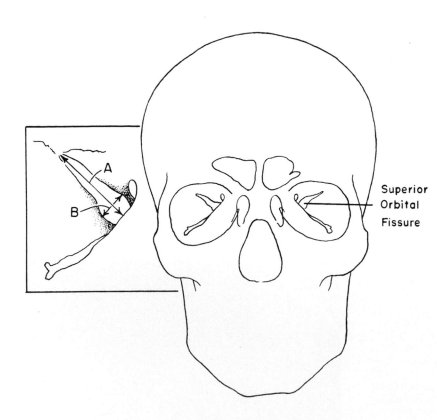

Superior Orbital Fissure

Figure 1 ▪ Measurement of the superior orbital fissure. A = greatest length, B = maximum width. See Table 1 for values.

Source ▪

These measurements were based on a study of 157 anatomic specimens.

REFERENCE

1. Kornblum K, Kennedy GR: AJR Am J Roentgenol 1942; 47:845.

▪▪ MEASUREMENT OF THE OPTIC FORAMINA[1]
▪ ACR Code: 222 (Optic Canal)

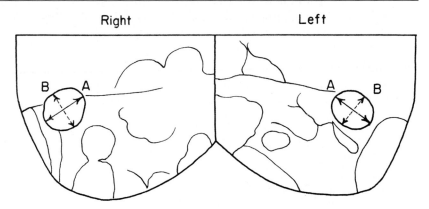

Right   Left

Figure 1 ▪ Measurement of the optic canal. A = width, B = height. See Table 1 for values.

Table 1 ▪ Optic Canal Dimensions: Measurements Corrected for Roentgenographic Distortion*†

	A (in mm)			B (in mm)		
	Max	Min	Av	Max	Min	Av
Right side	5.3	3.5	4.26	5.6	3.0	4.33
Left side	5.6	3.5	4.49	5.5	3.5	4.30

*Data from Goalwin HA: AJR 1925; 13:480; and Young BR: The Skull, Sinuses, Mastoids: A Handbook of Roentgen Diagnosis. Chicago, Year Book Medical Publishers, 1948.

†Neonate: average maximum diameter is 4 mm. Age 6 months: average maximum diameter is 5 mm. Optic foramina reach adult size at about 5 years.

Technique ▪

Central ray: Perpendicular to the film passing through the center of the orbit being examined. Pfeiffer method:[2] 37° to sagittal plane and 30° to canthomeatal plane.

Position: Rotate the head 53° from the true frontal position toward the orbit under study, so that the supraorbital ridge and zygomatic arch rest firmly on the plate. Pfeiffer method:[2] requires a V-shaped cassette tunnel to support the patient's head.

Target-film distance: Pfeiffer method:[2] 25 inches. Immaterial for adult measurements.

Measurements (Figure 1 and Table 1) ▪

A = Line from the superomesial margin of the canal to the inferolateral extremity, at an angle of 45°.

B = Line from the superolateral edge to the inferomesial border at a right angle to A.

Source ▪

These measurements were based on a radiographic study of 80 normal skulls and have been corrected for radiographic distortion.

REFERENCES

1. Goalwin HA: AJR Am J Roentgenol 1925; 13:480; and Young BR: The Skull, Sinuses, Mastoids: A Handbook of Roentgen Diagnosis. Chicago, Year Book Medical Publishers, Inc, 1948.
2. Evans RA, et al: Radiol Clin North Am 1963; 1:459. Contains description of Pfeiffer method.

⬚ PNEUMATIZATION OF THE PARANASAL SINUSES WITH AGE
▪ ACR Code: 23 (Paranasal Sinus)

Technique ▪

The article by Seuderi and associates is a pictorial essay based on the authors' clinical experience, supplemented by 4 references.[1] Simonson performed sagittal T1-weighted images of the brain (TR and TE not given) with a 0.5-T machine (Picker International, Highland Heights, OH) or a 1.5-T unit (General Electric, Milwaukee, WI).[2]

Measurements ▪

Figures 1, 2, and 3 show development of the paranasal sinuses during childhood in coronal, axial, and sagittal planes, respectively.[1] In the work of Simonson and colleagues, pneumatization of the sphenoid and frontal sinuses was graded subjectively by percentage, and this is shown in Figure 4.[2]

Source ▪

Simonson's study included 246 examinations of 238 patients (127 male, 119 female, aged newborn to 24 years), who also had no known condition affecting the marrow.[2] These subjects were divided into 8 age groups (range of n = 21–41, mean of n = 39) for analysis.[2]

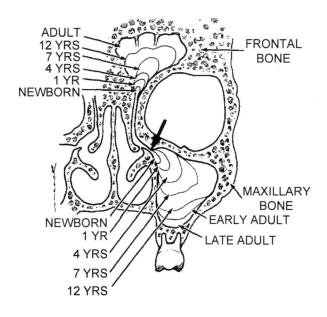

Figure 1 ▪ Development of maxillary and frontal sinus aeration from birth to adulthood. Composite drawing in the coronal plane. The large black arrow indicates the ethmoid infundibulum. (From Scuderi AJ, Harnsberger HR, Boyer RS: AJR Am J Roentgenol 1993; 160[5]:1101–1104. Used by permission.)

Figure 2 ▪ Development of ethmoid and sphenoid sinus aeration from birth to adulthood. Composite drawing in the axial plane. (From Scuderi AJ, Harnsberger HR, Boyer RS: AJR Am J Roentgenol 1993; 160[5]:1101–1104. Used by permission.)

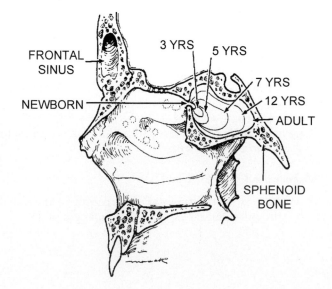

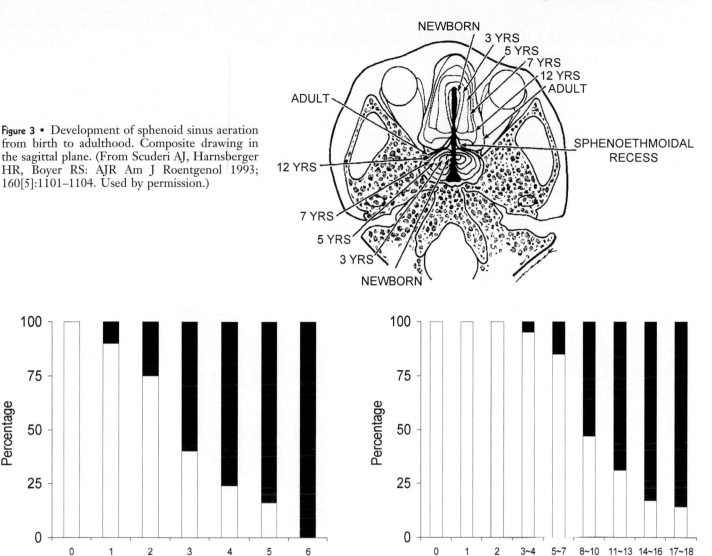

Figure 3 ▪ Development of sphenoid sinus aeration from birth to adulthood. Composite drawing in the sagittal plane. (From Scuderi AJ, Harnsberger HR, Boyer RS: AJR Am J Roentgenol 1993; 160[5]:1101–1104. Used by permission.)

Figure 4 ▪ Graph of sinus aeration percentages with age on MRI scans. (*A*) Sphenoid sinus; (*B*) frontal sinus. Black = air, white = marrow. (From Simonson TM, Kao SC: Pediatr Radiol 1992; 22[8].556–559. Used by permission.)

Comments ▪

Aeration of the sinuses progresses in the following order: maxillary (partly aerated at birth), ethmoid (partly aerated at birth, sphenoid (aeration as early as 2 years), frontal (aeration begins shortly after 2 years). Objective measurements of aeration of the sphenoid sinus with age are presented in a separate section.

REFERENCES

1. Scuderi AJ, Harnsberger HR, Boyer RS: Pneumatization of the paranasal sinuses: Normal features of importance to the accurate interpretation of CT scans and MR images. AJR Am J Roentgenol 1993; 160(5):1101–1104.
2. Simonson TM, Kao SC: Normal childhood developmental patterns in skull bone marrow by MR imaging. Pediatr Radiol 1992; 22(8):556–559.

▪: MEASUREMENT OF THE MAXILLARY, FRONTAL, AND SPHENOID SINUSES[1]
- ACR Code: 23 (Paranasal Sinuses)

Technique ▪

The charted measurements are actual anatomic dimensions.

Measurements (Figures 1 and 2; Tables 1, 2, and 3) ▪

A = Anteroposterior dimension of maxillary sinus.
B = Vertical height of maxillary sinus.
C = Width of maxillary sinus.
D = Distance of cupola of frontal sinus above nasion.
E = Height of frontal sinus.
F = Width of frontal sinus.
G = Length of frontal sinus.
H = Height of sphenoid sinus.
I = Width of sphenoid sinus.
J = Length of sphenoid sinus.

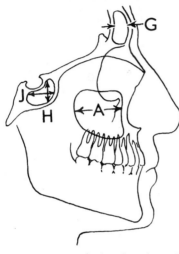

Figure 1 ▪ Sinus measurements depicted on lateral projection. See text for letter meanings and Tables 1–3 for values.

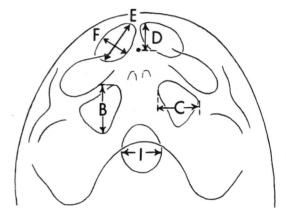

Figure 2 ▪ Sinus measurements depicted on base projection. See text for letter meanings and Tables 1–3 for values.

Table 1 ▪ Maxillary Sinuses (in millimeters)			
AGE	A	B	C
Newborn	7.0–8.0	4.0–6.0	3.0–4.0
9 mon	11.0–14.0	5.0–5.0	5.0–5.0
1 yr	14.0–16.0	6.0–6.5	5.0–6.0
2 yr	21.0–22.0	10.0–11.0	8.0–9.0
3 yr	22.0–23.0	11.0–12.0	9.0–10.0
6 yr	27.0–28.0	16.0–17.0	16.0–17.0
10 yr	30.0–31.0	17.5–18.0	19.0–20.0
15 yr	31.0–32.0	18.0–20.0	19.0–20.0
18 yr	31.0–33.0	20.0–21.0	19.0–21.0

Table 2 ▪ Frontal Sinuses (in millimeters)				
AGE	D	E	F	G
6–12 mon	2.0	2.0	2.0	3.5
1–2 yr	1.8	5.0	2.5	4.5
3–4 yr	2.5	7.0	4.0	5.5
7–8 yr	9.5	13.0	10.0	8.5
10–11 yr	12.5	16.0	10.0	9.0
13–14 yr	12.0	16.0	9.5	10.0
17–18 yr	15.0	18.0	20.0	16.0
19–20 yr	28.0	26.0	26.0	17.0

AGE (Yr)	SIDE	H	I	J
Table 3 ▪ Sphenoid Sinuses (in millimeters)				
1	R	2.5	2.5	1.5
	L	2.5	2.5	1.5
2	R	4.0	3.5	2.2
	L	4.0	3.5	2.2
5	R	7.0	6.5	4.5
	L	6.5	6.8	4.7
9	R	15.0	12.0	10.0
	L	14.5	11.5	11.0
14	R	14.0	9.0	12.0
	L	15.0	14.0	7.0

Source ▪

Actual anatomic measurements based on a study of more than 3000 specimens.

REFERENCE

1. Schaeffer JP: Pa Med J 1936; 39:395.

▪: MEASUREMENT OF PARANASAL SINUS MUCOUS MEMBRANE THICKNESS[1]
- ▪ ACR Code: 23 (Paranasal Sinuses)

Technique ▪

Central ray: Caldwell: To nasion.
Waters: To anterior nasal spine.
Anteroposterior basal: Perpendicular to base of skull and to midpoint of inferior orbitomeatal line on median plane.
Position: Caldwell projection.
Waters projection.
Anteroposterior basal.
Target-film distance: The measurements given below are anatomic thicknesses. Therefore, if sinus films are taken at a target-film distance of 36 inches, a correction should be made to a 72-inch target-film distance.

Measurements ▪

Frontal sinus: Caldwell projection. 0.06–0.5 mm
Ethmoid sinus: Caldwell projection. 0.08–0.45 mm

Sphenoid sinus: Anteroposterior basal projection. 0.07–0.6 mm
Maxillary sinus: Waters projection. Medial wall, 0.2–1.2 mm. Lateral wall, 0.1–0.5 mm

Average thickness in health varies from 0.6 mm for the medial wall of the maxillary sinus to 0.1 mm for the ethmoid, sphenoid, and frontal sinuses. Thicknesses varying from 2.0 to 6.0 mm are found in pathologic states.

Source ▪

Measurements were made of 3000 sinus specimens. The measurements given above are anatomic thicknesses.

REFERENCE

1. Schaeffer JP. Pa Med J 1936.39:395.

▪: NORMAL DEVELOPMENT OF THE SPHENOID DURING CHILDHOOD
- ▪ ACR Code: 234 (Sphenoid)

Technique ▪

All scans were done with a 1.5-T Gyroscan S unit (Philips, Netherlands). T1-weighted (200–800/20–50) sagittal images and T2-weighted (600–3500/29–70) axial images were chosen from each examination for review. When available, T1-weighted coronal images were evaluated as well.

Measurements ▪

Measurements of the aerated portion of the sphenoid sinus were done in three planes from the available images. Subjective grading of signal intensities was done by 3 radiologists by consensus. A scale of three grades was used as

follows: 1 = uniformly low signal, 2 = mixed signal intensity or uniformly high signal intensity, 3 = complete pneumatization or partial pneumatization with grade 2 findings. Figure 1 shows typical evolution of marrow signal with age. Figure 2 shows the relative percentages of each grade against age. Table 1 lists the dimensions of the pneumatized part of the sinus versus age.

Source ▪

Retrospective examination of 401 children (177 girls, 224 boys) who had MRI of the head for a variety of reasons (suspected congenital abnormality, vascular disease, devel-

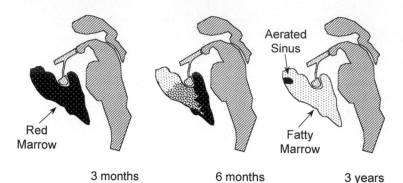

Red Marrow

Aerated Sinus

Fatty Marrow

3 months   6 months   3 years

Figure 1 ▪ Depiction of midsagittal T1-weighted MRI scans of children showing the sequence of marrow conversion in the sphenoid bone. This is shown for 3 months old, 4 months old, and 3 years old. Note the progression from uniformly low intensity to uniformly high intensity, moving from anterior to posterior. At 3 years, the sinus is beginning to be aerated as indicated. (From Szolar D, Preidler K, Ranner G, et al: Surg Radiol Anat 1994; 16[2]:193–198. Used by permission.)

Figure 2 ▪ Graphic representation of age-related changes in subjective grading of sphenoid marrow conversion. Conversion to fatty marrow is complete by 9 years of age, and the aerated portion continues to enlarge through 15 years of age. Percentage distributions of various signal intensities are shown. Black = low signal (hematopoietic), hatched = intermediate signal, white = high signal (fat). (From Szolar D, Preidler K, Ranner G, et al: Surg Radiol Anat 1994; 16[2]:193–198. Used by permission.)

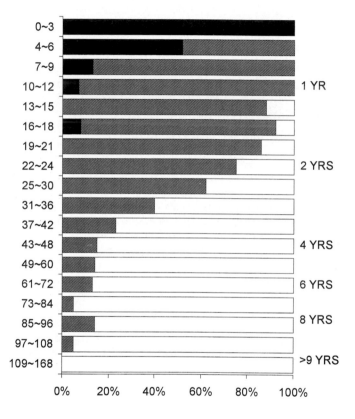

Table 1 ▪ Size of Pneumatized Portion of the Sphenoid Sinus with Age				
AGE (yr)	LENGTH (mm)	HEIGHT (mm)	WIDTH (mm)	VOLUME (cc)
0–1	—	—	—	
1–2	6.2	6.0	7.4	0.15
2–3	8.6	8.1	10.8	0.41
3–4	11.3	12.5	15.3	1.19
4–5	14.8	14.0	17.2	1.96
5–6	17.0	14.6	18.9	2.58
6–7	17.1	13.3	17.8	2.23
7–8	17.4	16.2	20.9	3.24
8–9	17.8	17.1	22.8	3.82
9–10	18.6	18.2	23.6	4.39
10–11	19.0	17.7	23.1	4.27
11–12	20.3	19.3	23.5	5.06
12–13	21.8	21.5	25.4	6.55
13–14	22.1	20.6	26.5	6.64

Volume was calculated as the product of the three axis measurements times 0.00055 (conversion to cc).
From Szolar D, Preidler K, Ranner G, et al: Surg Radiol Anat 1994; 16(2):193–198. Used by permission.

opmental delay, hydrocephalus, encephalitis, and brain tumor). None of the subjects had a history of sinus disease, bone marrow disorder, systemic disease, radiation to the area, or chemotherapy. The ages were roughly evenly distributed from infants through 15 years of age.

Comments ▪

Signal intensity started as uniformly low (grade 1) and gradually increased with age, indicating conversion from

hematopoietic marrow to fatty replacement. Pneumatization developed in a ventral to dorsal direction with onset near the choana, proceeding to the anterior and basal sphenoid and then to the occipitosphenoidal portion of the sinus.

REFERENCE

1. Szolar D, Preidler K, Ranner G, et al: The sphenoid sinus during childhood: Establishment of normal development standards by MRI. Surg Radiol Anat 1994; 16(2): 193–198.

▪: NORMAL LATERAL MEASUREMENTS OF THE SELLA TURCICA IN CHILDREN
▪ ACR Code: 122 (Sella Turcica)

Technique ▪

Central ray: Perpendicular to plane of the film centered over the midportion of the skull.
Position: Lateral.
Target-film distance: 5 feet.

Measurements ▪

The area of the pituitary fossa is measured with a compensating polar planimeter. Conversion to the metric system (square millimeters) is made by multiplying by the factor 6.45. The area is measured by tracing the contour from the tip of the dorsum sellae clockwise to the tuberculum

sellae and then following a straight line from the tuberculum sellae back to the point of origin. When the tip of the dorsum sellae can be visualized through the clinoid processes, the line of reference is drawn to the visual boundaries of the dorsum sellae, disregarding the superimposition of the clinoid processes.

The length (*L*, Figure 1) is the distance from the dorsum sellae to the tuberculum sellae corresponding to the position of the diaphragmatic sellae. The depth is a perpendicular line dropped to the deepest point (*D*, Figure 1). In the absence of a compensating polar planimeter, the measurements of the pituitary fossa are obtained as outlined. The tables for boys and girls (Tables 1 and 2) show the mean

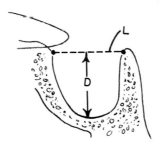

Figure 1 ▪ Measurement of the sella turcica. D = depth, L = length. See Tables 1 and 2 to obtain areas for boys and girls respectively.

LENGTH IN MM *(L)*	\multicolumn{8}{c}{DEPTH IN MM *(D)*}							
	3	4	5	6	7	8	9	10
5	14.5	15.0	13.0	—	—	—	—	—
6	14.1	18	19.0	—	—	—	—	—
7	17.8	20.2	25.5	35.7	36	61	—	—
8	17.2	22.3	30.0	36.8	47.4	55.9	61.0	—
9	13.0	27.3	34.2	42.0	51.4	60.2	69.9	—
10	—	31.7	38.1	46.7	55.8	65.0	74.8	87.5
11	—	29.0	41.9	51.7	60.9	69.9	81.9	85.3
12	—	45.0	47.0	57.6	64.3	72.9	81.3	92.3
13	—	—	43.9	55.2	69.7	78.1	87.3	95.0
14	—	—	61.0	66.8	73.6	81.0	87.6	97.0
15	—	—	—	58.0	71.3	90.6	103.3	97.0
16	—	—	—	—	84.0	90.0	96.7	—

Table 1 ▪ Mean Area of Pituitary Fossa for Given Combinations of Length and Depth (Boys)

Adapted from Silverman F: AJR Am J Roentgenol 1957; 78:451.

Table 2 ▪ Mean Area of Pituitary Fossa for Given Combinations of Length and Depth (Girls)

LENGTH IN MM (L)	DEPTH IN MM (D)							
	3	4	5	6	7	8	9	10
5	14.4	16.0	22.7	42.0	43.2	39.0	—	—
6	17.4	22.0	28.2	39.1	41.9	51.1	55.0	—
7	19.8	24.7	30.5	40.4	46.8	56.6	81.7	89.0
8	21.0	28.0	35.6	43.1	52.5	61.0	74.8	—
9	—	32.0	41.0	47.9	55.2	66.7	75.7	84.9
10	—	37.5	42.7	55.9	59.1	69.4	80.6	86.2
11	—	—	49.2	60.3	68.3	78.6	85.7	92.7
12	—	—	52.0	65.8	73.2	81.4	88.4	96.2
13	—	—	—	65.4	78.6	85.4	93.8	—
14	—	—	—	—	—	—	—	—
15	—	—	—	—	—	—	—	—
16	—	—	—	—	—	—	—	—

Adapted from Silverman F: AJR Am J Roentgenol 1957; 78:451.

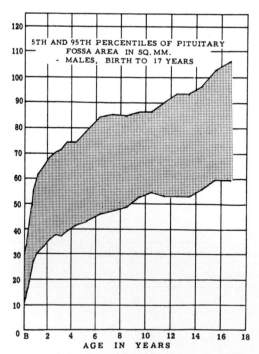

Figure 2 ▪ (From Silverman F: AJR Am J Roentgenol 1957; 78:451.)

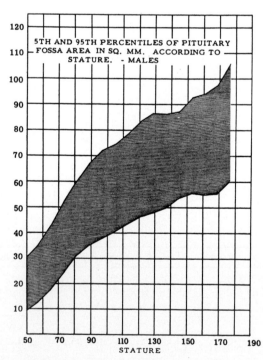

Figure 3 ▪ (From Silverman F: AJR Am J Roentgenol 1957; 78:451.)

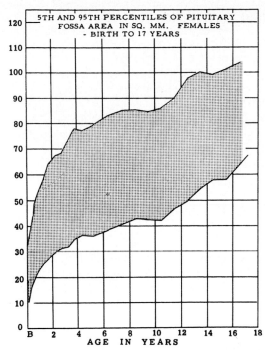

Figure 4 ▪ (From Silverman F: AJR Am J Roentgenol 1957; 78:451.)

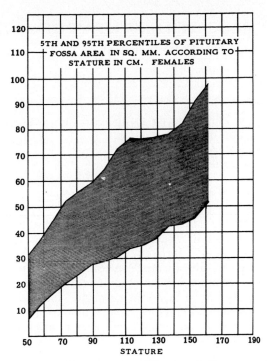

Figure 5 ▪ (From Silverman F: AJR Am J Roentgenol 1957; 78:451.)

areas. The mean figure is located on graphs where the area is plotted against age (Figures 2 and 3), or on graphs where the area is plotted against height (Figures 4 and 5). The height of the subject is probably a better standard than is age for evaluation of the pituitary fossa area. These graphs indicate the position of the pituitary fossa with respect to pituitary fossae from a group of normal children of the same age and the same height. A value for the area obtained from Table 1 or 2 that lies outside the 5th and 95th percentiles would have real significance with respect to indicating a deviation from the normal.

Note: The significance of the small sella turcica is open to question in the light of Di Chiro's work on the small sella turcica. See "Measurement of the Hard Palate in the Neonate" in this chapter.

Source ▪

These data are based on measurements of the pituitary fossa seen in lateral roentgenograms of the skull on 2137 films from 168 boys and on 1899 films from 152 girls, between the ages of 1 month and 18 years. The children were participants in the longitudinal growth study of the Fels Research Institute.

REFERENCE

1. Silverman F: AJR Am J Roentgenol 1957; 78:451.

⁝ NORMAL VOLUME MEASUREMENTS OF THE SELLA TURCICA
- ACR Code: 122 (Sella Turcica)

Children[1] ▪

Technique

Central ray: Perpendicular to plane of film, centered over midportion of the skull.
Positions: Posteroanterior; lateral.
Target-film distance: 60 inches.

Measurements (Figure 1)

The skull films were taken at a 60-inch (152.4 cm) source-to-film distance rather than the usual 34-inch (86.4 cm) to 40-inch (101.6 cm) distance used in clinical radiology. If the sella is about 3 inches (7.6 cm) from the film, a 60-inch source-to-film distance produces magnification of 5.2%. The volume will be magnified 16.6% and correspondingly 31.7% for a 34-inch distance and 26.3% for a 40-inch distance. Therefore, to obtain the "actual" sellar volume, measured volumes have been multiplied by the factor 1/1.17 or 0.86. To convert the volumes given in Figure 2 to observed sellar volume on a 34-inch film, multiply the values by the factor 1.32; for a 40-inch source-to-film distance, multiply by 1.26.

Source

Measurements were made on 960 sets of skull films of 427 children aged 6 to 16 years with no known neurologic, endocrine, or skeletal disease.

Adults ▪

Technique

Central ray: Posteroanterior: to glabella; lateral: to a point 1 inch anterior and 1 inch superior to the external auditory meatus.
Positions: Posteroanterior; lateral.
Target-film distance: 36 inches

Measurements (Figures 3, 4, and 5)

Source

These measurements were based on 60 cases[3] in a series that was later extended to 80 cases.[4] The sellar volume was calculated from posteroanterior and lateral roentgenograms and was compared with the volume determined by filling the sella turcica with dentist's wax. The method was then tested on 347 "normals."[4]

Di Chiro has pointed out that the sellar size cannot be reliably estimated from the lateral roentgenogram alone. If the three linear dimensions of the sella are known, it is possible to state pituitary gland size and sellar size so that 90% of the cases will be accurate within approximately 30%. The "best estimate" of pituitary gland volume from pituitary fossa measurements requires the use of regression analysis.[5]

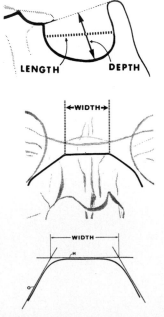

Figure 1 ▪ Diagrams illustrating method for measurement of sellar dimensions. The bottom figure indicates method of width measurement for the "rounded edge" sellar floor. (From Underwood E, et al: Radiology 1976; 119:651.)

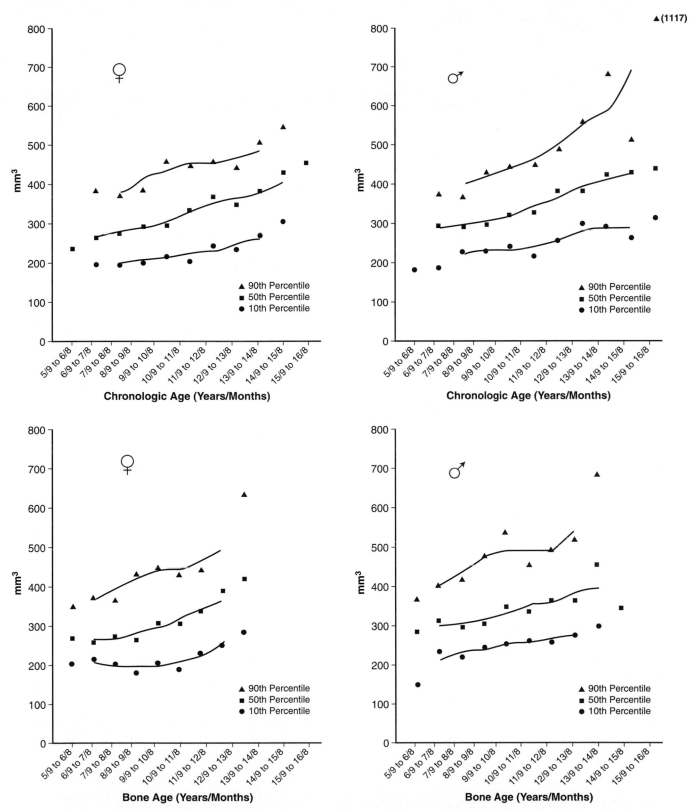

Figure 2 ▪ Volume of sella turcica corrected for magnification for boys and girls by chronologic age and bone age. Lines represent 10th, 50th, and 90th percentiles, calculated by a method of moving averages. (From Chilton LA, et al: AJR Am J Roentgenol 1983; 140:797. Used by permission.)

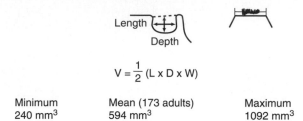

$$V = \frac{1}{2}(L \times D \times W)$$

Minimum	Mean (173 adults)	Maximum
240 mm³	594 mm³	1092 mm³

Accuracy
Prediction of sella size 83%
Prediction of pituitary size 87%

Figure 3 ▪ The volume of the sella turcica. (From Di Chiro G, Nelsen KB: AJR Am J Roentgenol 1962; 87:989. Used by permission.)

Figure 4 ▪ Sellar volumes of 347 "normal" controls. (From Fisher RL, Di Chiro G: AJR Am J Roentgenol 1964; 91:996. Used by permission.)

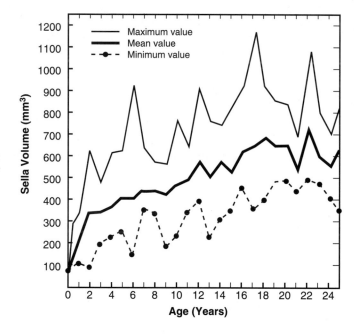

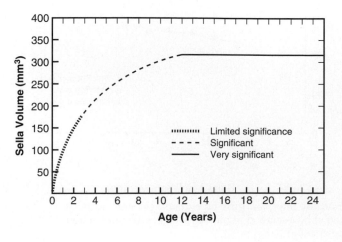

Figure 5 ▪ Minimal expected normal sellar volumes. (From Fisher RL, Di Chiro G: AJR Am J Roentgenol 1964; 91:996. Used by permission.)

REFERENCES

1. Underwood LE, Radcliffe WB, Guinto FC: New standards for the assessment of sella turcica volume in children. Radiology 1976; 119:651.
2. Chilton LA, Dorst JP, Garn SM: The volume of the sella turcica in children: New standards. AJR Am J Roentgenol 1983; 140:797.
3. Di Chiro G, Nelsen KB: AJR Am J Roentgenol 1962; 87:989.
4. Fisher RL, Di Chiro G: AJR Am J Roentgenol 1964; 91:996.
5. McLachlan MSF, Williams ED, Fortt RW, Doyle FH: Estimation of pituitary gland dimensions from radiographs of the sella turcica. A post-mortem study. Br J Radiol 1968; 41:323.

▪: MEASUREMENT OF THE HARD PALATE IN THE NEONATE[1]
- ▪ ACR Code: 262 (Palate)

Technique ▪

Central ray: Perpendicular to plane of film centered over the midportion of the skull.
Position: Lateral.
Target-film distance: 40 inches.

Measurements (Figure 1) ▪

Length of hard palate (*AB*) extends from the anterior maxillary process to posterior termination.

$D = 31$ mm $\pm$ 3 mm.

Note: In a newborn term infant, roentgenographic hard palate length of 26 mm or less is a sign of mongolism. Hard-palate length of 27 mm or 28 mm is indeterminate, and 29 mm or more is within normal limits.

Source ▪

One hundred eighty-two newborn full-term infants considered to be normal at birth.

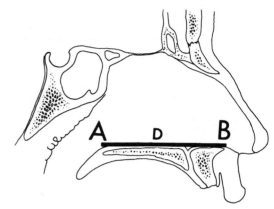

Figure 1 ▪ (Adapted from Austin JHM, et al: Radiology 1969; 92:775.)

REFERENCE

1. Austin JH, Preger L, Siris E, Taybi H: Short hard palate in newborn. Roentgen sign of mongolism. Radiology 1969; 92:775–776.

CHAPTER 3

Orbital Contents, Face, and Neck

∎: VOLUME OF ORBITAL STRUCTURES
∎ ACR Code: 22 (Orbit)

Technique ∎

Feldon and colleagues performed axial orbital scans at 1- to 5-mm intervals, using an unspecified CT scanner.[1] Forbes and colleagues obtained 1.5-mm axial scans of the orbits using a GE 8800 scanner (General Electric, Milwaukee, WI).[2,3] Peyster and associates used a GE 8800 CT scanner to make 1.5- to 5-mm axial scans through the orbits.[4] All scans were done at 0 to 10 degrees off the canthomeatal line, without contrast material.

Measurements ∎

Peyster and associates[4] used the volume measurement function from General Electric Display (GDIS) software (General Electric, Milwaukee, WI) running on the scanner whereas the other workers[1-3] transferred image data to stand-alone computers for off-line volume analysis. Forbes and associates used a combination of computer techniques, including automated tracing, region growing, and neighborhood sampling to trace the outlines of muscles (rectus, oblique, and levator) and fat on each slice.[2,3] Manual tracing of these structures on each slice was done by the other two groups.[1,4] In all four series, the areas of muscles and fat from each slice were summed with appropriate correction to obtain volumes.

The bony orbit was defined as a cone bounded by the lateral wall, the medial wall, the roof, and the floor.[1-4] The anterior border was defined by a line between the lateral wall and the medial nasal prominence[2-4] or by the globe and orbital septum.[1]

AUTHOR GROUP	NO. OF ORBITS	ORBITAL VOLUME (cc)	MUSCLE VOLUME (cc)	FAT VOLUME (cc)
Feldon				
−Ophthalm	70	23.15 ± 3.33	2.20 ± 0.80	
+Ophthalm	10	27.39 ± 7.27	4.76 ± 1.98	
Developed Ophthalm	16	26.98 ± 6.92	4.43 ± 1.72	
Forbes				
Normal male	24		4.79 ± 0.70	11.19 ± 1.41
Normal female	34		4.69 ± 0.75	10.10 ± 1.05
Forbes				
Normal	44		4.83 (3.07–6.80)	10.53 (8.22–14.00)
+Ophthalm	124		8.10 (3.80–21.57)	12.42 (6.05–22.63)
−Ophthalm	20		5.94 (3.50–9.10)	10.2 (3.77–16.39)
Peyster				
Normal	30	19.82 ± 3.68		8.16 ± 1.68
Proptosis	32	18.97 ± 2.00		11.04 ± 1.76

Table 1 ∎ Volumes of Orbital Fat, Muscle, and Total Soft Volume

Measurements given as mean ± standard deviation or mean and (range). −Ophthalm/+Ophthalm = without or with Graves ophthalmopathy; developed Ophthalm = developed ophthalmopathy later.[1-4]

Table 1 lists the total volume of the soft tissues in the globe, the muscle volume, and the fat volumes arranged by researcher and patient group. The normal values in the second paper by Forbes were divided by gender and side, and the data for Graves disease patients were divided by side; the range, rather than standard deviation, was reported for all groups.[3] These were combined by averaging to simplify in Table 1, which results in minimal error since the intergroup differences had a maximum of around 3%.

Source ■

Feldon's subjects included 48 patients with Graves disease, ranging in age from 11 to 81 years. There were 9 males and 40 females. Of these, 35 (70 orbits) had no signs or symptoms of ophthalmopathy, 5 (10 orbits) had clinical ophthalmopathy, and 8 (16 orbits) developed ophthalmopathy during follow-up.[1] Forbes and group studied 29 (58 orbits) patients referred for field cuts or scotomata who had normal scans. The age ranged from 6 months to 22 years, with 12 males and 17 females.[2] In a second study,

Forbes and groups evaluated 94 (188 orbits) subjects (48 women, 24 men; age range, 15–77 years). Of these, 22 (44 orbits) were normal, 10 (20 orbits) had Graves disease without eye findings on examination, and 62 (124 orbits) had ophthalmopathy.[3] Peyster and associates studied 15 (30 orbits) patients with clinical proptosis for various reasons, including Graves disease, Cushing disease/syndrome, or obesity, as well as 16 (32 orbits) normal controls. The age and gender distribution were not given.[4]

References

1. Feldon SE, Lee CP, Maramatsu SK, Weiner DPH: Quantitative computed tomography of Graves' ophthalmopathy. Arch Ophthalmol 1985; 103:213–215.
2. Forbes G, Gehring DG, Gorman CA, et al: Volume measurements of normal orbital structures by computed tomographic analysis. AJR Am J Roentgenol 1985; 145:149–154.
3. Forbes G, Gorman CA, Brennan MD, et al: Ophthalmopathy of Graves' disease: Computerized volume measurements of the orbital fat and muscle. AJNR Am J Neuroradiol 1986; 7:651–656.
4. Peyster RG, Ginsberg F, Silber JH, Adler LP: Exophthalmos caused by excessive fat: CT volumetric analysis and differential diagnosis. AJR Am J Roentgenol 1986; 146:459–464.

⁚ SIZE AND MR SIGNAL INTENSITY OF THE LACRIMAL GLAND
■ ACR Code: 223 (Lacrimal Apparatus)

Technique ■

All scans were done in the coronal plane with a 1.5-T Signa machine (General Electric Medical Systems, Milwaukee, WI), using T1 (500–600/20) spin echo sequences. Slice thicknesses were 1.5 or 3.0 mm, and a surface coil was used.[1]

Measurements ■

The thickness and area of the gland were measured on the section showing its maximal size (Figure 1). MR signal intensities (SI) were recorded from oval regions of interest (ROI) within the palpebral part of the lacrimal gland (lg), the vitreous body (vb), and surrounding air (sa). Mean and standard deviation (SD) of the SI were recorded from each ROI. An MR signal intensity ratio (SIR) was derived as follows: $SIR\% = (SI_{lg} - SI_{sa}) \times 100/(SI_{vb} - SI_{sa})$.

Figures 2 through 4 are scatterplots of the lacrimal gland thickness, area, SIR, and SD of the SIR related to age. Table 1 shows these data in tabular form.[1]

Source ■

The study population consisted of 45 males (mean age = 38.3 years; age range = 2 to 79 years) and 59 females (mean age = 46.6 years; age range = 3 to 78 years). All subjects had no history of disease or treatment that could affect the lacrimal gland.[1]

Comments ■

The lacrimal gland becomes smaller and brighter on T1-weighted images with aging in women, and these parameters remained the same in men with age.[1] The SIR changes

	SECOND DECADE (MEAN ± SD)	SEVENTH DECADE (MEAN ± SD)	LINEAR REGRESSION RESULTS (PARAMETER VERSUS AGE)			
			Multiplier (a)	Constant (b)	r value	p value
Males						
Thickness (mm)	4.9 ± 0.8	4.6 ± 1.0	−0.005	4.96	0.11	0.245
Area (sq mm)	68.5	60.5	−0.16	70.9	0.02	0.90
SIR (no units)	3.24	4.04	0.016	3.00	0.31	0.40
SD of SI	5.32	9.08	0.075	4.2	0.76	<0.001
Females						
Thickness (mm)	5.7 ± 1.2	4.3 ± 0.8	−0.032	5.95	0.62	<0.001
Area (sq mm)	89.93	66.68	−0.465	96.90	0.47	<0.001
SIR (no units)	2.69	3.99	0.026	2.30	0.48	<0.001
SD of SI	4.01	10.36	0.127	2.10	0.78	<0.001

Table 1 ■ Lacrimal Gland Measurements from MRI Versus Age

Predicted values of each parameter may by derived from the linear regression equations as follows: Expected value = a × Age (yr) + b.
SIR = signal intensity ratio (see text for equation); SD = standard deviation; SI = signal intensity.[1]

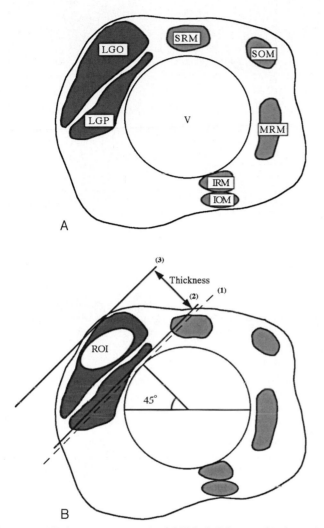

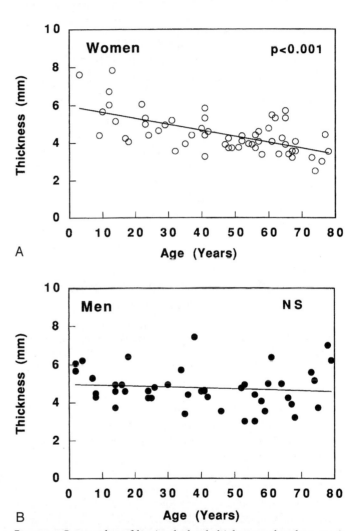

Figure 1 ▪ *(A)* Anatomy on sagittal MRI. LGO = orbital portion of the gland, LGP = palpebral portion of the gland; muscle abbreviations are standard. *(B)* Technique of measuring the thickness of the lacrimal gland from coronal images. A horizontal line was drawn through the center of the globe, then a second line 45 degrees to the first originating at the midglobe and passing through the lacrimal gland. The gland thickness is measured (including both palpebral and orbital portions) along the second line. The perimeter of the gland was traced for area determination. A region of interest (ROI) was placed within the LGO as shown for signal intensity measurements. (From Ueno H, Arije E, Izume M, et al: Acta Radiol 1996; 37:714–719. Used by permission.)

Figure 2 ▪ Scatterplot of lacrimal gland thickness related to age in women *(A)* and men *(B)*. Linear regression lines are shown. (From Ueno H, Arije E, Izume M, et al: Acta Radiol 1996; 37:714–719. Used by permission.)

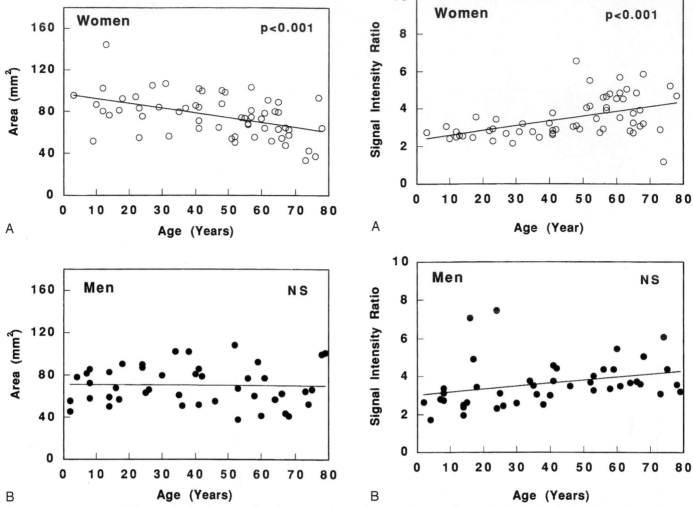

Figure 3 ▪ Scatterplot of lacrimal gland area related to age in women *(A)* and men *(B)*. Linear regression lines are shown. (From Ueno H, Arije E, Izume M, U et al: Acta Radiol 1996; 37:714–719. Used by permission.)

Figure 4 ▪ Scatterplot of lacrimal gland signal intensity ratio (SIR) related to age in women *(A)* and men *(B)*. Linear regression lines are shown. (From Ueno H, Arije E, Izume M, et al: Acta Radiol 1996; 37:714–719. Used by permission.)

were due to increased SI in the lacrimal gland as the SI in the lacrimal gland did not change with age. Both men and women exhibited an increase in variability of the SI in the lacrimal gland with age.

REFERENCE

1. Ueno H, Arije E, Izume M, et al: MR imaging of the lacrimal gland: Age-related and gender-dependent changes in size and structure. Acta Radiol 1996; 37:714–719.

▪: MEASUREMENT OF PROPTOSIS FROM AXIAL IMAGES
▪ ACR Code: 224 (Eyeball, Other Soft Tissue)

Technique ▪

Nugent and colleagues examined orbits with CT using a GE-9800 scanner (General Electric Medical Systems, Milwaukee, WI) in axial and direct coronal planes.[1] Contiguous scans were done with 3- or 5-mm thickness. Peyster and colleagues used a GE-8800 CT scanner (General Electric Medical Systems, Milwaukee, WI) to perform axial (0 to 10 degrees to the orbitomeatal line) images through the

orbits at 0.5- to 1.5-mm thickness.[2] Ozgen and Ariyurek used a Tomoscan SR 7000 CT unit (Philips, Eindhoven, Netherlands) and did axial scans (−10 to −15 degrees to the orbitomeatal line). Scan thickness was not given.[3]

Measurements ▪

In both series, the axial slice that showed the lenses to the best advantage was selected for measurement of proptosis,

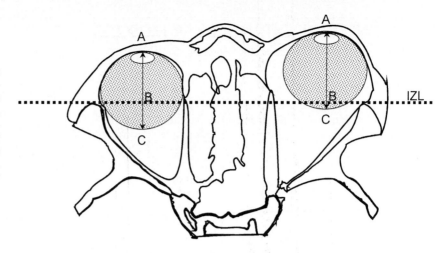

Figure 1 • Tracing of a representative axial CT slice through the lenses showing measurement of proptosis, with a normal right side and a proptotic left side. The interzygomatic line (*IZL*) is drawn between the anterior margins of the zygomas. Measurement is made either from the anterior margin of the globe to the IZL (*A–B*) or from the posterior margin to the IZL (*B–C*). Note that in marked proptosis the posterior globe margin may lie in front of the IZL.[1, 2]

Table 1 • Measurements of Globe Position in Normal Subjects and in Patients with Proptosis

AUTHOR/GROUP	NO. OF ORBITS	POSTERIOR GLOBE TO IZL DISTANCE	POSITION	ANTERIOR GLOBE TO IZL DISTANCE
Nugent et al				
Normal	40	9.9 ± 1.7	Behind IZL	
All Graves	142	2.3 ± 4.1	Behind IZL	
Graves − Neurop	124	3.0 ± 3.8	Behind IZL	
Graves + Neurop	18	2.6 ± 2.4	In front of IZL	
Ozgen and Ariyurek				
Normal	200	9.4 ± 1.7	Behind IZL	
Peyster et al				
Normal	32			15.4 ± 2.5
Proptosis	30			24.8 ± 2.5
Obesity	18			25.0 + 2.1
Graves	8			23.9 ± 3.9
Cushing	4			25.3 ± 1.0

All measurements are in millimeters (mean ± standard deviation). −Neurop/+Neurop = without or with neuropathy; IZL = interzygomatic line.[1, 2]

and a line was drawn with electronic calipers between the anterior margins of the zygomas (interzygomatic line = IZL). Nugent and Ozgen and associates measured the distance between the posterior margin of the globe to the IZL.[1, 3] Peyster and group measured the distance between the anterior margin of the globe to the IZL.[2] Figure 1 shows these measurements. Table 1 lists the average values of these measurements in normal and proptotic patients, as well as the suggested cut-off values.

Source •

Nugent's subjects included 71 (142 orbits) adults with Graves disease. Eighteen of the orbits were judged to have Graves neuropathy by clinical examination, and 124 had no evidence of neuropathy. Normal controls were 20 (40 orbits) adult patients referred for problems unrelated to the eyes.[1] Peyster and group studied 15 (30 orbits) patients with clinical proptosis for various reasons, including Graves disease (4), Cushing disease/syndrome (2), and gross obesity (9) with no endocrine abnormality.[2] A control group of 16 (32 orbits) patients had unilateral choroidal melanoma confined to the globe. Ozgen's subjects included 100 (200 orbits) adults referred for scans of the sinuses, with no orbital abnormality.[3]

Comments •

Nugent and colleagues state that clinical exophthalmos (proptosis) is likely when little or no globe lies posterior to the IZL.[1] From their data, 95% of normal subjects will have the posterior globe lying 6.5 mm or more behind the IZL (mean − 2 SD), and in 95% of Graves patients with clinical neuropathy and proptosis it will be no more than 2.2 mm (mean + 2 SD) behind the IZL. It seems that 5 mm behind the IZL is an appropriate cut-off value for the posterior globe margin. Nugent and group also state that if the anterior margin of the globe is more than 21 mm in front of the IZL, proptosis may be diagnosed. Peyster's data confirm this.[2]

REFERENCES

1. Nugent RA, Belkin RI, Neigel JM, et al: Graves orbitopathy: Correlation of CT and clinical findings. Radiology 1989; 177:675–682.
2. Peyster RG, Ginsberg F, Silber JH, Adler LP: Exophthalmos caused by excessive fat: CT volumetric analysis and differential diagnosis. AJR Am J Roentgenol 1986; 146:459–464.
3. Ozgen A, Ariyurek M: Normative measurements of orbital structures using CT. AJR Am J Roentgenol 1998; 170:1093–1096.

▪: THICKNESS OF EXTRAOCULAR MUSCLES
▪ ACR Code: 2246 (Extraocular Muscles)

Technique ▪

Nugent and colleagues examined orbits with CT using a GE-9800 scanner (General Electric Medical Systems, Milwaukee, WI) in axial and direct coronal planes.[1] Contiguous scans were done with 3- or 5-mm thickness. Demer and Kerman performed MRI of the orbits with a GE-Signa 1.5-T. machine (General Electric Medical Systems, Milwaukee, WI).[2] Coronal images at 3-mm thickness with T1 (550/15) weighting and no gap were attained through the orbits. Ohnishi and colleagues made sagittal orbital images of subjects using a 0.5-T MRT-50A machine (Toshiba, Tokyo, Japan), a 20-cm surface coil, 3-mm slices with 0.6-mm gap, and T1 (450/30) weighting.[3] Demer and Kerman also did A-mode echography of each studied orbit using an Ophthascan-S Mini-A unit (Alcon, Fort Worth, TX) with an 8-MHz transducer and an image sampling period of 40 nsec, yielding an axial resolution of 0.3 mm per dot.[2] Byrne and associates performed A-mode echography of the orbits, using the same machine and methods as did Demer.[4] Ozgen and Ariyurek used a Tomoscan SR 7000 CT unit (Philips, Eindhoven, Netherlands) for axial (−10 to −15 degrees to the orbitomeatal line) and coronal scans. Scan thickness was not given.[5]

Measurements ▪

Axial CT scans were used to measure the maximal thickness of the medial and lateral rectus muscle bellies.[1] The inferior rectus, superior oblique, and superior rectus/levator palpebrae complex were measured with electronic calipers, using the coronal CT image showing the muscle belly at its thickest point.[1] Coronal MRI images were transferred to an imaging workstation and used to measure the thickest part of the belly of four extraocular muscles (excluding the superior oblique).[2] Sagittal MRI images depicting the levator palpabrae muscle and electronic calipers were utilized for measurement of that structure at its thickest point, which was usually above the globe.[3] Ophthalmologic A-mode scanning was done in real time to find each extraocular muscle (excluding the superior oblique) at its widest point. The thickness was measured from frozen images, using calibrated electronic calipers.[2, 4] Figure 1 depicts the orbit in axial, coronal, and sagittal planes, with relevant muscle measurements shown.

Table 1 lists the diameters of the extraocular muscles for each group of patients studied.[1-5] Nugent and group calculated the sum of five extraocular muscle thicknesses, including the superior oblique.[1] The rest summed the rectus (and levator) muscle thicknesses.[2, 4, 5] Byrne and group's thickness data are for the right orbit only, with right versus left differences listed separately.[4] Ozgen's data include male, female, and combined measurements, as well as the 95th percentile of the right versus left difference.[5]

Source ▪

Nugent's subjects included 71 (142 orbits) adults with Graves disease. Eighteen of the orbits were judged to have Graves neuropathy by clinical examination, and 124 had no evidence of neuropathy. Normal controls were 20 (40 orbits) adult patients referred for problems unrelated to the eyes.[1] Demer and Kerman studied 20 (40 orbits)

	Table 1 ▪ Measurements of the Thickness of Extraocular Muscles								
AUTHOR (MODALITY)	SUBJECT GROUP	NUMBER ORBITS	MEDIAL RECTUS	LATERAL RECTUS	INFERIOR RECTUS	SUPERIOR COMPLEX	SUPERIOR OBLIQUE	SUM OF DIAMETERS	LEVATOR PALPEBRAE
Nugent									
CT	Normal	40	4.1 ± 0.5	2.9 ± 0.6	4.9 ± 0.8	3.8 ± 0.7	2.4 ± 0.4	18.1 ± 1.4	
CT	All Graves	142	6.0 ± 2.4	4.2 ± 1.4	7.3 ± 2.0	5.9 ± 1.9	2.7 ± 0.9	26.1 ± 7.7	
CT	Graves −Neurop	124	5.7 ± 2.1	4.0 ± 1.3	6.9 ± 2.4	5.6 ± 1.7	2.6 ± 0.9	24.8 ± 6.5	
CT	Graves +Neurop	18	8.2 ± 3.0	5.7 ± 1.4	10.3 ± 4.7	7.7 ± 2.1	3.1 ± 1.2	35.0 ± 9.4	
Ozgen									
CT	Normal male	88	4.3 ± 0.4	3.6 ± 0.8	5.1 ± 0.8	4.9 ± 0.8		18.0 ± 1.9	
CT	Normal female	112	4.1 ± 0.5	3.1 ± 0.7	4.6 ± 0.8	4.4 ± 0.6		16.0 ± 1.5	
CT	Normal all	200	4.2 ± 0.4	3.3 ± 0.8	4.8 ± 0.9	4.6 ± 0.8		16.9 ± 1.9	
CT	L/R difference (95th pctl)	100	0.5	0.7	1.1	0.9		1.4	
Ohnishi									
MRI	Normal	24							1.7 ± 0.3
MRI	All Graves	104							2.2
MRI	Graves −Ophthalm	64							1.7 ± 0.3
MRI	Graves +Ophthalm	40							3.1 ± 0.9
Demer									
MRI	Normal	40	4.5 ± 0.6	4.8 ± 0.7	4.8 ± 0.7	5.0 ± 1.0	—	19.1 ± 1.6	
U/S	Normal	40	4.7 ± 0.9	4.2 ± 0.6	3.9 ± 0.5	5.2 ± 0.5	—	18.0 ± 1.6	
Byrne									
U/S	Normal (right)	38	3.5 ± 0.6	3.0 ± 0.4	2.6 ± 0.5	5.3 ± 0.7	—	14.4 ± 1.3	
U/S	L/R difference	38	0.2 ± 0.2	0.1 ± 0.1	0.2 ± 0.2	0.3 ± 0.3	—	0.5 ± 0.5	

All measurements are in millimeters and show mean ± standard deviation. −Neurop/+ Neurop = without or with neuropathy; −Ophthalm/+Ophthalm = without or with ophthalmopathy; L/R difference = left to right difference, pctl = percentile.

Figure 1 ▪ Drawing of the orbit in axial *(A)*, coronal *(B)*, and sagittal *(C)* planes, with measurements of each muscle shown. ON = optic nerve, LR = lateral rectus, MR = medial rectus, IR = inferior rectus, SC = superior complex (rectus and levator), SO = superior oblique, LP = levator palpebrae, SR = superior rectus. Note that different coronal planes may be needed for each muscle as the thickest part of the bellies may not reside on the same scan.

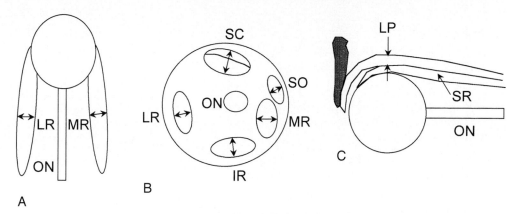

healthy adult volunteers with both MRI and echography.[2] Ohnishi and group examined 20 (40 orbits) adult patients who had Graves disease and class I ophthalmopathy, 32 (64 orbits) with Graves disease and no ophthalmopathy, and 12 (24 orbits) normal controls.[3] Byrne's subjects consisted of 38 adults with healthy orbital tissues.[4] Ozgen's subjects included 100 (200 orbits) adults referred for scans of the sinuses with no orbital abnormality.[5]

Graves neuropathy (Neurop in Table 1) was defined by Nugent and group as two or more of the following: reduced acuity, color vision abnormality, visual field defect, afferent pupillary defect.[1] Class I Graves ophthalmopathy (Ophthalm in Table 1) was defined by Ohnishi and group as eyelid retraction without proptosis.[3]

Comments ▪

Measurement of the levator palpabrae may be useful in mild (grade I) Graves ophthalmopathy, as involvement of

this muscle is thought to cause lid retraction without proptosis. The other muscles become involved later, and this (along with increased intraorbital fat volume) may lead to proptosis.

REFERENCES

1. Nugent RA, Belkin RI, Neigel JM, et al: Graves orbitopathy: Correlation of CT and clinical findings. Radiology 1989; 177:675–682.
2. Demer JL, Kerman BM: Comparison of standardized echography with magnetic resonance imaging to measure extraocular muscle size [see comments]. Am J Ophthalmol 1994; 118(3): 351–361.
3. Ohnishi T, Noguchi S, Murakami N, et al: Levator palpebrae superioris muscle: MR evaluation of enlargement as a cause of upper eyelid retraction in Graves disease. Radiology 1993; 188:115–118.
4. Byrne SF, Gendron EK, Glaser JS, et al: Diameter of normal extraocular recti muscles with echography. Am J Ophthalmol 1992; 112:706–713.
5. Ozgen A, Ariyurek M: Normative measurements of orbital structures using CT. AJR Am J Roentgenol 1998; 170:1093–1096.

▪▪ T2 MEASUREMENT OF EXTRAOCULAR MUSCLES
- ▪ ACR Code: 2246 (Extraocular Muscles)

Technique ▪

Ohnishi and colleagues performed MRI imaging of the orbits with a 0.5-T MRI-50A imager (Toshiba, Tokyo, Japan) and a surface coil.[1] Images were obtained in the coronal plane using T2-weighted (2000/30, 120) spin echo sequences, 5-mm section thickness, and a 1-mm gap. Hosten and colleagues used a 0.5-T Magnetom machine (Siemens, Erlangen, Germany) and a surface coil.[2] A single

midorbital T2 (1600, 30, 60, . . . 240)-weighted, eight-echo coronal sequence with 10-mm section thickness was used for T2 calculations.

Measurements ▪

Ohnishi and colleagues calculated T2 relaxation times (method not specified) of the superior, inferior, lateral, and medial rectus muscles as well as retrobulbar fat.[1] These

Table 1 ▪ T2 Relaxation Times of the Extraocular Muscles and Retrobulbar Fat

	NORMAL (Mean ± SD)	NORMAL (Range)	GRAVES −OPHTHALM (Mean ± SD)	GRAVES +OPHTHALM (Mean ± SD)
Number	24	24	54	164
Superior rectus	56.7 ± 4.02	49.7–62.5	53.9 ± 8.00	64.1 ± 15.22
Inferior rectus	58.2 ± 5.72	48.3–69.5	59.9 ± 10.23	72.3 ± 17.00
Medial rectus	61.4 ± 4.85	52.3–70.2	59.3 ± 7.08	68.5 ± 14.36
Lateral rectus	57.0 ± 4.92	41.3–65.7	58.4 ± 9.40	65.7 ± 10.94
Retrobulbar fat	76.0 ± 3.88	67.6–83.9	74.2 ± 4.04	73.8 ± 5.2

−Ophthalm/+Ophthalm = without or with ophthalmopathy.
From Ohnishi T, Noguchi S, Murakami N, et al: Radiology 1994; 190:857–862. Used by permission.

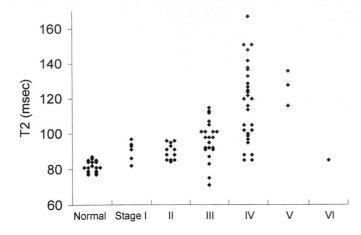

Figure 1 ▪ Scattergram of calculated T2 relaxation times of the inferior rectus muscles in normal orbits and in the orbits of patients with Graves disease who have various stages of ocular involvement (class I through class VI). (From Hosten N, Sander B, Cordes M, et al: Radiology 1989; 172:759–762. Used by permission.)

Table 2 ▪ **T2 Relaxation Times of the Extraocular Muscles and Retrobulbar Fat in Normal Subjects and Patients with Graves Disease**

	CONTROL	CLASS I	CLASS II	CLASS III	CLASS IV	CLASS V	CLASS VI
Number	24	26	8	56	64	2	8
Superior rectus	56.7 ± 4.02	54.4 ± 5.01	54.4 ± 8.66	59.9 ± 9.54	71.2 ± 17.10	56.6 ± 8.20	80.3 ± 22.24
Inferior rectus	58.2 ± 5.72	65.1 ± 9.94	61.3 ± 10.64	69.7 ± 14.62	77.8 ± 19.59	58.6 ± 4.95	85.2 ± 15.08
Medial rectus	61.4 ± 4.85	58.2 ± 5.47	62.4 ± 3.12	65.1 ± 10.62	74.2 ± 16.37	58.6 ± 4.53	85.2 ± 15.08
Lateral rectus	57.0 ± 4.92	60.0 ± 6.58	61.1 ± 5.18	63.6 ± 7.84	68.5 ± 12.21	70.6 ± 12.45	79.1 ± 17.24
Retrobulbar fat	76.0 ± 3.88	71.3 ± 4.39	69.3 ± 2.48	74.5 ± 6.00	74.7 ± 4.95	75.2 ± 1.63	72.9 ± 3.70

All measurements given as mean ± standard deviation.
From Ohnishi T, Noguchi S, Murakami N, et al: Radiology 1994; 190(3):857–862. Used by permission.

measurements were correlated with clinical staging. Hosten and colleagues calculated T2 relaxation times (method not specified) of the inferior rectus muscles and correlated them with clinical staging. Table 1 lists the T2 relaxation times for four rectus muscles and retrobulbar fat in normal subjects and those with Graves disease with and without ophthalmopathy.[1] Table 2 shows T2 relaxation times from the same structures, grouped by stage of Graves ophthalmopathy. Figure 1 is a scatterplot of T2 relaxation times in the inferior rectus muscles of Hosten's subjects, grouped by stage of Graves disease ocular involvement.[2]

Source ▪

Ohnishi's subjects consisted of 12 (24 orbits) normal controls, 27 (54 orbits) who had Graves disease without ophthalmopathy, and 82 (164 orbits) with Graves ophthalmopathy (class I through class VI) by clinical criteria defined by Werner.[3] Hosten and groups studied 9 (18 orbits) normal controls and 39 (48 orbits) patients with Graves disease having various stages of ophthalmopathy (class I through class VI) based on symptoms and ophthalmologic examination.[2]

Comments ▪

According to Ohnishi and group, the T2 relaxation times did not differ from normal in Class I and II disease.[1] The inferior and lateral rectus muscles were significantly longer in class III disease. All four measured muscles had longer T2 times in class IV and VI involvement (not enough in class V for statistical certainty). Hosten and group also performed visual evaluation of the extraocular muscles on T2-weighted images (TE 90 msec or more) and found bright areas in 12 of 23 patients with enlarged extraocular muscles when the TE was 90 msec or greater.[2] Bright areas were never seen in the lateral or superior rectus muscles.

REFERENCES

1. Ohnishi T, Noguchi S, Murakami N, et al: Extraocular muscles in Graves ophthalmopathy: Usefulness of T2 relaxation time measurements. Radiology 1994; 190(3): 857–862.
2. Hosten N, Sander B, Cordes M, et al: Graves ophthalmopathy: MR imaging of the orbits. Radiology 1989; 172:759–762.
3. Werner SC: Modification of the classification of the eye changes of Graves' disease. Am J Ophthalmol 1977; 83:725–727.

▪: NORMAL SEQUENCE OF MARROW CONVERSION IN THE MANDIBLE
▪ ACR Code: 243 (Mandible)

Technique ▪

A 1.5-T MRI unit (manufacturer not specified) was used to obtain T1 (500–600/20)-weighted axial and coronal images through the mandible, using a head coil.[1]

Measurements ▪

The mandible was divided into 4 regions (condyle, ramus, angle, and body), and the signal intensity in each region was compared with that of subcutaneous fat and masticatory muscles by two radiologists. They assigned each region a grade of 0, 1, 2, or 3, representing hematopoietic (lower or equal to muscle = 0) through fatty (equal to fat = 4) states. Figures 1, 2, and 3 represent images of the mandible in 1, 9, and 24 year old females. Figure 4 is a graphic depiction of marrow conversion during maturation. Figure 5 is a map of marrow signal distributions at various ages.[1]

Source ▪

A total of 45 patients (21 male and 24 female) ranging in age from 4 months to 25 years was included in the study. The subjects had no hematopoietic or bone marrow disease and were not taking any drugs expected to affect the bone marrow.[1]

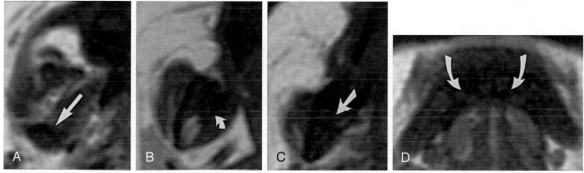

Figure 1 ▪ T1-weighted MR images in the axial plane of the mandible in a normal 1 year old girl. *A*, Condyle; *B*, ramus; *C*, angle; *D*, mental regions. (From Yamada M, Matsuzaka T, Uetani M, et al: AJR Am J Roentgenol 1995; 165[5]:1223–1228. Used by permission.)

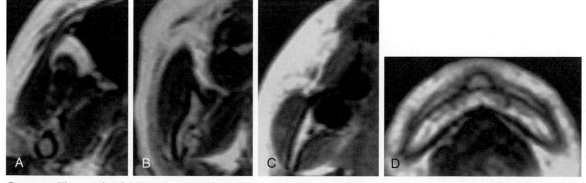

Figure 2 ▪ T1-weighted MR images in the axial plane of the mandible in a normal 9 year old girl. *A*, Condyle; *B*, ramus; *C*, angle; *D*, mental regions. (From Yamada M, Matsuzaka T, Uetani M, et al: AJR Am J Roentgenol 1995; 165[5]:1223–1228. Used by permission.)

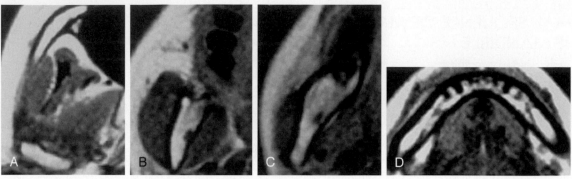

Figure 3 ▪ T1-weighted MR images in the axial plane of the mandible in a normal 24 year old woman. *A*, Condyle; *B*, ramus; *C*, angle; *D*, mental regions. (From Yamada M, Matsuzaka T, Uetani M, et al: AJR Am J Roentgenol 1995; 165[5]:1223–1228. Used by permission.)

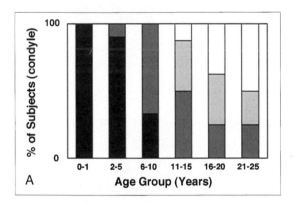

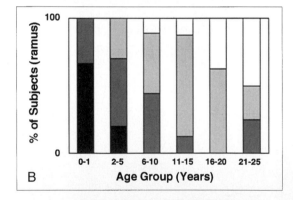

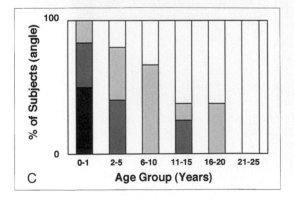

Figure 4 ▪ Bone marrow conversion with age in the mandible as assessed by two observers using a 0 to 3 grading scale. Black = 0, dark gray = 1, light gray = 2, white = 3. Graphs show scores from *A*, condyle, *B*, ramus, *C*, angle. (From Yamada M, Matsuzaka T, Uetani M, et al: AJR Am J Roentgenol 1995; 165[5]:1223–1228. Used by permission.)

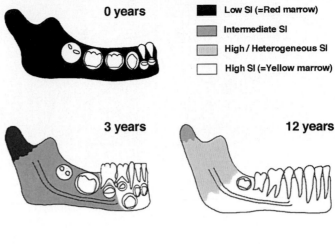

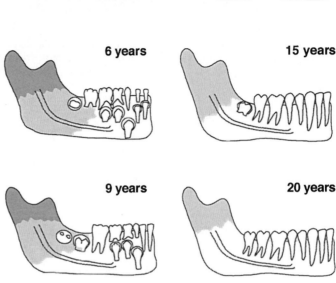

Figure 5 ▪ Map of conversion of marrow in the mandible on MR images with age. These are based on visual grades assigned by two observers viewing axial T1-weighted images. (From Yamada M, Matsuzaka T, Uetani M, et al: AJR Am J Roentgenol 1995; 165[5]:1223–1228. Used by permission.)

Comments ▪

This information should help in distinguishing diseases causing abnormal marrow signal from normal maturational heterogeneity in the mandible.[1]

REFERENCE

1. Yamada M, Matsuzaka T, Uetani M, et al: Normal age-related conversion of bone marrow in the mandible: MR imaging findings. AJR Am J Roentgenol 1995; 165(5): 1223–1228.

▪▪ MEASUREMENTS OF THE CHOANA AND VOMER IN CHILDREN
▪ ACR Code: 261 (Choana)

Technique ▪

Axial CT scans through the nasopharynx at 3- to 10-mm section width were made. The authors settled on 5-mm section thickness as being the best compromise as a result of the study.[1]

Measurements ▪

The best axial scan showing the vomer and choana was chosen. The transverse distance between the lateral wall of the nasal cavity and the vomer was measured on both sides (choanal air space = CAS). The width of the vomer (VW) was also measured. Figure 1 shows the measurement and Table 1 lists the results.[1]

Source ▪

Children undergoing head or facial CT scanning with normal scans for nonchoanal problems were included. There were 66 subjects ranging in age from newborn to 20 years of age.[1]

Comments ▪

In most cases the CAS was symmetric and where it was not, the difference was less than 1.0 mm. There was a strong positive correlation between the CAS and age (p < 0.001). Children with bony choanal atresia will have abnormally decreased (or absent) CAS, as well as a visible

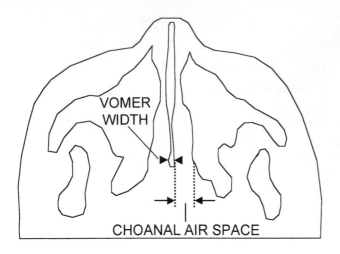

Figure 1 ▪ Measurement of the choanal air space from an axial scan through the mesopharynx. The distance between the vomer and the posterior lateral wall of the airway (*arrows*) was measured. The width of the vomer at the same level (*arrowheads*) was also recorded.

Table 1 ▪ Normal Values of the Choanal Air Space and Vomer Width with Age		
AGE (YR)	NUMBER	MEAN ± SD
CHOANAL AIR SPACE (mm)		
newborn	5	6.7 ± 1.70
>0–2	25	7.0 ± 1.65
>2–4	4	7.5 ± 1.70
>4–6	5	8.0 ± 1.70
>6–8	4	8.6 ± 1.65
>8–10	1	9.1 ± 1.70
>10–12	2	9.7 ± 1.65
>12–14	5	10.2 ± 1.65
>14–16	2	10.7 ± 1.70
>16–18	4	11.3 ± 1.65
>18–20	1	11.8 ± 1.65
VOMER WIDTH (mm)		
0–8	44	2.3 ± 0.55
>8–20	22	2.8 ± 1.35

From Slovis TL, Renfro B, Watts FB, et al: Radiology 1985; 155:345–348. Used by permission.

bony abnormality consisting of bowing and thickening of the lateral walls of the nasal cavity and thickening of the vomer. Children with membranous atresia often will have an abnormally small CAS measurement.[1]

REFERENCE

1. Slovis TL, Renfro B, Watts FB, et al: Choanal atresia: Precise CT evaluation. Radiology 1985; 155:345–348.

▪▪ MEASUREMENT OF ADENOIDAL SIZE IN CHILDREN[1]
▪ ACR Code: 263 (Nasopharynx, Adenoids)

Technique ▪

Central ray: Perpendicular to the plane of the film centered over the midskull.
Position: True lateral erect.
Target-film distance: Immaterial.

Measurements ▪

See Figure 1, *left side*, adenoidal measurement. A represents the distance from A^1, point of maximal convexity, along the inferior margin of the adenoid shadow to line B, drawn along the straight part of the anterior margin of the basiocciput. A is measured along a line perpendicular from point A^1 to its intersection with B.

See Figure 1, *right side*, nasopharyngeal measurement. N is the distance between C^1, the posterior superior edge of the hard palate, and D^1, the anteroinferior edge of the sphenobasioccipital synchondrosis. When synchondrosis is not clearly visualized, point D^1 can be determined as 5.6 of the crossing of the posteroinferior margin of the lateral pterygoid plates P and the floor of the bony nasopharynx. The AN ratio is obtained by dividing the measurement for A by the value for N (Table 1).

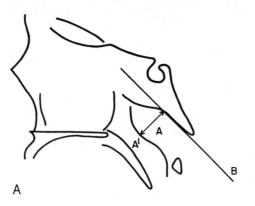
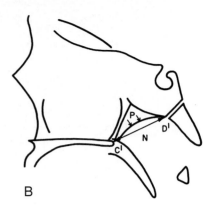

A   B

Figure 1 ▪ *A*, Adenoidal measurement. *B*, Nasopharyngeal measurement. (From Fujioka M, et al: AJR Am J Roentgenol 1979; 133:401. Used by permission.)

Table 1 ▪ Adenoidal-Nasopharyngeal Ratios (AN Ratio) in Infants and Children

MEDIAN AGES (yr, mon)	NO. OF CHILDREN (n = 1,398)	MEAN	SD
0, 1.5	33	0.329	0.1154
0, 4.5	51	.457	.1242
0, 9	74	.508	.1087
1, 3	56	.548	.1023
1, 9	45	.538	.0940
2, 6	78	.555	.0991
3, 6	82	.567	.1021
4, 6	85	.588	.1129
5, 6	79	.586	.1046
6, 6	98	.575	.1182
7, 6	85	.555	.1174
8, 6	73	.568	.1108
9, 6	74	.536	.1372
10, 6	79	.511	.1515
11, 6	93	.532	.1401
12, 6	81	.518	.1542
13, 6	84	.458	.1521
14, 6	85	.435	.1436
15, 6	63	.380	.1533

From Fujioka M, et al: AJR Am J Roentgenol 1979; 133:401. Used by permission.

Source ▪

Data were taken from 1398 children: 812 boys and 586 girls. Patients with sinus or lung abnormality were excluded.

REFERENCE

1. Fujioka M, Young LW, Sirdany, BR: Radiographic evaluation of adenoidal size in children: Adenoidal-nasopharyngeal ratio. AJR Am J Roentgenol 1979; 133:401.

▪: NORMAL LATERAL MEASUREMENTS OF THE ADULT NASOPHARYNX[1]

▪ ACR Code: 263 (Nasopharynx, Adenoids)

Technique ▪

Central ray: To the nasopharynx at the level of the posterior angle of the mandible.
Position: True lateral of the nasopharynx.
Target-film distance: 100 cm.

Measurements ▪

See Figure 1 and Tables 1 and 2.

Source ▪

Two hundred one normal Japanese adults (92 men and 109 women) from age 20 to 70+ years.[1]

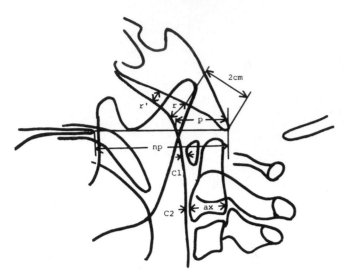

Figure 1 ▪ Measured section of the nasopharynx on the lateral view. r′ = middle third roof thickness; r = roof thickness; p = posterior wall thickness; C1 = c_1—postpharyngeal distance; C2 = c_2—postpharyngeal distance; ax = thickness of axis (c_1 vertebral body); np = depth of nasopharynx. (From Okimura T, et al: Nippon Acta Radiol 1977; 37:429. Used by permission.)

Table 1 ▪ Measurement of Thickness of Nasopharyngeal Soft Tissue

DIAMETER OF NASOPHARYNX	MALE (Mean ± SD mm)	FEMALE (Mean ± SD mm)
Middle third roof thickness (r′)	5.2 ± 1.6	4.8 ± 1.4
Roof thickness (r)	8.4 ± 2.4	7.0 ± 1.9
Posterior wall thickness (p)	19.2 ± 2.9	17.6 ± 2.9
C1-postpharyngeal space (C1)	4.5 ± 1.7	4.2 ± 1.3
C2-postpharyngeal space (C2)	2.9 ± 0.8	3.1 ± 0.8
Thickness of axis (ax)	19.2 ± 1.6	17.8 ± 1.2
Depth of nasopharynx (np)	50.0 ± 4.8	47.5 ± 3.5

From Okimura T, et al: Nippon Acta Radiol 1977; 37:429. Used by permission.

Table 2 ▪ Comparison of Thickness of Nasopharyngeal Tissue Measured by Three Investigators

	THICKNESS OF PHARYNX (mm)		
	Khoo[2]*	Eller[3]	Okimura[1]
MALE			
r′	8.4 ± 3.6 (7.5)	—	5.2 ± 1.6
r	—	11.5 ± 4.4	8.4 ± 2.4
p	17.2 ± 2.7 (16.9)	21.0 ± 3.8	19.2 ± 2.9
C1	3.9 ± 1.9 (3.8)	—	4.5 ± 1.7
C2	3.1 ± 0.9 (3.1)	—	2.9 ± 0.8
FEMALE			
r′	6.7 ± 3.0 (5.8)	—	4.8 ± 1.4
r	—	8.9 ± 3.6	7.0 ± 1.9
p	16.1 ± 2.3 (15.9)	19.0 ± 3.6	17.6 ± 2.9
C1	3.8 ± 1.6 (3.7)	—	4.2 ± 1.3
C2	2.8 ± 0.7 (2.8)	—	3.1 ± 0.8

*Parentheses show the mean for adults excluding minors in Khoo's measurements.

640 Chinese patients (355 males and 285 females) from age 10 to 70+ years.[2]

309 United States patients with an equal number of males and females from age 16 to 80 years. (Eller identified the patients as 4% black, 12% Hispanic, and 84% white.) Eller used a target-film distance of 36 inches.[3]

REFERENCES

1. Okimura T, Miyamura T, Kato S, et al: [Roentgenologic measurement of the normal nasopharynx in lateral roentgenograms of skull and face]. (authors translation). Nippon Acta Radial 1977; 37:429.
2. Khoo FY, Lee WS, Ng HW, Tye CY: Four diameters of the roof and posterior wall of the nasopharynx in the lateral neck radiograph. Br J Radiol 1974; 47:763.
3. Eller JL, Roberts JF, Ziter MH Jr: Normal nasopharyngeal soft tissue in adults; A statistical study. AJR Am J Roentgenol 1971; 112:537.

▪: MEASUREMENT OF NASOPHARYNGEAL SOFT TISSUES FOR THE DIAGNOSIS OF FRACTURES OF THE BASE OF THE SKULL[1]
▪ ACR Code: 263 (Nasopharynx, Adenoids)

Technique ▪

Central ray: Perpendicular to film centered over midportion of skull.
Position: True lateral, brow up.
Target-film distance: 115 cm.

Measurements (Figure 1) ▪

EA is the external auditory meatus, from which a line is drawn to *P*, the posterior end of the hard palate. The distance measured, *BS*, is from *B*, the skull base, to *S*, the anterior margin of the soft tissue. *PF* is the pituitary fossa, *SS* the sphenoid sinus, *O* the odontoid process, and *AA* the anterior arch of the atlas. The shaded area is the posterior nasopharyngeal air space.

The average measurement of *BS* (in millimeters) of adolescents was 10.68, ranging from 5 to 16. The average in adults was 10.03, ranging from 5 to 15. The measurement in patients with fractured bases of the skull was nearly twice normal.

Source ▪

Data are based on a study of 60 normal adults and 20 normal adolescents and compared with 45 patients with fractures.

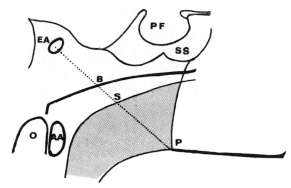

Figure 1 ▪ Measurements of nasopharyngeal soft tissues. (From Andrew WK: Clin Radiol 1978; 29:443.)

REFERENCE

1. Andrew WK: The soft tissue sign: A new parameter in the diagnosis of fractures of the base of the skull. Clin Radiol 1978; 29:443.

▪: ADENOID SIZE CORRELATED WITH EXCISED WEIGHT
▪ ACR Code: 263 (Nasopharynx, Adenoids)

Technique ▪

Lateral radiographs of the postnasal space were performed, using 7 kV and 60 mAs. The focus-film distance (FFD) was 6 feet, and the central beam was centered 2 inches behind the nasion. Care was taken to ensure that the orbitomeatal baseline was parallel to the floor.[1]

Measurements ▪

The outline of the adenoidal shadow was traced onto graph paper, using a line drawn through the posterior nasopharyngeal wall and continuing upward toward the anterior clinoid process (which it often intersected), as the posterior extent. The superior extent was taken to be the base of the skull, and the anterior margin was the junction of the adenoidal shadow with the airway. The area was calculated in square centimeters. The distance in centimeters between the anteriormost extent of the adenoidal shadow and the posterior wall of the maxillary sinuses was measured perpendicular to the tangent on the adenoid at this point. This was called the airway width.[1] Figure 1 depicts a radiograph with these measurements indicated.

The excised specimens were washed, dried, and weighed. These weights were correlated with the radiographic measurements. Figures 2 and 3 are scatterplots of the adenoid area measured on radiograph and excised weight. Figures 4 and 5 are scatterplots of the airway width and excised weight. These data were shown in the original paper as log/log plots (Figures 2 and 4), and we have adapted them into linear plots (Figures 3 and 5).

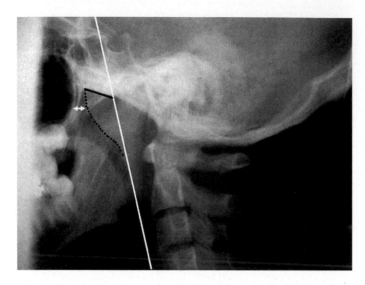

Figure 1 ▪ Measurement of adenoid area and airway width (at the adenoids) from a lateral radiograph. The adenoid area is defined by a line (*white*) continuing the posterior pharyngeal wall upward toward the anterior clinoid. The superior extent is the base of the skull (*black line*), and the anterior margin is the limits of the shadow (*dotted black line*). The airway width (*white line with arrowheads*) is measured between the anteriormost aspect of the adenoid and the posterior wall of the maxillary sinus.

Figure 2 ▪ Scatterplot of log 10 x-ray area versus log 10 adenoid weight. The regression given by the authors (see text for equation) is shown. (From Hibbert J, Whitehouse GH: Clin Otolaryngol 1978; 3:43–47. Used by permission.)

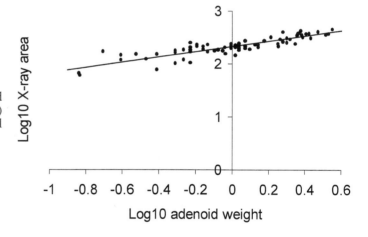

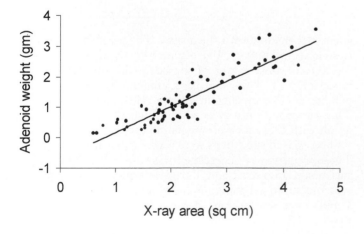

Figure 3 ▪ Scatterplot of adenoid weight (grams) versus x-ray area (square centimeters). Linear regression (see text for equation) is shown.

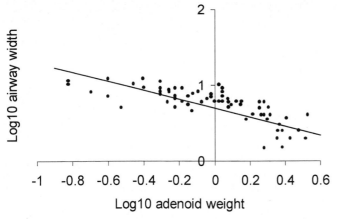

Figure 4 ▪ Scatterplot of log 10 adenoid weight versus log 10 airway width. The regression given by the authors (see text for equation) is shown. (From Hibbert J, Whitehouse GH: Clin Otolaryngol 1978; 3:43–47. Used by permission.)

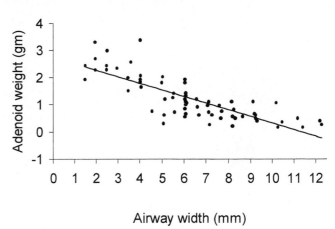

Airway width (mm)

Figure 5 ▪ Scatterplot of adenoid weight (grams) versus airway width (millimeters). Linear regression (see text for equation) is shown.

Source ▪

The study group consisted of 50 boys (age range: 2 years, 11 months to 10 years, 9 months; median age, 6 years, 9 months) and 26 girls (age range: 4 years, 10 months to 10 years, 10 months; median age, 7 years, 6 months). The radiographs were made the day before adenoidectomy in all subjects.[1]

Comments ▪

The authors gave the following logarithmic equations for adenoid weight:

$$\text{Log 10 (x-ray area)} = 2.33 + 0.50 \times \text{log 10 (adenoid weight), } r = 0.88.$$

$$\text{Log 10 (airway width)} = 0.73 - 0.56 \times \text{log 10 (adenoid weight), } r = 0.78.$$

Based on the linear regressions from Figures 3 and 5 (calculated by us based on scatterplot data in the paper), the adenoid weight might be more easily calculated from x-ray area and airway width as follows:

$$\text{Adenoid weight (gm)} = 0.85 \times \text{x-ray area (square cm)} - 0.68, r = 0.89.$$

$$\text{Adenoid weight (gm)} = 2.75 - 0.24 \times \text{airway width, } r = 0.79.$$

REFERENCE

1. Hibbert J, Whitehouse GH: The assessment of adenoidal size by radiological means. Clin Otolaryngol 1978; 3:43–47.

▪: MRI OF THE PAROTID GLAND FOR GRADING SJÖGREN SYNDROME
▪ ACR Code: 2641 (Parotid)

Technique ▪

All imaging was done with a 1.5-T Signa unit (General Electric Medical Systems, Milwaukee, WI). Axial T1 (500/20), T2 (2000/80), and fat saturation inversion recovery (IR) (100/20/120) sequences were done on each subject.[1] All images were made with 5-mm section thickness. Imaging results were correlated with labial gland biopsy in 35 of 40 patients with Sjögren syndrome (SS) and sialography, using standard techniques on 37 of 40 patients with SS and 10 of 10 patients with parotid inflammation. Biopsy grading was based on the criteria of Greenspan,[2] and sialography was graded according to Rubin.[3]

Measurements ▪

For qualitative analysis of the parotid gland, T1-weighted images through the midsection of the parotid gland were selected. A region of interest (ROI) with a constant area (0.87 cm^2) was placed posterior to the retromandibular gland (Figure 1) on the left side for controls, the left side for SS patients, and on the affected side for patients with parotid inflammation. The standard deviation (SD) of signal intensity within each ROI was recorded as a measure of glandular heterogeneity. For qualitative grading, two radiologists reviewed all three sequences on all patients and assigned a numeric grade from 0 to 4. The scores were based on the heterogeneity of signal and amount of high signal on each sequence and are detailed in Table 1 and illustrated in Figure 2.

Figure 3 gives the results of quantitative grading of parotid gland signal heterogeneity (SD) on T1-weighted images grouped by patient category. There were significant differences between patients with proved or suspected SS and normal subjects or those with inflammatory conditions. Table 2 indicates that the relationship between subjective scores, labial gland biopsy, and sialography demonstrates good correlation, especially with higher scores.

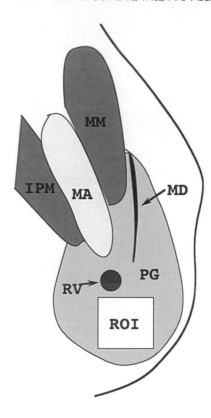

Figure 1 ▪ Placement of region of interest (*ROI*) on T1-weighted axial image through the parotid gland (*PG*) for standard deviation measurement. The square ROI has an area of 0.87 square cm. Shown are the retromandibular vein (*RV*), main duct (*MD*), internal pterygoid muscle (*IPM*), mandible (*MA*), and masseter muscle (*MM*). (From Izumi M, Eguchi K, Ohki M, et al: AJR Am J Roentgenol 1996; 166[6]:1483–1487. Used by permission.)

Table 1 ▪ Subjective Grading Scale for Parotid Gland Involvement with Sjögren Syndrome

MRI GRADE	SIGNAL ON T1-WEIGHTED IMAGE	EXAMPLE FROM FIGURE 2	SIGNAL ON T2-WEIGHTED IMAGE	EXAMPLE FROM FIGURE 2
0	homogeneous	A	low to moderate	E
1	sparse high signal	B	low to moderate	E
2	sparse high signal	B	high signal areas	F
3	moderate high signal	C	high signal areas	F
4	diffuse high signal	D	low to moderate	E

Reference (by letter) is made to appearances shown in Figure 2.[1]

Table 2 ▪ Correlation of Subjective Grade of T1 and T2 Signal Intensities in the Parotid, with Results of Labial Gland Biopsy and Sialography

SUBJECTIVE MRI GRADE	QUANTITATIVE HETEROGENEITY (Mean ± SD)	GRADING ON LABIAL GLAND BIOPSY					GRADING ON SIALOGRAPHY				
		0	1	2	3	4	0	1	2	3	4
0	14.0 ± 1.1	4	1	—	—	—	7	—	—	—	—
1	19.0 ± 3.8	—	2	3	—	—	4	1	—	—	—
2	23.5 ± 5.4	—	—	3	1	3	1	7	4	—	—
3	32.1 ± 9.3	—	—	—	2	5	—	—	—	7	—
4	29.6 ± 6.5	—	—	2	—	7	—	—	—	—	6

Numbers of patients in each category are listed.
From Izumi M, Eguchi K, Ohki M, et al: AJR Am J Roentgenol 1996; 166(6):1483–1487. Used by permission.

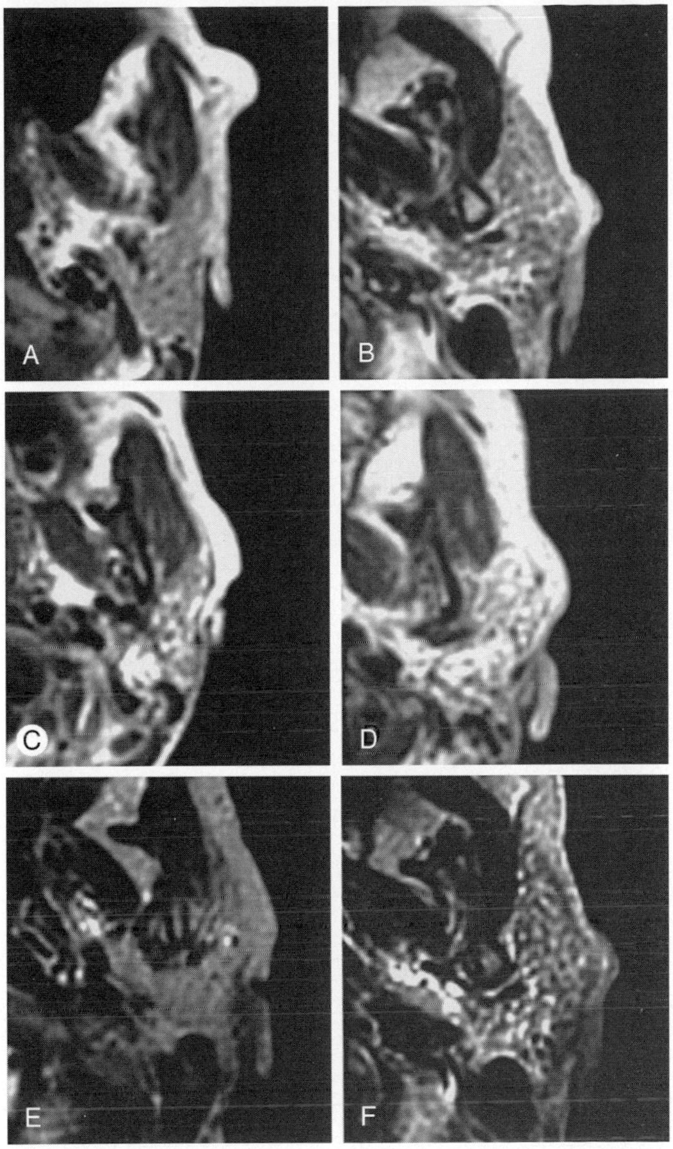

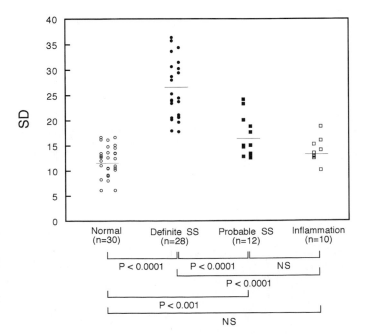

Figure 2 ▪ Illustration of subjective grading of the parotid gland. *A–D*: T1-weighted images with increasing amount of high signal. *E*: T2=weighted image with no focal high signal areas. *F*: T2=weighted image with focal high signal areas. (From Izumi M, Eguchi K, Ohki M, et al: AJR Am J Roentgenol 1996; 166[6]:1483–1487. Used by permission.)

Figure 3 ▪ Correlation of quantitative measurement of parotid gland signal inhomogeneity on T1-weighted images (*SD*) and parotid gland involvement with Sjögren syndrome as well as inflammatory processes. The statistical significance of differences in mean SD is shown below the graph. (From Izumi M, Eguchi K, Ohki M, et al: AJR Am J Roentgenol 1996; 166[6]:1483–1487. Used by permission.)

Source ▪

The study population consisted of 40 patients with suspected or confirmed SS, ranging in age from 23 to 74 years (mean = 53 years). There were 37 women and 3 men. There were also 10 subjects with parotid inflammation (7 women and 3 men), ranging in age from 18 to 56 years (mean = 46 years). A control group of 30 subjects was included who had no parotid disease and who ranged in age from 25 to 68 years (mean = 56 years). There were 27 women and 3 men in the control group.

REFERENCES

1. Izumi M, Eguchi K, Ohki M, et al: MR imaging of the parotid gland in Sjogren's syndrome: A proposal for new diagnostic criteria. AJR Am J Roentgenol 1996; 166(6):1483–1487.
2. Greenspan JS, Daniels TE, Talal N, Sylvester RA: The histopathology of Sjogren's syndrome in labial salivary gland biopsies. Oral Surg Oral Med Oral Pathol 1974; 37:217–230.
3. Rubin P, Holt J: Secretory sialography in disease of the major salivary glands. AJR Am J Roentgenol 1957; 77:575–598.

▪: NORMAL ANTERIOR COMMISSURE OF THE GLOTTIS
- ACR Code: 271 (Larynx)

Technique ▪

CT scans through the neck at 1.5-mm thickness were done with a field of view of 12 cm. Intravenous contrast was not administered.

Measurements ▪

Magnified (× 3.2) images through the true vocal cords were displayed, with a window setting of 350 and level of 40. Electronic calipers were used to measure the anterior-to-posterior thickness of the anterior commissure. Figure 1 shows how to take the measurement, and Figure 2 is a histogram of distribution of thickness measurements in normal subjects.

Source ▪

Thirty-eight patients referred for cervical CT myelography were included. None had any history of abnormality of the head and neck other than cervical radiculopathy. All scans were felt to be normal as far as the larynx was concerned. There were 26 men and 12 women, whose ages ranged from 24 to 70 years (mean = 51 years).

Comments ▪

The width of the anterior commissure was 1.02 +/− 0.56 mm (mean/SD). The width was less than or equal to 1.7 mm in 92% of subjects. An upper limit of 2.1 mm would include just over 95% of patients. In staging CT scans for staging of cancer of the true cord, it is very important

Figure 1 ▪ Measurement of the anterior commissure of the glottis on thin-section axial CT. The measurement is taken between the arrowheads on a scan done through the true cords. The vocalis muscles are indicated (vm). (From Kallmes DF, Phillips CD: AJR Am J Roentgenol 1997; 168:1317–1319. Used by permission.)

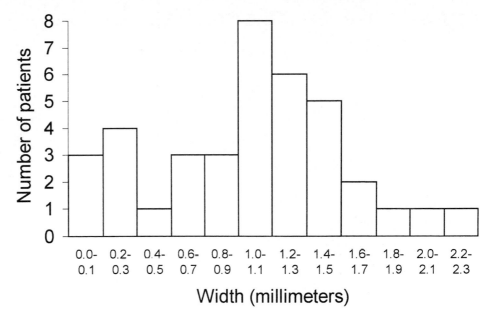

Figure 2 ▪ Distribution of thickness of the anterior commissure of the glottis in 38 normal adults on axial CT scans. Thicknesses are plotted against the number of times each was observed. (From Kallmes DF, Phillips CD: AJR Am J Roentgenol 1997; 168:1317–1319. Used by permission.)

to ascertain whether the lesion has crossed the midline. Measurement of the anterior commissure of greater than 2.0 mm should raise the suspicion of tumor extension across the midline.

REFERENCE

1. Kallmes DF, Phillips CD: The normal anterior commissure of the glottis. AJR Am J Roentgenol 1997; 168:1317–1319.

▪▪ ARYEPIGLOTTIC FOLD WIDTH TO DIAGNOSE EPIGLOTTITIS
▪ ACR Code: 2711 (Epiglottis)

Technique ▪

Lateral soft tissue detail neck radiographs were done. Technique and distances were not provided.[1]

Measurements ▪

The aryepiglottic fold thickness was measured directly from the radiographs at the midpoint (site 1), just behind the epiglottis (site 2), and at the junction with the arytenoid cartilage (site 3). These are shown in Figures 1 and 2. Mean thickness (millimeters), standard deviation (SD), and ranges were calculated for each site in each group of subjects. Receiver operating characteristic (ROC) analysis was performed on the measurements at each site with disease-positive being clinical epiglottitis. Table 1 shows the measured thicknesses, area under the ROC curve, sensitivity, and specificity for epiglottitis at each site.[1]

Source ▪

Children with clinically diagnosed epiglottitis (n = 38; ages: 8 months to 5 years, mean, 3 years); groups with

Table 1 ▪ Measurements of the Aryepiglottic Fold Width

Site	1	2	3
Location	Midpoint	Behind Epiglottis	Base of Folds
Control patients			
Mean ± SD	1.8 ± 0.7	1.7 ± 0.8	6.6 ± 1.8
Range	0.8 ± 3.0	0.8 ± 4.0	3.0 ± 11.0
Croup patients			
Mean ± SD	1.9 ± 0.9	1.5 ± 0.7	6.3 ± 1.6
Range	0.5–4.0	0.5–4.0	3.5–10.0
Epiglottitis patients			
Mean ± SD	5.8 ± 1.8	5.1 ± 1.7	9.2 ± 2.0
Range	2.0–11.0	2.5–11.0	5.0–14.0
Area under ROC			
Curve	0.99	0.98	0.84
Specificity	95%	95%	82%
Sensitivity	98%	97%	74%

Measurements are in millimeters. ROC = receiver operating characteristics.
From John SD, Swischuk LE, Hayden CK Jr, Freeman DH Jr: Radiology 1994; 190:123–125.

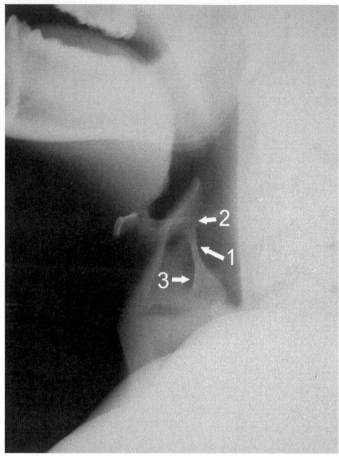

Figure 1 ▪ Lateral soft tissue radiograph of the neck showing the sites of measurement (*1, 2, 3*) of the aryepiglottic fold width corresponding to Figure 2.[1]

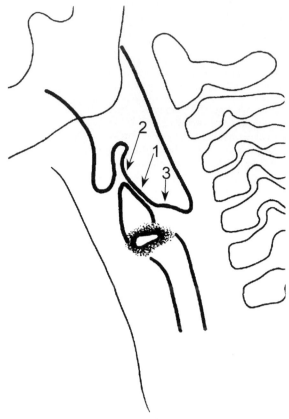

Figure 2 ▪ Sites of measurement of the aryepiglottic fold width from lateral neck radiographs. Measurements are taken at the midpoint (*site 1*), just behind the epiglottis (*site 2*), and at the junction with the arytenoid cartilage (*site 3*). (From John SD, Swischuk LE, Hayden CK Jr, Freeman DH Jr: Radiology 1994; 190:123–125. Used by permission.)

croup (n = 100; ages: 6 months to 11 years, mean, 2.5 years), and normal controls (n = 100; ages: 2 months to 12 years, mean, 4.2 years).[1]

Comments ▪

The authors state that they did not intend to establish normal values or cut-off thickness measurements; rather, the goal of the study was to determine the best site for

measurement. The best location was determined to be just behind the epiglottis (site 2), with the next best location being in the midportion of the structure (site 1).[1]

REFERENCE

1. John SD, Swischuk LE, Hayden CK Jr, Freeman DH Jr: Aryepiglottic fold width in patients with epiglottitis: Where should measurements be obtained? Radiology 1994; 190:123–125.

▪: MEASUREMENTS OF THE EPIGLOTTIS IN CHILDREN AND ADULTS
▪ ACR Code: 2711 (Epiglottis)

Technique ▪

Standard lateral soft tissue detail radiographs of the neck were performed on patients with epiglottitis at the time of diagnosis. The control group had similar radiographs obtained during the same time period.[1]

Measurements ▪

The epiglottic width (EW), epiglottic height (EH), aryepiglottic width (AEW), and C3 width (C3W) were measured from all radiographs by three residents in emergency medicine blinded to the clinical status of the subject.[1] Figure 1

shows these measurements. For purposes of analysis, each measurement was treated separately, so a total of 75 measurements were available for children with epiglottitis and their controls, as well as 18 measurements from adults with epiglottitis and the controls (total measurements = 150).

Table 1 details the mean and standard deviations (SD) of these measurements, expressed as ratios (EW/C3W, AEW/C3W, EW/EH) for each of the adults, children, and all subjects grouped by clinical status (with or without epiglottitis). Suggested cut-off levels for each ratio are also given, along with sensitivity and specificity for detecting epiglottitis in children and adults.

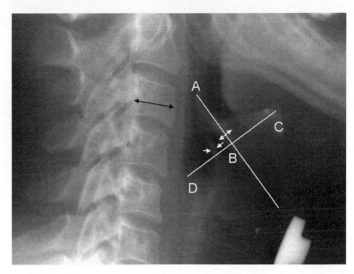

Figure 1 ▪ Lateral radiograph of the neck showing measurements of the epiglottis and aryepiglottic folds. A line is drawn from the apex of the epiglottis *(A)* through the base *(B)*. A second line *(CD)* is drawn perpendicular to the first at the level of the valeculae. The epiglottic height (EH) is measured from the apex of the structure to the second line *(AB)*. The epiglottic width (EW) is measured parallel to line CD at the widest point above that line *(double arrowhead, white line)*. The aryepiglottic width is measured at the midpoint of the structure *(between white arrows)*. The width of C3 (C3W) also is shown *(black line with arrowheads)*.[1]

Table 1 ▪ Epiglottis and Aryepiglottis Ratio Measurements

GROUP	NO. OF PATIENTS	NO. MEASURED	EPIGLOTTIC WIDTH/ C3 WIDTH	ARYEPIGLOTTIC WIDTH/C3 WIDTH	EPIGLOTTIS WIDTH/ EPIGLOTTIS HEIGHT
Adults with epiglottitis	6	18	1.20 ± 0.54	1.03 ± 0.35	1.81 ± 0.69
Normal adults	6	18	0.41 ± 0.16	0.21 ± 0.06	0.40 ± 0.27
Children with epiglottitis	25	75	1.12 ± 0.34	0.76 ± 0.24	1.75 ± 0.79
Normal children	25	75	0.34 ± 0.09	0.25 ± 0.10	0.41 ± 0.20
All with epiglottitis	31	93	1.17 ± 0.44	0.81 ± 0.28	1.76 ± 0.77
All normal subjects	31	93	0.39 ± 0.15	0.24 ± 0.10	0.41 ± 0.22
Suggested cut-off			0.5	0.35	0.6
Sensitivity/specificity for adults			100%/100%	100%/100%	100%/100%
Sensitivity/specificity for children			100%/87%	100%/96%	87%/100%

Ratios are given as mean ± standard deviation.[1]

Source ▪

Forty-one patients with the diagnosis of epiglottitis confirmed by direct visualization were included in the study. These included 6 adults (ages 18 to 60 years) and 25 children (ages 7 months to 9 years). All these patients had good-quality radiographs taken before intubation or other intervention. Age and gender-matched controls were selected from computerized records of lateral soft tissue radiographs done during the study interval, and none had clinical evidence of epiglottitis, croup, or other causes of soft tissue swelling at the time of the examination.[1]

Comments ▪

The same cut-offs can be used for children and adults with 100% sensitivity/specificity in adults for detecting epiglottitis and somewhat reduced specificity in children, with sensitivity maintained at 100%. These are EW/C3W > 0.5, AEW/C3W > 0.35, and EW/EH > 0.6.[1]

REFERENCE

1. Rothrock SG, Pignatiello GA, Howard RM: Radiologic diagnosis of epiglottitis: Objective criteria for all ages. Ann Emerg Med 1990; 19:978–982.

▪: VOLUME AND THICKNESS OF THE THYROID GLAND
▪ ACR Code: 273 (Thyroid Gland)

Technique ▪

Vade and colleagues performed ultrasound of the neonatal thyroid using model 128 and XP/10 scanner (Acuson, Mountain View, CA), with 7.0 MHz linear and sector transducers in the transverse and longitudinal planes.[1] Ueda used an SSD-650 unit (Aloka Co, Japan) with 5.0- and 7.5-MHz transducers and a stand-off pad.[2] Scans were done in transverse and longitudinal orientation over the thyroid

glands of children. Hegedus and colleagues performed transverse scans of adult thyroid glands with a 4.0-MHz transducer and a model 3401 compound scanner (Bruel and Kjaer, Norum, Denmark).[3]

Measurements ▪

Frozen images of the midgland in the transverse plane and each side in the longitudinal plane were used to obtain

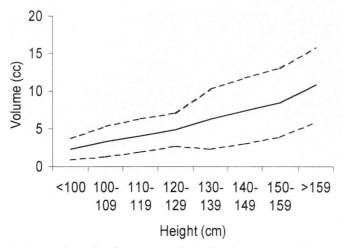

Figure 1 ▪ Thyroid volume versus body height. Mean (solid line) as well as +/−2 standard deviations (dashed lines) is shown.[2]

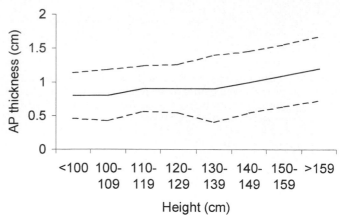

Figure 2 ▪ Anteroposterior (AP) thickness of the thyroid versus body height. Mean (solid line) as well as +/−2 standard deviations (dashed lines) is shown.[2]

anteroposterior (AP), transverse (TRV), and cephalocaudal (CC) dimensions of the right and left lobes with electronic calipers.[1, 2] The volume of each lobe was calculated using the formula for a prolate ellipse (AP × TRV × CC × 0.523) and summed. In the study of children, the same three dimensions were obtained from frozen longitudinal and transverse images of the isthmus, and a volume was calculated as for adults, which was added to the total thyroid volume.[2] In Hegedus's study, sequential transverse images at 5-mm intervals were obtained in adults from the top through the bottom of the gland. The outline of the thyroid was traced from these images and the areas summed to form a volume measurement.[3]

For children and adults, each subject's weight in kilo-

grams was divided into the volume of the thyroid in cubic centimeters and reported as a volume-to-weight ratio.[1, 2] We were able to calculate this ratio from reported data for neonates.[3] Ueda found that the AP measurement of each lobe correlated strongly with the volume and developed a model (volume = [6.91 × RAP] + [3.05 × LAP] − 3.48) for calculating thyroid volume from the AP dimension of each (RAP = right, LAP = left) lobe.[2] We used this model to back-calculate the AP dimensions of adult glands (not reported) from Hegedus's data, assuming the right and left AP dimensions to be equal.[3] Ueda did not report the children's weights, and these were calculated from volume and V/W ratio data.

Vade reported results of all neonates in a single group,[1]

Table 1 ▪ Thyroid Measurements with Ultrasound						
	NUMBER	SUBJECT WEIGHT (kg)	THYROID VOLUME (cc)	RIGHT AP DIMENSION (cm)	LEFT AP DIMENSION (cm)	V/W (cc/kg)
Neonates	68	3.49 ± 0.46	0.95 ± 0.24	0.76 ± 0.09	0.75 ± 0.10	0.272 ± 0.08*
Children (by Height in cm)						
<100	16	12.9*	2.3 ± 0.7	0.8 ± 0.17	0.8 ± 0.18	0.178 ± 0.060
100–109	34	16.8*	3.3 ± 1.0	0.8 ± 0.19	0.8 ± 0.21	0.196 ± 0.055
110–119	35	21.4*	4.1 ± 1.1	0.9 ± 0.17	0.9 ± 0.19	0.192 ± 0.053
120–129	45	24.5*	4.9 ± 1.1	0.9 ± 0.18	0.9 ± 0.20	0.200 ± 0.047
130–139	36	31.2*	6.3 ± 2.0	0.9 ± 0.25	1.0 ± 0.25	0.202 ± 0.071
140–149	42	38.1*	7.4 ± 2.2	1.0 ± 0.23	1.0 ± 0.23	0.194 ± 0.053
150–159	59	48.6*	8.5 ± 2.3	1.1 ± 0.23	1.1 ± 0.24	0.175 ± 0.050
>159	20	54.5*	10.9 ± 2.5	1.2 ± 0.24	1.2 ± 0.25	0.200 ± 0.040
Adult males (by Age in Years)						
14–29	47	68.9 ± 9.9	16.8 ± 4.4	2.04*	2.04*	0.249 ± 0.057
30–49	35	76.3 ± 11.5	21.0 ± 4.9	2.46*	2.46*	0.275 ± 0.050
50–69	42	76.5 ± 9.3	21.3 ± 3.6	2.49*	2.49*	0.279 ± 0.042
72–91	15	70.1 ± 10.6	20.4 ± 4.1	2.40*	2.40*	0.293 ± 0.048
Adult females (by Age in Years)						
13–29	40	58.0 ± 8.4	15.6 ± 3.9	1.92*	1.92*	0.269 ± 0.061
30–49	36	61.1 ± 8.5	17.7 ± 4.5	2.13*	2.13*	0.288 ± 0.060
50–69	36	67.9 ± 10.1	17.9 ± 3.2	2.15*	2.15*	0.267 ± 0.043
71–91	20	65.2 ± 10.1	20.5 ± 4.1	2.41*	2.41*	0.319 ± 0.068

*Calculated values.
Mean and standard deviation (when available) are given. AP = anteroposterior; V/W = thyroid volume divided by patient weight.[1–3]

Ueda divided the children in his population into 8 groups by weight in kilograms,[2] and Hegedus and group divided their subjects into 4 age groups, as well as by gender.[3] Table 1 lists the number of subjects, body weight, thyroid volume, right and left AP dimensions, and the V/W ratio from each of these groups. Mean values are shown for all categories, and standard deviation (SD) is given if reported, but not for calculated values. Figures 1 and 2 show thyroid volume and AP thickness by body height from Ueda.[2]

Source ▪

Vade's subjects were 68 near-term healthy neonates (37 to 41 weeks' gestational age) with birth weights between 2570 and 4790 gm.[1] Ueda studied 287 children ranging in age from 8 months to 15 years.[2] None had clinical or laboratory evidence of thyroid disease. Hegedus and colleagues evaluated 111 healthy adult volunteers whose age ranged from 13 to 90 years.[3]

Comments ▪

Hegedus also measured thyroid volume with ultrasound in 39 patients within 24 hours of thyroidectomy (not included

in normative data) and compared the results with excised volume.[3] Linear regression yielded good correlation (r = 0.99, p < 0.001). Rasmussen and Yokoyama and associates used similar methods (summed transverse areas) to measure thyroid volume with ultrasound and found equally good correlation with excised thyroid volume and weight, respectively.[4, 5] We do not know of any studies comparing linear three-axis-measurement thyroid volume estimation with surgical volume or weight, but presumably this method would be somewhat less accurate.

REFERENCES

1. Vade A, Gottschalk ME, Yetter EM, Subbaiah P: Sonographic measurements of the neonatal thyroid gland. J Ultrasound Med 1997; 16:395–399.
2. Ueda D: Normal volume of the thyroid gland in children. J Clin Ultrasound 1990; 18:455–462.
3. Hegedus L, Perrild H, Poulsen LR, et al: The determination of thyroid volume by ultrasound and its relationship to body weight, age, and sex in normal subjects. J Clin Endocrinol Metab 1983; 56:260–263.
4. Rasmussen SN, Hjorth L: Determination of thyroid volume by ultrasonic scanning. J Clin Ultrasound 1974; 2:143–147.
5. Yokoyama N, Nagayama Y, Kakezono F, et al: Determination of the volume of the thyroid gland by a high resolution ultrasonic scanner. J Nucl Med 1986; 27:1475–1479.

▪▪ MEASUREMENT OF SIZE OF CERVICAL AND RETROPHARYNGEAL LYMPH NODES BY CT[1]

▪ ACR Code: 276 (Other Soft Tissues of the Neck; Lymph Nodes)

Technique ▪

1. Studies performed on a Siemens Somatom II and a Philips 300 CT scanner.
2. Position: Supine.
3. Section thickness varied between 4 and 8 mm. All studies were contrast enhanced.

Table 1 ▪ Size and Frequency of Visualization of Normal Cervical and Retropharyngeal Nodes

GROUP	NO. PATIENTS IN WHICH IT WAS SEEN	SIZE RANGE (mn)	NO. PATIENTS WITH NODES AT UPPER LIMIT OF RANGE
Occipital	0/30	—	—
Mastoid	0/30	—	—
Facial	0/30	—	—
Lingual	0/30	—	—
Parotid	7/30	3–5	1/7
Retropharyngeal			
Median	0/30	—	—
Lateral	20/30	3–7	2/20
Submental-submandibular	28/30	3–10	3/28
Internal jugular			
Superior	30/30	3–10	6/30
Middle	30/30	3–10	2/30
Inferior	30/30	3–5	5/30
Anterior jugular:			
juxtavisceral-scalene	0/30	—	—
Spinal accessory	28/30	3–5	5/28

From Mancuso AA, et al: Radiology 1983; 148:709–714. Used by permission.

Measurement ▪

Nodes were measured using cursors. The largest cross-sectional diameter of the node was recorded. Nodes smaller than 3 mm were assigned a measurement of 3 mm. The size range of nodes in the various anatomic sites is shown in Table 1.

Source ▪

Data were derived from a CT study of 30 patients.

REFERENCE

1. Mancuso AA, Harnsberger HR, Muraki AS, Stevens MH: Computed tomography of cervical and retropharyngeal lymph nodes; normal anatomy, variants of normal, and applications in staging head and neck cancer. Part I: normal anatomy. Radiology 1983; 148:709–714.

▪: SIZE OF CERVICAL LYMPH NODES BY CT
▪ ACR Code: 276 (Soft Tissue of Neck; Lymph Nodes)

Technique ▪

Steinkamp performed helical CT of the node-bearing regions of the neck, using a Somatom Plus-S machine (Siemens, Erlangen, Germany) with 2-mm section thickness, table feed of 2 mm, and dynamic technique. Ultravist (Schering, Berlin, Germany), 100 to 120 ml, was injected intravenously at 3 to 4 ml/sec.[1] Delay times were between 25 and 50 seconds.

Measurements ▪

Coronal, axial, paraxial, and sagittal reconstructions were made, and each visible node was displayed in the optimal plane for measuring minimal axial diameter, maximal axial diameter, and the longitudinal dimension (length) with electronic calipers. The length divided by the maximal transverse diameter (L/T ratio) was calculated for each node. The presence or absence of central low attenuation and rim enhancement was also noted. Table 1 lists the histologic status in individual nodes grouped by various CT criteria.

Source ▪

Seventy patients were included in the study, all but one (breast cancer) of whom had head and neck tumors with clinical suspicion of nodal metastasis.[1] There were 46 men and 51 women. The average age was 51 years (range = 20 to 78 years). Histologic confirmation was obtained by fine-needle biopsy (2 patients), excisional biopsy (7 patients), or neck dissection (61 patients). A total of 164 individual nodes was thus characterized, and results were correlated with CT measurements.

Comments ▪

The L/T ratio < 2 was the most accurate in differentiating malignant nodes from reactive change, followed by minimal nodal diameter > 8 mm and central low attenuation with rim enhancement. The maximal axial diameter is the easiest measurement to obtain though it was the least accurate in this study.[1] It is generally accepted that nodes > 10 mm should be considered suspicious in all regions except submandibular and jugulodigastric, where > 15 mm serves as the cut-off.[2–4] Groups of 3 or more contiguous nodes with

Table 1 ▪ Correlation of Enhanced Helical CT with Histologic Examination of 164 Individual Cervical Lymph Nodes

	L/T RATIO	MAXIMAL NODE DIAMETER		MINIMAL NODE DIAMETER	CENTRAL LOW ATTENUATION AND RIM ENHANCEMENT
Cut-off value	<2	>10 mm	>15 mm	>8 mm	—
Metastatic nodes	94	91	66	83	75
Reactive nodes	66	5	42	61	68
False-positive nodes (%)	2 (3)	63 (93)	26 (31)	7 (11)	0
False-negative nodes (%)	2 (3)	5 (5)	30 (38)	13 (13)	21 (22)
Sensitivity (%)	97	95	69	87	78
Specificity (%)	97	7	62	89	100*
Accuracy (%)	97	61	66	88	86

Note—Numbers in parentheses are percentages.
*Based solely on differentiation of reactively enlarged lymph nodes and metastases. Other cervical lymph node enlargements (lateral cysts of the neck, lymph node tuberculosis, abscesses) also demonstrate central low attenuation and rim enhancement.
From Steinkamp HJ, Hosten N, Richter C, et al: Radiology 1994; 191:795–798. Used by permission.

a maximal axial diameter of 8 to 15 mm or minimal axial diameter of 8 to 10 mm, especially in the drainage pattern of the primary tumor, are suspicious.[3]

REFERENCES

1. Steinkamp HJ, Hosten N, Richter C, et al: Enlarged cervical lymph nodes at helical CT. Radiology 1994; 191:795–798.
2. Som PM: Lymph nodes of the neck. Radiology 1987; 165:593–600.
3. Som PM: Detection of metastasis in cervical lymph nodes: CT and MR criteria and differential diagnosis. AJR Am J Roentgenol 1992; 158:961–969.
4. van den Brekel MW, Castelijns JA, Snow GB: Detection of lymph node metastases in the neck: Radiologic criteria. Radiology 1994; 192:617–618.

▪: SIZE CRITERIA FOR MALIGNANCY IN CERVICAL NODES BY CT AND MRI
▪ ACR Code: 276 (Soft Tissue of Neck; Lymph Nodes)

Technique ▪

CT scans (unspecified machines) were done through the neck (occlusal plane through clavicles) during intravenous contrast administration, using dynamic technique. Section thickness was from 2 to 4 mm; and section interval was no more than 5 mm. MRI (unspecified machines) was done in the axial plane through the neck with T2 (2000/30,80)-weighted spin echo sequences, using 5-mm section thickness and 1-mm intersection gap. T1 (650/20) images of the neck were done in the sagittal plane with 5-mm section thickness. Following intravenous gadolinium, T1 (800/200)-weighted axial images were repeated with 3- to 4-mm section thickness and no more than 5-mm section interval.[1]

Measurements ▪

Each scan was graded by 8 radiologists with respect to maximum nodal dimension in millimeters and nodal appearance on a 5-point scale (0 = definitely normal through 4 = definitely abnormal). Appearance scores were considered abnormal (higher numbers) based on low central attenuation and enhancement by CT and inhomogeneous/hyperintense nodal architecture by MRI. The neck was divided into 4 zones, as shown in Figure 1, and each zone was graded according to the largest single node and/or the most abnormal-appearing node within that zone on each scan. Correlation with histologic status of excised nodes was done by zone, with any positive (for cancer) node in that zone being considered disease-positive. Table 1 gives a breakdown of dissections by side and zone, with disease-positive percentages shown.[1]

An aggregate imaging score for each zone (hybrid) was developed to combine size and appearance criteria (numbered from 0 to 32) for the purposes of receiver operating characteristic (ROC) analysis. Table 2 shows areas under ROC curves for CT and MRI using size alone and a combination of size and abnormal appearance (hybrid score) in each zone. For purposes of sensitivity, specificity, negative predictive value (NPV), and positive predictive value (PPV) calculation, size and appearance were combined as follows: an appearance score of 3 or 4 was considered test-positive regardless of size; otherwise, the specified size cut-off was used. Table 3 shows sensitivity, specificity, NPV, and PPV for CT and MRI in zones II and III combined.[1]

Source ▪

A total of 276 patients (150 men, 63 women, mean age = 59 yrs; age range = 18 to 84 yrs) with squamous cell carcinoma (SCCA) of the aerodigestive tract was included in the study. None had been treated with surgery or radiation and all had neck dissection following CT and MRI

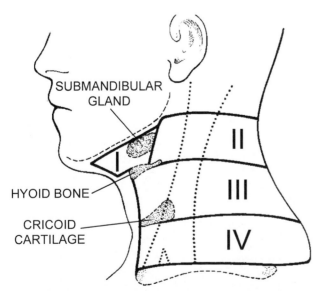

Figure 1 ▪ Diagram of lymph node drainage regions used for interpretation of CT and MR scans of the neck. Note that the spinal accessory (posterior) region is not considered to be separate, as is often done in other studies. (From Curtin HD, Ishwaran H, Mancuso AA, et al: Radiology 1998; 207:123–130. Used by permission.)

Table 1 ▪ Listing of Numbers of Node Dissections by Side and Zone				
ZONE	RIGHT SIDE OF NECK	LEFT SIDE OF NECK	TOTAL NO. NECK DISSECTIONS	TOTAL NO. PATIENTS
I	75 (17)	78 (26)	153 (22)	121 (26)
II	139 (34)	130 (33)	269 (34)	196 (40)
III	136 (24)	130 (25)	266 (24)	194 (27)
IV	100 (14)	91 (13)	191 (14)	151 (15)

Percentages of histologically positive zones in surgical specimens are shown in parentheses.

From Curtin HD, Ishwaran H, Mancuso AA, et al: Radiology 1998; 207:123–130. Used by permission.

Table 2 ▪ Area Under the ROC Curves for CT and MRI in Each Nodal Zone

	SIZE ALONE		
ZONE	CT	MRI	p VALUE
I	0.67 ± 0.06	0.72 ± 0.05	0.13
II	0.73 ± 0.06	0.70 ± 0.05	0.15
III	0.71 ± 0.04	0.72 ± 0.04	0.66
II & III	0.77 ± 0.03	0.73 ± 0.03	0.04
	SIZE AND NODAL APPEARANCE		
ZONE	CT	MRI	p VALUE
I	0.76 ± 0.06	0.72 ± 0.05	0.38
II	0.77 ± 0.06	0.71 ± 0.05	0.02
III	0.72 ± 0.04	0.72 ± 0.04	0.91
II & III	0.80 ± 0.03	0.75 ± 0.03	0.008

Mean and standard error are given, as well as an estimate of significance of the difference between CT and MRI (p value).
ROC = receiver operating characteristic.
From Curtin HD, Ishwaran H, Mancuso AA, et al: Radiology 1998; 207:123–130. Used by permission.

Table 3 ▪ Performance of CT and MRI of Cervical Nodes

SIZE (mm)	SENSITIVITY	SPECIFICITY	NPV	PPV	SENSITIVITY	SPECIFICITY	NPV	PPV
MRI: Size Alone					MRI: Size and Appearance			
5	0.92	0.20	0.77	0.44	0.92	0.20	0.77	0.44
7	0.90	0.23	0.77	0.45	0.90	0.23	0.77	0.45
8	0.87	0.31	0.77	0.47	0.87	0.31	0.77	0.47
9	0.83	0.41	0.78	0.50	0.84	0.41	0.79	0.50
10	0.81	0.48	0.79	0.52	0.82	0.48	0.79	0.52
11	0.70	0.65	0.76	0.58	0.73	0.63	0.77	0.58
12	0.66	0.72	0.75	0.62	0.70	0.69	0.77	0.61
15	0.51	0.86	0.72	0.72	0.60	0.81	0.75	0.69
CT: Size Alone					CT: Size and Appearance			
5	0.98	0.13	0.90	0.44	0.98	0.13	0.90	0.44
7	0.97	0.17	0.88	0.44	0.97	0.17	0.89	0.45
8	0.95	0.22	0.86	0.45	0.95	0.21	0.86	0.45
9	0.92	0.31	0.85	0.48	0.93	0.31	0.86	0.48
10	0.88	0.39	0.83	0.50	0.90	0.38	0.84	0.50
11	0.80	0.56	0.81	0.56	0.84	0.53	0.83	0.55
12	0.74	0.67	0.79	0.61	0.80	0.63	0.83	0.61
15	0.56	0.84	0.73	0.71	0.71	0.78	0.80	0.69

Figures are for zones II and III combined. NPV = negative predictive value, PPV = positive predictive value.
From Curtin HD, Ishwaran H, Mancuso AA, et al: Radiology 1998; 207:123–130. Used by permission.

scans of the neck (right side = 158, left side = 153, total = 311).

Comments ▪

In their conclusion, the authors state that the addition of nodal appearance improves test performance for CT at higher nodal sizes (greater than 1 cm) and gives no significant improvement over size alone for MRI. Overall, CT performed slightly better than MRI at virtually all size cut-off levels. For CT, a maximum size cut-off of 5 mm gives a NPV of 90% and a PPV of 44%. With a cut-off of 1 cm, the NPV is 84% and PPV is 50%. MRI did not achieve an NPV of 90% with any interpretive criteria.[1]

REFERENCE

1. Curtin HD, Ishwaran H, Mancuso AA, et al: Comparison of CT and MR imaging in staging of neck metastases. Radiology 1998; 207:123–130.

▪: AXIAL MEASUREMENTS OF LYMPH NODES IN THE NECK WITH ULTRASOUND
▪ ACR Code: 276 (Soft Tissue of Neck; Lymph Nodes)

Technique ▪

Van den Brekel and colleagues used real-time linear array 7.5-MHz transducers and an SSD-650 machine (Aloka, Tokyo, Japan) for examination of the neck from submandibular to supraclavicular levels.[1] Takashima's group used a 5-MHz linear array transducer and real-time ultrasound unit (Yokagawa Medical Systems, Tokyo, Japan) to perform ultrasound of the neck.[2]

Measurements ▪

Van den Brekel measured the minimal diameter of all visible lymph nodes in the axial plane from frozen images with electronic calipers to the nearest millimeter.[1] The location of each node was carefully noted, using standard nomenclature as shown in Figure 1.[3] All patients subsequently underwent radical or selective neck dissection and histopathologic examination of all nodes contained in the specimens. Correlation of the nodal status and location was made with ultrasound findings to derive sensitivity and specificity. Table 1 (top) lists these numbers for various sizes of single nodes and for groups of three or more nodes (up to 2 mm smaller). The subdigastric nodes were allowed to be 1 mm larger and still considered to be test negative. Groups of three or more nodes were considered positive even when their minimum axial diameters were up to 2 mm smaller than the cut-off size.

In Takashima's study, the minimal and maximal axial diameter of each node under study was measured with electronic calipers prior to the fine-needle aspiration biopsy (FNAB).[2] Nodal location was noted, using standard nomenclature.[3] Histopathologic confirmation of metastatic malignancy from various primary sites was obtained in 66 (73%) of the 91 lesions by surgery (n = 61) or autopsy (n = 5). The remaining 25 lesions were presumed to be benign since they shrank or disappeared on follow-up. Correlation of the ratio of minimal to maximal diameter in individual nodes with pathologic/clinical status expressed as sensitivity and specificity is contained in Table 1 (bottom).

Source ▪

Van den Brekel and colleagues studied 107 adults (age and gender distribution not given) with head and neck squamous cell carcinoma (SCCA).[1] Ultrasound-guided FNAB was done in 57 cases. Takashima and colleagues evaluated 1120 adult patients with various diseases of the neck.[2] A total of 91 nodes from 70 patients also had ultrasound-guided FNAB.[2]

Comments ▪

In both series, all patients had negative physical examinations with respect to palpable cervical adenopathy. The accuracy of ultrasound using minimal axial diameter for detecting local nodal metastases was 70% compared with FNAB at 89%.[1] The accuracy of the axial diameter ratio in diagnosing metastatic cervical adenopathy from local or distant sites was 80% compared with 88% for FNAB.[2]

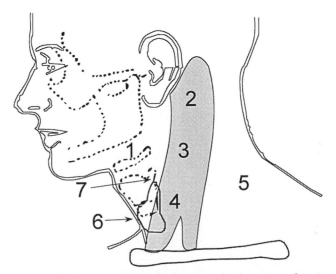

Figure 1 ▪ Drawing of the neck showing the location of various numbered nodal groups in what has become a standard nomenclature:[3]
1) Submandibular and sublingular; 2) internal jugular (upper); 3) internal jugular (middle); 4) internal jugular (lower); 5) posterior triangle; 6) juxta-thyroid; 7) tracheoesophageal groove.

Table 1 ▪ Sensitivity and Specificity of Size Criteria for Determining Whether Cervical Lymph Nodes Are Malignant

	SENSITIVITY (%)	SPECIFICITY (%)
Minimal Axial Diameter (mm)		
≥4	89	33
≥5	85	44
≥6	81	59
≥7	60	77
≥8	42	85
≥9	26	95
≥10	15	97
Min/Max Axial Diameter Ratio		
≥0.40	100	13
≥0.50	96	45
≥0.55	92	63
≥0.60	81	66
≥0.70	49	84
≥0.80	38	95
≥0.90	21	95
≥0.95	8	100

Min/Max = minimum divided by maximum axial diameters.[1,2]

REFERENCES

1. van den Brekel MWM, Castalijns JA, Stel HV, et al: Occult metastatic neck disease: Detection with US and US-guided fine-needle aspiration cytology. Radiology 1991; 180:457–461.

2. Takashima S, Sone S, Nomura M, et al: Nonpalpable lymph nodes of the neck: Assessment with US and US-guided fine-needle aspiration biopsy. J Clin Ultrasound 1997; 25:283–292.

3. Som PM: Lymph nodes of the neck. Radiology 1987; 165:593–600.

▪: SHAPE OF CERVICAL LYMPH NODES WITH ULTRASOUND (THE L/T RATIO)
▪ ACR Code: 276 (Soft Tissue of Neck; Lymph Nodes)

Technique ▪

Bruneton and colleagues used a 13-MHz sector transducer and a real-time ultrasound scanner (Esaote Biomedica, Genoa, Italy) to examine the necks of subjects and identify and measure all visible lymph nodes.[1] Na's group used 5- to 10-MHz linear transducers with UM-9 or HDI-3000 machines (Advanced Technology Laboratories, Bothell, WA) for examination and characterization of cervical nodes.[2] Tohnosu and colleagues used 3.75- to 7.5-MHz convex and linear transducers and an SSA-90A unit (Toshiba) for detection and measurement of nodes in the supraclavicular area and the neck.[3]

Measurement ▪

In all three series, the entire neck, and in one study[3] the supraclavicular region, was scanned. Visible lymph nodes were identified and counted separately for statistical purposes. The greatest longitudinal and transverse diameters of each node were measured with electronic calipers and recorded. The longitudinal diameter divided by the transverse diameter (L/T ratio) of each studied node was calculated.[1-3] Figure 1 shows measurement of nodes to obtain the L/T ratio. Table 1 gives combined results from Bruneton (nodes found in normal volunteers) and Na (benign and malignant pathology) with respect to the L/T ratio.[1, 2] Note that tuberculous and malignant nodes tend to have lower L/T ratios whereas normal benign nodes have higher L/T ratios. Table 2 gives percentages of malignant nodes from Tohnosu divided into categories by greatest longitudinal dimension and L/T ratio.[3]

Source ▪

One thousand healthy volunteers (355 men and 645 women), with 431 being under 50 years of age and 569 being 50 or older, were studied by Bruneton and groups.[1] Na and colleagues evaluated patients with cervical adenopathy (n = 148, ages not given), with clinical and pathologic diagnoses of reactive adenopathy, tuberculosis, lymphoma, and metastatic disease.[2] The numbers of patients and nodes

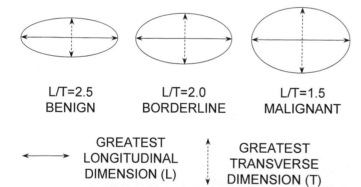

L/T=2.5 BENIGN   L/T=2.0 BORDERLINE   L/T=1.5 MALIGNANT

GREATEST LONGITUDINAL DIMENSION (L)   GREATEST TRANSVERSE DIMENSION (T)

Figure 1 ▪ Depiction of a lymph node in the longitudinal axis, showing measurement of the longitudinal dimension (L) and transverse dimension (T). The L/T ratio is calculated by division of the two measurements. Shown are lymph nodes with L/T ratios of 2.5 (benign), 2.0 (borderline), and 1.5 (malignant).

Table 1 ▪ Distribution of L/T Ratios in Normal Subjects[1] and Various Pathologic Conditions[2]

NODAL SHAPE	NORMAL NODES (BRUNETON)	BENIGN ADENITIS	TUBERCULOUS ADENITIS	LYMPHOMA	METASTASIS
L/T < 1.5	8 (1.2)	4 (12)	4 (24)	9 (64)	31 (60)
L/T 1.5–2.0	85 (12.6)	5 (14)	7 (31)	3 (21)	13 (25)
L/T ≤ 2.0	93 (13.8)	9 (26)	11 (65)	12 (86)	44 (85)
L/T ≥ 2.0	583 (86.2)	25 (74)	6 (35)	2 (14)	8 (15)
Total nodes	676	34	17	14	52
Number of patients	1000	28	17	14	46
Diameter of nodes (mm)	1–8		10–40 (mean = 22.0)		

The number and percent (in parentheses) of total in each nodal category are shown. The range of largest transverse diameters is given on the bottom row (combined for adenopathy).

Table 2 ▪ Histologic Results of Excised Cervical Lymph Nodes

LONG AXIS (mm)	L/T > 2.0	L/T ≤ 2.0	ANY L/T
< 5	—	—	1/30 (3)
5–10	2/40 (5)	6/47 (13)	8/87 (9)
11–15	1/11 (9)	7/15 (47)	8/26 (31)
16–20	0/2 (0)	6/6 (100)	6/8 (75)
> 5	3/53 (6)	24/73 (33)	27/126 (21)
> 10	1/13 (8)	18/26 (69)	19/39 (49)
> 20	0	5/5 (100)	5/5 (100)

Numbers are malignant/total (percentage in parentheses).[3]

in each category are shown in Table 1. Tohnosu's subjects all had esophageal cancer (n = 58, ages not given), and nodal status was determined by histologic examination of excised specimens.[3]

Comments ▪

In the study of 1000 normal subjects, 676 (67.6%) had visible nodes, and all the nodes were less than 8 mm in diameter ranging in length from 5 to 21 mm.[1] For determination of malignant adenopathy by L/T ratio, Na and colleagues found that a cut-off of 2.0 had a sensitivity of 85% and a specificity of 61%. They also found that an abnormal hilum (deformed or absent) and peripheral vascularity at color Doppler sonography were correlated with malignant pathology.[2] Tohnosu and group conclude that a cervical node with a longitudinal dimension of more than 10 mm and an L/T ratio of less than 2.0 strongly suggests metastasis.[3]

REFERENCES

1. Bruneton JN, Balu-Maestro C, Marcy PY, et al: Very high frequency (13 MHz) ultrasonographic examination of the normal neck: Detection of normal lymph nodes and thyroid nodules. J Ultrasound Med 1994; 13(2): 87–90.
2. Na DG, Lim HK, Byun HS, et al: Differential diagnosis of cervical lymphadenopathy: Usefulness of color Doppler sonography. AJR Am J Roentgenol 1997; 168:1311–1316.
3. Tohnosu N, Onoda S, Isono K: Ultrasonographic evaluation of cervical lymph node metastasis in esophageal cancer with special reference to the relationship between the short-to-long axis ratio and the cancer content. J Clin Ultrasound 1989; 17:101–106.

▪: DOPPLER WAVEFORMS IN CERVICAL LYMPH NODES
▪ ACR Code: 276 (Soft Tissue of Neck; Lymph Nodes)

Technique ▪

Choi and colleagues used an XP/10 ultrasound machine (Acuson, Mountain View, CA) with a 7-MHz linear transducer to evaluate cervical lymph nodes with color and duplex Doppler.[1] Na's group used 5- to 10-MHz linear transducers with UM-9 or HDI-3000 machines (Advanced Technology Laboratories, Bothell, WA) for examination, measurement, and Doppler characterization of cervical nodes.[2]

Measurements ▪

Using minimal pressure, each node under study was examined first with color Doppler imaging. The dominant color flow regions were then sampled with duplex Doppler. The maximum peak systolic velocity (PSV), end-diastolic velocity (EDV), resistive index (RI = [PSV − EDV]/PSV), and

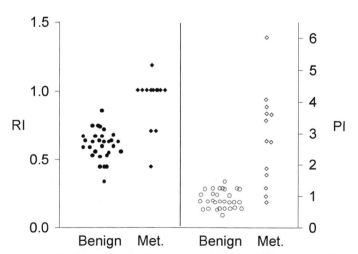

Figure 1 ▪ Scatterplot showing resistive index (RI) and pulsatility index (PI) of benign and malignant (Met.) lymph nodes. Note that while there is definite grouping of malignant nodes at higher values of each measure, there is significant overlap between the two groups. (From Choi MY, Lee JW, Jang KJ: AJR Am J Roentgenol 1995; 165:981–984. Used by permission.)

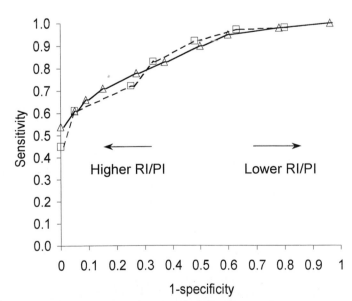

Figure 2 ▪ Receiver operating characteristic curves for resistive index (RI, squares and dotted line) and pulsatility index (PI, triangles and solid line) in detecting malignancy in cervical nodes. (From Na DG, Lim HK, Byun HS, et al: AJR Am J Roentgenol 1997; 168:1311–1316. Used by permission.)

Table 1 ▪ Resistive Index, Pulsatility Index, and Peak Systolic Velocity from Cervical Lymph Nodes of Various Categories

AUTHOR/ NODE TYPES	RESISTIVE INDEX	PULSATILITY INDEX	PEAK SYSTOLIC VELOCITY	NO. OF NODES
Choi et al				
Benign adenitis	0.59 ± 0.11	0.90 ± 0.23	24.0 ± 16.0	30
Metastasis	0.92 ± 0.23	2.66 ± 1.59	25.0 ± 11.7	13
Na et al				
Benign adenitis	0.57 ± 0.10	0.85 ± 0.22	30.77 ± 13.35	34
Tuberculosis	0.64 ± 0.09	1.03 ± 0.24	20.44 ± 8.24	16
Lymphoma	0.70 ± 0.15	1.20 ± 0.42	20.07 ± 9.96	14
Metastasis	0.83 ± 0.15	1.62 ± 0.52	22.65 ± 14.0	52

All measurements are given as mean ± standard deviation. Peak systolic velocity in cm/sec.[1,2]

Table 2 ▪ Performance of Various Cut-off Values for Resistive Index and Pulsatility Index for Discriminating Benign from Malignant Cervical Nodes[2]

	SENSITIVITY %	SPECIFICITY %
RESISTIVE INDEX		
> 0.5	98	20
> 0.6	92	51
> 0.7	72	75
> 0.8	45	100
PULSATILITY INDEX		
> 0.6	100	4
> 0.8	95	40
> 1.0	83	63
> 1.2	71	85
> 1.4	61	95

pulsatility index (PI = [PSV − EDV]/average velocity over one cardiac cycle) were measured, using software on each ultrasound machine, from frozen duplex images, and recorded for each node. These measurements were correlated with the known pathologic and clinical status of the node in question. Table 1 lists the reported measurements for benign adenitis, metastasis, tuberculosis, and lymphoma.[1,2] Table 2 gives performance statistics of RI and PI in diagnosing malignant (metastasis and lymphoma) nodes from Na and group.[2] Figure 1 is a scatterplot of these data. Figure 2 depicts combined receiver operating characteristic (ROC) curves for Doppler resistive index and pulsatility index, with disease-positive being metastasis or lymphoma.[1]

Source ▪

Choi's subjects were 43 consecutive untreated patients with palpable lymph nodes. All but two (one inguinal, one axillary) of the nodes studied were cervical.[1] Pathologic diagnosis was obtained in 24 (43 nodes). In 19 subjects with suspected non-neoplastic disease, clinical follow-up was done for 1 to 7 months. Of the biopsied nodes, 13 were involved with metastatic malignancy. In all the patients who had clinical follow-up, the nodes resolved completely or decreased in size. Na and colleagues evaluated patients with cervical adenopathy (n = 148, ages not given) with clinical and pathologic diagnosis of reactive adenopathy, tuberculosis, lymphoma, and metastatic disease.[2]

Comments ▪

Peak systolic velocity does not seem to be particularly useful. Resistive and pulsatility indices do differ between benign and malignant nodes but have significant overlap of recorded values. Cut-offs of 0.7 for resistive index and 1.2 for pulsatility index yield reasonable sensitivity and specificity, as shown in Table 2.

REFERENCES

1. Choi MY, Lee JW, Jang KJ: Distinction between benign and malignant causes of cervical, axillary, and inguinal lymphadenopathy: Value of Doppler spectral waveform analysis. AJR Am J Roentgenol 1995; 165:981–984.
2. Na DG, Lim HK, Byun HS, et al: Differential diagnosis of cervical lymphadenopathy: Usefulness of color Doppler sonography. AJR Am J Roentgenol 1997; 168:1311–1316.

▪: PREVERTEBRAL SOFT TISSUE THICKNESS IN SUSPECTED CERVICAL TRAUMA

▪ ACR Code: 276 (Soft Tissues of the Neck, Prevertebral)

Technique ▪

Eight studies that included measurements of normal prevertebral soft tissue widths are included here.[1–8] In each series, lateral cervical spine films were evaluated to determine the normal thickness of the prevertebral soft tissue (PVST). Focus-to-film distance varied from 40 to 70 inches. In all cases the patient was placed as close to the film as possible. Two of these studies and one additional series evaluated trauma patients with respect to prediction of fracture based on various PVST criteria.[5, 7, 8]

Measurement ▪

In all cases the PVST was measured to the nearest millimeter from the films, with a transparent ruler, and recorded. Figure 1 is a lateral cervical spine radiograph with the measurement locations indicated. Table 1 shows the reported normal values for PVST at C2–C4 and at C6.[1–7] A "combined" mean, standard deviation (SD), and range is also included for each level, with these values having been calculated from all available data. Values for the C5 PVST were not reported except in Templeton's work.[5] The C5 PVST value shows greater variation than at other levels because the cervical esophagus may or may not be included. Table 2 lists various combinations of cut-off values for PVST and their utility in predicting cervical spine fracture.[5, 7, 8]

Source ▪

Patients presenting with trauma, neck pain, cervical neuropathy, or other complaints were included in the various studies. All were adults, and the numbers of subjects are stated in Tables 1 and 2. Patients included in calculations of normal PVST thickness values had no radiographic or clinical evidence of fracture or ligamentous injury at the time the radiographs were obtained or on follow-up.

Comments ▪

Matar and Doyle suggest using a PVST cut-off value at C2 or C3 of > 7 mm.[7] The mean + 2 SD derived from our combined values at C2 and C3 are 6.7 and 7.1 mm, respectively. Thus, the suggested cut-off falls at the 95th percentile of reported normal values. Matar and Doyle go on to suggest a cut-off PVST of > 21 mm at C6 or C7. This is at odds with the combined mean + 2 SD of 14.2

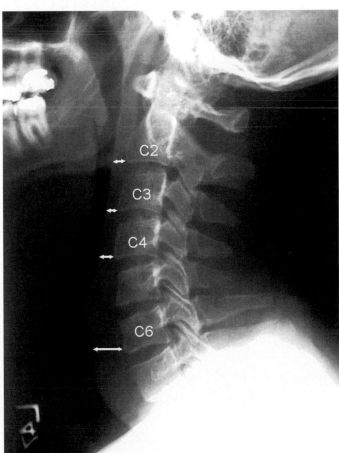

Figure 1 ▪ Lateral cervical spine radiograph with appropriate locations for measuring the prevertebral soft tissue from C2 to C6 (*arrows*).

Table 1 ▪ Table of Normal Values of the Prevertebral Soft Tissue Thickness at C2–4 and C6

AUTHOR	NUMBER	C2 MEAN ± SD	C2 RANGE	C3 MEAN ± SD	C3 RANGE	C4 MEAN ± SD	C4 RANGE	C6 MEAN ± SD	C6 RANGE
Wholey	600	3.5	(2.0–7.0)					7.9	(5.0–14.0)
Oon	150							12.4 ± 1.9	(8.0–17.0)
Weir	360	3.7	(2.6–4.8)	3.1 ± 0.7	(1.5–4.5)				
Penning	50	3.2	(1.0–5.0)	3.4	(2.0–7.0)	5.1	(2.0–7.0)	15.1	(11.0–20.0)
Templeton	236	4.7 ± 1.5		5.0 ± 1.5		6.4 ± 2.0			
Sistrom	227	4.7 ± 1.2	(2.0–8.0)	5.0 ± 1.5	(2.0–15.0)	8.2 ± 3.6	(2.0–21.0)		
Matar	79	4.5 ± 1.2		4.7 ± 1.1				15.5 ± 2.7	
Combined	1702	3.9 ± 1.4	(1.0–8.0)	4.5 ± 1.3	(1.5–15.0)	7.1 ± 2.9	(2.0–21.0)	9.8 ± 2.2	(5.0–20)

All measurements are in millimeters.[1-7]

Table 2 ▪ Performance of Various Single or Combined Cut-offs for Predicting Cervical Fracture

AUTHOR/ CERVICAL LEVEL	+ FRACTURE/ − FRACTURE	CRITERIA FOR ABNORMAL (mm)	TRUE POSITIVES (%)	FALSE POSITIVES (%)
Templeton[5]				
C2	51/236	> 7	18	5
C3	"	> 4	83	60
C3 or C4	"	> 5	75	66
C3 or C4	"	> 8	33	13
Matar[7]				
C2 or C3	57/79	> 5	62	33
C2 or C3	"	> 6	51	13
C2 or C3	"	> 7	40	3
C6 or C7	"	> 19	62	41
C6 or C7	"	> 20	42	24
C6 or C7	"	> 21	33	7
Miles[8]				
C2, C3, C5, C6	41/17	C2 > 7, C3 > 5,	49	17
Any abnormal		C5 > 22, C6 > 17		

+ Fracture/ − Fracture = Numbers of patients with and without cervical fracture.

mm, at C6 from the studies of normal patients. Note the relatively low mean value of PVST at C6 from Wholey and colleagues, which tends to decrease the combined mean because of the large number. If we do not include Wholey's data, the combined mean becomes 13.8 and the 95th percentile would be 19.2 mm (using Matar's SD of 2.7).

REFERENCES

1. Wholey MH, Brunwer AJ, Baker HI: The lateral roentgenogram of the neck (with comments on the atlanto odontoid-basion relationship). Radiology 1958; 77:350–356.
2. Oon CL: Some sagittal measurements of the neck in normal adults. Br J Radiol 1964; 674–677.
3. Weir DC: Roentgenographic signs of cervical injury. Clin Orthop Rel Res 1975; 109:9–17.
4. Penning L: Prevertebral hematoma in cervical spine injury: Incidence and etiologic significance. AJR Am J Roentgenol 1981; 136:553–561.
5. Templeton PA, Young JW, Mirvis SE, Buddemeyer EU: The value of retropharyngeal soft tissue measurements in trauma of the adult cervical spine. Skeletal Radiol 1987; 16:98–104.
6. Sistrom CL, Southall EP, Peddada SD, Schaffer HA: Factors affecting the thickness of the cervical prevertebral soft tissues. Skeletal Radiol 1993; 22:167–171.
7. Matar LD, Doyle AJ: Prevertebral soft-tissue measurements in cervical spine injury. Australas Radiol 1997; 41:229–237.
8. Miles KA, Finlay D: Is prevertebral soft tissue swelling a useful sign in injury of the cerebral spine? Injury 1988; 19:177–179.

▪: SOFT TISSUES OF THE NECK: RATIO METHOD
▪ ACR Code: 276 (Soft Tissues of the Neck, Prevertebral)

Technique ▪

Lateral radiographs of the cervical spine/neck were done in neutral position.[1, 2] Chen and Bohrer specified that their subjects were upright and that the target-film distance was 40 inches.[2]

Measurements ▪

Four measurements may be made in the midcervical region. All are expressed as ratios of the anterioposterior (AP) dimension of the C5 vertebral body. Figure 1 shows the measurement locations. Table 1 lists the normal values expressed as multiples of the C5 AP dimension.[1, 2] The AP diameter of the trachea at the point of greatest construction equals $1.2 \times$ C5 AP. Ardran and Kemp found that in children the thickness of the soft tissue between the pharyngeal lumen and the vertebra should be about three fourths of the diameter of the adjacent vertebra.[3]

Source ▪

Hay studied 50 normal adults and 25 normal infants and children.[1] Bohrer and Chen evaluated radiographs from 54 adults (men = 19, women = 34) with no cervical injury or other abnormality that would alter the soft tissues.[2] Ardran and Kemp studied 100 individuals aged 0.5 to 5 years.[3]

Comments ▪

Direct measurement of the retropharyngeal soft tissues as a sign of cervical trauma is of limited usefulness due to large overlap in measurement of normal and abnormal patients. The ratio method provides a way of mitigating this problem and may be useful.

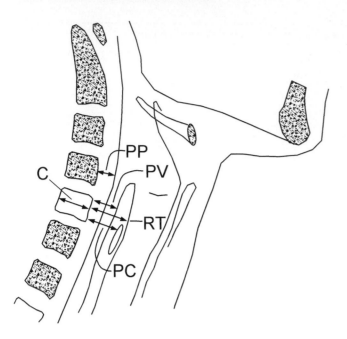

Figure 1 ▪ Measurements of precervical soft tissues from a neutral lateral cervical spine radiograph.

PP = Postpharyngeal soft tissue, measured at a point where the soft tissues run parallel to the vertebra.

PV = Postventricular soft tissue for use in children when the cricoid is not visible. The distance is measured between the posterior commissure of the larynx and the nearest portion of the cervical spine.

RT = Retrotracheal soft tissue, measured between the posterior wall of the trachea and the anterior surface of the adjacent cervical vertebra.

PC = Postcricoid soft tissue, measured between the posterior surface of the cricoid cartilage and the anterior surface of the adjacent cervical vertebra.

C = Anterior to posterior dimension of the C5 vertebral body at its middle.

(From Hay PD: Paul B Hoeber, Inc., New York, 1939, vol 9. Used by permission.)

Table 1 ▪ **Prevertebral Soft Tissues in the Midcervical Spine**

RESEARCHER	GROUP	POSTPHARYNGEAL (PP)	POSTVENTRICULAR (PV)	POSTCRICOID (PC)	RETROTRACHEAL (RT)
Hay[1]	0–1 yr	1.5	2.0		
	1–2 yr	0.5	1.5		
	2–3 yr	0.5	1.2		
	3–6 yr	0.4	1.2		
	6–14 yr	0.3	1.2		
Hay[1]	Adult male	0.3		0.7	
	Adult female	0.3		0.6	
Chen/Bohrer[2]	Adult male			0.50 ± 0.14	0.81 ± 0.20
	Adult female			0.57 ± 0.12	0.81 ± 0.16
	Adult (both)			0.55 ± 0.13	0.81 ± 0.17
	Range (both)			0.28 ± 0.82	0.47 ± 1.15

All measurements expressed as multiples of the C5 AP dimension (measurement/C5).

PP = Postpharyngeal soft tissue, measured at a point where the soft tissues run parallel to the vertebra.

PV = Postventricular soft tissue for use in children when the cricoid is not visible. The distance is measured between the posterior commissure of the larynx and the nearest portion of the cervical spine.

PC = Postcricoid soft tissue, measured between the posterior surface of the cricoid cartilage and the anterior surface of the adjacent cervical vertebra.

RT = Retrotracheal soft tissue, measured between the posterior wall of the trachea and the anterior surface of the adjacent cervical vertebra.

REFERENCES

1. Hay PD: Annals of Roentgenology. Paul B Hoeber, Inc., New York, 1939, vol 9.

2. Chen MYM, Bohrer SP: Radiographic measurement of prevertebral soft-tissue thickness on lateral radiographs of the neck. Skeletal Radiology 1999; 44:26–38.

3. Ardran GM, Kemp FH: The mechanism of changes in form of the cervical airway in infancy. Med Radiogr Photogr 1968; 44:26–38.

▪: MEASUREMENT OF THE LATERAL THORACIC INLET[1]

▪ ACR Code: 29 (Thoracic Inlet)

Technique ▪

Central ray: Perpendicular to the plane of the film directed to the level of the seventh cervical and first thoracic vertebrae.
Position: True lateral.
Target-film distance: 72 inches.

Measurements (Figure 1) ▪

D_1 = Minimum distance between the posterior cortex of the manubrium and spine.
D_2 = Minimum distance between the trachea and spine.

Sagittal inlet (D_1): average = 6.2 cm; range = 5.0 to 8.7 cm.

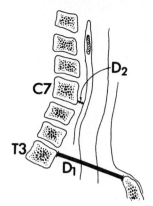

Figure 1 ▪ (From Kendall BE, Aschroft K, Whiteside CG: Br J Radiol 1962; 35:769. Used by permission.)

Distance from spine to trachea (D_2): average = 1.3 cm; range = 0.5 to 2.5 cm.

Source ▪

Sixty-seven patients who had routine barium swallows.

Note: A narrow thoracic inlet may cause compression of the esophagus by the trachea. This compression is seen as a smooth, crescent-shaped defect of the barium-filled esophagus at the C7 to T3 level. The defect usually is on the right side of the esophagus in the PA projection.

REFERENCE

1. Kendall BE, Aschroft K, Whiteside CG: Br J Radiol 1962; 35:769.

CHAPTER 4

Spine and Contents

∙∙
∙

∙∙ MEASUREMENT OF SCOLIOSIS[1, 2]
∙ ACR Code: 3 (Spine)

Technique ∙

Central ray: Perpendicular to plane of film centered over dorsolumbar junction.
  Position: Anteroposterior.
  Target-film distance: Immaterial.

Measurements (Figures 1 and 2) ∙

The secondary curvatures function to bring the head erect over the pelvis and keep the body in balance in the erect posture. When the primary curve is not definitely identified, examination is made with the patient seated with the pelvis elevated 4 inches (by sandbag or otherwise) on the side of the convexity of the lumbar curve. No support is allowed the patient. In this posture the muscles at the convex aspect of the lumbar curve cause marked straightening throughout that curve if it is compensatory but little or no straightening (except possibly at the end of the curve) if it is primary (Figure 3).

The Ferguson and Cobb methods are two systems for measurement of scoliosis. The Scoliosis Research Society

has selected the Cobb system as the standard method of measurement.[3] The Ferguson method should be used for curves under 50°. The Cobb method should be used for curves over 50°.

Method of Ferguson (Figure 1)

1. Locate the end vertebrae: the vertebra at each end of a curve that is the least rotated and lies between the two curves.
2. Locate the apex vertebra: the most rotated vertebra at the peak of the curve.
3. In each of these three vertebrae, the *center* of the *outline* of the *body* is marked with a dot.
4. Lines are drawn from the apex to each end vertebra. The angle of the curve is the divergence of these two lines from 180°.

Method of Cobb (Figure 2)

1. Locate the top vertebra of the curve: the highest one whose superior surface tilts to the side of the concavity of the curve to be measured.

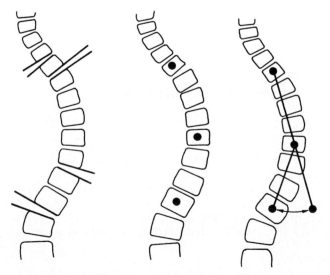

Figure 1 ∙ Method of Ferguson. (Adapted from Kittleson AC, Lim LW: AJR Am J Roentgenol 1970; 108:775.)

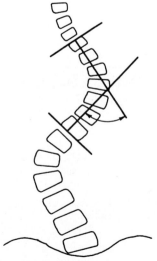

Figure 2 ∙ Method of Cobb. (Adapted from Kittleson AC, Lim LW: AJR Am J Roentgenol 1970; 108:775.)

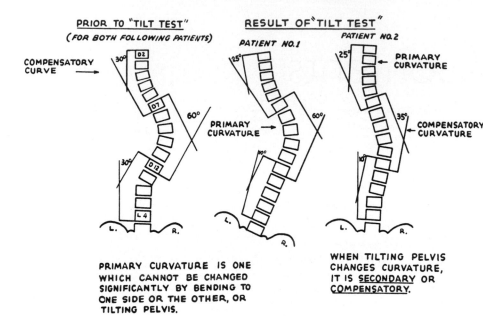

DETERMINATION OF PRIMARY AND SECONDARY CURVATURES IN DORSAL SCOLIOSIS

Figure 3 ▪ (From Meschan I: Roentgen Signs in Clinical Diagnosis. Philadelphia, WB Saunders Co, 1956, p 453.)

2. Locate the bottom vertebra: the lowest one whose inferior surface tilts to the side of the concavity of the curve to be measured.
3. Erect intersecting perpendiculars from the superior surface of the top and the inferior surface of the bottom vertebrae of the curve. The selection of the end vertebrae and the top and bottom vertebrae is aided by a study of the disc spaces. All the vertebrae in a given curve will show widening of the disc space on the convex side of the curve.
4. The angle formed by these perpendiculars is the angle of the curve.

Source ▪

Original observations from the clinical work of Ferguson and from Cobb.

REFERENCES

1. Cobb JR: Am Acad Orthop Surg 1948; 5:261.
2. Ferguson AB: Roentgen Diagnosis of Extremities and Spine. Paul B. Hoeber, Inc., New York, 1949.
3. Kittelson AC, Lim LW: Measurement of scoliosis. AJR Am J Roentgenol 1970; 108:775.

⁛ NORMAL INTERPEDICULATE DISTANCES IN CHILDREN AND ADULTS
▪ ACR Code: 3 (Spine)

Technique ▪

Central ray: Perpendicular to the plane of the film, centered over the midportion of the segment of spine being examined.
Position: Anteroposterior.
Target-film distance: 40 inches.

Measurements ▪

Interpediculate distance is the shortest distance between the medial surfaces of the pedicles of a given vertebra.

Figures 2 to 9 from Hinck and associates[1] contain a shaded area for each graph, which indicates the 90% tolerance range. These tolerance ranges are the high and low limits within which the central 90% of "normals" may be expected to fall.

Figure 1 from Schwarz[2] shows the "extreme upper limits" for the normal spinal canal in neonates to adults.

Source ▪

Hinck used 474 radiographs, including 353 children (under age 19 years) and 121 adults. Radiographs were selected

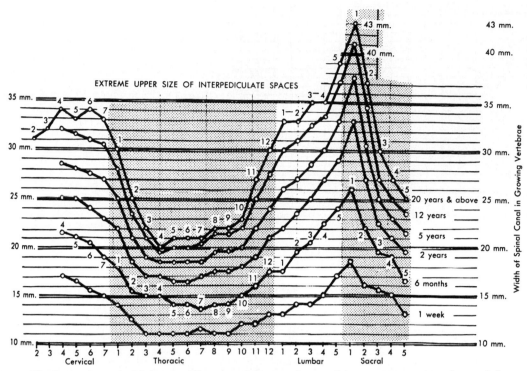

Figure 1 ▪ Newborn through 20 years. All curves delineate the maximum measurement observed for a given vertebra at the age designated. (Adapted from Schwarz GS: AJR Am J Roentgenol 1956; 76:476.)

Figure 2 ▪ (From Hinck VC, et al: AJR Am J Roentgenol 1966; 97:141. Used by permission.)

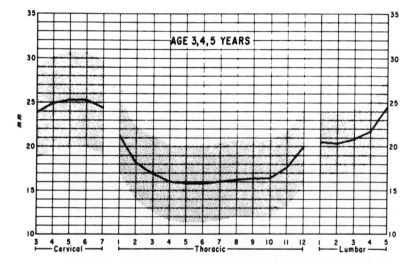

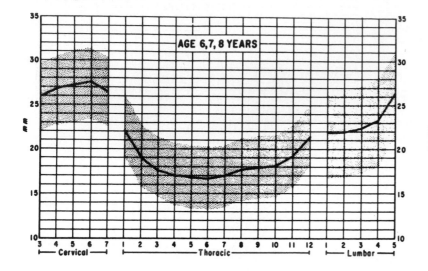

Figure 3 ▪ (From Hinck VC, et al: AJR Am J Roentgenol 1966; 97:141. Used by permission.)

Figure 4 ▪ (From Hinck VC, et al: AJR Am J Roentgenol 1966; 97:141. Used by permission.)

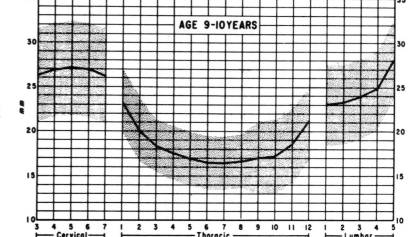

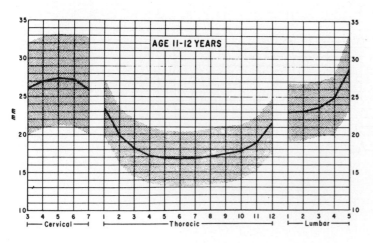

Figure 5 ▪ (From Hinck VC, et al: AJR Am J Roentgenol 1966; 97:141. Used by permission.)

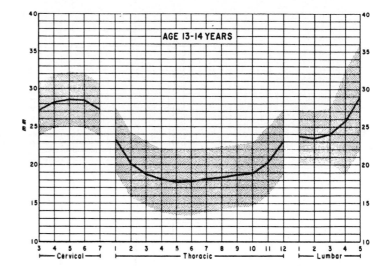

Figure 6 ▪ (From Hinck VC, et al: AJR Am J Roentgenol 1966; 97:141. Used by permission.)

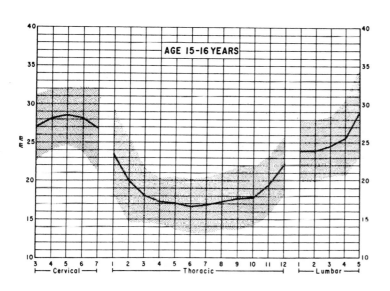

Figure 7 ▪ (From Hinck VC, et al: AJR Am J Roentgenol 1966; 97·141. Used by permission.)

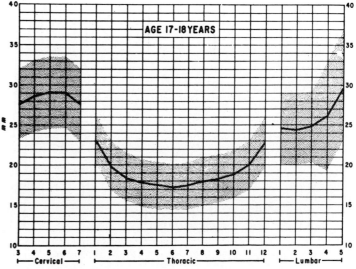

Figure 8 ▪ (From Hinck VC, et al: AJR Am J Roentgenol 1966; 97:141. Used by permission.)

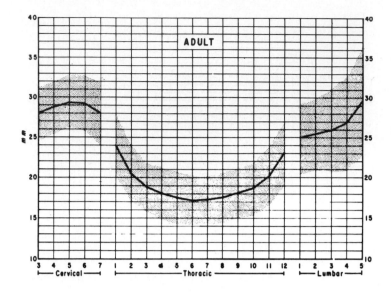

Figure 9 ▪ (From Hinck VC, et al: AJR Am J Roentgenol 1966; 97:141. Used by permission.)

from the files of the University of Oregon Medical School, and an attempt was made to eliminate subjects with significant anomalies and problems likely to influence growth and development.

Schwarz used radiographs of 200 patients.

REFERENCES

1. Hinck VC, Clark WM, Hopkins CE: Normal interpediculate distances (minimum and maximum) in children and adults. AJR Am J Roentgenol 1966; 97:141.
2. Schwarz GS: AJR Am J Roentgenol 1956; 76:476.

▪: MEASUREMENT OF THE NORMAL SPINAL CORD IN CHILDHOOD[1]
▪ ACR Codes: 341, 351, 361 (Spinal Cord)

Technique ▪

Air myelography with tomography.

Central ray: Perpendicular to plane of film.
Position: Anteroposterior and lateral.
Target-film distance: Immaterial.

Measurements (Figure 1) ▪

The spinal cord and subarachnoid space are measured in the sagittal diameter of the midvertebral level, at right angles to the long axis of the cord, and in the transverse diameter at interpedicular level. The cord/subarachnoid space (cord/sas) ratio is calculated.

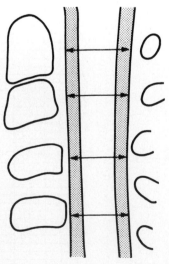

Figure 1 ▪ Measurement of the sagittal width of the subarachnoid space. (From Boltshauser E, Hoare RD: Neuroradiology 1976; 10:235. Used by permission.)

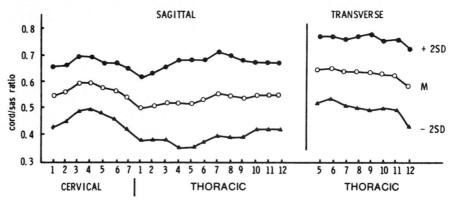

Figure 2 • Mean and two standard deviations of cord subarachnoid space ratio in sagittal and transverse planes. (From Boltshauser E, Hoare RD: Neuroradiology 1976; 10:235. Used by permission.)

Normal values are given in Figure 2. The values are independent of gender. These measurements are of use in evaluating cord atrophy.

Source •

Based on a study of 110 normal air myelograms in children aged 1 month to 15 years.

REFERENCE

1. Boltshauser E, Hoare RD: Radiographic measurements of the normal spinal cord in childhood. Neuroradiology 1976; 10:235–237.

▪: MEASUREMENT OF ATLAS-ODONTOID DISTANCE
▪ ACR Codes: 31 (Cervical Spine)

Technique •

Central ray: Perpendicular to the plane of the film centered at the level of thyroid cartilage.
Position: Lateral. Patient sitting with head in "neutral" position.
Target-film distance: 72 inches.

Measurements (Figure 1) •

Measurement is made between the posteroinferior margin of the anterior arch of the atlas and the anterior surface of the odontoid process.

This measurement is useful in the diagnosis of minimum atlantoaxial subluxation. Normal range

1. Adult (average normal in mm)[1]:
   Female: $D_F = 1.238 - (0.0074 \times$ age in years) $\pm$ 0.900 mm
   Between ages of 20 and 80 years.
   Male: $D_M = 2.052 - (0.0192 \times$ age in years) $\pm$ 1.00 mm.
   Between ages of 30 and 80 years.
2. Children (average normal in mm)[2]:
   D = 2.0; 99% of patients will be between 1 mm and 4 mm. Maximum distance found in a normal patient was 5 mm.

There is a significant difference between measurements in extension and in neutral position, but there is a negligible difference between flexion and neutral position.[1] Ninety-five percent of normal adults will have an atlas-odontoid distance in flexion of between 0.3 and 1.8 mm, in neutral position between 0.4 mm and 2.0 mm, and in extension between 0.3 and 2.2 mm.[1] Neutral position is recommended for children.

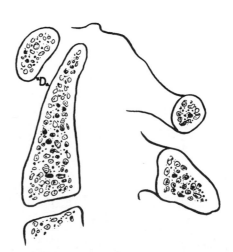

Figure 1 • Atlas-odontoid distance.[1]

Source ▪

Hinck studied 25 adult men (aged 30 to 80 years) and 25 adult women (aged 20 to 80 years).

Locke studied 200 children whose ages ranged from 3 to 15 years.[2] Lateral roentgenograms were made in neutral, flexion, and extension positions at target-film distances of 72 inches (patient sitting) and 40 inches (patient supine). Neutral position is recommended because flexion at both 72- and 40-inch distances tends to increase the atlas-odontoid distance, as does extension at a 40-inch distance.

REFERENCES

1. Hinck VC, Hopkins CE: AJR Am J Roentgenol 1960; 84:945.
2. Locke GR, Gardner JI, Van Epps EF: Atlas-dens interval (ADI) in children: A survey based on 200 normal cervical spines. AJR Am J Roentgenol 1966; 97:135.

▪: ATLANTOAXIAL JUNCTION IN DOWN SYNDROME
▪ ACR Code: 31 (Cervical Spine)

Technique ▪

Pueschel and Scola performed lateral cervical spine radiographs in neutral, flexion, and extension positions. The target-to-film distance was 72 inches.[1] White and colleagues also performed lateral cervical spine radiographs in neutral (17/17) and flexion (14/17) positions, with 72-inch target-to-film distance.[2] Additionally, White and group performed MRI of the cervical spine with a 1.5-T Signal unit (GE Medical Systems, Milwaukee, WI) in flexion (17/17) and extension (13/17) positions. In flexion, spin echo T1 (500/15) and gradient echo (500/15/20°) sagittal and axial images were made. In extension, T1 (500/15) sagittal images were done. All sequences were performed with a 3-mm section thickness and 1-mm gap.[2]

Measurements ▪

In both studies, the atlanto-dens interval (ADI) and the spinal canal width at C1 (SCW) were measured from the radiographs.[1, 2] These measurements are shown in Figure 1. White and colleagues measured the width of the cord and the width of the neural canal in the plane of C1. The subarachnoid space width (SAW) was calculated by subtracting the cord width from the neural canal width.[1] Correlation was done between radiographically measured ADI and SCW and MRI-derived SAW.

Table 1 lists population mean and standard deviations for ADI and SCW at C1 in neutral, flexion, and extension from Pueschel's data. The percentage of subjects having ADI > 5 mm and SCW < 16 mm are also shown for each position.[1] White and colleagues found that there was poor correlation (R = .21) between ADI and SAW and good correlation (R = .88) between SCW and SAW.

Source ▪

Pueschel's subjects included 400 children and young adults (age range = 1 to 30 years; male = 231, female = 173) with Down syndrome.[1] White and colleagues examined 17 children (age range = 3 to 15 years; boys = 7, girls = 10) with Down syndrome.[2]

Table 1 ▪ Atlanto-Dens Interval (ADI) and Spinal Canal Width (SCW) at C1 in Down Syndrome

PARAMETER	GENDER	NUMBER	NEUTRAL	FLEXION	EXTENSION
ADI	Males	231	3.0±1.4	3.3±1.5	2.4±1.1
"	Females	173	2.9±1.7	3.1±1.7	2.5±1.7
"	Both	404	2.9±1.5	3.2±1.6	2.5±1.4
ADI ≥ 5.0 mm	Both	404	39 (9.6%)	50 (12.4%)	22 (5.4%)
SCW	Males	231	19.3±3.1	19.4±3.0	19.3±3.0
"	Females	173	17.7±3.0	18.1±3.1	17.8±3.0
"	Both	404	18.6±3.1	18.9±3.1	18.7±3.1
SCW < 16.0 mm	Both	404	62 (15.2%)	44 (11.0%)	61 (15.0%)

All measurements are in millimeters and are given as mean ± standard deviation. ADI = Atlanto-dens interval, SCW = sagittal canal width. Numbers of patients with ADI of 5 mm or more and SCW of less than 16 mm are given as percentages.
From Pueschel SM, Scola FH: Pediatrics 1987; 80:555–560. Used by permission.

Table 2 ▪ Lower Limit of Normal (90% Tolerance) of the Spinal Canal Width at C1 in Normal Subjects and in Patients with Down Syndrome[1, 4]

AUTHOR (POPULATION)	POSITION	AGE	MALE	FEMALE
Hinck et al (normal subjects)	Neutral	3	15.2	12.9
	"	8	15.7	13.9
	"	13	16.4	14.9
	"	18	17.0	15.8
Pueschel (Down syndrome)	Neutral	1–30	14.2	12.8
	Flexion	"	14.5	13.0
	Extension	"	14.4	12.9

ADI

SCW

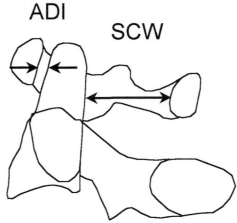

Figure 1 ▪ Measurement of the atlanto-dens interval (*ADI*) and spinal canal width (*SCW*) at C1 from lateral radiographs of the cervical spine.

Comments ▪

The Committee on Sports Medicine of the American Academy of Pediatrics gives the following recommendations concerning children with Down syndrome wishing to participate in sports activities:[3]

1. All children with Down syndrome who wish to participate in sports that involve possible trauma to the head and neck should have lateral-view roentgenograms of the cervical region in neutral, flexion, and extension positions within the patient's tolerance before beginning training or competition. This recommendation applies to all participants in the high-risk sports who have not previously had normal findings on cervical roentgenograms.
2. When the distance between the odontoid process of the axis and the anterior arch of the atlas exceeds 4.5 mm or the odontoid is abnormal, there should be restrictions on sports that involve trauma to the head and neck, and the patient should be followed-up at regular intervals.
3. At the present time, repeated roentgenograms are not indicated for those who have previously had normal findings. Indications for repeated roentgenograms will be defined by research.
4. Persons with atlantoaxial subluxation or dislocation and neurologic signs or symptoms should be restricted in all strenuous activities, and operative stabilization of the cervical spine should be considered.
5. Persons with Down syndrome who have no evidence of atlantoaxial instability may participate in all sports. Follow-up is not required unless musculoskeletal or neurologic signs or symptoms develop.

White and colleagues state that the most important determinate of risk of cord injury is the SAW, and since the correlation between ADI and SAW is poor, he recommends measuring the SCW as well as the ADI.[1] They further recommend that lower 90% tolerance limits from Hinck's study of SCW of normal children be used, and these are shown in Table 2.[4] It seems that Pueschel's data which are derived from a large study of Down patients, might provide an additional source for cut-off values, and these are included in Table 2 as calculated by mean $-1.64 \times$ SD.[1]

REFERENCES

1. Pueschel SM, Scola FH: Atlantoaxial instability in individuals with Down syndrome: Epidemiologic, radiographic, and clinical studies. Pediatrics 1987; 80:555–560.
2. White KS, Ball WS, Prenger EC, et al: Evaluation of the craniocervical junction in Down syndrome: Correlation of measurements obtained with radiography and MR imaging. Radiology 1993; 186(2):377–382.
3. Pueschel SM: Atlantoaxial instability and Down syndrome. Pediatrics 1988; 81:879–880.
4. Hinck VC, Hopkins CE, Savara BS: Sagittal diameter of the cervical spinal canal in children. Radiology 1962; 79:97–108.

▪: DETECTION OF ANTERIOR ATLANTO-OCCIPITAL DISLOCATION[1]
▪ ACR Code: 31 (Cervical Spine)

Technique ▪

Central ray: Perpendicular to plane of film centered over the midcervical spine.
Position: True lateral.
Target-film distance: Immaterial.

Measurement (Figure 1) ▪

B = Basion
O = Opisthion of the occipital bone

A = Anterior arch of the atlas
C = Posterior arch of the atlas

The ratio BC/OA is used to determine anterior atlanto-occipital dislocation. BC/OA is equal to or greater than 1 in all cases of atlanto-occipital dislocation. Ratios less than 1 are normal. This relationship is valid only in the absence of associated fractures of the atlas.

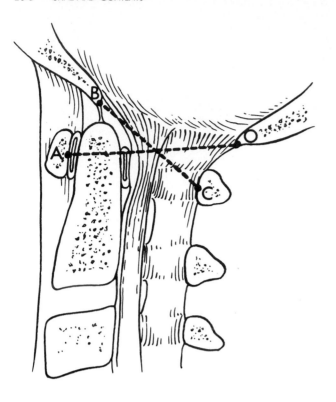

Figure 1 ▪ Normal relationship between the occipital and atlas vertebra. (From Powers B, et al: Neurosurgery 1979; 4:12. Used by permission.)

Source ▪

Normal criteria were determined from a series of 100 normal adult and 50 normal pediatric cervical spine examinations. Criteria were tested against four cases of dislocation.

REFERENCE

1. Powers B, Miller MD, Kramer RS, et al: Traumatic atlanto-occipital dislocation. Neurosurgery 1979; 4:12–17.

▪▪ ATLANTO-OCCIPITAL JUNCTION, THE X-LINE
▪ ACR Code: 31 (Cervical Spine)

Technique ▪

Cross-table lateral radiographs of the cervical spine were performed in the emergency department.[1]

Measurements ▪

A line is drawn from the basion to the midpoint of the C2 spinolaminar line (BC2SL), and a second line is drawn from the opisthion to the posterior inferior corner of the C2 vertebral body (C2O). Figure 1 shows these lines and their ideal relationships with the dens and the C1 spinolaminar line (C1SL). Of the 150 normal subjects, the BC2SL and the C2O lines were tangential to the posterosuperior dens and the C1SL in 28%, the BC2SL was within 5.0 mm behind or 3.0 mm in front of the dens, and the C2O line was tangential to the C1SL in 58%, whereas in 14% the BC2SL line was perfectly aligned with the dens and the C2O line fell within 3.0 mm of the C1SL.[1] In the nine patients with dislocation, there were three types of abnormality of the relationship of the BC2SL and C2O lines: anterior (two patients), posterior (four patients), and longitudinal (three patients). These are shown in Figure 2.

Source ▪

The radiographs of 12 patients with atlanto-occipital dislocation, 100 normal adults, and 50 normal children were evaluated.[1]

Comments ▪

The authors propose that if both lines are out of alignment, atlanto-occipital dislocation be suspected. In their 12 patients with proved atlanto-occipital dislocation, one had a rotatory dislocation rendering the method invalid, two were normal, and nine (75%) had both lines displaced.[1]

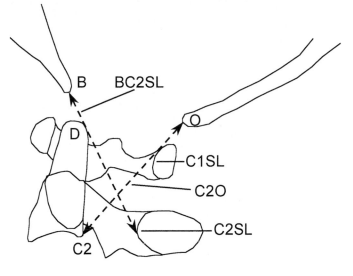

Figure 1 ▪ The X-line method for diagnosing atlanto-occipital dislocation. The ideal relationships of the basion-C2 spinolaminar line (*BC2SL*) and the C2-basion (*C2O*) line with the dens and the C1 spinolaminar line (*C1SL*) are shown. The basion (*B*), opisthion (*O*), posterior inferior C2 vertebral body (*C2*), and the dens (*D*) are indicated.

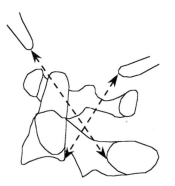

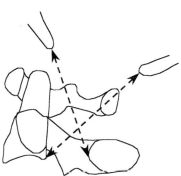

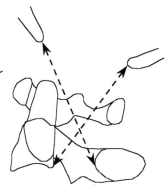

Figure 2 ▪ Three types of atlanto-occipital dislocation and associated patterns of displacement of the diagnostic X-lines.

ANTERIOR   POSTERIOR   LONGITUDINAL

The authors also state that the X-line method does not work well in children and suggest that Kaufman's method of direct measurement of the atlanto-occipital joint be used. They suggest a cut-off of 5 mm rather than 10 mm.[1]

REFERENCE

1. Lee C, Woodring JH, Goldstein SJ, et al: Evaluation of traumatic atlanto-occipital dislocations [see comments]. AJNR Am J Neuroradiol 1987; 8(1):19–26.

▪: THE BASION-DENS INTERVAL
▪ ACR Code: 31 (Cervical Spine)

Technique ▪

Horizontal beam, cross-table lateral radiographic technique was used to examine the cervical spine and craniocervical junction.[1–4] The target-to-film distance was listed as 40 inches in the study by Harris.[3]

Measurements ▪

In all four studies the basion-dens interval (BDI) was measured directly from the films with a ruler between the tip of the odontoid to the basion.[1–4] Figure 1 shows this measurement. Table 1 lists the number of cases in which the landmarks were visible, normal measurements, and suggested cut-off values.[1–4]

Source ▪

Bulas and colleagues evaluated 156 pediatric trauma patients. The mean age of these children was 8.5 years, and the age ranged from newborn to 16 years. None had radiographic or clinical evidence of cervical injury.[1] Lee and colleagues studied 100 adults and 50 children seen in the emergency department, who had normal films and no clinical sequelae.[2] Harris and colleagues used cervical spine films from 400 adult patients evaluated for trauma, with

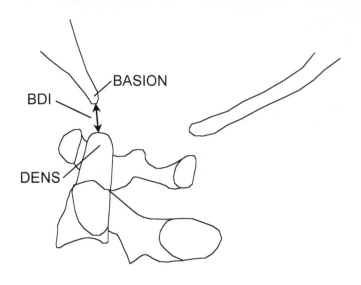

Figure 1 ▪ Measurement of the basion-dens interval (*BDI*) was performed between the tip of the odontoid and the basion from cross-table lateral cervical spine radiographs.

Table 1 ▪ **Basion-Dens Interval in Adults and Children**

RESEARCHER/GROUP	NUMBER	BDI MEAN ± SD	BDI RANGE	BDI CUT-OFF
Bulas[1]				
Children (NB–7 yrs.)	46	9.1 ± 4.0	3.0–12.0	12.5
Children (8–16 yrs.)	64	7.7 ± 2.0	—	—
Children (NB–16 yrs.)	110	8.3 ± 4.2	—	—
Lee[2]				
Children	50	5.0	2.0–11.0	12.0
Adults	100	7.0	2.0–15.0	15.0
Harris[3]				
Adults	374	7.5 ± 4.3	2.0–15.0	12.0
Powers[4]				
Children	50	9.0 ± 3.6		
Adults	100	9.0 ± 3.6		

All measurements are in millimeters. BDI = basion-dens interval, NB = newborn.

normal radiographic findings and no clinical evidence of cervical injury.[3] Powers evaluated radiographs of 100 normal adults and 50 normal children.[4]

Comments ▪

The main use of this measurement is to detect atlanto-occipital dislocation. It was first described by Wholey, and colleagues who gave the average adult measurement of 5.0 mm and an upper limit of 10.0 mm in infants and children.[5] The measurement may be difficult in children when the odontoid is partly developed or in any case if the landmarks are not visible due to technical factors. Harris and group did not attempt to measure the BDI in children and was able to measure it in 374 of 400 (94%) adults.[3] Bulas and colleagues were able to measure the BDI in 110 of 156 (71%) children.[1] Based on these data a cut-off of 12.0 mm would seem to be useful and may be combined with the Powers ratio method,[4] Lee's X-line method,[2] the Harris

basion-axial interval,[3] and Kaufman's direct measurement of the joint.[6]

REFERENCES

1. Bulas DI, Fitz CR, Johnson DL: Traumatic atlanto-occipital dislocation in children. Radiology 1993; 188:155–158.
2. Lee C, Woodring JH, Goldstein SJ, et al: Evaluation of traumatic atlanto-occipital dislocations [see comments]. AJNR Am J Neuroradiol 1987; 8(1):19–26.
3. Harris JH, Carson GC, Wagner LK: Radiologic diagnosis of traumatic occipitovertebral dissociation: 1. Normal occipitovertebral relationships on lateral radiographs of supine subjects. AJR Am J Roentgenol 1994; 162:881–886.
4. Powers B, Miller MD, Kramer RS, et al: Traumatic anterior atlanto-occipital dislocation. Neurosurgery 1979; 4:12–17.
5. Wholey MH, Brunwer AJ, Baker HI: The lateral roentgenogram of the neck (with comments on the atlanto-odontoid-basion relationship). Radiology 1958; 77:350–356.
6. Kaufman RA, Carroll CD, Buncher CR: Atlanto-occipital junction: Standards for measurement in normal children. AJNR Am J Neuroradiol 1987; 8:995–999.

•: THE BASION-AXIAL INTERVAL
- ACR Code: 31 (Cervical Spine)

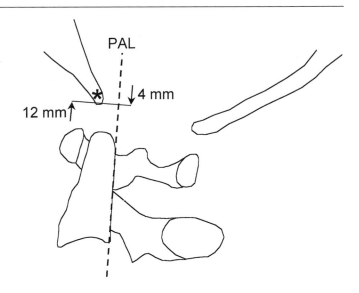

Figure 1 • Measurement of the basion-axial interval on a lateral radiograph of the cervical spine. Shown are the posterior axial line (*PAL*), basion (*asterisk*), and upper limits of normal distances (*arrows*). In the vast majority of normal adults and in all children, the basion lies anterior to the PAL.[1]

Technique •

Horizontal beam, cross-table lateral radiographic technique (target-to-film distance = 40 inches) was used to examine the cervical spine and craniocervical junction.[1, 2]

Measurements •

A line is drawn through the posterior margin of C2 extending rostrally into the cranium, called the posteroaxial line (PAL). If the cortex was less than 1 mm, the line was drawn over it. When the thickness of the posterior cortex of the C2 vertebral body exceeded 1 mm (anatomic variation or due to rotation), the line was drawn to coincide with the vertical midplane between the anterior and posterior margins. The distance between this line and the basion in millimeters was defined as the basion-axial interval (BAI). Figure 1 shows these relationships.

Of the 400 normal adult subjects, the BAI was 0 to 6 mm anterior to the PAL in 322 (80%), 7 to 12 mm anterior to the PAL in 70 (18%), and 0 to 12 anterior to the PAL in 392 (98%). In 8 (2%) of the adults, the BAI was 1 to 4 mm posterior to the PAL. In the 50 children, the BAI was 0 to 6 mm anterior to the PAL in 36 (72%), and 7 to 12 mm anterior to the PAL in 14 (28%). The BAI was between 0 and 12 mm anterior to the PAL in all the children.[1]

Source •

Cervical spine films from 400 adult and 50 pediatric patients were evaluated for trauma, with normal radiographic findings and no clinical evidence of cervical injury.[1] In a companion study, 37 patients (age range not given) with clinical suspicion of atlanto-occipital dislocation were evaluated. Of these, 23 had frank dislocation, 8 had incomplete dislocation, and 6 were neurologically normal and had normal radiographic findings.[2]

Comments •

The BAI in combination with the basion-dens interval (BDI) was 100% accurate in detecting all 31 cases of atlanto-occipital dislocation.[2] The suggested cut-off values are no greater than 12.0 mm for both BAI (anterior) and BDI and no more than 4.0 mm posterior for the BDI.[2] Harris makes a strong argument for use of the BAI/BDI measurements in the clinical setting of suspected atlanto-occipital dislocation as opposed to other methods, based on the fact that the other measurements may not be possible due to poor visualization of the opisthion and the spinal laminar line, as well as significant false-positive and false-negative rates.[1, 2] The BDI and other measurement techniques are covered in separate sections of this work.

REFERENCES

1. Harris JH, Carson GC, Wagner LK: Radiologic diagnosis of traumatic occipitovertebral dissociation: 1. Normal occipitovertebral relationships on lateral radiographs of supine subjects. AJR Am J Roentgenol 1994; 162:881–886.
2. Harris JH Jr, Carson GC, Wagner LK, Kerr N: Radiologic diagnosis of traumatic occipitovertebral dissociation: 2. Comparison of three methods of detecting occipitovertebral relationships on lateral radiographs of supine subjects. AJR Am J Roentgenol 1994; 162:887–892.

❄ ATLANTO-OCCIPITAL JUNCTION

▪ ACR Code: 31 (Cervical Spine)

Technique ▪

Cross-table lateral radiographs of the skull were made, with 40-inch target-to-film distance and an 8:1 grid.[1]

Measurements ▪

The atlanto-occipital joint was defined as the top of the C1 facet and the bottom of the occipital condyles. These landmarks were traced onto transparent film and the joint was measured at five evenly spaced points denoted as 1 through 5, going from anterior to posterior with a hand lens micrometer in millimeters. Figure 1 shows these measurement points and landmarks. Table 1 shows the results, including number and percentage of cases measurable at each point; the mean, standard deviation, and range of measurement for 100 normal subjects and 8 patients with distraction injury. In 16% of normal subjects, the measurement could not be obtained at any point, whereas at least one point was measurable in all patients with injury.

The normal subjects were separated into three age groups, and statistical testing of age-dependence of the measured distance showed a marginal effect (p = 0.0465) at point 4 and no significant differences elsewhere. Based on their data, the researchers suggest a cut-off of 4.5 mm to discriminate between normal and abnormal, with 4.5 to 5.0 mm being considered borderline. There is a 7% chance that a normal child will have a measurement of greater than 4.5 mm at one point and a 1.2% chance of having a greater than 4.5-mm measurement at two points (almost always points 2 and/or 3). No normal child had borderline measurements at more than two points, and none had a measurement of more than 5.0 mm. As for patients with atlanto-occipital distraction, the authors state that most will have at least one measurement that exceeds 5.0 mm and that the few that fall in the borderline range of 4.5 to 5.0 mm will do so throughout the whole joint. They suggest repeating the lateral radiograph and adding an antero-posterior view in problem cases.[1]

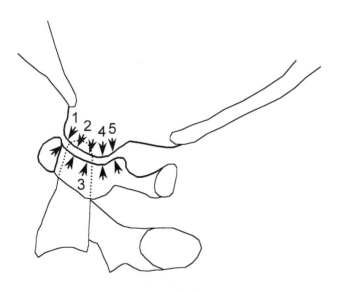

Figure 1 ▪ Measurement of the atlanto-occipital joint on a lateral skull film in children. Five measurement points are defined (*1–5, anterior to posterior*) between the occipital condyle and the upper margin of the C1 facet.[1]

Table 1 ▪ Measurements of the Atlanto-Occipital Joint			
MEASUREMENT POSITION	**MEASURABLE (%)**	**MEAN ± SD**	**RANGE**
NORMAL SUBJECTS (N = 100)			
1	65 (77)	2.22 ± 0.70	1.0–3.5
2	64 (76)	2.63 ± 1.02	1.0–5.0
3	58 (69)	2.52 ± 0.95	1.0–5.0
4	63 (75)	2.13 ± 0.70	1.0–4.0
5	60 (71)	1.96 ± 0.65	1.0–4.0
ATLANTO-OCCIPITAL DISTRACTION INJURY (N = 8)			
1	8 (100)	6.44 ± 1.43	4.5–8.0
2	8 (100)	8.12 ± 2.20	5.5–11.0
3	6 (75)	7.50 ± 1.70	5.0–9.5
4	6 (75)	7.67 ± 2.09	5.0–10.0
5	3 (38)	6.33 ± 3.01	3.5–9.5

All measurements are in millimeters.
From Kaufman RA, Carroll CD, Buncher CR: AJNR Am J Neuroradiol 1987; 8:995–999. Used by permission.

REFERENCE

1. Kaufman RA, Carroll CD, Buncher CR: Atlanto-occipital junction: Standards for measurement in normal children. AJNR Am J Neuroradiol 1987; 8:995–999.

Source ▪

Normal subjects comprised 63 boys and 37 girls, ranging in age from 1 to 15 years, radiographed for various chronic complaints or minor trauma. None were read as abnormal, and no neurologic abnormalities were noted clinically. Eight cases of proven atlanto-occipital distraction injury were also analyzed.[1]

▪▪ POSTERIOR ATLANTOAXIAL RELATIONSHIPS
▪ ACR Code: 31 (Cervical Spine)

Technique ▪

Lateral cervical spine radiographs (distance not given) were done with the subject in maximal flexion.

Measurements ▪

The height of the posterior arch of C1 at the spinolaminar line (SLL) was measured to the nearest millimeter, and the flexion interspinous distance (FID) between C1 and C2 was measured to the nearest millimeter.[1] Figure 1 shows these measurements, and Table 1 gives the normal values in women, men, and all patients combined. The ratio of the two (FID/SLL) is also given. Figure 2 is a scatterplot of FID/SLL values against age and shows that there is no change with advancing age.[1]

Source ▪

Healthy volunteers (n = 100) with no spinal abnormalities were chosen, consisting of 56 men (age range = 20 to 69 years) and 44 women (age range = 20 to 64 years).[1]

Comments ▪

The ratio between the flexion interspinous distance and the C1 spinolaminar line (FID/SLL) width was quite constant,

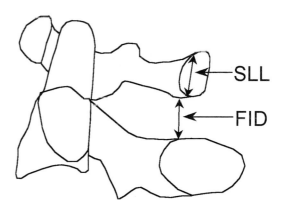

Figure 1 ▪ Diagram of lateral upper cervical spine radiograph with measurements of the C1 spinolaminar line (*SLL*) and the flexion interspinous distance (*FID*) shown.

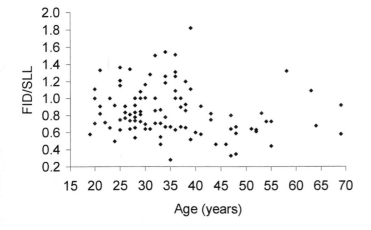

Figure 2 ▪ Scatterplot of the flexion interspinous distance divided by the height of the posterior arch of C1 at the spinolaminar line (*FID/SLL*) related to age. Note the lack of correlation with age and that the value of the ratio does not exceed 2.0 mm. (From Lovelock JE, Schuster JA: Skeletal Radiol 1991; 20(2):121–123. Used by permission.)

Table 1 ■ Normal Posterior Atlantoaxial Relationships in Flexion

	MEN	WOMEN	TOTAL
Number	56	44	100
Mean FID (mm)	10.69	8.79	9.86
Range FID (mm)	5–20	4–15	4–20
Mean SLL (mm)	12.64	11.18	12.0
Mean ± SD FID/SLL	0.85 ± 0.29	0.79 ± 0.27	0.82 ± 0.28
Range FID/SLL	0.36–1.82	0.29–1.33	0.29–1.82

FID = flexion interspinous distance, SLL = height of C1 at the spinolaminar line, SD = standard deviation.
From Lovelock JE, Schuster JA: Skeletal Radiol 1991; 20(2):121–123. Used by permission.

whereas the individual measurements varied considerably within individuals and between genders. If the FID/SLL exceeds 2.0 mm in flexion, posterior ligamentous injury may be suspected.[1]

REFERENCE

1. Lovelock JE, Schuster JA: The normal posterior atlantoaxial relationship. Skeletal Radiol 1991; 20(2): 121–123.

⁞ DIFFERENTIATION BETWEEN TRUE AND PSEUDOSUBLUXATION OF C2 ON C3 IN CHILDREN: THE POSTERIOR CERVICAL LINE[1]

■ ACR Code: 31 (Cervical Spine)

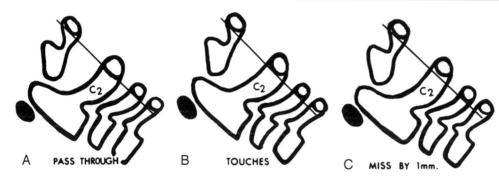

A PASS THROUGH **B** TOUCHES **C** MISS BY 1mm.

Figure 1 ■ Normal positions of the posterior cervical line. (From Swischuk LE: Radiology 1977; 122:759. Used by permission.)

Technique ■

Central ray: Perpendicular to plane of film centered over cervical spine.
Position: True lateral.
Target-film distance: Immaterial.

Measurements ■

In Figure 1, the line is drawn through the anterior cortex of the posterior arches of C1, C2, and C3. In the normal situation, or in pseudosubluxation, the line is normal if it: (1) passes through or just behind the anterior cortex of the posterior arch of C2; (2) touches the anterior aspect of the cortex of C2; or (3) comes within 1 mm of the cortex of C2.

In pathologic dislocation of C2 on C3, the posterior cervical line misses the posterior arch of C2 by 2 mm or more. If the line misses the arch by 1.5 mm, one should be suspicious, but if the distance is 2 mm or more, true dislocation should be assumed unless further tests show that there is no dislocation.

Source ■

Based on a study of 500 children up to the age of 14 years.

REFERENCE

1. Swischuk LE: Anterior displacement of C2 in children; Physiologic or pathologic? Radiology 1977; 122: 759–763.

▪: INTERSPINOUS DISTANCE FOR THE DETECTION OF ANTERIOR CERVICAL DISLOCATION IN THE SUPINE FRONTAL PROJECTION[1]
▪ ACR Code: 31 (Cervical Spine)

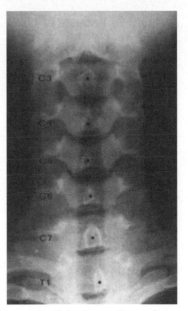

Figure 1 ▪ Measurement of the interspinous distances in a normal supine frontal projection. (From Naidich JB, et al; Radiology 1977; 123:113. Used by permission.)

Technique ▪

Central ray: Perpendicular to plane of film centered over midcervical spine.
Position: Anteroposterior projection, supine.
Target-film distance: Immaterial.

Measurements (Figure 1) ▪

The interspinous distance (ISD) (Figure 1) is measured from the center of the spinous process above to the center of the spinous process below. A widened interspinous distance, which measures more than 1½ times the ISD above and more than 1½ times the ISD below, indicates the presence of an anterior cervical dislocation at the level of the abnormal widening.

This measurement is particularly useful in patients in whom the lower cervical spine cannot be visualized because of obscuration by the shoulders.

Source ▪

Based on a study of 500 patients with normal cervical spines and 14 patients with documented anterior cervical dislocations.

REFERENCE

1. Naidich JB, Naidich TP, Garfein C, et al: The widened interspinous distance: A useful sign of anterior cervical dislocation in the supine frontal projection. Radiology 1977; 123:113–116.

▪: SAGITTAL DIAMETER OF THE CERVICAL SPINAL CANAL IN INFANTS[1]
▪ ACR Code: 34 (Cervical Spinal Canal and Contents)

Table 1 ▪ Sagittal Diameter of Spinal Canal	
VERTEBRAL LEVEL	MEAN DIAMETER (mm)
C2	12.5
C3	11.5
C4	11.5
C5	12.2
C6	12.6
C7	12.1

Standard deviation is 0.7 mm.
From Naik DR: Clin Radiol 1970; 21:323. Used by permission.

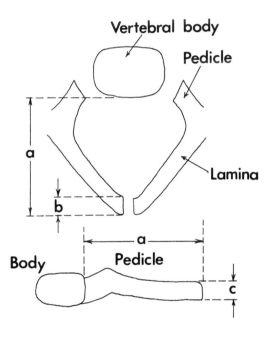

Figure 1 ▪ Cervical spinal canal in infants. a = Distance from posterior border of vertebral body to tip of the spinous process; b = thickness (in dissected specimen) of the spinous process; c = height (on lateral radiograph) of the spinous process. At this age, b = c. (Adapted from Naik DR: Clin Radiol 1970; 21:323. Used by permission.)

Technique ▪

Central ray: Projected to the seventh cervical vertebra.
Position: True lateral.
Target-film distance: 90 cm.

Measurements (Figure 1 and Table 1) ▪

The sagittal diameter can be determined by measuring from the posterior border of the vertebral body to the posterior end of the laminae (distance a) and subtracting the height (c) of the laminae. Sagittal diameter of the spinal canal = $a - c$.

Source ▪

Twenty-five normal spines of infants under 12 months of age were studied postmortem.

REFERENCE

1. Naik DR: Cervical spinal canal in normal infants. Clin Radiol 1970; 21:323–326.

⁚ SAGITTAL DIAMETER OF THE CERVICAL SPINAL CANAL IN ADULTS[1]

▪ ACR Code: 34 (Cervical Spinal Canal and Contents)

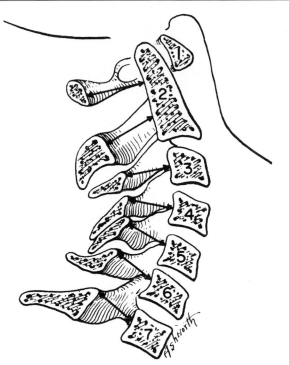

Figure 1 ▪ (From Hinck VC, Hopkins CE, Savara BS: Radiology 1962; 79:97. Used by permission.)

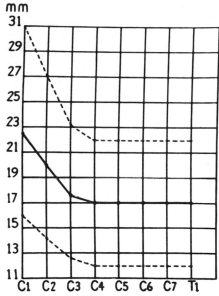

Figure 2 ▪ Curves for average, maximal, and minimal sagittal measurements of cervical spinal canal in adults. Plotted values are uncorrected measurements from lateral neck films taken at 72-inch target–table top distance. True measurements are 1.5 mm less than those shown. (From Wolf BS, Khilnani M, Malis L: J Mt Sinai Hosp 1956; 23:283. Used by permission.)

Technique ▪

Central ray: Projected through the fourth cervical vertebra.
Position: True lateral. Patient seated with the head in neutral position.
Target-film distance: 73.8 inches. Target to table top distance was 72 inches, and table top to film in Bucky tray was 1.8 inches.

Measurements (Figures 1 and 2) ▪

The sagittal diameter was measured from the middle of the posterior surface of the ventral body to the nearest point on the ventral line of the cortex, seen at the junction of spinous processes and laminae (arrows).

Source ▪

Measurements were made on 200 adults with no known neurologic disturbance and showing no obvious bone or joint changes on the films.

REFERENCE

1. Wolf BS, Khilnani M, Malis L: J Mt Sinai Hosp 1956; 23:283.

⁚ SAGITTAL DIAMETER OF THE CERVICAL SPINAL CANAL IN CHILDREN

▪ ACR Code: 34 (Cervical Spinal Canal and Contents)

Technique ▪

Lateral upright neutral radiographs of the cervical spine, with target to film distance of 60 inches.[1,2]

Measurements ▪

In both studies, the sagittal diameter of the spinal canal was measured from the midportion of each vertebral body to the closest point of the corresponding spinal laminar line.[1,2] At C1, the dorsal aspect of the dens was used as the anterior margin of the spinal canal. The measurements were taken directly from the films with a Bolton-Broadbent cephalometer[1] or a slide caliper.[2] Figure 1 shows the measurement sites at each cervical level. Figure 2 shows Hinck's longitudinal data as 90% confidence intervals by age and level. Figure 3 depicts the differences between adjacent

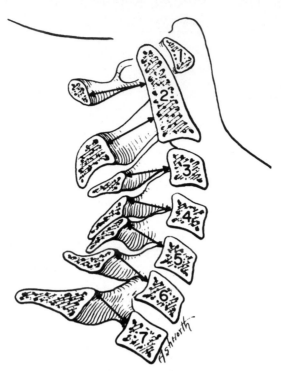

Figure 1 ▪ Measurement of the sagittal diameter of the cervical spinal canal. Arrows show site of measurement at each level from C1 to C7.[1]

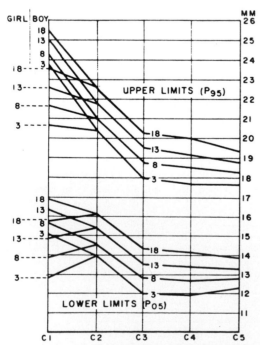

Figure 2 ▪ Ninety percent confidence intervals for the sagittal diameter of the spinal canal from C1 to C5 in children from 3 to 18 years of age.[1]

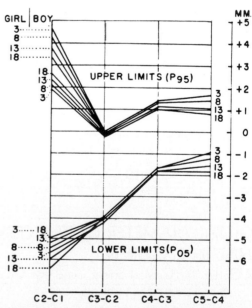

Figure 3 ▪ Ninety percent confidence intervals for differences in the sagittal diameter of the spinal canal between vertebrae from C1 to C5 in children from 3 to 18 years of age.[1]

Table 1 ▪ Sagittal Diameter of the Cervical Spinal Canal in Children from 3 to 14 Years of Age

AGE	3–6 yr		7–10 yr		11–14 yr	
NUMBER	40		40		40	
	Mean ± SD	90% CI	Mean ± SD	90% CI	Mean ± SD	90% CI
Level						
C1	19.9 ± 1.3	17.8–22.0	20.6 ± 1.3	18.5–22.7	21.3 ± 1.4	19.0–23.6
C2	17.9 ± 1.3	15.8–20.0	18.8 ± 1.0	17.2–20.4	19.4 ± 1.1	17.6–21.2
C3	16.0 ± 1.3	13.9–18.1	17.2 ± 1.0	15.6–18.8	17.8 ± 1.0	16.2–19.4
C4	15.8 ± 1.3	13.7–17.9	16.9 ± 0.9	15.4–18.4	17.3 ± 0.9	15.8–18.8
C5	15.7 ± 1.3	13.6–17.8	16.7 ± 0.9	15.2–18.2	17.0 ± 0.9	15.5–18.5
C6	15.6 ± 1.2	13.6–17.6	16.4 ± 0.9	14.9–17.9	16.7 ± 0.9	15.2–18.2
C7	15.3 ± 1.1	13.5–17.1	16.0 ± 0.9	14.5–17.5	16.2 ± 0.9	14.7–17.7

All measurements are in millimeters. SD = standard deviation, CI = confidence interval.
From Markuske H: Pediatr Radiol 1977; 6:129–131. Used by permission.

levels.[1] Table 1 lists Markuske's data in tabular form with mean, standard deviation (SD), and 90% confidence intervals (CI) for each level.[2]

Source ▪

Hinck and colleagues studied 48 children with annual radiographs from ages 3 to 18.[1] Markuske's work included 120 normal children ranging in age between 3 and 14 years, with an equal number of boys and girls in each age group.[2]

Comments ▪

Hinck and associates found significant differences between genders only at C1 and Markuske found no significant gender differences.[1, 2]

REFERENCES

1. Hinck VC, Hopkins CE, Savara BS: Sagittal diameter of the cervical spinal canal in children. Radiology 1962; 79:97–108.
2. Markuske H: Sagittal diameter measurements of the bony cervical spinal canal in children. Pediatr Radiol 1977; 6:129–131.

▪: CERVICAL SPINAL CANAL: VERTEBRAL BODY RATIO METHOD
▪ ACR Code: 34 (Cervical Spinal Canal and Contents)

Technique ▪

Lateral cervical spine radiographs in neutral position were performed. The target-to-film distances were not specified.[1]

Measurements ▪

The sagittal spinal canal diameter (SCD) was measured from C3 through C6, from the middle of the posterior surface of the vertebral body to the nearest point on the corresponding spinal laminar line. The sagittal diameter of the C3 through C6 vertebral bodies was measured at the midpoint. A sagittal canal ratio (SCR) was calculated by dividing the sagittal canal diameter by the vertebral body diameter for each segment.[1] Figure 1 shows these measurements. Table 1 gives values for normal males, normal females, and symptomatic patients.

Table 1 ▪ Cervical Spinal Canal Measurements

	MALE CONTROLS (n = 49)		FEMALE CONTROLS (n = 25)		SYMPTOMATIC PATIENTS (n = 23)	
	Mean ± SD	Range	Mean ± SD	Range	Mean ± SD	Range
SAGITTAL CANAL DIAMETER						
C3	19.24 ± 0.188	(13.7–23.5)	17.19 ± 0.151	(13.3–20.0)	15.91 ± 0.297	(9.50–23.5)
C4	18.56 ± 0.195	(14.3–23.5)	16.92 ± 0.134	(13.7–20.4)	15.43 ± 0.241	(9.00–19.5)
C5	18.71 ± 0.183	(14.7–23.5)	17.04 ± 0.138	(14.8–19.6)	14.87 ± 0.247	(8.50–19.0)
C6	19.03 ± 0.193	(15.0–23.5)	17.52 ± 0.144	(15.2–20.1)	14.82 ± 0.221	(10.00–18.5)
C3–6 average	18.9	(13.7–23.5)	17.2	(13.3–20.4)	15.22	(8.50–23.5)
SAGITTAL CANAL RATIO						
C3	1.008 ± 0.118	(0.69–1.27)	1.018 ± 0.106	(0.81–1.25)	0.725 ± 0.166	(0.33–1.18)
C4	0.973 ± 0.110	(0.76–1.19)	1.011 ± 0.071	(0.85–1.18)	0.703 ± 0.118	(0.32–0.86)
C5	0.975 ± 0.091	(0.80–1.17)	1.016 ± 0.057	(0.89–1.15)	0.683 ± 0.112	(0.31–0.90)
C6	0.978 ± 0.104	(0.80–1.23)	1.016 ± 0.078	(0.87–1.26)	0.662 ± 0.094	(0.36–0.85)
C3–6 average	0.98	(0.69–1.27)	1.02	(0.81–1.26)	0.69	(0.31–1.18)

Canal diameter measurements are in millimeters, and the ratios are dimensionless.[1]

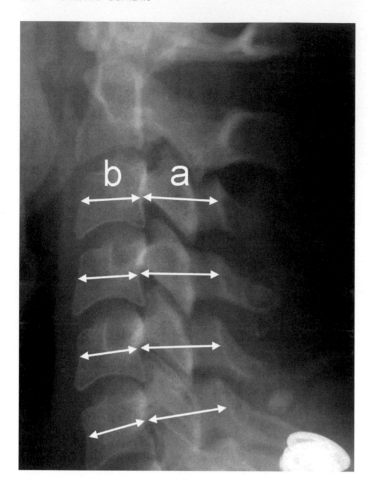

Figure 1 ▪ The sagittal canal diameter (SCD) was measured from the midpoint of the posterior vertebral body to the nearest point of the corresponding spinal laminar line (*a*). The sagittal diameter of the vertebral body was measured at the midpoint (*b*). The sagittal canal ratio (SCR) was calculated with the formula a/b. The normal ratio is about 1.0, and 0.8 serves as a cut-off for spinal stenosis.[1]

Source ▪

Control subjects (49 male and 25 female) with no neurologic abnormalities, whose ages ranged from 15 to 38 years, were studied. A group of 23 patients with documented transient neuropraxia were also included. These were all male athletes, and the ages ranged from 15 to 32 years.[1]

Comments ▪

The authors calculated receiver operating curves for SCD and SCR from the control and symptomatic populations, with disease-positive being a history of neuropraxia. The SCR method was 2.5 times more accurate than the SCD method for diagnosing symptomatic spinal stenosis. At SCR operating points of .76, .8, and .82, the sensitivities were 70%, 80%, and 92%, respectively, and the specificities were 98%, 96%, and 94%, respectively. In a previous work, the authors propose a cut-off point of .8, with those falling below being considered to have significant spinal stenosis.[2] Bey and associates recommend the use of the SCR method (with a cut-off of .8) to aid in triage of patients with neurologic symptoms and no fractures.[3]

REFERENCES

1. Pavlov H, Torg JS, Robie B, Jahre C: Cervical spinal stenosis: Determination with vertebral body ratio method. Radiology 1987; 164:771–775.
2. Torg JS, Pavlov H, Genuario SE, et al: Neuropraxia of the cervical spinal cord with transient quadriplegia. J Bone Joint Surg Am 1986; 68:1354–1370.
3. Bey T, Waer A, Walter FG, et al: Spinal cord injury with a narrow spinal canal: Utilizing Torg's ratio method of analyzing cervical spine radiographs. J Emerg Med 1998; 16:790–782.

▪: SIZE OF THE CERVICAL CORD, DURAL SAC, AND SPINAL CANAL
▪ ACR Code: 34 (Cervical Spinal Canal and Contents)

Technique ▪

Yone and colleagues performed T1-weighted axial images (parameters and machine type not given), with a 5-mm slice thickness of the cervical spine.[1] Okada'a group obtained T1 (500/20–30)-weighted axial images using an MRI-50A machine (Toshiba, Tokyo, Japan) and 10 mm slice thickness.[2] A cervical coil was used in both studies.

Measurements ▪

The anteroposterior diameter of the spinal cord was measured on sagittal images at each midvertebral body level and each disc space.[1] The cross-sectional area of the cord, dural sac, and spinal canal was measured with a computer-linked digitizer from axial images from C3 through C7.[2]

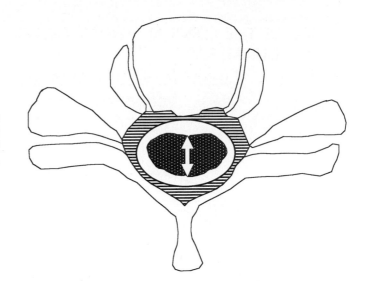

Figure 1 ▪ Cervical spine in the axial plane showing boundaries of the cord (*dark gray*), dural sac (*white*), and spinal canal (*horizontal hatching*) for area measurements. The anteroposterior diameter of the cord is also shown (*double arrow*), though in the cited study this was actually measured from sagittal images.

Table 1 ▪ Normal Values of Cervical Cord, Dural Sac, and Spinal Canal Measurements

LEVEL	AP DIAMETER (mm)	SPINAL CORD AREA (mm²)	DURAL SAC AREA (mm²)	SPINAL CANAL AREA (mm²)	OCCUPYING RATIO (%)
C2–C3		79.4 ± 6.9	218.8 ± 31.4		
C3	7.8 ± 2.4	80.5 ± 7.1	200.8 ± 25.4	248.9 ± 30.3	33.0 ± 4.4
C3–C4	7.6 ± 2.8	82.9 ± 7.2	192.6 ± 21.9		
C4	7.7 ± 2.6	84.6 ± 6.2	193.0 ± 21.6	236.1 ± 29.0	36.4 ± 4.1
C4–C5	7.5 ± 2.8	85.8 ± 7.2	189.8 ± 20.3		
C5	7.5 ± 2.4	83.2 ± 6.2	188.9 ± 21.2	238.8 ± 30.6	35.5 ± 4.4
C5–C6	7.3 ± 2.4	81.2 ± 7.2	186.0 ± 20.3		
C6	7.3 ± 1.9	76.1 ± 7.3	191.7 ± 24.2	248.5 ± 30.1	30.8 + 3 9
C6–C7	7.1 ⊥ 1.7	69.3 ± 8.0	186.6 ± 22.0		
C7	7.0 ± 1.6	60.9 ± 7.5	196.5 ± 24.4	254.8 ± 32.7	23.7 ± 3.4

All measurements are given as mean ± standard deviation.
From Okada Y, Ikata T, Katoh S, Yamada H: Spine 1994; 19(20):2331–2335. Used by permission.

Figure 1 depicts these measurements in the axial plane. Table 1 lists the reported values as well as the occupying ratio (area of cord/area of canal × 100).

Source ▪

Yone and colleagues examined 31 healthy adult volunteers (age and gender not given). Okada studied 54 men and 42 women (mean age = 46.5 years, range = 21 to 73 years).

Comments ▪

Both groups studied patients with cervical spondylotic myelopathy (CSM), and Yone and colleagues also evaluated patients with ossification of the posterior longitudinal ligament (OPLL). The anteroposterior diameter of the cord was significantly smaller than normal at one or more levels in symptomatic patients with OPLL; there was no significant difference in the cord diameter between CSM patients and normal subjects.[1] In CSM patients, the cord area and canal-occupying ratio at the level of involvement was significantly smaller than normal and was inversely correlated with the severity of symptoms.[2]

REFERENCES

1. Yone K, Sakou T, Yanase M, Ijiri K: Preoperative and postoperative magnetic resonance image evaluations of the spinal cord in cervical myelopathy. Spine 1992; 17(10 Suppl):S388–392.
2. Okada Y, Ikata T, Katoh S, Yamada H: Morphologic analysis of the cervical spinal cord, dural tube, and spinal canal by magnetic resonance imaging in normal adults and patients with cervical spondylotic myelopathy. Spine 1994; 19(20):2331–2335.

⁚ SIZE OF THE CERVICAL AND THORACIC SPINAL CORD AND DURAL SAC

▪ ACR Code: 34 (Cervical Spinal Canal and Contents)

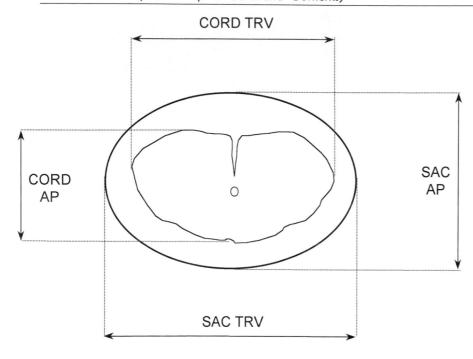

Figure 1 ▪ Linear measurements of the spinal contents, including transverse (*TRV*) and anteroposterior (*AP*) measurements of the spinal cord and dural sac.

Table 1 ▪ Spinal Cord and Dural Sac Dimensions and Size of Dorsal and Ventral CSF Spaces

LEVEL	SPINAL CORD		DURAL SAC	
	AP	TRV	AP	TRV
C4	7.3 ± 0.6	13.6 ± 1.1	13.3 ± 1.4	20.4 ± 2.0
C5	6.9 ± 0.6	13.4 ± 1.1	13.4 ± 1.5	20.6 ± 2.0
C6	6.7 ± 0.6	13.0 ± 1.1	13.4 ± 1.4	20.7 ± 2.1
T5	5.9 ± 0.6	8.5 ± 0.7	13.4 ± 1.7	14.8 ± 1.9
T6	5.9 ± 0.7	8.3 ± 0.6	13.2 ± 1.8	14.8 ± 1.9
T11	6.7 ± 0.7	9.1 ± 0.7	14.5 ± 1.6	17.8 ± 1.9
T12	7.0 ± 0.5	9.1 ± 0.7	16.0 ± 1.7	20.1 ± 2.0

All measurements are in millimeters (mean ± standard deviation). TRV = transverse, AP = anteroposterior.
From Holsheimer J, den Boer JA, Struijk JJ, Rozeboom AR: AJNR Am J Neuroradiol 1994; 15:951–959. Used by permission.

Technique ▪

Turbo spin echo T2 (4000/168)-weighted axial images were made with a spine coil, 5-mm section thickness, and a 0.5-mm interscan gap through the cervical and thoracic spine. A dedicated spine coil was used for both sequences. The thoracic scans were repeated with the subjects prone, to assess change in cord position within the dural sac.[1]

Measurements ▪

The transverse (TRV) and anteroposterior (AP) diameters of the spinal cord and the dural sac were measured. The width of the CSF spaces ventral and dorsal to the cord were also measured. The contours of the cord and dural sac at T11 and T12 with the subjects supine were traced onto transparent film and overlaid on corresponding prone images.[1] Figure 1 shows the measurements. Table 1 lists the measurements at three cervical and three thoracic levels, including mean and standard deviation (SD). The dorsal dural space increased by 2.2 mm when subjects were scanned in the prone position at T11 and by 3.4 mm at T12.

Source ▪

Twenty-six healthy male volunteers (age range = 19 to 38 years) were examined.

REFERENCE

1. Holsheimer J, den Boer JA, Struijk JJ, Rozeboom AR: MR assessment of the normal position of the spinal cord in the spinal canal. AJNR Am J Neuroradiol 1994; 15:951–959.

▪: NORMAL SPINAL CORD IN INFANTS AND CHILDREN BY CT METRIZAMIDE MYELOGRAPHY[1]
▪ ACR Code: 341 (Cervical Spinal Cord)

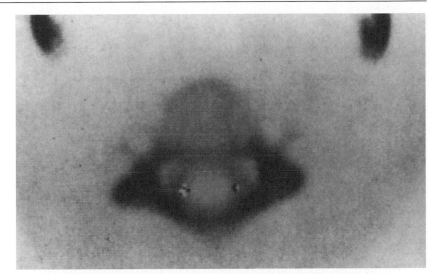

Figure 1 ▪ Diameter of the cervical cord. Transverse diameter, 11.1 mm. (From Resjo IM, et al: Radiology 1979; 130:691. Used by permission.)

Table 1 ▪ Range of Cord Measurements by Age Group (Millimeters)[1]

AGE GROUP	CERVICAL		MIDTHORACIC		CONUS	
	Sagittal Diameter	Transverse Diameter	Sagittal Diameter	Transverse Diameter	Sagittal Diameter	Transverse Diameter
0–3 mon	4.5 5	4.5–7	2.5–5	3–4	4	5
3–18 mon	5–7	7–12	4.5–6	5 7.5	5.5–7	6.5–7
1½–6 yr	7–7.5	10.5–12	5–6.5	6–7	6.5–7	6.5–9
Older than 6 yr	7.5–9	10–14	5–6.5	7–8.5	6.5–9	8–11

From Resjo IM, et al: Radiology 1979; 130:691–696.

Technique ▪

1. Technicare Delta 50 scanner, with 256 matrix and scan circles of 20 to 40 cm. Thirteen-millimeter slice collimation and table indexing 26 mm.
2. Scan localization with radiopaque ruler and anteroposterior radiograph. Most patients were scanned in the supine position.
3. Two- to 16-ml metrizamide (140- to 250-mg iodine/ ml). Head flexion and Trendelenburg position for a few minutes improved visualization about the upper cord. For CT without routine myelogram filming, a smaller amount of metrizamide is better.

Measurements (Figure 1 and Table 1) ▪

Sagittal and transverse measurements of the cord were performed with electronic calipers.

It is important to use high window-width settings and a low concentration of metrizamide to obtain the true size of the cord. Low-window settings and dense metrizamide underestimate cord size.

Source ▪

Measurements were taken from normal cords in 25 infants and children and from four children with well-localized abnormality at a distance from the normal measurements.

REFERENCE

1. Resjo IM, Harwood-Nash DC, Fitz CR, Chuang S: Normal cord in infants and children examined with computed tomographic metrizamide myelography. Radiology 1979; 130:691–696.

▪: MEASUREMENT OF THE SAGITTAL DIAMETER OF THE CERVICAL SPINAL CORD IN ADULTS[1]

▪ ACR Code: 341 (Cervical Spinal Cord)

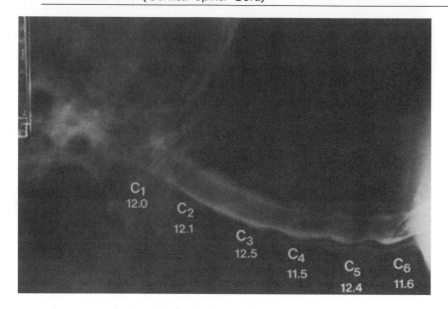

Figure 1 ▪ Myelogram indicating cord atrophy, especially at C4. (From Devkota J, et al: South Med J 1982; 75:1363. Used by permission.)

Table 1 ▪ Anteroposterior Diameter of the Normal Cervical Spinal Cord

	MEAN (2:1 MAGNIFICATION) (mm)	VARIANCE	CORRECTED (1.1:1 MAGNIFICATION) (mm)	VARIANCE	NO. PATIENTS
C1	15.94	1.94	8.767	.587	100
C2	15.72	2.21	8.646	.669	100
C3	15.07	2.48	8.288	.750	100
C4	14.54	3.90	7.997	1.180	100
C5	14.33	2.94	7.881	.889	55
C6	14.02	2.13	7.711	.774	55

Technique ▪

Metrizamide myelography:

Central ray: Centered to midcervical spine.
Position: Prone: cross-table lateral.
Target-film distance: 40 inches.

Measurements (Figure 1 and Table 1) ▪

Measurement of the anteroposterior diameters of the cervical cord were made at the middle of the posterior aspect of each vertebral body.

Source ▪

Measurements are based on 100 selected cervical myelograms of patients without long-tract signs.

REFERENCE

1. Devkota J, El Gammal T, Lucke JF: Measurement of the normal cervical cord by metrizamide myelography. South Med J 1982; 75:1363–1365.

▪: MEASUREMENT OF NORMAL CERVICAL SPINAL CORD IN ADULTS BY CT METRIZAMIDE MYELOGRAPHY[1]

▪ ACR Code: 341 (Cervical Spinal Cord)

Figure 1 ▪ *A*, Normal frontal diameter of cervical cord. Mean value ± 2 SD; n = 20. *B*, Normal sagittal diameter of cervical cord. Mean value ± 2 SD; n = 20. (From Thijssen HOM, et al: Neuroradiology 1979; 18:57. Used by permission.)

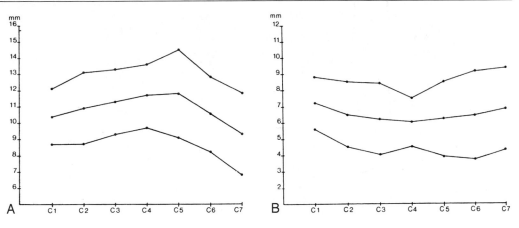

Table 1 ▪ Normal Mean Frontal and Sagittal Diameter (±2 SD) of Cervical Cord

	FRONTAL DIAMETER (mm)	SAGITTAL DIAMETER (mm)
C1	10.4 ± 1.7	7.2 ± 1.6
C2	10.9 ± 2.2	6.5 ± 2.0
C3	11.3 ± 2.0	6.2 ± 2.2
C4	11.7 ± 1.9	6.0 ± 1.5
C5	11.8 ± 2.7	6.2 ± 2.3
C6	10.5 ± 2.3	6.4 ± 2.7
C7	9.3 ± 2.5	6.8 ± 2.5

From Thijssen HOM, et al: Neuroradiology 1979; 18:57. Used by permission.

Technique ▪

1. Technicare Delta 50-FS with 13-mm slice collimation and the gantry angulation perpendicular to the longitudinal axis of the spinal column.
2. Localization with radiopaque catheters and AP radiograph made before scanning. Patients scanned in supine position.
3. Nineteen millimeters of metrizamide (170-mg iodine/ml) in the lumbar subarachnoid space. After completion of the myelogram, the patient is placed in lateral decubitus position for 1 hour to mix the cervical region.

Measurements (Table 1 and Figure 1) ▪

Transverse and sagittal diameters are measured with electronic calipers. Window level of 200 HU and window widths of 400 to 600 HU.

Source ▪

Measurements were taken of 20 patients undergoing lumbar myelography because of suspected herniated disc. There was no clinical suspicion of cervical pathology.

REFERENCE

1. Thijssen HOM, Keyser A, Horstink MW, Meijer E: Morphology of the cervical spinal cord on computed myelography. Neuroradiology 1979; 18:57–62.

▪: MEASUREMENT OF THORACIC KYPHOSIS[1]

▪ ACR Code: 32 (Thoracic Spine)

Technique ▪

Central ray: Perpendicular to plane of film centered over midchest.
Position: True lateral, standing with arms above shoulders.
Target-film distance: Immaterial.

Measurements (Figure 1; Tables 1 and 2) ▪

The upper and lower vertebral bodies defining the curve were selected and lines drawn extending along the superior border of the upper-end vertebra, as well as along the inferior border of the lower-end vertebra. Perpendiculars

Table 1 ▪ Degree of Normal Kyphosis in Males by Age

AGE (YR)	NO. CASES	KYPHOSIS (DEGREE)			
		Mean	SD	Minimum	Maximum
2–9	26	20.88	7.85	5	40
10–19	28	25.11	8.16	8	39
20–29	37	26.27	8.12	13	48
30–39	26	29.04	7.93	13	49
40–49	20	29.75	6.93	17	44
50–59	10	33.00	6.46	25	45
60–69	9	34.67	5.12	25	62
70–79	3	40.67	7.57	32	66

Table 2 ▪ Degree of Normal Kyphosis in Females by Age

AGE (YR)	NO. CASES	KYPHOSIS (DEGREE)			
		Mean	SD	Minimum	Maximum
2–9	23	23.87	6.67	8	36
10–19	22	26.00	7.43	11	41
20–29	24	26.83	7.98	7	40
30–39	26	28.42	8.63	10	42
40–49	32	32.66	6.72	21	50
50–59	17	40.71	9.88	22	53
60–69	7	44.86	7.80	34	54
70–79	6	41.67	9.00	30	56

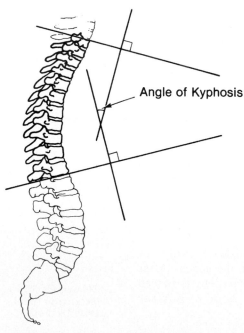

Angle of Kyphosis

Figure 1 ▪ Method of measuring kyphosis. (From Fon GT, et al: AJR Am J Roentgenol 1980; 134:979. Used by permission.)

were drawn from these two lines, and the angle was measured at the intersection.

Source ▪

Thoracic kyphosis was measured in 316 normal subjects, 159 males and 157 females, ranging in age from 2 to 77 years.

REFERENCE

1. Fon GT, Pitt MJ, Thies AC Jr: Thoracic kyphosis; Range in normal subjects. AJR Am J Roentgenol 1980; 134:979–983.

▪: MEASUREMENT OF THORACIC SPINE LENGTH ON CHEST FILMS OF NEWBORN INFANTS[1]

▪ ACR Code: 32 (Thoracic Spine)

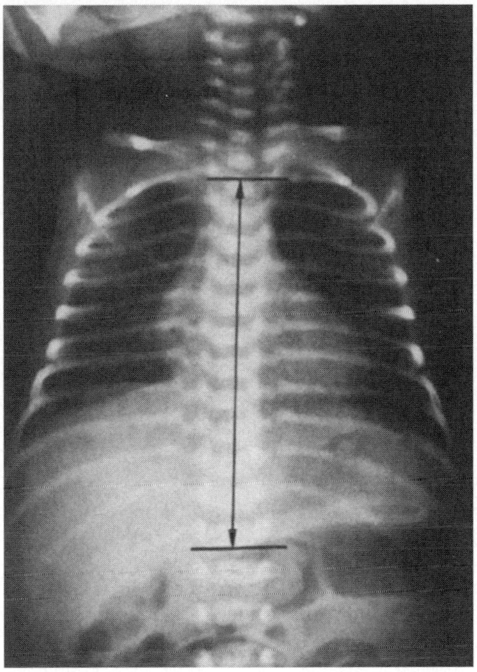

Figure 1 ▪ Measurement of thoracic spine length. (From Kuhns LR, Holt JF: Radiology 1975; 116:395.)

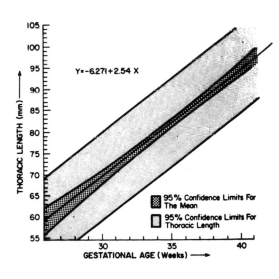

Figure 2 ▪ Plot of linear regression model of thoracic spine length and gestational age. (From Kuhns LR, Holt JF: Radiology 1975; 116:395. Used by permission.)

Technique ▪

Central ray: Perpendicular to plane of film centered over midchest.
Position: Anteroposterior, supine.
Target-film distance: 40 inches (102 cm).

Measurements (Figure 1) ▪

The length of the thoracic spine is taken as the distance from the superior edge of the first thoracic vertebra to the inferior edge of the twelfth thoracic vertebral body. Normal dimensions are shown in Figure 2. If the gestational age is known, a markedly lengthened thoracic spine suggests that the mother is diabetic, whereas a markedly shortened thoracic spine suggests retarded intrauterine growth.

Source ▪

Data based on a study of 88 normal neonates.

REFERENCE

1. Kuhns LR, Holt JF: measurement of thoracic spine length on chest radiographs of newborn infants. Radiology 1975; 116:395.

❝❞ MEASUREMENT OF THORACIC SPINE LENGTH ON CHEST FILMS FROM BIRTH TO 16 YEARS[1]

▪ ACR Code: 32 (Thoracic Spine)

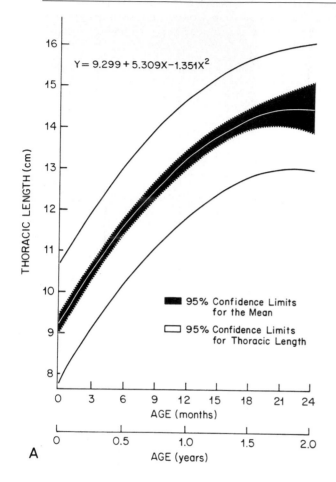

$$Y = 9.299 + 5.309X - 1.351X^2$$

95% Confidence Limits for the Mean

95% Confidence Limits for Thoracic Length

A

$$Y = 13.067 + 0.9989X$$

95% Confidence Limits for the Mean

95% Confidence Limits for Thoracic Length

B

Figure 1 ▪ *A*, Results of statistical analysis in children from birth to 2 years and *B*, in children from 2 to 16 years. The predicted values for the mean are indicated by the *center curve*, and the 95% confidence limits for the mean by the *shaded area*. The boundaries of the *unshaded area* (outside curves) denote the calculated 95% confidence limits for thoracic length for an individual child. In the equations shown in these figures, *Y* is the thoracic length in centimeters, and *X* is the age in years. (From Currarino G, Williams B, Reisch JS: Skeletal Radiol 1986; 15:628–630. Used by permission.)

Technique ▪

Central ray: Perpendicular to plane of film.
Position: Children under 2 years: supine, AP projection.
  Children over 2 years: upright, PA projection.
Target-film distance: Under 2 years: 100 cm; over 2 years:
  180 cm.

Measurement ▪

The length of the thoracic spine was measured in the frontal projection from the superior edge of the first thoracic vertebral body to the lower edge of the twelfth vertebral body.

The results of the statistical analysis of these data are shown in Figure 1.

Source ▪

Data are based on a study of 331 children from birth to 16 years without thoracic or vertebral anormalies.

REFERENCE

1. Currarino M, Williams B, Reisch JS: Linear growth of the thoracic spine in chest roentgenograms from birth to 16 years. Skeletal Radiol 1986; 15:628–630.

▪: MEASUREMENT OF NORMAL THORACIC SPINAL CORD AND SUBARACHNOID SPACE IN ADULTS BY CT METRIZAMIDE MYELOGRAPHY[1]

▪ ACR Code: 35 (Thoracic Spinal Canal and Contents)

Technique ▪

1. GE 8000 CT/T scanner. Slice thickness not stated.
2. Scan localization with scout view film. Supine or prone position for scanning.
3. Unstated volume of metrizamide (170- to 300-mg iodine/ml). A time delay between injection and scanning is not critical as long as it does not exceed 6 hours.

Trendelenburg position is used at some time before scanning to opacify the thoracic region.

Measurements (Figures 1 and 2; Table 1) ▪

Sagittal and transverse measurements of the cord and subarachnoid space are made with electronic calipers.

Window width is 1000 HU, and window level is set so

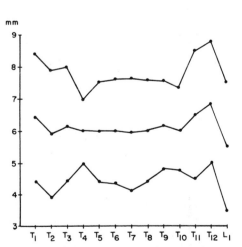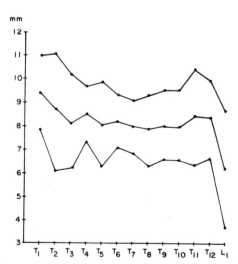

Figure 1 ▪ CT sagittal *(left)* and coronal *(right)* diameters of normal thoracic spinal cord in vivo (n = 28). *Center line* = plot of mean values at each level; *upper line* = mean + 2 SD; *lower line* = mean − 2 SD. (From Gellad F, et al: AJNR Am J Neuroradiol 1983; 4:614. Used by permission.)

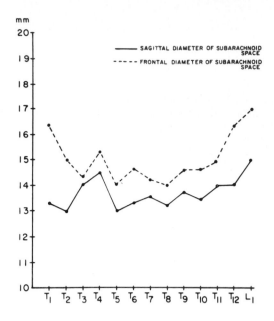

Figure 2 ▪ Mean CT sagittal and frontal diameters of normal subarachnoid space in vivo (n = 28). (From Gellad F, et al: AJNR Am J Neuroradiol 1983; 4:614. Used by permission.)

Table 1 ▪ CT Diameters (Mean ± 2 SD) of Normal Thoracic Cord and Subarachnoid Space in Vivo (n = 28)

	THORACIC CORD		SUBARACHNOID SPACE	
	Sagittal Diameter	Frontal Diameter	Sagittal	Frontal
T1	6.4 ± 2	9.4 ± 1.6	13.3 ± 2.5	16.4 ± 1.8
T2	5.9 ± 2	8.7 ± 2.5	13.0 ± 2.4	14.9 ± 2.5
T3	6.2 ± 1.8	8.2 ± 2	14.0 ± 2.8	14.1 ± 2.4
T4	6.0 ± 1	8.5 ± 1.2	14.5 ± 2.2	15.7 ± 2.5
T5	6.0 ± 1.6	8.1 ± 1.8	13.0 ± 3.4	13.9 ± 2.8
T6	6.0 ± 1.7	8.2 ± 1.1	13.3 ± 3.2	14.6 ± 2.2
T7	5.9 ± 1.8	8.0 ± 1.2	13.5 ± 3.0	14.2 ± 3.3
T8	6.0 ± 1.6	7.8 ± 1.5	13.2 ± 2.6	13.9 ± 2.7
T9	6.2 ± 1.4	8.0 ± 1.5	13.7 ± 2.8	14.5 ± 2.6
T10	6.0 ± 1.3	8.0 ± 1.5	13.4 ± 2.8	14.4 ± 2.8
T11	6.5 ± 2	8.4 ± 2	14.0 ± 3.4	14.9 ± 3.1
T12	6.8 ± 1.8	8.3 ± 1.7	14.0 ± 3.5	16.3 ± 3.4
L1	5.5 ± 2	6.2 ± 2.5	15.0 ± 3.6	17.0 ± 3.2

From Gellad F, et al: AJNR Am J Neuroradiol 1983; 4:614. Used by permission.

that densities of the cord and metrizamide lie within the gray-scale range of the viewer.

Source ▪

Measurements were taken from 28 patients with symptoms related to the cervical or lumbar spine. The mean dimensions correlate well with postmortem measurements obtained from 10 patients dying from illnesses other than spinal disease.

REFERENCE

1. Gellad F, Rao KC, Joseph PM, Vigorito RD: Morphology and dimensions of the thoracic cord by computer assisted metrizamide myelography. AJNR Am J Neuroradial 1983; 4:614–617.

▪: LUMBAR FACET ANGLES
▪ ACR Code: 33 (Lumbosacral Spine)

Technique ▪

Boden and colleagues performed axial MRI scans (machine type and sequence parameters not given) through L2–3 to L5–S1.[1] Noren and colleagues performed CT (machine type not given) of the L3–4 to L5–S1 interspaces using 4-mm slice thickness.[2] Van Schaik and colleagues did axial CT scans with a Tomoscan (Phillips Medical Systems, Irvine, CA) through L3–4 to L5 with 3- to 4.5-mm slice thickness.[3] In all three series, the scans were angled parallel to the lower end-plate at each disc level.[1–3]

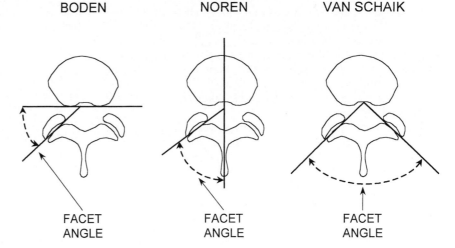

BODEN   NOREN   VAN SCHAIK

FACET ANGLE   FACET ANGLE   FACET ANGLE

Figure 1 ▪ Methods of measuring facet angles on axial scans through the lumbosacral facets. Each author's method is shown, and Boden's and Van Schaik's numbers have been normalized to Noren's method as detailed in the text.[1–3]

Table 1 ▪ **Facet Angles (with Respect to the Sagittal Plane) at L2–3 through L5–S1**

AUTHOR/CRITERIA	L2–3	L3–4	L4–5	L5–S1
Boden et al				
Number	16	66	66	63
Right angle (± SD)	31.0 ± 14.0	39.0 ± 8.9	48.0 ± 10.6	51.0 ± 10.3
Left angle (± SD)	34.0 ± 12.8	41.0 ± 10.6	50.0 ± 11.4	53.0 ± 9.5
Mean	32.5	40.0	49.0	52.0
95% confidence intervals (combined R&L)	23.5–40.8	36.8–43.4	45.4–52.4	48.6–55.5
Noren et al				
Number		46	46	35
Mean		39.6	48.4	53.9
Range		17.6–57.0	30.0–64.5	29.0–77.5
Van Schaik et al				
Number		70	71	71
Mean		37.1	48.2	53.1
Range		17.0–57.0	29.5–75.0	36.0–70.0
Combined mean	33	39	49	53
Suggested cut-off (lower)	23	36	45	48

Mean, standard deviations, 95% confidence intervals, and ranges are all given in degrees.[1–3]

Table 2 ▪ **Facet Angle Trophism in the Lumbosacral Spine**[1, 2]

AUTHOR/ CRITERIA	L2–3	L3–4	L4–5	L5–S1
Boden				
Number	16	66	66	63
50th percentile	6	7	5	6
75th percentile	10	11	8	11
95th percentile	16	15	15	18
Noren				
N > 5°/total N		11/31	20/32	13/25
(%)		(35)	(63)	(52)

Measurements ▪

In all three papers, scans through a disc level were discarded if they were not parallel to the lower end-plate, if the landmarks were not adequately visualized, or if there was significant asymmetry of morphology. The numbers of segments measured and included at each level for each paper are shown in Table 1. The measurements were made through the midfacet (mid-disc or lower end-plate level), and the method differed somewhat in each study, as is shown in Figure 1. Briefly, Boden[1] measured each facet angle with respect to a coronal line drawn through the posterior vertebral body; Noren[2] measured the facet angle with respect to a sagittal line through the vertebral body and spinous process; and Van Schaik[3] drew tangential lines through each facet and measured the angle at their inter-

section. The angles listed in Table 1 have all been normalized to the method of Noren. From Boden's work,[1] the mean angles were calculated from those given for right and left, and the standard deviations were back-calculated from the listed number of subjects and standard error of the mean. Combined means were calculated from all three series, and suggested cut-offs were taken from Boden's[1] lower 95th percentiles.

Boden and Noren and associates also calculated the difference between angles (trophism) at each disc level.[1, 2] These data are presented in Table 2. Boden's[1] trophism data are given as the cut-off angles for the upper three quartiles at each level, and Noren's[2] data are given in terms of numbers of patients having more than 5 degrees of difference at each level.

Source ▪

Boden's subjects included 67 asymptomatic adult volunteers aged from 20 to 79 years (mean age = 42 years), with the gender distribution not given.[1] Noren studied 46 patients with back pain, in age ranging from 15 to 49 years (mean age = 32.5 years). There were 23 men and 23 women.[2]

Van Schaik scanned 123 adult patients with low back problems; the age/gender parameters were not given.[3]

Comments ▪

The facet angles at each level are quite consistent between MRI and CT and among studies, with a tendency to be more sagittally oriented as one moves caudad. In general, more sagittally oriented joints (suggested cut-offs given in Table 1) were significantly associated with facet degeneration and degenerative spondylolisthesis.[1–3] Increased trophism (difference of 6 to 7 degrees or more) was significantly associated with disc herniation[1] or degeneration.[2]

References

1. Boden SD, Riew KD, Yamaguchi K, et al: Orientation of the lumbar facet joints: Association with degenerative disc disease. J Bone Joint Surg Am 1996; 78(3):403–411.
2. Noren R, Trafimow J, Andersson GB, Huckman MS: The role of facet joint tropism and facet angle in disc degeneration. Spine 1991; 16:530–532.
3. Van Schaik JP, Verbiest H, Van Schaik FD: The orientation of laminae and facet joints in the lower lumbar spine. Spine 1985; 10:59–63.

▪▪ MEASUREMENT OF THE NORMAL WEDGING OF THE DORSOLUMBAR VERTEBRAE[1]
▪ ACR Code: 32 (Thoracic Spine), 33 (Lumbosacral Spine)

Technique ▪

Central ray: Perpendicular to plane of film.
Position: Lateral.
Target-film distance: Immaterial.

Measurements (Figure 1) ▪

The heights of the anterior (*a*) and posterior (*p*) aspects were measured at a distance of 2 mm from the midpoint of the vertebral margins to avoid the edges, which are

Table 1 ▪ Degree of Vertebral Wedging in the Male and Female Groups

| | CONFIDENCE LIMITS | | | | |
VERTEBRAE	80%	90%	95%	97.5%	TOTAL
Men					
Th8	0.81	0.77	0.75	0.72	62
Th9	0.84	0.81	0.78	0.76	67
Th10	0.86	0.83	0.80	0.78	67
Th11	0.85	0.81	0.79	0.76	66
Th12	0.84	0.81	0.79	0.77	63
L1	0.86	0.84	0.82	0.80	68
L2	0.90	0.88	0.86	0.84	68
L3	0.95	0.92	0.90	0.88	67
Women					
Th8	0.86	0.84	0.82	0.80	94
Th9	0.90	0.88	0.85	0.84	95
Th10	0.91	0.89	0.87	0.85	95
Th11	0.87	0.85	0.82	0.80	94
Th12	0.89	0.87	0.85	0.84	96
L1	0.90	0.88	0.86	0.84	95
L2	0.94	0.92	0.90	0.89	95
L3	0.96	0.94	0.92	0.90	95

From Lauridsen KN, De Carvalho A, Andersen AH: Acta Radiol Diagn 1984; 25:29–32. Used by permission.

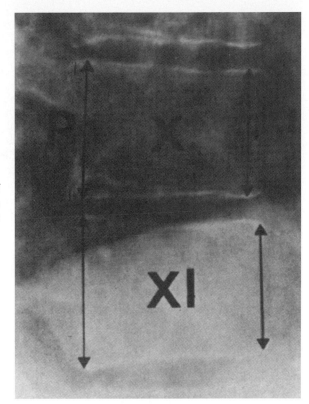

Figure 1 ▪ Degree of wedging measured as the ratio between the heights of the anterior (*a*, to the right) and the posterior (*p*, to the left) aspects. (From Lauridsen KN, De Carvalho A, Andersen AH: Acta Radiol Diagn 1984; 25:29–32. Used by permission.)

difficult to define. The mean a/p ratios were calculated and are shown in Table 1.

Source ▪

Data are based on a study of 164 persons: 96 women aged 25 to 59 years and 68 men aged 17 to 59 years. Subjects were selected at random, and those with fractures were excluded.

Reference

1. Lauridsen KN, De Carvalho A, Andersen AH: Degree of vertebral wedging of the dorso-lumbar spine. Acta Radiol Diagn 1984; 25:29–32.

▪▪ LUMBAR VERTEBRAL BODY INDEX
▪ ACR Code: 33 (Lumbosacral Spine)

Technique ▪

Saraste and colleagues studied lateral lumbar spine radiographs. Patient position and distances were not given.[1–3] Ulmer and colleagues performed MRI of the lumbo-sacral spine with a surface coil on a 1.5-T machine (manufacturer not given). Sagittal images with 4-mm spacing and T1 (600/15)-weighting were made.[4]

Measurements ▪

Using radiographs or sagittal MRI, the posterior height (PH) and anterior height (AH) of the vertebral body in

AUTHOR/STATISTIC	NORMAL	GRADE 0	GRADE I	GRADES II–IV	GRADES 0–IV
Saraste[3]					
Number	170	30	86	43	159
Mean ± SD	0.86 ± 0.06	0.84 ± 0.09	0.78 ± 0.08	0.68 ± 0.06	0.76 ± 0.10
Ulmer[4]					
Number		13	42	11	66
Mean ± SD		0.84 ± 0.09	0.75 ± 0.09	0.64 ± 0.11	0.75 ± 0.11
Range		0.68–95	0.55–1.00	0.50–0.81	0.50–1.00

Table 1 ▪ **Lumbar Index for Normal Subjects and Patients with Spondylolysis**

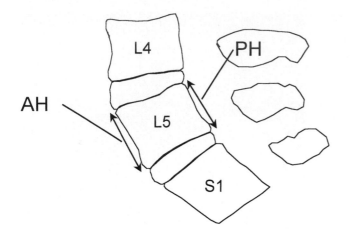

LUMBAR INDEX (LI) = PH / AH

Figure 1 ▪ Measurement of the lumbar index at L5–S1. The posterior height (*PH*) and anterior height (*AH*) of the vertebral body are measured, and a lumbar index (*LI*) is formed as shown. This method is similar for radiographs and sagittal MRI and can be done at any affected level.

question were measured, and a ratio (lumbar index = LI) was calculated as follows: LI = PH/AH. Figure 1 shows these measurements. Table 1 lists the values of the LI for normal subjects (at L5–S1) and patients with spondylolysis (mostly L5 on S1).

Source ▪

Saraste and colleagues evaluated 170 normal subjects (68 men, 102 women) and 202 patients with spondylolysis at L5–S1.[1-3] Ulmer's subjects included 64 individuals with spondylolysis at 66 levels (L5 = 59, other levels = 7). There were 16 females and 48 males, whose ages ranged from 12 to 77 years, with a mean age of 41 years.[4] In both studies, the degree of anterior subluxation (spondylolisthesis) at the affected level was graded, with Ulmer's group using a standard 0 to IV system and Saraste's group using a 0 to II scale. In both scales, 0 corresponds to no significant slippage. Saraste's grade I corresponds to the standard grade I (< 25% subluxation), and her grade II corresponds to the standard grades II to IV (> 25% subluxation). We shall use the standard convention for the severest group (II to IV).

Comments ▪

Saraste and colleagues followed their spondylolysis patients for 25 years, with repeat radiographs and clinical evaluation.[3] The LI did not change during the time of observation and was strongly correlated (p < 0.001) with the degree of subluxation at the time of diagnosis. This obtained a cut-off level of 0.75. Progression of slipping and age at time of diagnosis showed no significant differences in groups above and below an LI of 0.75.[3] Ulmer also found significant (p < 0.01) correlation between the LI and grade of spondylolisthesis.[1]

REFERENCES

1. Saraste H, Bronstrom LA, Aparisi T: Radiographic assessment of anatomic deviations in lumbar spondylolysis. Acta Radiol 1984; 25(4):317–323.
2. Saraste H, Bronstrom LA, Aparisi T: Prognostic radiographic aspects of spondylolisthesis. Acta Radiol 1984; 25:427–432.
3. Saraste H: Long-term clinical and radiological follow-up of spondylolysis and spondylolisthesis. Pediatr Orthop 1987; 7:631–638.
4. Ulmer JL, Mathews VP, Elster AD, et al: MR imaging of lumbar spondylolysis: The importance of ancillary observations. AJR Am J Roentgenol 1997; 169:233–239.

▪▪ MEASUREMENT OF THE LUMBOSACRAL ANGLE[1]
▪ ACR Code: 33 (Lumbosacral Spine)

Technique ▪

Central ray: Perpendicular to plane to film. Upright spot films of L5–S1 intervertebral space centered 1 inch below iliac crest.
Position: True lateral with patient standing.
Target-film distance: 40 inches.

Measurements (Figures 1 and 2) ▪

The line of inclination in Figure 1 is the plane of the first sacral surface. The horizontal line is drawn parallel to the bottom margin of the film.

The lumbosacral angle is φ. The mean lumbosacral angle = 41.1°. SD = 7.7°. Ninety-five percent of all values will lie between 25.7° and 56.5°.

Values in the study approximated a normal distribution.

By using the graph (Figure 2), it is possible to find the percentage of individuals above or below a given value. For example, an angle of 50° shows 92% of individuals with less than that angle and 8% greater.

When supine and standing views are compared, there is usually an increase in the lumbosacral angle of 8° to 12° in the standing position.

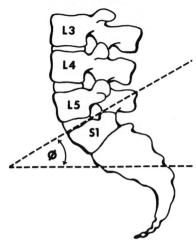

Figure 1 ▪ Measurement of the lumbosacral angle. See text for description.[1]

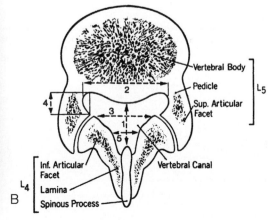

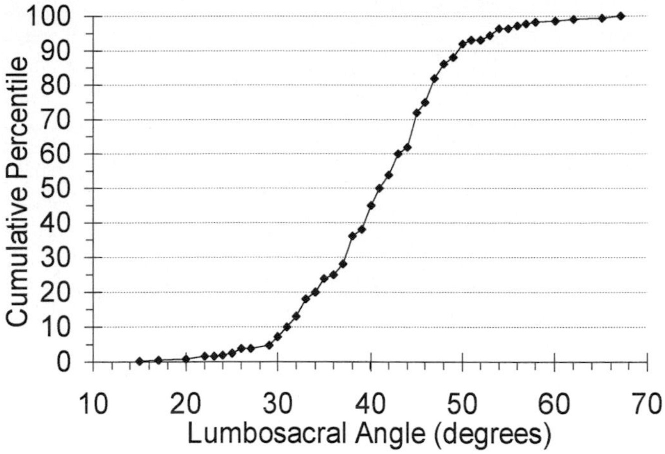

Figure 2 ▪ Cumulative percentage plot of the normal lumbosacral angle.[1]

Source ▪

Hellems and Keats used 319 normal men, ranging in age from 17 to 58 years, who had lumbosacral spine films made as part of a routine preemployment examination.

REFERENCE

1. Hellems HK, Keats TE: Measurement of the normal lumbosacral angle. AJR Am J Roentgenol 1971; 113:642–645.

▪: MEASUREMENT OF DEPTH OF THE LATERAL RECESSES OF THE LUMBOSACRAL SPINE[1]
▪ ACR: 33 (Lumbosacral Spine)

Technique ▪

1. Anteroposterior measurements corrected for magnification.
2. Measured on plain lateral radiographs, polytomograms, CT scans, and myelograms.

Measurements (Figures 1 and 2) ▪

The normal lateral recess reduces in size, proceeding from L2 to S1. The lateral recess syndrome occurred most frequently at L5–S1.

Figure 1 ▪ Measurement of the depth of the lateral recess shown on an axial CT section (*A, arrows*) and diagrammatically (*B, 4*). Some additional measurements are depicted in the diagram (*B*) and are not included herein. (From Mikhael MA, et al: *Radiology* 1981; 140:97. Used by permission.)

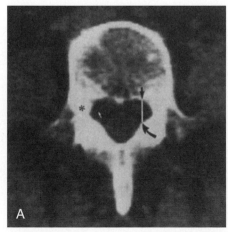

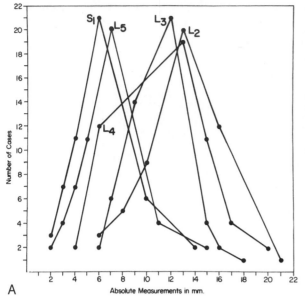

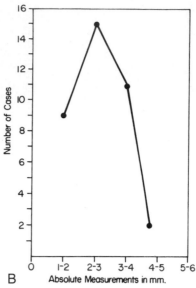

Figure 2 ▪ *A*, Normal range of the absolute depth of the lateral recess as measured on CT scans and polytomograms at L2–L5 and S1 in 50 asymptomatic patients. *B*, Absolute depth of the lateral recess as measured on CT scans and polytomograms in 35 patients with surgically proved lateral recess syndrome. (From Mikhael MA, et al: Radiology 1981; 140: 97. Used by permission.)

Source ▪

Measurements on 50 asymptomatic patients and 35 with lateral recess syndrome surgically confirmed.

Reference

1. Mikhael MA, Ciric I, Tarkington JA, Vick NA: Neuroradiological evaluation of lateral recess syndrome. Radiology 1981; 140:97–107.

▪▪ MEASUREMENT OF NORMAL INTERVERTEBRAL DISC HEIGHTS[1]
▪ ACR Code: 336 (Lumbar Intervertebral Disc)

Technique ▪

Central ray: Perpendicular to plane of film.
Position: Upright in neutral position.
Target-film distance: Measurements corrected for magnification.

Measurements (Figure 1) ▪

A nondimensional index of disc shape was calculated from the height and depth measurements to indicate how the wedged shape of the disc varied at different levels. This index was calculated as:

$$\frac{\text{Anterior disc height} - \text{Posterior disc height} \times 100\%}{\text{Disc depth}}$$

The individual measurements and disc shapes are shown in Table 1.

Table 1 ▪ True Mean Disc Heights, Depths, and Shapes for Each Level of the Lumbar Spine in the Upright Position for the 11 Normal Subjects*

LEVEL	ANTERIOR DISC HEIGHT		POSTERIOR DISC HEIGHT		DISC DEPTH		DISC SHAPE	
	Mean	Range (mm)	Mean	Range (mm)	Mean	Range (mm)	Mean	Range (%)
L1–L2	8	6–11	4	2–6	34	29–37	12	3–25
L2–L3	11	8–13†	4.5	2–6	34	29–38	19	8–25†
L3–L4	12.5	11–15	4.5	3–6	33	29–36‡	23	18–29
L4–L5	14	11–16‡	5.5	3–8	33	29–36	26	19–38
L5–S1	13	9–16	4.5	3–6‡	31	27–34†	27	14–46

*Statistically significant differences between one level and the next superior level.
† = p < 0.01.
‡ = p < 0.05.
From Tibrewal SB, Pearcy MJ: Spine 1984; 10:452–454. Used by permission.

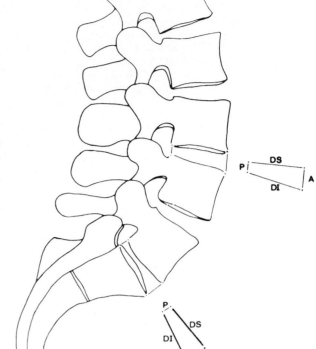

Figure 1 ▪ Tracing of a lateral radiograph of a lumbar spine in the upright position, showing the position of the marks used for taking measurements. *A* = anterior disc height; *P* = posterior disc height; *DS* = superior disc depth; *DI* = inferior disc depth. (From Tibrewal SB, Pearcy MJ: Spine 1984; 10:452–454. Used by permission.)

Source ▪

Data based on a study of 11 normal men, ranging in age from 25 to 36 years.

REFERENCE

1. Tibrewal SB, Pearcy MJ: Lumbar intervertebral disc heights in normal subjects and patients with disc herniation. Spine 1985; 10:452–454.

▪▪ MEASURED HEIGHT OF THE LUMBOSACRAL DISC WITH AND WITHOUT TRANSITIONAL VERTEBRAE[1]

▪ ACR Code: 336 (Lumbar Intervertebral Disc)

Technique ▪

Central ray: Perpendicular to plane of film.
Position: Anteroposterior and lateral horizontal.
Target-film distance: Disregarded because of differences in pelvic width.

Measurements (Figure 1) ▪

The average disc height was measured at each lumbar level between adjacent end-plates at the midpoint between the anterior and posterior margins of the vertebra. The height of the lumbosacral intervertebral disc was expressed as a proportion of the sum of the disc heights of the other four levels, and the differences are presented as 95% confidence limits.

The results are given in Table 1.

The lumbosacral intervertebral disc is significantly narrower than its counterpart in nontransitional spines. Even in normal spines the lumbosacral disc is significantly nar-

	NORMAL (46)	TRANSITIONAL (48)	SIGNIFICANCE
L1:L2	11.13 ± 1.78	10.4 ± 2	NS
L2:L3	12.21 ± 1.84	13.0 ± 2.5	NS
L3:L4	12.93 ± 2.01	12.5 ± 2	NS
L4:L5	12.98 ± 2.11*	12.0 ± 2.5	NS
L5:S1	10.37 ± 2.05*	8.2 ± 2.5	p < 0.001

Table 1 ▪ Disc Height Measurements (mm) in Normal and Transitional Lumbar Spines (mean ± sem)

*Significant difference: p < 0.001.
From Nicholson AA, et al: Br J Radiol 1988; 61:454–455. Used by permission.

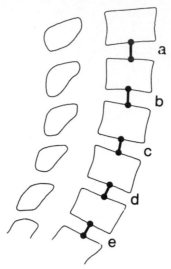

Figure 1 ▪ Disc height measurements. In the two groups of patients studied, the 95% confidence limits were derived from the formula (average e/average [a + b + c + d]) × 100. (From Nicholson AA, et al: Br J Radiol 1988; 61:454–455. Used by permission.)

rower than discs at higher levels. This narrowing does not imply disc degeneration.

Source ▪

Data are based on radiographic examination of 46 young adults with transitional vertebrae and 48 age- and gender-matched subjects without transitional segmentation. All subjects were under age 40 years.

REFERENCE

1. Nicholson AA, Roberts GM, Williams LA: The measured height of the lumbosacral disc in patients with and without transitional vertebrae. Br J Radiol 1988; 61:454–455.

▪▪ VERTEBRAL BODY AND INTERVERTEBRAL DISC INDEX (TWELFTH THORACIC TO THIRD LUMBAR)[1]
▪ ACR Code: 336 (Lumbar Intervertebral Disc)

Technique ▪

Central ray: Projected through first lumbar vertebra.
Position: True lateral projection with Bucky table.
Target-film distance: 110 cm. However, indices are independent of target-film distance.

Measurements (Figure 1; Tables 1 and 2) ▪

$$I_{vb} = \text{Vertebral body index} = \frac{v}{s} = \frac{\text{Height of vertebral body}}{\text{Sagittal diameter of vertebral body}}$$

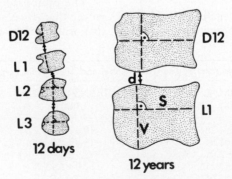

Figure 1 ▪ Measurement of the vertebral body to intervertebral disc ratio. See text for description. (Adapted from Brandner ME: AJR Am J Roentgenol 1970; 110:618. Used by permission.)

Table 1 · I_{vb} (v/s) of Vertebral Bodies

VERTEBRAL BODY	AGE GROUP	NO.	MEAN v/s
D12	0–1 mon	13	0.81
	2–18 mon	26	0.91
	19–36 mon	22	0.86
	4–12 yr (F)	18	0.86
	4–12 yr (M)	35	0.78
	13 yr and over (F)	7	0.93
	13 yr and over (M)	20	0.84
L1	0–1 mon	16	0.87
	2–18 mon (F)	11	1.02
	2–18 mon (M)	16	0.96
	2–18 mon (M & F)	27	0.98
	19–36 mon	23	0.89
	4–12 yr (F)	20	0.87
	4–12 yr (M)	40	0.80
	13 yr and over (F)	19	1.03
	13 yr and over (M)	27	0.87
L2	0–1 mon	10	0.92
	2–18 mon	21	1.01
	19–36 mon	20	0.91
	4–12 yr	49	0.82
	13 yr and over (F)	15	1.03
	13 yr and over (M)	25	0.88
L3	0–1 mon	11	0.95
	2–18 mon	17	0.98
	19–36 mon	16	0.88
	4–12 yr	35	0.79
	13 yr and over (F)	11	1.00
	13 yr and over (M)	17	0.87

F = female; M = male.
Adapted from Brandner ME. AJR Am J Roentgenol 1970; 110:618.

Table 2 · I_d (d/v) of Intervertebral Disc and Vertebral Body

VERTEBRAL SEGMENT	AGE GROUP	NO.	MEAN d/v
D11/12	0–1 mon	12	0.37
	2–18 mon	26	0.30
	19–36 mon	19	0.25
	4–12 yr	49	0.24
	13 yr and over	21	0.18
D12/L1	0–1 mon	17	0.35
	2–18 mon	27	0.28
	19–36 mon	20	0.26
	4–12 yr	53	0.25
	13 yr and over	37	0.19
L1/2	0–1 mon	15	0.35
	2–18 mon	26	0.26
	19–36 mon	19	0.27
	4–12 yr	44	0.28
	13 yr and over	37	0.20
L2/3	0–1 mon	9	0.38
	2–18 mon	18	0.28
	19–36 mon	15	0.30
	4–12 yr	32	0.30
	13 yr and over	22	0.21

Adapted from Brandner ME: AJR Am J Roentgenol 1970; 110:618.

Height is the largest vertical measurement of the body. Sagittal diameter is the smallest anteroposterior measurement of the body.

$$I_d = \text{Intervertebral disc index} = \frac{d}{v} =$$

$$\frac{\text{Intervertebral disc thickness}}{\text{Height of vertebral body}}$$

Upper disc and lower vertebral body are compared.

Note: Additional work by Brandner,[2] based on a study of adults, indicates that the intervertebral disc index *d/v* in adults is comparable to the results obtained in children.

Source ▪

Brandner studied 187 roentgenograms of dorsal and lumbar spines, from neonates to adolescents.

REFERENCES

1. Brandner ME: Normal values of the vertebral body and intervertebral disc index during growth. AJR Am J Roentgenol 1970; 110:618–627.
2. Brandner ME: Normal values of the vertebral body and intervertebral disc index in adults. AJR Am J Roentgenol 1972; 114:411–414.

▪▪ LUMBAR DISC SPACES: FARFAN RATIO
▪ ACR Code: 336 (Lumbar Intervertebral Disc)

Technique ▪

Cohn and colleagues evaluated lateral lumbar spine radiographs centered on the iliac crest with a film-screen distance of 40 inches and phototimed technique. MRI scans of the lumbar spine were done on a 1.5-T Magnetom unit (Siemens, Erlangen, Germany), with T1 (500/14–15)-weighted sagittal and axial sequences as well as turbo T2 (3500/103)-weighted sagittal and axial images.[1] Murata and colleagues performed upright lateral lumbar spine radiography (distances not given) and sagittal T2 (2000–2200/80–100) images using 1.5-T Magnetom H15 (Siemens, Erlangen, Germany) or 1.0-T SMT 100 (Shimadzu, Japan) machines.[2]

Measurements ▪

Cohn and colleagues measured the anterior disc height (ADH) and posterior disc height (PDH) at the lumbosacral junction between the respective corners of the adjacent vertebral bodies. The lumbosacral angle (LSA) was measured by drawing intersecting lines through the inferior end-plate of L5 and the superior end-plate of S1, then

Table 1 ▪ Lumbosacral Disc Space Measurements

FINDINGS AT MRI	NUMBER	POSTERIOR HEIGHT Mean ± SD	POSTERIOR HEIGHT 95% CI	ANTERIOR HEIGHT Mean ± SD	ANTERIOR HEIGHT 95% CI	LUMBOSACRAL ANGLE Mean ± SD	LUMBOSACRAL ANGLE 95% CI
Normal	35	6.8±2.7	5.9–7.7	17.3±5.2	15.5–19.0	14.6±4.1	12.6–16.7
Mild DDD	45	5.9±2.1	5.3–6.5	16.5±5.4	14.9–18.1	12.8±5.2	11.2–14.3
Severe DDD	20	4.6±2.0	3.7–5.4	14.6±5.4	12.2–16.9	12.4±5.7	10.0–14.9

SD = standard deviation, CI = confidence interval, DDD = degenerative disk disease. Measurements of heights are in millimeters and the lumbosacral angle in degrees. From Cohn EL, Maurer EJ, Keats TE, et al: Skeletal Radiol 1997; 26:161–166. Used by permission.

Table 2 ▪ Farfan Ratio Correlated with Disc Disease at MRI

RESEARCHER/ LEVEL	DISK DEGENERATION	NO.	FARFAN RATIO Mean ± SD	FARFAN RATIO 95% CI
Cohn et al			Mean ± SD	95% CI
L5–S1	Normal	35	0.57±14	0.52–0.61
	Mild	45	0.49±0.12	0.46–0.53
	Severe	20	0.42±0.14	0.36–0.48
Murata et al			Mean	Range
L3–4	Normal	7	0.57	0.49–0.65
	Mild-mod.	89	0.55	0.36–0.72
	Severe	13	0.47	0.31–0.63
L4–5	Normal	4	0.60	0.53–0.64
	Mild-mod.	82	0.60	0.38–0.81
	Severe	21	0.45	0.17–0.66
L5–S1	Normal	5	0.63	0.47–0.84
	Mild-mod.	56	0.62	0.33–0.90
	Severe	32	0.52	0.17–0.85

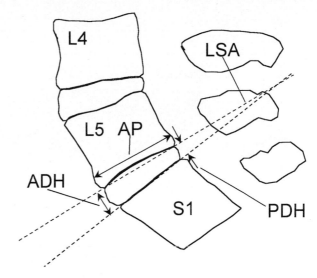

Figure 1 • Measurement of the lumbosacral disc space. Anterior disc height (*ADH*), posterior disc height (*PDH*), anteroposterior width of the L5 inferior end plate (*AP*), lumbosacral angle (*LSA*). Farfan ratio is calculated by (ADH + PDH)/AP and the technique is the same at other disc levels.

measuring the angle subtended by them.[1] Both groups measured Farfan ratio[3] at L5–S1 as follows:

$$\text{Ratio} = (ADH + PDH)/AP$$

where AP was the anterior-to-posterior width of the lower end-plate of the vertebral body.[1, 2] Murata and colleagues also measured the ratio at L3–4 and L4–5.[2] Figure 1 shows these measurements at L5–S1, and the technique is essentially the same at other levels.

Disc degeneration was evaluated visually on the MRI images of the L5–S1 interspace and graded as normal, mild, or severe in Cohn's work.[1] Murata and colleagues used a 5-step subjective grading scale for disc degeneration, with 1 being normal, 2–3 being mild-moderate, and 4–5 being severe.[2] Table 1 lists the ADH, PDH, and LSA divided into groups based on severity of disc disease as assessed by MRI.[1] Table 2 lists Farfan ratio segregated by disc level and severity of disc degeneration by MRI.[1, 2]

Source •

Cohn's subjects included 100 adult patients with low back pain or leg pain: 48 men and 52 women whose mean age was 45.5 years.[1] Murata studied 109 adult patients with low

back pain and/or sciatica: 60 men and 49 women ranging in age from 14 to 82 years, with a mean age of 48.6 years.[2]

Comments •

Cohn and colleagues determined that the PDH and Farfan ratio were significantly correlated with severity of disc disease whereas the ADH and LSA showed no significant correlation. A PDH of less than 5.5 mm on a lateral lumbar spine radiograph predicts the presence of disc degeneration whereas a PDH of more than 7.6 predicts its absence.[1] Murata and colleagues also found significant differences in Farfan ratio between groups with different degrees of disc degeneration.[2] Patients with low back symptoms and a Farfan ratio of less than .5 might benefit from MRI to evaluate the discs for degenerative changes.

REFERENCES

1. Cohn EL, Maurer EJ, Keats TE, et al: Plain film evaluation of degenerative disk disease at the lumbosacral junction. Skeletal Radiol 1997; 26:161–166.
2. Murata M, Morio Y, Kuranobu K: Lumbar disc degeneration and segmental instability: A comparison of magnetic resonance images and plain radiographs of patients with low back pain. Arch Orthop Trauma Surg 1994; 113(6):297–301.
3. Farfan HF: Mechanical Disorders of the Low Back. Lea and Febiger, Philadelphia, 1973, pp 523–526.

•: MEASUREMENT OF THE SAGITTAL DIAMETER OF THE LUMBAR SPINAL CANAL IN CHILDREN AND ADULTS[1]

■ ACR Code: 36 (Lumbosacral Spinal Canal and Contents)

Technique •

Central ray: Perpendicular to plane of film centered at level of third lumbar vertebral body.
Position: Lateral lumbar spine.
Target-film distance: 40 inches.

Measurements (Figure 1 and Table 1) •

The sagittal diameter of the spinal canal is measured at the level of each lumbar vertebra. The sagittal diameter is the shortest midline perpendicular distance from the posterior

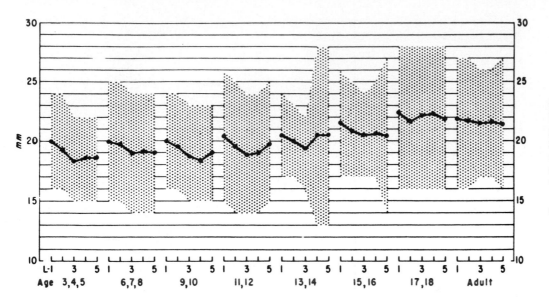

Figure 1 ▪ Age group means and 90% tolerance limits for the sagittal diameter of the spinal canal of each lumbar vertebra, male and female combined. (From Hinck VC, Hopkins CE, Clark WM: Radiology 1965; 85:929. Used by permission.)

Table 1 ▪ Age-Group Means and Standard Deviations by Gender (mm)

VERTEBRA	MALE			FEMALE			MALE			FEMALE		
	No.	Mean	SD	No.	Mean	SD	No.	Mean	SD	No.	Mean	SD
	AGE 3, 4, 5 YR						AGE 6, 7, 8 YR					
L1	15	20.3	1.8	9	19.8	1.2	14	20.3	1.9	10	19.3	2.6
2	15	19.6	1.2	9	18.9	1.4	15	19.9	1.7	9	19.5	1.6
3	15	18.4	1.4	9	18.1	1.4	15	19.1	1.8	10	18.4	1.6
4	15	18.8	1.1	9	18.0	1.5	15	19.0	1.7	10	19.1	1.8
5	14	19.0	1.6	9	17.5	1.4	15	19.0	2.4	10	19.1	2.3
	AGE 9, 10 YR						AGE 11, 12 YR					
L1	8	20.1	1.0	4	19.8	1.9	5	22.6	2.0	11	19.6	1.1
2	8	19.6	1.0	5	19.6	1.7	5	21.2	2.7	11	18.9	1.7
3	8	18.8	1.6	5	18.9	1.3	5	19.9	2.9	11	18.4	1.4
4	8	18.6	1.7	5	18.6	1.2	5	18.8	3.0	11	19.1	1.7
5	8	19.1	1.9	5	18.9	1.1	5	19.7	2.7	11	19.8	2.4
	AGE 13, 14 YR						AGE 15, 16 YR					
L1	14	20.5	1.5	10	20.8	1.4	10	21.6	2.2	18	21.6	2.2
2	14	19.7	1.4	10	20.1	0.9	11	20.8	2.1	18	20.9	1.8
3	14	18.9	1.7	10	20.0	1.3	11	20.5	1.6	18	20.7	1.6
4	14	20.4	4.1	10	20.2	2.5	11	20.0	1.7	18	21.0	2.1
5	14	20.8	4.2	10	20.1	3.2	10	20.1	2.9	18	20.8	3.4
	AGE 17, 18 YR						ADULT					
L1	11	23.9	1.9	17	21.7	1.7	22	22.2	3.1	25	21.3	2.3
2	11	22.4	2.3	17	21.3	1.9	23	22.3	2.7	26	21.2	2.1
3	12	22.6	2.3	18	22.0	3.1	23	21.7	2.6	26	21.3	2.1
4	12	22.9	2.8	18	21.9	2.6	23	21.8	2.4	26	21.3	1.9
5	12	22.6	3.4	18	21.4	2.2	21	22.6	2.7	25	20.4	2.4

From Hinck VC, Hopkins CE, Clark WM: Radiology 1965; 85:929. Used by permission.

surface of the vertebral body to the inner surface of the neural arch.

Source ▪

Films were selected on the basis of readability, and an attempt was made to eliminate subjects who showed significant anomalies and other problems likely to influence growth and development. The number of subjects in each group is shown in Table 1.

REFERENCE

1. Hinck VC, Hopkins CE, Clark WM: Sagittal diameter of the lumbar spinal canal in children and adults. Radiology 1965; 85:929.

▪: MEASUREMENT OF THE LUMBAR SPINAL CANAL FOR DETECTION OF THE NARROW SPINAL CANAL[1]

- ▪ ACR Code: 36 (Lumbosacral Spinal Canal and Contents)

Technique ▪

Central ray: Perpendicular to plane of film centered over the midlumbar spine.
Position: Anteroposterior and lateral.
Target-film distance: Immaterial.

Measurements (Figure 1) ▪

Measurements of the canal are related proportionately to the size of the adjacent vertebra. The AP measurement of the canal is made on the lateral projection and is taken from the middle of the posterior edge of the vertebral body to the base of the spinous process. The transverse measurement, taken from the frontal film, is the interpedicular distance.

Measurement of the vertebral body is made from the midpoint of the lateral margin of the vertebral body in the AP film and between the midpoints of the anterior and posterior surfaces of the vertebral body in the lateral projection.

The AP canal measurement is multiplied by the interpedicular distance and is used as the numerator in a ratio, with product of AP and transverse diameters of the vertebral body as the denominator.

The total range of normals was found to be:

L3 and L4: 1:3.0 to 1:6.0
L5: 1:3.2 to 1:6.5

The higher values represent narrower lumbar spine canals.

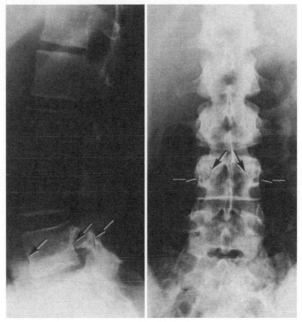

Figure 1 ▪ Measurement of the normal lumbar spinal canal. (From Williams RM: Australas Radiol 1975; 19:356. Used by permission.)

Source ▪

Data based on a study of 100 Australian patients.

REFERENCE

1. Williams RM: The narrow lumbar spinal canal. Australas Radiol 1975; 19:356–360.

▪: MEASUREMENTS OF LUMBAR SPINAL CANAL BY CT IN NORMAL ADULTS[1]

- ▪ ACR Code: 36 (Lumbosacral Spinal Canal and Contents)

Technique ▪

1. CT was performed on Ohio Nuclear 50-FS with 18-second scan time, 13-mm collimation, and 36- or 42-cm scan circle diameter displayed on 256 × 256 matrix.
2. *Measurements:* Directly on the CT video display using computer functions. Images were enlarged four times for cursor placement.

Measurements (Figures 1 and 2) ▪

Each vertebral level was divided into four major zones: upper, middle, and lower vertebral body, and disc space.

Anteroposterior spinal cord and interpedicular diameters were measured with the typical window of 800 HU and the lower window limit at the bone–soft tissue interface value of 115 HU. Electronic calipers measured the diameter.

Spinal canal cross-sectioned areas were outlined with an irregular region of interest, using the windows set in paragraph 2. Windows were reset with the upper limit of 115 HU and number of pixels within the region of interest less than the limit totaled. Multiplying this total by known area per pixel yields the cross-sectional area of the spinal canal. Figure 1 gives normal spinal canal measurements.

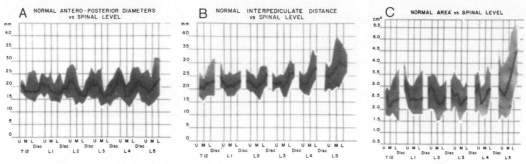

Figure 1 ▪ (From Ullrich CG, et al: Radiology 1980; 134:137. Used by permission.)

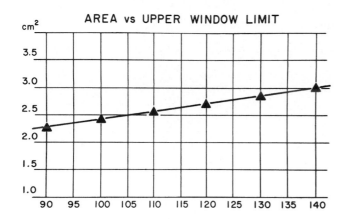

Figure 2 ▪ Variation of calculated cross-sectional area with change in the upper window limit. By selecting progressively higher upper window limits, progressively larger calculated areas are obtained. This is because the higher upper window limit allows more pixels to fall within the window and be counted. Data from four different images of the same vertebral body were plotted, and the best straight line was drawn using the least squares linear regression method (correlation coefficient: 0.84). (From Ullrich CG, et al Radiology 1980; 134:137. Used by permission.)

Note that cross-sectional area measurements are directly related to the setting of the upper window limits, and 115 HU gave a "true canal area" on a spinal phantom.

Source ▪

Thirty men 18 to 74 years of age and 30 women 27 to 74 years of age, who were undergoing abdominal CT studies for other reasons. Anteroposterior radiographs and CT scans were normal. Minor degenerative changes were allowed if there was no encroachment upon the spinal cord.

REFERENCE

1. Ullrich CG, Binet EF, Sanecki MG, Kieffer SA: Quantitative assessment of the lumbar spinal canal by computed tomography. Radiology 1980; 134:137–143.

▪▪ LUMBAR SAGITTAL CANAL RATIO FOR SPONDYLOLISTHESIS
▪ ACR Code: 36 (Lumbosacral Spinal Canal and Contents)

Technique ▪

Sagittal MRI images (machine type not given) were done with surface coils at 1.5 T, 5-mm section thickness without gap, and T1 (600/15)-weighting.[1] A subset of patients (with spondylolisthesis) had CT and/or conventional radiography with oblique views to assess the pars inarticularis. Conventional radiography was also done on all control subjects.

Measurements ▪

The lumbar canal width was measured on the midsagittal image by drawing a line parallel and tangent to the posterior margin of each lumbar veterbral body. A second line was drawn, parallel to the first, at the most anterior aspect of the corresponding lamina. The distance between these lines (in millimeters) was taken to be the lumbar canal width. The ratio of the measurement at each level, divided by that at L1, was calculated and termed the sagittal canal ratio (SCR). Figure 1 shows these measurements at L1 and L5, and the SCR for L5 would be the L5 sagittal diameter divided by the L1 sagittal diameter (shown to be 1 in this illustration). Table 1 gives the normal sagittal diameters and the SCR at each lumbar level. Measurements in isthmic and degenerative spondylolisthesis are also shown. Figure 2 depicts patients with degenerative and isthmic spondylolisthesis at L5–S1.

Source ▪

The study included 53 patients with CT (n = 14) or plain film (n = 48) evidence of isthmic (n = 35, 26 men, 9 women, age range, 17 to 78 years) or degenerative (n = 18, 3 men, 15 women, age range, 42 to 83 years) spondylolisthesis of the lower lumbar spine (n = 22) or the lumbosacral junction (n = 34). One hundred age-matched (range 18 to 84 years) control subjects with radiographic evidence of normal pars inarticularis at all levels were examined with MRI.

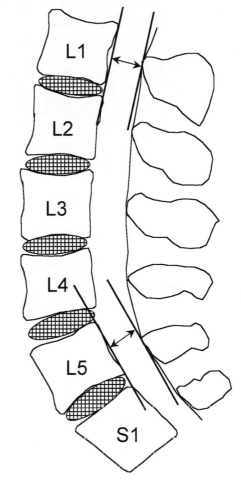

Figure 1 ▪ Measurement of the anteroposterior diameter of the lumbar spinal canal on midsagittal MR images. Measurements at L1 and L5 are shown and the same method is used at each level. The sagittal canal ratio is simply the diameter at the level in question divided by that at L1.

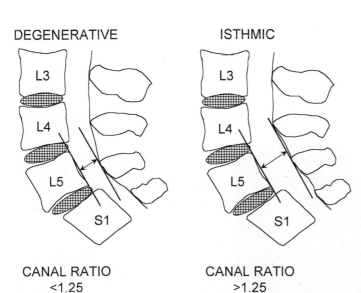

Figure 2 ▪ Drawing of midsagittal images of the lumbosacral junction with degenerative and isthmic spondylolisthesis at L5–S1. Note the "wide canal sign" of the isthmic variety (SCR > 1.25) at the level of the pars inarticularis defects.

Table 1 ▪ Lumbar Spinal Canal Measurements in Normal Subjects and Spondylolisthesis

GROUP/LEVEL NORMAL (n = 100)	AP DIAMETER (mm)		SAGITTAL CANAL RATIO	
	Mean ± SD	Range	Mean ± SD	Range
L1	17 ± 1.5	13–21	1.00	
L2	16 ± 1.5	12–20	0.95 ± 0.05	0.87–1.06
L3	16 ± 1.6	12–20	0.93 ± 0.07	0.77–1.14
L4	16 ± 2.3	12–21	0.96 ± 0.08	0.83–1.24
L5	17 ± 2.0	13–22	0.99 ± 0.10	0.78–1.25
Spondylolisthesis				
Degenerative (n = 18)			1.00 ± 0.13	0.75–1.20
Isthmic (n = 35)			1.56 ± 0.20	1.13–2.00

From Ulmer JL, Elster AD, Mathews VP, King JC: AJR Am J Roentgenol 1994; 163(2):411–416. Used by permission.

Comments ▪

Although the pars defect of isthmic spondylolisthesis often can be seen on MRI, it may be missed owing to several factors, as was true in 10% of cases in this study that involved expert neuroradiologists. At L4 or L5 (where more than 90% of spondylolisthesis occurs), an SCR of greater than 1.25 is 97% sensitive and 100% specific in detecting isthmic spondylolisthesis. There were no cases of spondylolisthesis at L2–3 and L4–5, but the expected SCR cut-offs would be 1.07 and 1.15, respectively.

REFERENCE

1. Ulmer JL, Elster AD, Mathews VP, King JC: Distinction between degenerative and isthmic spondylolisthesis on sagittal MR images: Importance of increased anteroposterior diameter of the spinal canal ("wide canal sign"). AJR Am J Roentgenol 1994; 163(2):411–416.

▪: MEASUREMENT OF THE NORMAL SACRAL SAC IN ADULTS[1]
▪ ACR Code: 36 (Lumbosacral Spinal Canal and Contents)

Technique ▪

Myelography with only contrast agent:

Central ray: Perpendicular to plane of film.
Position: Anteroposterior and lateral erect.
Target-film distance: 45 cm. Magnification for lateral views is 1.25 to 1.30 and for AP views is 1.30 to 1.36.

Measurements (Figure 1 and Table 1) ▪

An interpedicular line was drawn between the midpoints of the medial borders of the pedicles of the first sacral segment. A line at right angles to this was taken as perpendicular. The width of the sac was measured at the mid-point between the interpedicular line and the tip of the sac (b).

On the lateral view, the upper margin of the body of the first sacral segment was projected backward to the posterior margin of the vertebral canal. A line was drawn at right angles to the tip of the sac. Measurements were made of the distance along this line from the upper border of the sacrum to the tip of the sacral sac (Y). The sagittal diameter was measured at the midpoint of the line between

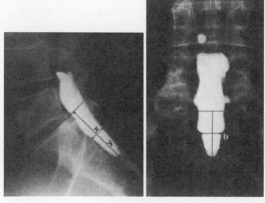

Figure 1 ▪ Points of measurement of sacral sac. (From Evison G, et al: Br J Radiol 1979; 52:777. Used by permission.)

Table 1 ▪ Measurements of Sacral Sac

	AP VIEW: WIDTH AT THE MIDPOINT			LATERAL VIEW: SAGITTAL DIAMETER			SACRAL LEVEL OF TERMINATION			
	<1 cm	1–2 cm	>2 cm	<1 cm	1–2 cm	>2 cm	S1	S2	S3	S4
n	1	99	60	6	137	17	28	111	20	1
%	0.6	61.9	37.5	3.8	85.6	10.6	17.5	69.4	12.5	0.6

From Evison G, et al: Br J Radiol 1979; 52:777. Used by permission.

the upper border of the sacrum and the tip of the sac (X).

Source ▪

Based on myelograms of 335 patients.

REFERENCE

1. Evison G, Windsor P, Duck F: Myelographic features of the normal sacral sac. Br J Radiol 1979; 52:777–780.

▪▪ LEVEL OF THE CONUS MEDULLARIS
▪ ACR Code: 361 (Conus Medullaris)

Technique ▪

Wilson and Prince performed MRI scans of the lower thoracic and lumbar spine with 0.5-T S5 Gyroscan (Philips, Shelton, CT), 1.5-T S15 Gyroscan (Philips, Shelton, CT), or 1.5-T Signa (General Electric, Milwaukee, WI) machines. Sagittal images were done with T1-weighting (350–600/20–30) and 3-mm or 5-mm slice thickness. Coronal images were also obtained with T1-weighting (same parameters as sagittal) in some subjects.[1] DiPietro performed real time ultrasound over the spine with 5.0- or 7.5-MHz linear array transducers (Acuson, Mountain View, CA or Acoustic Imaging, Phoenix, AZ) in the longitudinal and transverse planes.[2]

Measurements ▪

On MRI scans, the level of the conus medullaris was located with respect to the lumbosacral junction (assuming five lumbar levels in each case). The intervertebral disc or midpoint of a vertebral body closest to the conus tip was taken to be the level and recorded.[1] Longitudinal ultrasound was used to mark the level of the conus on the skin in infants (less than 3 months of age) with incomplete ossification of the posterior elements. After ossification, transverse ultrasound scans through the disc levels were used to locate and mark the conus level. If the conus tip could not be seen at a disc space, the level was taken to be between the space where cord and cauda equina were visible. A metallic marker was secured to the skin prior to the radiographic study. The conus was also related to the lowest rib for determination of the vertebral level by ultrasound alone. Subsequent anteroposterior radiographs were used to establish the vertebral level of the conus by means of locating the metallic marker.[2]

Figure 1 shows the mean and range of the conus level at MRI for each age group.[1] Figure 2 shows the mean and range of the level of the conus marked with ultrasound and determined by radiograph for various ages.[2]

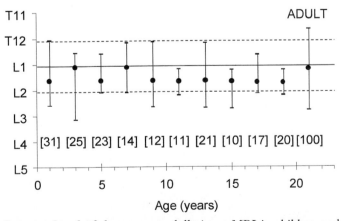

Figure 1 ▪ Level of the conus medullaris on MRI in children and young adults. The mean (*solid circle*) and range (*error bars*) of the vertebral level where the conus is found for each age is indicated. The number of subjects for each age group is given in brackets. The overall mean (*solid line*) and range (*dashed lines*) are also shown. (From Wilson DA, Prince JR: AJR Am J Roentgenol 1989; 152:1029–1032. Used by permission.)

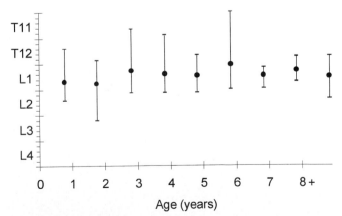

Figure 2 ▪ Level of the conus medullaris at ultrasound. The mean (*solid circle*) and range (*error bars*) at each age group are shown. (From DiPietro MA: Radiology 1993; 188:149–153. Used by permission.)

Source •

Wilson's subjects were 184 infants, children, and adolescents (92 females and 92 males) ranging in age from 5 days to 20 years. The patients were scanned for various reasons (99 for possible tethered cord), and all had their scans interpreted as being normal by the radiologist of record. An additional group of young adults (37 women and 63 men) with normal scans was included. The ages ranged from 21 to 40 years, with a mean age of 32 years.[1] DiPietro scanned 161 children (117 girls and 44 boys) ranging in age from 4 days to 13 years, with a mean age of 3 years 7 months. These patients were all scheduled to have radiographic studies of the abdomen and were recruited for the ultrasound study prior to their procedure.[2]

Comments •

Ultrasound was able to depict the conus in 161 of 163 (98.7%) infants and children, and determination of its position by ultrasound alone was within 1 vertebral level in 90% and within 1.5 levels in 97% compared to the concurrent radiograph.[2]

REFERENCES

1. Wilson DA, Prince JR: MR imaging determination of the location of the normal conus medullaris throughout childhood. AJR Am J Roentgenol 1989; 152:1029–1032.
2. DiPietro MA: The conus medullaris: Normal US findings throughout childhood. Radiology 1993; 188:149–153.

CHAPTER 5

Upper Extremity

:: MEASUREMENT OF THE ACROMIOHUMERAL DISTANCE[1]

- ACR Code: 41 (Shoulder Girdle and Arm)

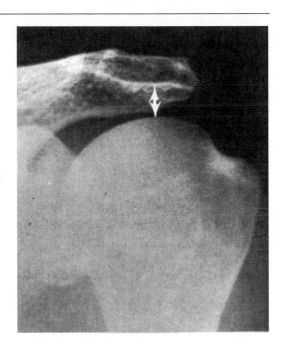

Figure 1 ▪ Acromiohumeral distance measurement. (From Alexander C: Proc Coll Radiol Aust 1959; 3:102. Used by permission.)

Technique ▪

Central ray: Perpendicular to the plane of the film centered over the humeral head.
Position: Anteroposterior: arm in adduction and neutral rotation.
Target-film distance: 36 inches.

Measurements (Figure 1) ▪

The measured distance is the minimum one between the inferior surface of the acromion tangential to the x-ray beam and the articular cortex of the humerus.

The range of normal measurement is 7 to 11 mm; the mean distance is 9.3 mm. A reduction of distance below 7 mm is believed to be a reliable indication of degenerative disease of the supraspinatus tendon.

Source ▪

Measurements were made in 53 shoulders that showed no clinical evidence of rotator cuff abnormality or bursitis.

REFERENCE

1. Alexander C. Proc Coll Radiol Aust 1959; 3:102.

▪: MEASUREMENT OF THE ACROMIOCLAVICULAR JOINT[1]
▪ ACR Code: 413 (Acromioclavicular Joint)

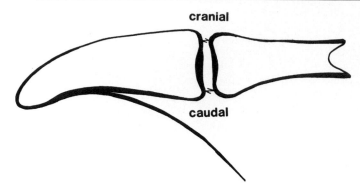

Figure 1 ▪ Cranial and caudad measuring sites for the acromioclavicular joint. (From Petersson CJ, Redlund-Johnell I: Acta Orthop Scand 1983; 54:431. Used by permission.)

Table 1 ▪ Acromioclavicular Joint Space in Various Measuring Sites			
	CRANIAL	CAUDAD	INTEGRAL
Men	3.8 ± 1.0	2.7 ± 0.6	3.3 ± 0.8
Women	3.5 ± 1.0	2.4 ± 0.6	2.9 ± 0.8
Common	3.7 ± 1.0	2.6 ± 0.6	3.1 ± 0.8

Measurements in millimeters, average ± 1 SD.
From Petersson CJ, Redlund-Johnell I: Acta Orthop Scand 1983; 54:431. Used by permission.

Technique ▪

Central ray: Perpendicular to the plane of the film, centered over the shoulder.
Position: Anteroposterior, with the patient supine.
Target-film distance: 110 cm.

Measurements (Figure 1) ▪

The joint space is measured at the superior and inferior borders, and an average of the two measurements made. Normal measurements are shown in Table 1.

There is no right-left difference in either gender. The joint space is wider in men than in women, and in both men and women there is a reduction in joint space with age.

Source ▪

One hundred fifty-one images were reviewed, 75 of men and 76 of women. There were 10 to 11 patients in each 10-year group between ages 20 and 90 years.

REFERENCE

1. Peterson CJ, Redlund-Johnell I: Radiographic joint space in normal acromioclavicular joints. Acta Orthop Scand 1983; 54:431–433.

▪: SCAPULAR CLAVICULAR RELATIONSHIPS
▪ ACR Code: 41 (Shoulder Girdle and Arm)

Technique ▪

Anteroposterior (AP) radiographs that included both shoulders, with the beam centered on the jugular vein, were performed using a film-focus distance of 2 meters.[1] Films were taken in neutral position, with the shoulders relaxed and with hanging wrist weights. The weights were 5.0 kg when the subject's body weight was below 75 kg and 7.5 kg when the body weight was 75 kg or more.

Measurements ▪

Five different linear measurements between various parts of the scapula and clavicle were made from each radiograph (Figure 1). Two radiologists performed all measurements from each film.[1] Table 1 lists the mean and standard deviation (SD) for the measured distances in all 56 joints without stress. The mean distances from 32 joints at two measurement locations, as well as the acromioclavicular joint space, are given with and without stress (hanging weights).

Source ▪

The study population consisted of 28 healthy volunteers (gender not given) whose age ranged from 21 to 33 years (mean age 27 years). All subjects (56 joints) had nonstress views and 16 (32 joints) had acceptable stress views.

Comments ▪

Stress caused the lateral portion of the clavicle (measurement *B* in Figure 1) to be depressed, probably reflecting

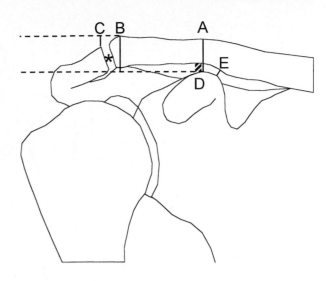

Figure 1 • Measurement of five distances between the clavicle and scapular structures, as well as the acromioclavicular (AC) joint space. *A* is the distance between the coracoid and the upper clavicle. *B* is the distance between the upper lateral clavicle and a line projected from the coracoid. *C* is the distance between the upper aspects of the acromion and the clavicle. *D* is the vertical distance between the coracoid and the lower clavicle. *E* is the shortest distance between the coracoid and the clavicle. The AC joint space *(asterisk)* was also measured. (From Vaatainen U, Pirinen A, Makela A: Skeletal Radiol 1991; 20(2):115–116. Used by permission.)

Table 1 • Normal Scapula-Clavicle Relationships

DESCRIPTION	LOCATION ON FIGURE 1	ALL SHOULDERS (n = 56) (mean ± SD)	NONSTRESS (n = 32) (mean)	STRESS (n = 32) (mean)
Coracoid—upper clavicle (vertical)	A	21.31 ± 0.36	21.81	22.61
Coracoid—upper clavicle (lateral)	B	20.66 ± 0.29	21.46	20.81
Upper acromion—upper clavicle	C	8.45 ± 0.28	—	—
Coracoid—lower clavicle (vertical)	D	8.16 ± 0.31	—	—
Coracoid—lower clavicle (shortest)	E	8.33 ± 0.17	—	—
Acromioclavicular joint space	Asterisk	—	3.56	4.12

All measurements are in millimeters. SD = standard deviation.[1]

postural changes. The coracoid to upper clavicle distance (measurement *A* in Figure 1) seemed to be the least affected by projection errors and had the smallest differences between the two radiologists' measurements. The researchers suggest that a stress-induced change in this distance of more than 3.0 mm is abnormal. As far as the acromiocla- vicular joint space itself is concerned, a distance exceeding 6.5 mm was considered to be abnormal.[1]

REFERENCE

1. Vaatainen U, Pirinen A, Makela A: Radiological evaluation of the acromioclavicular joint. Skeletal Radiol 1991; 20(2):115–116.

•: AXIAL RELATIONSHIPS OF THE SHOULDER[1]
- ACR Code: 414 (Shoulder Joint)

Technique •

Central ray: Perpendicular to the plane of the film centered over the shoulder.
Position: Anteroposterior: external rotation (anatomic posi- tion) for axial angle; internal or external rotation for joint space.
Target-film distance: 36–40 inches for joint space. Immaterial for axial angle.

Measurements (Figure 1) •

Axial angle:

AB: Axis of the shaft is drawn between two points, each measured to lie in the midline of the diaphysis.
CD: Axis of the head is drawn between the apex of the greater tuberosity to the junction of the shaft with the distal extremity of the articular surface of the head (the point where the medial cortex changes from a band to a line).

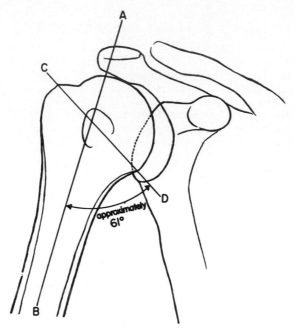

Figure 1 ▪ Axial angle. Average for adult females, 62°. Average for adult males, 60°.

Source ▪

Data on the axial angle were derived from a study of 50 normal subjects, equally divided between men and women and ranging in age from 17 to 72 years.

REFERENCE

1. Keats TE, Teeslink R, Diamond AE, Williams JH: Normal axial relationships of the major joints. Radiology 1966; 87:904–907.

▪: MEASUREMENT OF THE JOINT SPACE OF THE SHOULDER[1]
▪ ACR Code: 414 (Shoulder Joint)

Technique ▪

Central ray: Perpendicular to the plane of the film centered over the shoulder.
Position: Anteroposterior with patient supine, arm in zero adduction and outward rotation.
Target-film distance: 110 cm.

Measurements (Figure 1) ▪

The projection of the joint surface to the humeral head forms a half-circle, the diameter of which is the line joining the two terminal points of the joint surface projection. The midpoint of this line is determined with a ruler. With the ruler aimed at this point and perpendicular to the joint surface of the head of the humerus, the joint space is measured at three sites: *a*, *b*, and *c*. Point *a* is the superior edge of the glenoid surface and point *c* the inferior edge. Point *b* is the midpoint. The three measurements are averaged.

The average was found to be between 4 and 5 mm. The value does not change with age, except in women, in whom it increases slightly.

Source ▪

A total of 175 images were reviewed, 88 of men and 87 of women. There were 10 to 11 patients in each 10-year age group between 10 and 90 years of age.

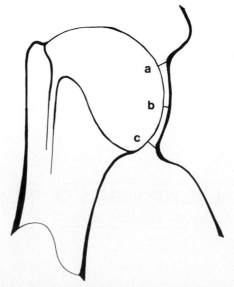

Figure 1 ▪ Measuring technique. (From Petersson CJ, Redlund-Johnell I: Acta Orthop Scand 1983; 54:274. Used by permission.)

REFERENCE

1. Petersson CJ, Redlund-Johnell I: Joint space in normal gleno-humeral radiographs. Acta Orthop Scand 1983; 54:274–276.

▪: LOCATION OF HILL-SACHS LESION AND ANATOMIC GROOVE ON THE HUMERAL HEAD

▪ ACR Code: 415 (Proximal End of Humerus)

Technique ▪

Axial MRI was performed of the shoulder with T1-weighted (parameters not given) sequences and 3- to 4-mm section thickness, using a variety of machines.[1]

Measurements ▪

A circular reference frame was constructed over the humeral head on the section showing the longest-length articular surface (usually 12- to 16- mm distal to the proximal humeral tip). The anterior margin of the articular surface was defined as 0 degrees and the posterior margin as 180 degrees. This scale was superimposed over the more cephalic and caudal images to define the position of the midpoint (in degrees) and extent (in degrees of arc) of the Hill-Sachs defect (HSD) and the normal anatomic groove (NAG) in the posterior humeral head. Additionally, the depth of the HSD or NAG and the distance between its upper extent and the proximal tip of the humeral head was measured.[1] Figures 1 and 2 show the measurements and Table 1 lists the results.

Source ▪

Normal subjects consisted of 17 men and 4 women volunteers ranging in age from 28 to 53 years (mean age 38 years). Patients with arthroscopically proved Hill-Sachs lesions were also studied. These were all men (n = 28) ranging in age from 19 to 44 years with an average age of 25 years.[1]

Comments ▪

All 21 asymptomatic volunteers and 27 of 28 patients with HSD exhibited the NAG on axial T1-weighted shoulder MRI. It is important to differentiate a true HSD from the ubiquitous NAG, as the former predicts 33% increased risk of subsequent shoulder dislocation. The researchers found a significant difference in the radial position (in degrees) of the midpoints of the two types of indentations ($p < .001$), with the NAG occurring more posteriorly than the HSD. However, there was considerable overlap in the ranges. There was no significant difference in the depth or width of the HSD or NAG. The most reliable means of distin-

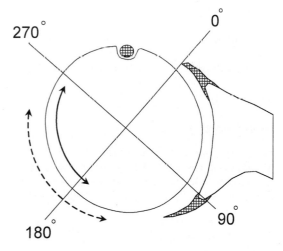

Figure 1 ▪ Measurement of the position of Hill-Sachs defects (HSD) and normal anatomic grooves (NAG) in the humeral head. A radial reference frame is constructed on the axial MRI slice, showing the longest-length humeral articular surface by defining 0 degrees as the anterior articular margin, as shown. The range of positions of each are shown, with the HSD being from 170 to 260 degrees (*solid arc*) and the NAG lying between 140 and 230 degrees (*dashed arc*). (From Richards RD, Sartoris DJ, Pathria MN, Resnick D: Radiology 1994; 190:665–668. Used by permission.)

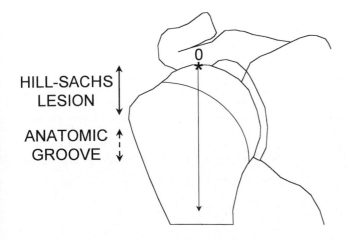

Figure 2 ▪ Measurement of the position of Hill-Sachs defects (HSD) and normal anatomic grooves (NAG) along the long axis of the humerus. Zero mm is defined as the proximal tip of the humeral head (*asterisk*). The approximate ranges of locations of the upper margins of the HSD (*solid line*) and NAG (*dashed line*) are shown. (From Richards RD, Sartoris DJ, Pathria MN, Resnick D: Radiology 1994; 190:665–668. Used by permission.)

Table 1 ▪ Data for MR Imaging of Hill-Sachs Lesions and Normal Anatomic Grooves

PARAMETER	HILL-SACHS LESION		ANATOMIC GROOVE	
	Mean	Range	Mean	Range
Arc midpoint (degrees)	209 ± 14	170–260	183 ± 10	140–230
Arc length (degrees)	52 ± 13	30–85	53 ± 11	—
Proximal endpoint (mm)	1.0 ± 2.0	0–18	24.9 ± 3.4	20–38
Depth (mm)	4	2–6	3	—

guishing the two is in the position of the upper margin along the long axis of the humerus (p < .001). The HSD usually will be found on the uppermost (21/28 = 75%) slice with all the remaining lesions on the next slice down, whereas the NAG will be found on more caudal sections.[1]

REFERENCE

1. Richards RD, Sartoris DJ, Pathria MN, Resnick D: Hill-Sachs lesions and normal humeral groove: MR imaging features allowing their differentiation. Radiology 1994; 190:665–668.

▪▪ BICIPITAL GROOVE AND TENDON
▪ ACR Code: 415 (Proximal End of Humerus)

Technique ▪

Bicipital groove radiographs were made with the subject supine and the shoulder in maximal external rotation and adducted. The cassette was placed above the shoulder perpendicular to the long axis of the humerus. The x-ray beam is directed cephalad parallel to the humerus in the coronal plane and angled 15 degrees medially.[1,2] Cadaver specimens were radiographed in the same orientation.[1] Ultrasound of the biceps tendon was done with high frequency linear transducers and scanning done perpendicular to the long axis of the tendon. The transducer may be angled up and down to best visualize the tendon as an echogenic circle or ellipse.[3] Figure 1 shows the radiographic positioning.

Measurements ▪

From radiographs, the angle of the medial wall of the groove with respect to the superior margins of the tuberosities, the width of the top of the groove, and the depth of the groove were measured.[1,2] These measurements are shown in Figure 2. The thickness of the biceps tendon was measured with electronic calipers from frozen ultrasound images, as shown in Figure 3.[3] Table 1 lists the angle and linear dimensions of the biceps groove measured from radiographs, and Table 2 lists the ultrasound-derived thickness of the biceps tendon bilaterally.

Source ▪

Cone and colleagues evaluated 100 radiographs made from adult patients with shoulder symptoms and no radiologic or clinical evidence of biceps abnormality, as well as 54 cadaver specimens.[1] Levinsohn and Santelli measured radiographs made during shoulder arthrography of 55 adults. Of these, seven had medial dislocation of the biceps tendon at arthrography.[2] Van Holsbeeck and Introcaso performed ultrasound of the biceps tendon on 96 adults separated by lifestyle (sedentary or athletic) and gender.[3]

Comments ▪

Levinsohn and Santelli state that a medial angle measured from the biceps groove radiograph of 30 degrees or less is

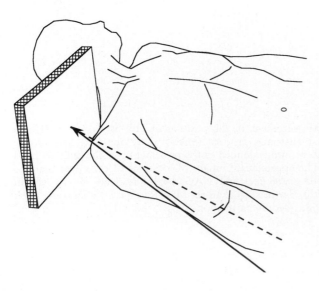

Figure 1 ▪ Positioning for a bicipital groove radiograph. The cassette is positioned above the shoulder perpendicular to the humerus. The shoulder is externally rotated and adducted. The x-ray beam *(arrow)* is parallel to the long axis of the humerus (in the coronal plane) and directed medially by 15 degrees.[1,2]

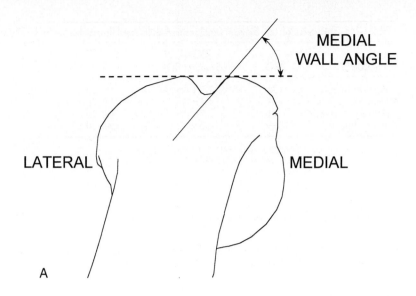

Figure 2 ▪ Measurement of the medial wall of the bicipital groove. *A*, An angle is measured between lines connecting the anterior aspects of the two trochanters *(dotted)* and parallel to the medial wall of the groove *(solid)*. *B*, Measurement of the width *(arrows)* and depth *(arrowheads)* of the bicipital groove.[1]

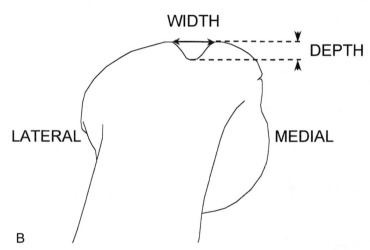

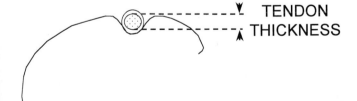

Figure 3 ▪ Measurement of the thickness of the biceps tendon from a frozen ultrasound image made perpendicular to the long axis of the tendon.[3]

Table 1 ▪ Measurements of Adult Bicipital Groove from Radiographs[1, 2]

MEASUREMENT	AUTHOR	SOURCE	NO.	MEAN ± SD	RANGE
Medial wall angle (degrees)	Cone	Specimens	54	56	25–90
	Cone	Normal	100	48	10–90
	Levinsohn	Normal	55	40.9 ± 12.9	18–80
	Levinsohn	Dislocated	7	22.1 ± 3.3	17–27
Width of groove (mm)	Cone	Specimens	54	8.8	5–14
	Cone	Normal	100	11	6–23
	Levinsohn	Normal	55	11.9 ± 2.2	7–18
	Levinsohn	Dislocated	7	15.4 ± 2.8	12–19
Depth of groove (mm)	Cone	Specimens	54	4.3	2–7
	Cone	Normal	100	4.6	2–8
	Levinsohn	Normal	55	3.9 ± 1.1	1–6
	Levinsohn	Dislocated	7	2.6 ± 0.8	2–4

Table 2 ▪ Thickness of the Biceps Tendon in Adults by Ultrasound

SUBJECTS	NO.	RIGHT (mean ± SD)	LEFT (mean ± SD)
Sedentary men	22	3.2 ± 0.5	3.3 ± 0.4
Male athletes	24	3.5 ± 0.4	3.7 ± 0.5
Sedentary women	21	2.7 ± 0.3	3.0 ± 0.3
Female athletes	19	3.0 ± 0.3	3.2 ± 0.3

All measurements are in millimeters. SD = standard deviation.
From van Holsbeeck MV, Introcaso JH: Mosby–Year Book, St. Louis, 1991, vol 1, pp 315–319. Used by permission.

associated with medial biceps tendon dislocation (7 of 12 = 58%). When the angle was greater than 30 degrees, there were no cases of dislocation.[2] Cone and colleagues suggest that subluxation/dislocation of the tendon may be associated with a shallow groove, as evidenced by lower than normal (3 mm or less) depth measurement.[1] Cone and group also found good correlation between the depth of the groove and the medial wall angle in patients, which would support this contention.[1] Ultrasound can directly visualize displacement of the tendon out of the groove, as well as detecting fluid in the sheath.

REFERENCES

1. Cone RO, Danzig L, Resnick D, Goldman AB: The bicipital groove: Radiographic, anatomic, and pathological study. AJR Am J Roentgenol 1983; 141:781–788.
2. Levinsohn EM, Santelli ED: Bicipital groove dysplasia and medial dislocation of the biceps brachii tendon. Skeletal Radiol 1991; 20:419–423.
3. van Holsbeeck MV, Introcaso JH: Appendix: Table of Normal Values. In van Holsbeeck MV, Introcaso JH (eds): Musculoskeletal Ultrasound. Mosby–Year Book, St. Louis, 1991, vol 1, pp 315–319.

▪: DETECTION OF SUPRACONDYLAR FRACTURES OF THE HUMERUS[1]
▪ ACR Code: 421 (Distal End of Humerus)

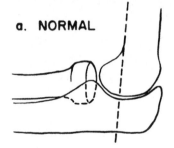

a. NORMAL

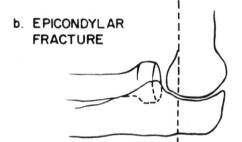

b. EPICONDYLAR FRACTURE

Figure 1 ▪ Use of an anterior humeral cortical line in detection of supracondylar fracture. (From Nelson SW: Radiol Clin North Am 1966; 4:241. Used by permission.)

Technique ▪

Central ray: Perpendicular to plane of film.
Position: True lateral with elbow flexed.
Target-film distance: Immaterial.

Measurements (Figure 1) ▪

In the normal lateral projection, a line drawn along the anterior cortex of the humerus and extended through its condyles will intersect a substantial portion of the condyles anteriorly and only a small portion posteriorly. When a supracondylar fracture is present, the anterior cortical line will intersect only a small portion of the condyles anteriorly and a larger portion posteriorly.

Source ▪

None given. Based on Nelson's extensive experience in this field.

REFERENCE

1. Nelson SW: Some important diagnostic and technical fundamentals in the radiology of trauma, with particular emphasis on skeletal trauma. Radiol Clin North Am 1966; 4:241–259.

▪: MEASUREMENT OF THE AXIAL ANGLES AT THE ELBOW[1]
- ▪ ACR Code: 422 (Elbow Joint)

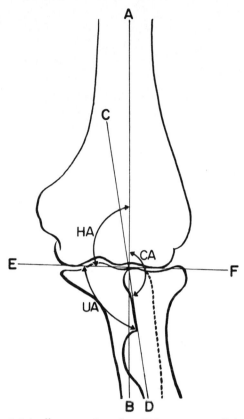

Figure 1 ▪ Axial elbow angles. See "Measurements" in text for explanation.

Technique ▪

Central ray: Perpendicular to plane of film.
Position: Arm fully extended, with the two epicondyles perfectly flat with respect to the film.
Target-film distance: Immaterial.

Table 1 ▪ Axial Angles of the Elbow			
ANGLE	MIN	MAX	AVERAGE
Men			
CA	154°	178°	169°
HA	77°	95°	85°
UA	74°	99°	84°
Women			
CA	158°	178°	167°
HA	72°	91°	83°
UA	72°	93°	84°

From Keats TE, et al: Radiology 1966; 87:904–907. Used by permission.

Measurements (Figure 1; Table 1) ▪

AB = Line of axis of the shaft of the humerus.
CD = Line of axis of the shaft of the ulna.
EF = Transverse line drawn tangentially to the most distal points of the articular surfaces of the trochlea and capitellum.
CA = The carrying angle formed by the intersection of *AB* and *CD*, measured on the radial side.
HA = The humeral angle formed by the intersection of *AB* and *EF*.
UA = The ulnar angle formed by the intersection of *CD* and *EF*.

Source ▪

The data were derived from a study of 50 normal subjects, equally divided between men and women and ranging in age from 21 to 66 years.

REFERENCE

1. Keats TE, Teeslink R, Diamond AE, Williams JH: Normal axial relationships of the major joints. Radiology 1966; 87:904–907.

⁝ DETECTION OF DISLOCATION OF THE RADIAL HEAD[1]
▪ ACR Code: 424 (Proximal End of Radius)

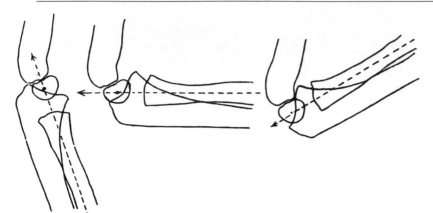

Figure 1 ▪ Normal relationships between the radius and the capitellum at the elbow. (From Storen G: Acta Chir Scand 1959; 116:144. Used by permission.)

Technique ▪

Central ray: Perpendicular to plane of film centered over joint.
Position: Lateral with elbow flexed.
Target film-distance: Immaterial.

Measurements (Figure 1) ▪

In the lateral projection, a line extending the radial axis should pass through the center of the capitellum in all stages of flexion of the elbow. This relationship is particularly useful in children, in whom the epiphyseal ossification centers have not yet appeared, the gap between the bone ends is wide, and the relationships between the bone ends are difficult to determine.

Source ▪

The data are based on the study of approximately 40 patients.

REFERENCE

1. Storen G: Acta Chir Scand 1959; 116:144.

⁝ ULNAR VARIANCE IN CHILDREN
▪ ACR Code: 432 (Distal End of Ulna)

Technique ▪

Posteroanterior (PA) radiographs of the wrist in the neutral position.[1]

Measurements ▪

The ulnar variance was measured in two ways. Method *A* involved measuring the distance between the most proximal point of the distal metaphysis of the ulna and radius. Method *B* consisted of measuring the distance between the most distal aspects of the ulnar and radial metaphysis.[1] Figure 1 shows the two methods. Table 1 lists the measurements by age for each of the two methods. Figure 2 shows the mean and 95% confidence intervals (+/- 2 SD) by age.[1]

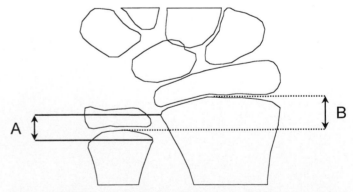

Figure 1 ▪ Measurement of ulnar variance in children. In method *A*, the distance between lines *(solid)* drawn between the proximalmost points of the distal radial and ulnar metaphyses is measured. Method *B* involves measuring the distance between lines *(dotted)* drawn through the distalmost aspects of the radial and ulnar metaphyses.

Source ▪

A total of 535 children (259 girls, 276 boys), ranging in age from 1.5 to 15.5 years, were studied with approximately 20 boys and 20 girls of each year. This was part of a ten-state (USA) survey.[1]

Comments ▪

Linear regression on variance versus age gave the following formulas for each method:

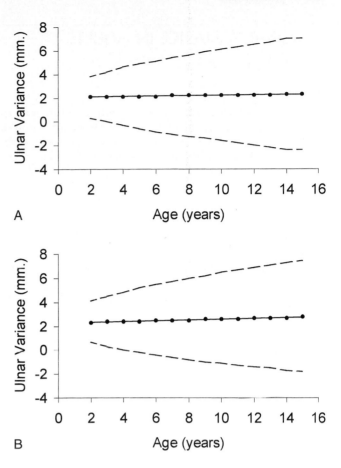

Figure 2 • Ulnar variance in children by age. *A*, Measurements made between the proximalmost point of the distal metaphyses of the radius and ulna. *B*, Measurements made between the distal aspects of the radial and ulnar metaphyses. Mean values *(circles)*, linear regression on the mean *(solid lines)*, and 95% confidence intervals *(dashed lines)* are shown. (From Hafner R, Poznanski AK, Donovan JM: Skeletal Radiol 1989; 18:513–516. Used by permission.)

Table 1 • Ulnar Variance in Children

AGE GROUP (yr)	METHOD A (PROXIMAL)		METHOD B (DISTAL)	
	Mean ± SD	95% CI	Mean ± SD	95% CI
2	2.1 ± 0.9	0.3–3.8	2.0 ± 0.9	0.7–4.1
3	2.1 ± 1.1	0.0–4.2	2.0 ± 1.1	0.3–4.5
4	2.1 ± 1.2	−0.3–4.6	2.0 ± 1.2	0.0–4.8
5	2.1 ± 1.4	−0.6–4.9	2.4 ± 1.4	−0.2–5.2
6	2.1 ± 1.5	−0.9–5.1	2.5 ± 1.5	−0.4–5.5
7	2.2 ± 1.6	−1.1–5.4	2.5 ± 1.6	−0.6–5.7
8	2.2 ± 1.7	−1.3–5.6	2.5 ± 1.7	−0.8–6.0
9	2.2 ± 1.8	−1.4–5.9	2.6 ± 1.8	−1.0–6.2
10	2.2 ± 1.9	−1.6–6.1	2.6 ± 1.9	−1.1–6.5
11	2.2 ± 2.0	−1.8–6.3	2.6 ± 2.0	−1.3–6.7
12	2.2 ± 2.1	−2.0–6.5	2.7 ± 2.1	−1.4–6.9
13	2.2 ± 2.2	−2.2–6.7	2.7 ± 2.2	−1.5–7.1
14	2.3 ± 2.4	−2.4–7.0	2.7 ± 2.3	−1.7–7.3
15	2.3 ± 2.4	−2.4–7.0	2.8 ± 2.3	−1.8–7.5

All measurements are in millimeters. SD = standard deviation, CI = confidence intervals.
From Hafner R, Poznanski AK, Donovan JM: Skeletal Radiol 1989; 18:513–516. Used by permission.

Method *A* ulnar variance (mm) =
$2.04 + (0.015 \times$ age in years), $r^2 = 0.82$

Method *B* ulnar variance (mm) =
$2.25 + (0.034 \times$ age in years), $r^2 = 0.96$

The authors state that method *A* may be superior because outliers are more symmetric about the regression line.[1]

REFERENCE

1. Hafner R, Poznanski AK, Donovan JM: Ulnar variance in children; Standard measurements for evaluation of ulnar shortening in JRA, hereditary multiple exostosis, and other bone or joint disorders in childhood. Skeletal Radiol 1989; 18:513–516.

▪: ULNAR VARIANCE IN ADULTS

▪ ACR Code: 432 (Distal End of Ulna)

Technique ▪

Posteroanterior (PA) radiographs, with the forearm and hand flat on the cassette (neutral), the elbow and shoulder at 90 degrees, and the beam centered on the wrist with 0 degrees angulation, were used to measure ulnar variance.

Measurements ▪

Three methods of measuring ulnar variance were described by Steyers and Blair.[1] These include the "project a line method," the "method of perpendiculars," and the "concentric circle technique." The latter, described by Palmer and colleagues, seems to be the most frequently used.[6]

Figure 1 shows these three methods. Figure 2 is a template for use in Palmer's concentric circle technique. Figure 3 depicts the three types of relationships (minus, zero, and plus variance). Table 1 lists the mean values, standard deviations (SD), and ranges determined in normal adult wrists.[2-5]

Source ▪

Steyers and Blair used radiographs of 9 adult cadavers (18 wrists) to compare methods of measuring ulnar variance.[1] The four studies from which ulnar variance values are cited were all done using radiographs from adults with no injury or disease involving the measured wrist.[2-5] The mean age

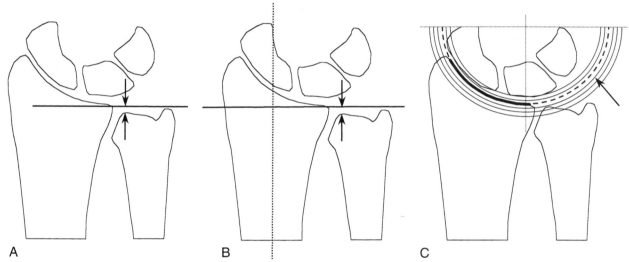

A   B   C

Figure 1 ▪ Methods of measuring ulnar variance. *A,* The "project a line technique" involves drawing a solid line from the ulnar side of the articular surface of the distal radius and measuring between it and the carpal surface of the ulna *(arrows). B,* The "method of perpendiculars" is performed by first drawing a line *(dotted)* through the central axis of the radius and a perpendicular *(solid)* line through the distal ulnar aspect of the radius. The distance between this line and the distal cortex of the ulna is the variance. *C,* The "concentric circle technique" is done with a template, and the circle most closely approximating the curve of the distal radius *(heavy line)* is placed over its contour. The variance is measured by counting between it *(dotted line)* and the line that intersects the ulnar head *(arrow).*[1]

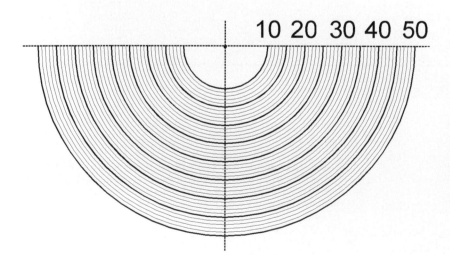

10 20 30 40 50

Figure 2 ▪ A template for measuring ulnar variance with the "concentric circle technique" described by Palmer. This consists of concentric semicircles ranging from 10 to 50 mm in diameter. This template has been printed to scale, and your template may be made by copying this figure onto transparent film.[6]

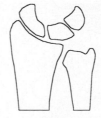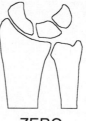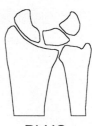

MINUS   ZERO   PLUS

Figure 3 • Depiction of the relationships between the distal radius and ulna. When the distal ulna is proximally located with respect to the radius, measurement is negative *(minus)*. When they are at the same level, a measurement of *zero* is obtained. If the articular surface of the ulna lies distal to that of the radius, the measurement is positive *(plus)*.

Table 1 • Ulnar Variance in Adults

AUTHOR	GENDER	NATIONALITY	NO.	MEAN ± SD	RANGE
Altissimi et al	Both	USA	233	0.3 ± 1.4	—
Chen and Shih	Both	Taiwan	1000	0.31 ± 1.27	−5.0–5.0
Kristensen et al	Both	Sweden	100	−0.60 ± 1.38	−4.0–2.0
Nakamura et al	Male	Japan	203	−0.14 ± 1.34	—
	Female	Japan	122	0.77 ± 1.27	—
	Both	Japan	325	0.20 ± 1.39	−4.0–5.0

All measurements are in millimeters. SD = standard deviation.
All measurements were done with Palmer's methods of concentric circles except those given by Altissimi, who used the "project a line" technique.[2–5]

of subjects ranged from 36 to 55 years, and the numbers of subjects are given in the data table. In all cases the growth plates were fused.

Comments •

Steyers and Blair compared measurements made using each method by three observers on the cadaveric radiographs and found a high degree of intra- and interobserver reliability. The differences in values obtained by each method were significant though small (< 0.40 mm), and they conclude that any method may be used.[1] Two of the studies cited herein also included measurements of ulnar variance of adults with Kienböck disease and found significantly different mean values of −2.04 and −1.22.[3, 4]

REFERENCES

1. Steyers CM, Blair WF: Measuring ulnar variance: A comparison of techniques. J Hand Surg Am 1989; 14:607–612.
2. Altissimi M, Antenuccu R Fiacca C, Mancini GB: Long-term results of conservative treatment of fractures of the distal radius. Clin Orthop 1986; 206:202–210.
3. Chen WS, Shih CH: Ulnar variance and Kienböck's disease: An investigation in Taiwan. Clin Orthop 1990; 255:124–127.
4. Kristensen SS, Thomassen E, Christensen F: Ulnar variance determination. J Bone Joint Surg Br 1986; 11:255–257.
5. Nakamura R, Tanaka Y, Imaida T, Miura T: The influence of age and sex on ulnar variance. J Hand Surg Br 1991; 16:84–88.
6. Palmer AK, Glisson RR, Werner FW: Ulnar variance determination. J Hand Surg Am 1982; 7:376–379.

•: MEASUREMENT OF CARPAL LENGTH IN CHILDREN
• ACR Code: 433 (Carpal Bone)

Technique •

Central ray: Perpendicular to plane of film.
Position: Posteroanterior.
Target-film distance: Immaterial.

Measurements (Figure 1) •

RM = A line from the point on the third metacarpal to the midgrowth plate of the radius. The point on the metacarpal is defined as the intersection of the central axis of this bone with the proximal end. The midportion of the distal radius can be determined by observation or by using a bisected triangle superimposed on the distal radial growth plate. The intersection of the bisection of the angle with the growth plate determines the point.

W = A line joining the most radial point on the base of the second metacarpal and the most ulnar point on the base of the fifth metacarpal.
M2 = The maximum length of the second metacarpal.

The nomogram (Figure 2) is used for determining relationships between *W* versus *RM* and *M2* versus *RM*. To determine how deviant a specific child is from the mean, a ruler is placed between the two points on the scales that correspond to these measures in the child in question. The intersection of the line with the central scales will give the number of standard deviations that this relationship deviates from the mean. Note that there are separate scales for boys and girls. For example, in evaluating *RM* against *W*, if, in a boy's wrist, *W* measures 36 mm and *RM* 28 mm, this wrist is quite small, being 4 standard deviations outside

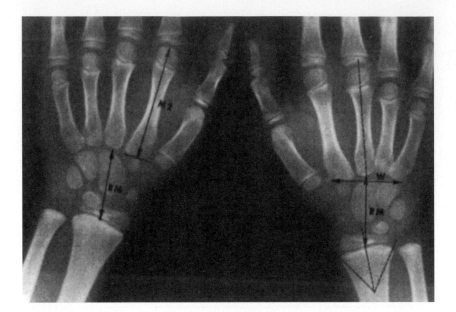

Figure 1 ▪ Measurement used in evaluating carpal and metacarpal size. (From Poznanski AK, et al: Radiology 1978; 129:661. Used by permission.)

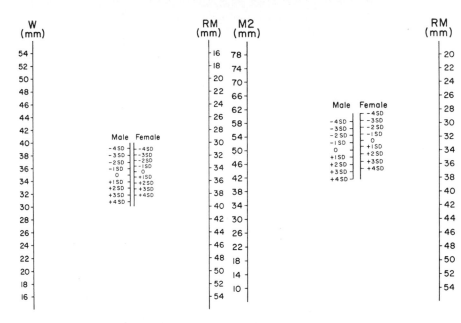

Figure 2 ▪ Nomogram for determining relationships. (From Poznanski AK, et al: Radiology 1978; 129:661. Used by permission.)

the normal limits. On the other hand, if both *W* and *RM* each measured 36 mm in a boy, then this child is exactly at the mean of the normal range.

These measures (or ratios) are useful in evaluating patients with juvenile rheumatoid arthritis and congenital malformation syndromes, because shortening of the carpus occurs in multiple epiphyseal dysplasia, the otopalatodigital syndromes, Turner syndrome, and arthrogryposis.

Source ▪

Five hundred thirty-nine hand radiographs of 280 boys ranging in age from 1.5 to 15.4 years and 259 girls ranging in age from 1.5 to 14.5 years.

REFERENCE

1. Poznanski AK, Hernandez RJ, Guire KE, et al: Carpal length in children. Radiology 1978; 129:661.

⁖ SCAPHOLUNATE DISTANCE

■ ACR Code: 433 (Carpal Bone)

Technique ■

Cautilli and Wehbe and Leicht and colleagues posteroanterior (PA) radiographs of the wrist with zero tube angulation and the wrist flat.[1, 2] Kindynis and colleagues made PA wrist radiographs of cadavers with the tube angled 10 degrees toward the ulnar side.[3] Moneim performed PA wrist radiography with a 20-degree foam wedge placed under the fingers and the thumb flat on the cassette with 0 degree tube angulation.[4] The tube-to-film distances were not given, and in all studies the beam was centered on the midportion of the proximal carpus.[1–4] Figure 1 shows these techniques for wrist radiography.

Measurements ■

Cautilli, Leicht, and Kindynis and their associates measured the transverse distance between the scaphoid and lunate proximally.[1–3] Kindynis and colleagues also measured the joint in its mid and distal portions.[3] Moneim did not specify where the measurement was taken.[4] Figure 2 shows these measurement positions. Table 1 lists the distances in children[2] and adults.[1, 3, 4]

Source ■

Cautilli and Wehbe evaluated radiographs from 32 men (44 wrists) and 40 women (56 wrists), with ages not given.[1]

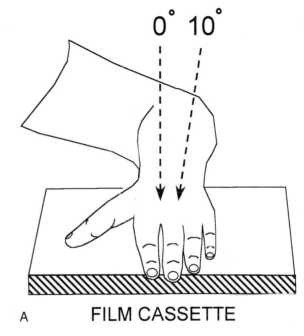

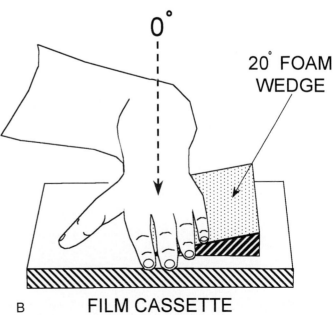

Figure 1 ■ Techniques for PA radiography of the scapholunate space. *A*, hand flat on the cassette with 0- and 10-degree (toward the ulnar side) tube angulation. *B*, 20-degree foam wedge placed under the fingers, with the thumb on the cassette and no tube angulation.

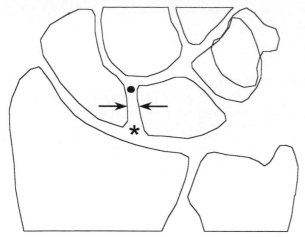

Figure 2 ▪ Measurement of the scapholunate space from a PA radiograph. The distance between the medial border of the scaphoid and the lateral border of the lunate most often has been measured proximally *(asterisk)* but may be measured in the midportion *(arrows)* or distally *(dot)*.

Leicht and colleagues examined the uninjured side in 79 children from 0 to 15 years of age presenting for unilateral wrist trauma.[2] Kindynis and colleagues studied 14 cadaveric wrists, discarding one with scapholunate dissociation.[3] Moneim's subjects included six men and two women volunteers, ranging in age from 26 to 40 years.[4]

Comments ▪

Scapholunate dissociation may result in an abnormally widened distance between the two bones. Cautilli and Wehbe found that in individual adults the distance can vary from side to side in up to 48% but never more than by 1 mm.[1] Moneim also found individual side-to-side variation that was not quantified.[4] Therefore, in adults comparison views of the noninjured wrist may not be helpful. Leicht and colleagues recommend comparison radiography of the normal side in cases of pediatric wrist trauma.[2]

Cautilli and Wehbe reviewed the literature and found cut-off values for diagnosing scapholunate dissociation

AUTHOR	MEASUREMENT LOCATION	AGE (yr)	NUMBER	DISTANCE (mm)
Leicht et al	Proximal	7	3	9.0 (7–11)
		8	5	8.0 (5–12)
		9	7	6.0 (4–9)
		10	8	4.0 (2–7)
		11	12	5.0 (4–8)
		12	8	4.5 (2–6)
		13	17	4.0 (2–6)
		14	10	3.0 (2–7)
		15	9	3.0 (2–5)
		7–15	79	4.6 (2–12)
Cautilli & Wehbe	Proximal	Adult	100	3.7 ± 0.6
Male			44	4.0 ± 0.5
Female			56	3.6 ± 0.5
Kindynis et al	Proximal	Adult	13	1.88 (1.5–2.0)
	Middle		13	1.66 (1.0–2.0)
	Distal		13	1.33 (1.0–2.0)
Moneim	Not given	26–40	8	1.6 (0.0–2.0)

Table 1 ▪ Scapholunate Distance in Children and Adults

Variance is shown by (range) or ± standard deviation. Radiographs taken with the wrist flat and no tube angulation except by Kindynis (10-degree ulnar tube tilt) and Moneim (20-degree ulnar wedge).[1-4]

ranging from 2 to 4 mm and conclude that from the data the distance (as measured proximally on neutral radiographs) may be up to 5 mm.[1] Kindynis and group and Moneim suggest that the upper limit of normal (on oblique or angled views) should be 2 mm.[3, 4] No recommendations for cut-off values in children were made by Leicht and group.[2]

References

1. Cautilli GP, Wehbe MA: Scapho-lunate distance and cortical ring sign. J Hand Surg Am 1991; 16:501–503.
2. Leicht P, Mikkelsen JB, Larsen CF: Scapholunate distance in children. Acta Radiol 1996; 37:625–626.
3. Kindynis P, Resnick D, Kang HS, et al: Demonstration of the scapholunate space with radiography. Radiology 1990; 175:278–280.
4. Moneim MS: The tangential posteroanterior radiograph to demonstrate scapholunate dissociation. J Bone Joint Surg Am 1981; 63:1324–1326.

▪: MEASUREMENT OF THE CARPAL AXES FOR THE DETECTION OF LIGAMENTOUS INSTABILITIES OF THE WRIST[1]

▪ ACR Code: 433 (Carpal Bone)

Technique ▪

Central ray: Perpendicular to plane of film.
Position: True lateral, neutral position, and extremes of flexion and extension.
Target-film distance: Immaterial.

Measurements (Figure 1) ▪

A line parallel to the center of the radial shaft is its axis. The lunate axis is a line drawn perpendicular to the anterior and posterior distal lunate poles. The scaphoid axis is determined by a line drawn connecting the proximal and distal

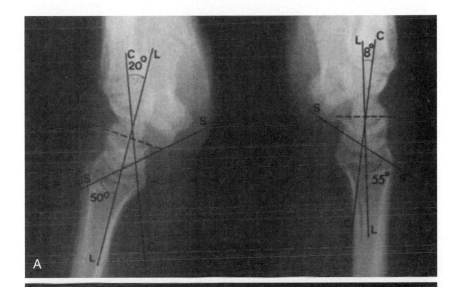

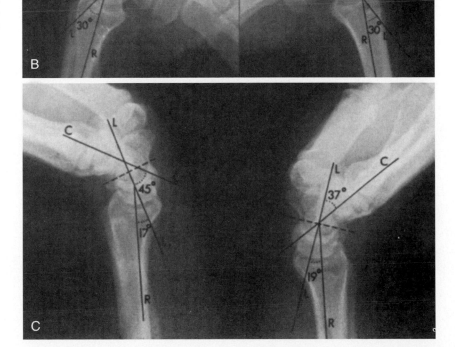

Figure 1 ▪ *A*, Lateral views of the "instability series." Scaphoid (navicular) *(S)*, lunate *(L)*, and capitate *(C)* axes are drawn on these lateral neutral views. *B*, Lateral flexion and *C*, lateral extension (dorsiflexion) views. The right wrist is to the reader's right. (From Gilula LA, Weeks PM: Radiology 1978; 129:641. Used by permission.)

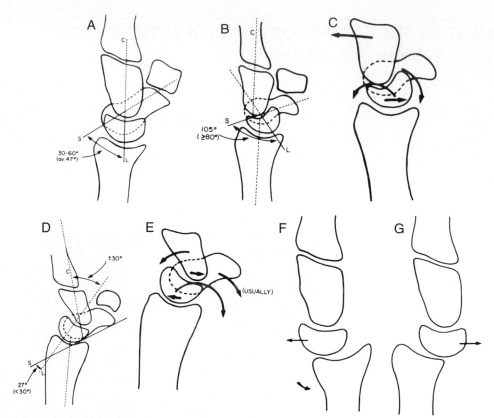

Figure 2 ▪ The axes of the carpal bone. *A,* The axes of the capitate *(C),* lunate *(L),* and scaphoid *(S)* bones are represented by the *solid* and *dashed* straight lines. A normal scapholunate angle is 30° to 60°, with an average angle of 47°. The radius, capitate, and lunate axes in this diagram coincide. *B,* Dorsiflexion instability can be diagnosed radiographically when the scapholunate angle is 80° or more. *C,* In dorsiflexion instability, the lunate has rotated or tilted so that its distal articular surface faces dorsally and the capitate is dorsal to the midplane of the radius. The scaphoid (navicular) stays in normal position, or its distal palmar tip moves toward the radius (tilts palmarly or ventrally). *Curved arrows* show the path of the carpal bone rotary motion. The *straight arrows* indicate the direction of bone movement or displacement.

D, Palmar flexion instability is diagnosed when the capitolunate angle is 30° or more or when the scapholunate angle is less than 30°. *E,* With palmar flexion instability, the distal articular surface of the lunate faces palmarly (ventrally), and the scaphoid usually tilts palmarly with the lunate. The central axis of the capitate lies palmar to the central radial axis, and the capitate may tilt dorsally. The *curved arrows* represent carpal bone rotation. *Straight arrows* indicate direction of bone movement or displacement.

F, Dorsal carpal subluxation exists when all the carpal bones lie dorsal to the center of the distal radial articular surface. The *curved arrow* indicates an impacted fracture deformity of the distal dorsal radius; the *straight arrow* indicates dorsal movement of the carpus (carpal bones). *G,* Palmar carpal subluxation would exist when the lunate and other carpal bones lie palmar to the central axis of the radius. The *arrow* indicates palmar movement of the carpal bones. (From Gilula LA, Weeks PM: Radiology 1978; 129:641. Used by permission.)

ventral convexities of the bone. The capitate axis is identified by passing a line from the center of its head through the center of its distal articular surface or the third metacarpal base.

The application of these data for the detection of ligamentous instabilities is shown in Figure 2.

Reference

1. Gilula LA, Weeks PM: Post-traumatic ligamentous instabilities of the wrist. Radiology 1978; 129:641–651.

▪ MEASUREMENT OF WRIST FLEXION AND EXTENSION[1]

- ACR Code: 434 (Joint of Wrist)

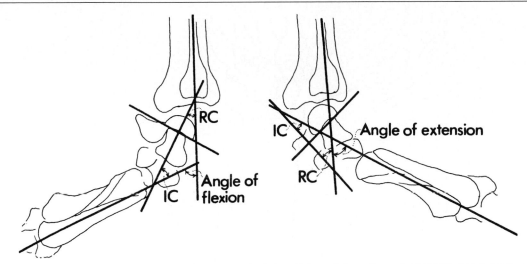

Figure 1 ▪ Measurement of radiocarpal and intercarpal angles. (Adapted from Brumfield RH Jr, Nickel VL, Nickel E: South Med J 1966; 59:909. Used by permission.)

	EXTENSION	FLEXION	TOTAL MOTION	RADIOCARPAL	INTERCARPAL
			Table 1 ▪ Average Values		
Men	72°	79°	151°	60°	77°
Women	72°	84°	156°	65°	82°

From Brumfield RH Jr, Nickel VL, Nickel E: South Med J 1996; 59:909. Used by permission.

Technique ▪

Central ray: Perpendicular to the plane of the film projected over the navicular bone:

Position: True lateral in full flexion, neutral, and full extension.

Target-film distance: Immaterial.

Measurements ▪

1. The longitudinal axes of the radius and second metacarpal are drawn. The angles are measured as shown in Figure 1. Total wrist motion is flexion plus extension.
2. The main axes of the lunate are determined by a line on the intercarpal face and a second line drawn at 90° to the first line.
3. The radiocarpal angle *(RC)* and intercarpal angle *(IC)* are drawn as shown in Figure 1.
4. Average values are listed in Table 1.

Source ▪

Ten healthy adults between 25 and 35 years of age.

REFERENCE

1. Brumfield RH Jr, Nickel VL, Nickel E: Joint motion in wrist flexion and extension. South Med J 1966; 59:909–910.

⁝ MEASUREMENT OF THE CARPAL ANGLE
▪ ACR Code: 434 (Joint of Wrist)

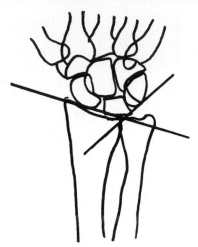

Figure 1 ▪ Measurement of the carpal angle.

Table 1 ▪ Age Trends, Gender, and Race Differences in Carpal Angle Percentiles

		CARPAL ANGLE IN DEGREES						
		Percentiles				Percentiles		
AGE GROUPS (yr)	Sample Size	5th	50th	95th	Sample Size	5th	50th	95th
		WHITE MALES				WHITE FEMALES		
4–6	10	116.0	122.0	132.5	13	120.0	126.5	143.0
6–8	36	111.0	124.0	153.5	25	115.0	130.5	147.5
8–10	25	122.0	133.5	147.0	15	115.5	129.5	139.5
10–12	24	155.5	133.0	143.0	19	123.0	134.0	152.5
12–14	24	117.0	132.0	142.5	24	116.0	130.0	143.0
14–24	49	119.0	134.0	149.5	58	115.0	129.0	139.5
24–40	30	114.0	136.0	145.5	42	112.0	130.5	142.5
40–83	33	113.5	134.0	146.5	34	113.0	130.5	149.0
		BLACK MALES				BLACK FEMALES		
4–6	9	124.0	131.0	143.0	16	116.5	130.5	140.5
6–8	32	119.0	128.5	147.5	22	121.0	133.0	145.6
8–10	31	128.0	139.0	142.0	16	125.0	139.5	155.0
10–12	28	121.0	138.0	152.5	23	125.5	138.5	151.0
12–14	32	125.5	141.0	143.0	28	123.0	141.0	153.5
14–24	52	125.0	146.0	139.5	67	123.0	139.0	150.0
24–40	14	128.0	136.0	142.5	18	127.0	136.5	151.0
40–83	32	125.5	140.0	149.0	46	126.5	140.5	153.5

From Harper HAS, et al: Invest Radiol 1974; 9:217–221. Used by permission.

Technique ▪

Central ray: Perpendicular to plane of film.
Position: Posteroanterior with hand in neutral position.
Target-film distance: Immaterial.

Measurements (Figure 1) ▪

The carpal angle is defined by the intersection of two tangents, one touching the proximal contour of the navicular and lunate bones and the second touching the triangular and lunate bones. Normal measurements for black and white populations are given in Table 1.

Source ▪

Data derived from hand films of 928 individuals randomly selected. The age distributions are given in Table 1.

REFERENCE

1. Harper Has, Poznanski AK, Garn SM: The carpal angle in American populations. Invest Radiol 1974; 9:217–221.

▪: VARIOUS MEASUREMENTS OF THE WRIST

▪ ACR Code: 434 (Joint of Wrist)

Technique ▪

Mann and colleagues performed a review of the literature concerning measurements of the wrist on radiographs for detecting congenital, developmental, and acquired abnormalities.[1]

Measurements ▪

The carpal height ratio (Figure 1) is used to quantify carpal collapse and is defined as the carpal height divided by the length of the third metacarpal.[1] An alternative method (Figure 2) involves dividing the height of the midcarpus by

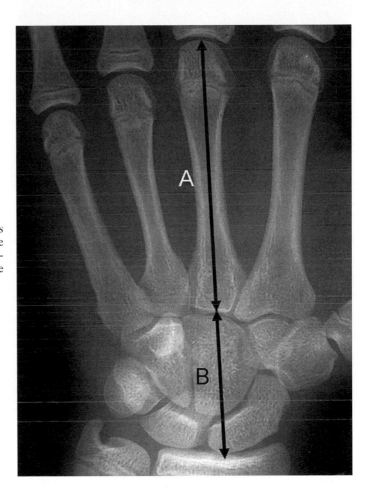

Figure 1 ▪ Carpal height ratio. The third metacarpal length *(A)* is measured along its central axis from proximal to distal cortex. The carpal height *(B)* is measured between the proximal third metacarpal cortex and the subchondral cortex of the distal radius. The ratio is equal to B/A and has a normal value of 0.54±0.03.[1]

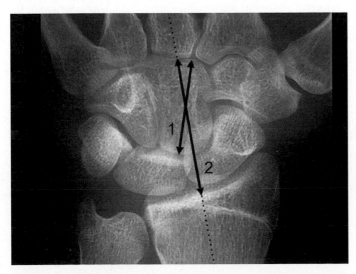

Figure 2 ▪ Alternative carpal height ratio. The height of the capitate *(1)* is measured from the distal cortex adjacent to the junction of the bases of the second and third metacarpals through the center of the capitate head to the proximal cortex. The carpal height *(2)* is measured from the proximal cortex of the third metacarpal to the distal radial cortex along the axis of the third metacarpal *(dotted line)*. The normal value is 1.57±0.05.[1,2]

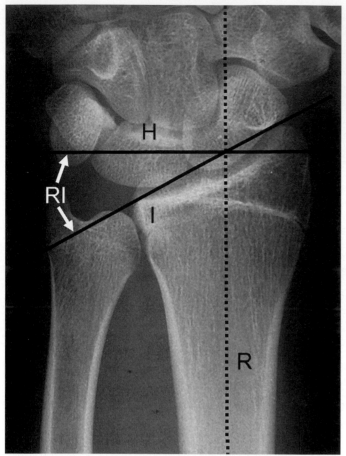

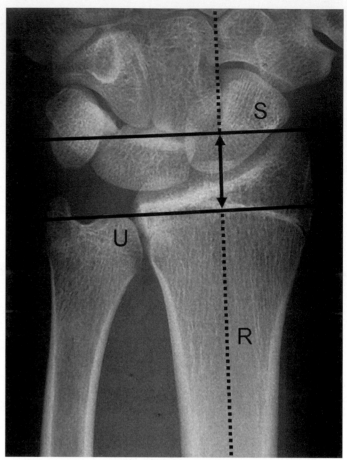

Figure 3 ▪ Radial inclination (RI). A line *(I)* is drawn between the distal tip of the radial styloid and the ulnar corner of the lunate fossa. The angle is measured between *(I)* and a horizontal line *(H)* to the central axis of the radius *(dotted line = R)*. The normal value is 25.4±2.2 degrees and the side-to-side difference should not exceed 1 degree.[1, 3]

Figure 4 ▪ Radial length. Lines perpendicular to the axis of the radius *(dotted line = R)* are drawn through the tip of the radial styloid *(S)* and the distal articular cortex of the ulna *(U)*. The radial length is measured between lines *S* and *U* and is normally 13.5±3.8 mm.[1, 5]

Table 1 ▪ Normal Measurements of the Wrist from Radiographs

MEASUREMENT	RADIOGRAPHIC TECHNIQUE	UNITS	MEAN VALUES	RANGE	SIDE-TO-SIDE VARIATION
Carpal height ratio	Neutral PA	none	0.54±0.03		
Alternate carpal height ratio	Neutral PA	none	1.57±0.05		
Carpal height index	Neutral PA	none	1.00±0.015		
Radial inclination	Neutral PA				
	May angle tube proximally (10°)	degrees	25.4±2.2	16–28	±1
Radial length	Neutral PA	mm	13.5±3.8		
Palmar tilt	Neutral lateral	degrees	14.5±4.3	0–22	
Men*			9.3±0.5		
Women*			12.4±0.6		
Radial shift	Neutral PA	mm			±1

Mean values given as mean ± standard deviation. PA = posteroanterior, mm = millimeters.
*The normal values for men and women are from a different study than those given for adults.
From Mann FA, Wilson AJ, Gilula LA: Radiology 1992; 184(1):15–24. Used by permission.

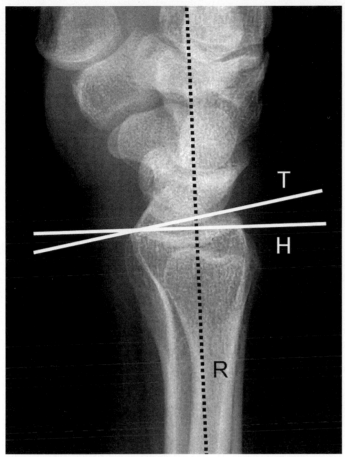

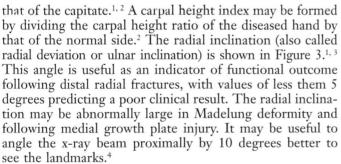

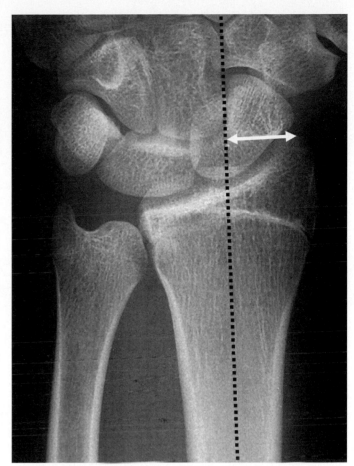

Figure 5 • Palmar tilt. A line *(T)* is drawn between the dorsal and palmar rims of the distal radius. The angle is measured between line *T* and horizontal line *(H)* passing through the palmar rim and perpendicular to the long axis of the radius *(dotted line = R)*. The normal value in adults is 14.5 ± 4.3 degrees.[1, 3, 6]

Figure 6 • Radial shift. This is measured *(white arrows)* between the distal tip of the radial styloid and the long axis of the radius *(dotted line)*. The side-to-side difference should not exceed 1 mm.[1, 5]

that of the capitate.[1, 2] A carpal height index may be formed by dividing the carpal height ratio of the diseased hand by that of the normal side.[2] The radial inclination (also called radial deviation or ulnar inclination) is shown in Figure 3.[1, 3] This angle is useful as an indicator of functional outcome following distal radial fractures, with values of less them 5 degrees predicting a poor clinical result. The radial inclination may be abnormally large in Madelung deformity and following medial growth plate injury. It may be useful to angle the x-ray beam proximally by 10 degrees better to see the landmarks.[4]

The radial length (also called radial height) is shown in Figure 4.[1, 5] Abnormally low measurements reflect distal radial shortening resulting from fractures or developmental abnormality. It is important to compare the side in question with the normal wrist since the radial length is influenced by ulnar variance.[1] The palmar tilt (also called volar tilt, volar inclination, or palmar slope) is depicted in Figure 5.[1-6] More than half of patients having palmar tilt of greater than 15 degrees after fracture will suffer decreased grip strength and endurance.[3, 5] A tilt of more than 20 to 25 degrees may indicate a form of midcarpal instability called the adaptive carpus.[5] The radial shift (also called radial width) is shown in Figure 6. This distance is used to

quantify offset of distal radial fracture fragments by comparing measurements between the injured wrist and the contralateral side.[1, 5]

Table 1 lists the normal values of all the measurements just described.[1-6]

Source •

See references.

REFERENCES

1. Mann FA, Wilson AJ, Gilula LA: Radiographic evaluation of the wrist: What does the hand surgeon want to know? Radiology 1992; 184(1):15–24.
2. Stahelin A, Pfeiffer K, Sennwald G, Segmuller G: Determining carpal collapse: An improved method. J Bone Joint Surg Am 1989; 71:1400–1405.
3. Altissimi M, Antenuccu R, Fiacca C, Mancini GB: Long-term results of conservative treatment of fractures of the distal radius. Clin Orthop 1986; 206:202–210.
4. Friberg S, Lundstrom B: Radiographic measurements of the radiocarpal joint in normal adults. Acta Radiol 1976; 17:249–256.
5. Jupiter JB: Current concepts review: Fractures of the distal end of the radius. J Bone Joint Surg Am 1991; 73:461–469.
6. Mann FA, Kang SW, Gilula LA: Normal palmar tilt: Is dorsal tilting really normal? J Hand Surg Br 1992; 17:315–317.

": CARPAL TUNNEL DIMENSIONS AND AREA
- ACR Code: 43 (Wrist and Hand)

Technique •

Cobb and colleagues performed MRI of the wrist in the axial plane using a 1.5-T Magnetom SP machine (Siemens Medical Systems, Erlangen, Germany). T2 (2000/20,80) sequences with 3-mm thickness and 1.5-mm gap were done.[1] Yoshioka and colleagues did axial MRI of the wrist at 1.5-T using a Signa unit (General Electric, Milwaukee, WI) with T1-weighted (250-500/14) slices with 3-mm, thickness. Examinations were done with each wrist in flexion, neutral, and extended positions.[2] In a more recent study, Cobb and colleagues used a 1.5-T Signa unit to perform axial T1 (400-600/minimum TE) and T2 (2000/30,60) images through the wrist.[3]

Measurements •

Cobb's measurements were done from the axial MRI slice containing the largest part of the hook of the hamate bone.[1, 3] Yoshioka and group used the section through the hook of the hamate as well as the slice showing the pisiform clearly.[2] In all studies, the carpal canal was outlined by hand, with the anterior border being the flexor retinaculum and the rest corresponding to the bony canal and the cross-

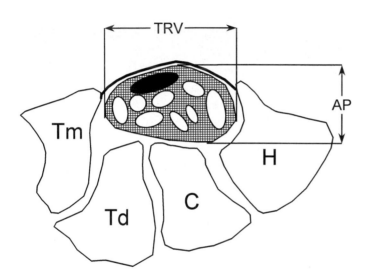

Figure 1 • Measurements of the carpal tunnel from an axial MRI slice through the level of the hook of the hamate. The anteroposterior *(AP)* and transverse *(TRV)* dimensions are shown. Also depicted are the areas of the tunnel *(cross-hatched)*, tendons *(white)*, and median nerve *(black)*. H = hamate, C = capitate, Td = trapezoid, Tm = trapezium.

Table 1 • Carpal Tunnel Areas

RESEARCH GROUP	NO.	CARPAL CANAL (cm²)	CARPAL CONTENTS (cm²)	RATIO (Contents/Canal)
Cobb et al (Cadavers)				
Direct	5	1.56±0.11	0.82±0.10	0.53±0.04
MRI	5	1.78±0.09	0.96±0.05	0.54±0.02
Cobb				
Normals	7	1.83±0.42	0.92±0.25	0.50±0.07
CTS	7	1.85±0.33	1.09±0.19	0.59±0.04

All measurements are given as mean ± standard deviation. CTS = carpal tunnel syndrome.

Table 2 • Carpal Tunnel Measurements in Different Positions (Normal Subjects)

LEVEL/ POSITION	NO.	CARPAL CANAL AREA (cm²)	CARPAL CANAL AP (mm)	CARPAL CANAL TRV (mm)
Hamate				
Neutral	25	1.58±0.13	9.1±0.5	21.1±0.9
Flexion	28	1.38±0.12	8.8±0.5	20.9±0.8
Extension	18	1.87±0.15	9.3±0.6	22.4±1.0
Pisiform				
Neutral	36	1.73±0.09	9.6±0.5	22.2±0.7
Flexion	31	1.46±0.01	9.2±0.5	20.8±0.7
Extension	27	1.52±0.11	7.8±0.5	23.4±0.8

All measurements given as mean ± standard deviation. AP = anteroposterior, TRV = transverse.

sectional area calculated with built-in software. This is termed the carpal tunnel area (CTA). Cobb and group outlined the tendons and the median nerve within the canal and summed the areas to obtain the carpal tunnel contents (CTC) area and calculated a ratio (CTC/CTA) called the carpal contents ratio.[1, 3] Yoshioka and colleagues measured the maximum anteroposterior (AP) and transverse (TRV) dimensions of the carpal tunnel.[2] After scanning the cadaver wrists, Cobb sliced them, photographed them, and traced the carpal tunnel, tendons, and median nerve to obtain area measurements.[1]

Figure 1 shows these measurements at the level of the hook of the hamate bone. Table 1 lists CTA, CTC, and the carpal contents ratios.[1, 3] Table 2 shows the measured CTA as well as the AP and TRV dimensions in neutral, flexion, and extension.[2]

Source ▪

Cobb and colleagues examined five upper extremities harvested from four cadavers, seven adults with clinically diagnosed carpal tunnel syndrome (CTS), and seven matched controls.[1, 3] Yoshioka evaluated the wrists of eight male and eight female volunteers with no wrist or hand problems. The ages ranged from 20 to 38 years, with a mean age of 27.8 years.[2].

Comments ▪

The measurement that seems most likely to be reproducible is the carpal contents ratio, and there was a significant difference between normal subjects and patients with CTS, with a p value of .01.[3] Yoshioka's work shows that there are significant differences in area and linear measurements of the carpal tunnel caused by different wrist positions, with p values from .05 to .01.[2] These are all rather small series, and further work will help determine whether the carpal contents ratio can be used to predict accurately which patients will enjoy symptomatic relief following decompressive surgery.

REFERENCES

1. Cobb TK, Dalley BK, Posteraro RH, Lewis RC: Establishment of carpal contents/canal ratio by means of magnetic resonance imaging. J Hand Surg Am 1992; 17(5):843–849.
2. Yoshioka S, Okuda Y, Tamai K, et al: Changes in carpal tunnel shape during wrist joint motion. MRI evaluation of normal volunteers [see comments]. J Hand Surg Br 1993; 18:620–623.
3. Cobb TK, Bond JR, Cooney WP, Metcalf BJ: Assessment of the ratio of carpal contents to carpal tunnel volume in patients with carpal tunnel syndrome: A preliminary report. J Hand Surg Am 1997; 22(4):635–639.

▪: THE MEDIAN NERVE IN THE CARPAL TUNNEL
▪ ACR Code: 43 (Wrist and Hand)

Technique ▪

Mesgarzadeh and colleagues performed axial MRI of the wrist with a 0.3-T Beta 300 unit (Fonar, Melville, NY), using 3-mm sections and T1 (500-700/28)-weighting.[1] Buchberger and colleagues did axial MRI of the wrist with a 1.5-T Magnetom machine (Siemens, Erlangen, Germany), using T1 (450-500/15)-weighting and 3- to 4-mm slice thickness.[2] Buchberger also performed axial real-time ultrasound of the wrist with 7.5-MHz linear probes, using a Picker LSC 9500 unit (Hitachi Medical Corp., Tokyo, Japan) and a stand-off pad.[2, 3] Cobb and Middleton and colleagues used 1.5-T Signa MRI units (General Electric, Milwaukee, WI) to perform axial T1 (400-600/20-30)-scans through the wrist with 3-mm slice thickness and surface coils.[4, 5]

Measurements ▪

The median nerve was identified and measured on axial ultrasound and MRI sections at the level of the distal radius, the pisiform, and the hook of the hamate. Figure 1 depicts the median nerve at each of these levels. Mesgarzadeh and Buchberger and groups measured the major axis (MA) and minor axis (MI) of the median nerve and calculated a flattening radio (FR) as follows: FR = MA/MI.[1–3] Buchberger and colleagues used the axis measurements from both ultrasound and MRI to calculate the area of the median nerve, assuming an ellipse as follows: Nerve area = Pi × MA/2 × MI/2.[2, 3] Middleton and colleagues also measured (and reported) the axes of the median nerve and calculated the area as above.[5] Cobb and group traced the median nerve to obtain the area and did not obtain linear dimensions.[4]

Figure 1 ▪ Median nerve *(black ellipse)* in the carpal tunnel at the distal radius, pisiform, and hamate levels. R = radius, L = lunate, US = ulnar styloid, S = scaphoid, T = triquetral, P = pisiform, Tm = trapezium, Td = trapezoid, C = capitate, H = hamate.

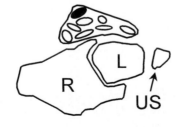

Distal Radius

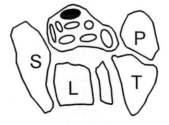

Pisiform

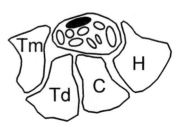

Hamate

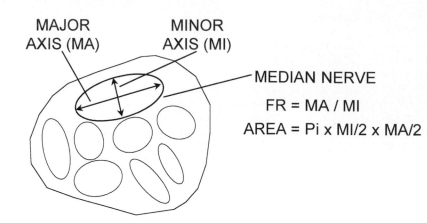

MAJOR AXIS (MA)

MINOR AXIS (MI)

MEDIAN NERVE

FR = MA / MI

AREA = Pi x MI/2 x MA/2

Figure 2 ▪ Measurements of the median nerve in the carpal tunnel from axial ultrasound and MR images. Linear measurements of the *minor axis (MI)* and *major axis (MA)* are combined to form a flattening ratio *(FR)* and the area as shown. In one study by Cobb,[4] the perimeter of the nerve was traced on MR images to obtain the area.

Table 1 ▪ Flattening Ratios of the Median Nerve in the Carpal Tunnel

RESEARCHER	MODALITY	LOCATION	SUBJECT CATEGORY	NO.	MEAN ± SD	RANGE
Mesgarzadeh et al	MRI	Distal radius	Normal	17	2.5 ± 1.0	1.4–5.4
		Pisiform	Normal	17	3.3 ± 1.1	1.0–4.8
		Hamate	Normal	17	2.9 ± 0.9	1.1–4.1
Middleton et al	MRI	Pisiform	Normal	18	2.3	1.2–3.8
		Hamate	Normal	18	2.3	1.3–4.5
Buchberger	MRI	Hamate	CTS	20	4.1 ± 0.8	2.5–5.6
	U/S	Distal radius	Normal	28	3.0 ± 0.5	1.6–3.9
		Pisiform	Normal	28	3.0 ± 0.5	1.7–4.0
		Hamate	Normal	28	3.2 ± 0.5	2.3–4.3
		Distal radius	CTS	28	3.1 ± 0.4	2.5–3.8
		Pisiform	CTS	28	3.2 ± 0.8	2.3–6.2
		Hamate	CTS	28	5.6 ± 0.8	3.3–6.7
		Distal radius	CTS	20	2.7 ± 0.4	2.2–3.1
		Pisiform	CTS	20	2.7 ± 0.4	2.0–3.7
		Hamate	CTS	20	4.6 ± 0.5	3.1–6.5

All measurements without units (ratio). CTS = carpal tunnel syndrome, SD = standard deviation.

Table 2 ▪ Median Nerve Cross-Sectional Areas in the Carpal Tunnel

RESEARCHER	MODALITY	LOCATION	SUBJECT CATEGORY	NO.	MEAN ± SD	RANGE
Cobb	MRI	Hamate	Normal	7	12.4 ± 3.8	8.0–17.0
		Hamate	CTS	7	15.3 ± 5.7	9.0–26.0
Middleton	MRI	Pisiform	Normal	18	7.0 ± 1.4	5.3–9.7
		Pisiform	Normal	18	8.0 ± 1.9	4.2–10.8
Buchberger	MRI	Hamate	CTS	20	14.3 ± 3.7	9.6–20.5
	U/S	Distal radius	Normal	28	7.9 ± 1.1	5.4–7.7
		Pisiform	Normal	28	8.1 ± 1.3	6.7–12.8
		Hamate	Normal	28	7.7 ± 1.1	6.3–11.6
		Distal radius	CTS	28	11.1 ± 1.8	7.9–15.0
		Pisiform	CTS	28	19.4 ± 7.1	9.0–37.3
		Hamate	CTS	28	13.6 ± 3.8	7.3–22.9
		Distal radius	CTS	20	10.0 ± 2.0	7.2–14.8
		Pisiform	CTS	20	14.5 ± 3.8	8.8–20.5
		Hamate	CTS	20	10.3 ± 2.5	5.9–15.9

All measurements are in square millimeters. SD = standard deviation, CTS = carpal tunnel syndrome.

Figure 2 shows these measurements. Table 1 lists the FR as reported[1-3] and calculated FR from Middleton's linear dimension data.[5] Table 2 lists the reported median nerve areas.[2-5] Note that Cobb's normal median nerve areas are larger, and this may be due to the different method of measurement. Middleton's normal median nerve dimensions are as follows: at the pisiform level, 2.0 mm (range 1.6 to 2.8 mm) by 4.5 mm (range 3.4 to 6.0 mm); and at the level of the hook of the hamate, 2.1 mm (range 1.4 to 2.6 mm) by 4.9 mm (range 3.4 to 6.3 mm). Standard deviations were not given.[5]

Source ▪

Mesgarzadeh and colleagues studied 17 normal adult volunteers with no wrist problems.[1] Buchberger evaluated 20 wrists in 18 adult patients who had clinical carpal tunnel syndrome (CTS) with both ultrasound and MRI.[2] They also performed ultrasound only on 28 wrists from 25 adult patients (17 women, 8 men, mean age 61 years) affected with CTS and 28 wrists of 14 asymptomatic adult volunteers, of whom 9 were women and 5 were men.[3] Cobb and colleagues studied seven adults with CTS and seven control wrists.[4] Middleton and colleagues scanned 18 wrists in 9 normal adult volunteers.[5]

Comments ▪

Buchberger and associates found good correlation between ultrasound and MRI measurements of FR (r = 0.86) and calculated median nerve area (r = 0.94) with p = .001 for both.[2] They further found significant differences between normal subjects and patients with CTS for both FR and median nerve area (p = .001), with the nerve being flattened and swollen in CTS compared with normal.[2, 3] These changes were most marked at the level of the hamate. Cut-off values of 4.5 for FR and 10 mm for the median nerve area (at the hamate) might prove useful for diagnosis of suspected CTS.

References

1. Mesgarzadeh M, Schneck CD, Bonakdarpour A: Carpal tunnel: MR imaging. Part I. Normal anatomy. Radiology 1989; 171(3):743–748.
2. Buchberger W, Judmaier W, Birbamer G, et al: Carpal tunnel syndrome: Diagnosis with high-resolution sonography. AJR Am J Roentgenol 1992; 159(4):793–798.
3. Buchberger W, Schon G, Jungwirth W: High-resolution ultrasonography of the carpal tunnel. J Ultrasound Med 1991; 10(10):531–537.
4. Cobb TK, Bond JR, Cooney WP, Metcalf BJ: Assessment of the ratio of carpal contents to carpal tunnel volume in patients with carpal tunnel syndrome: A preliminary report. J Hand Surg Am 1997; 22(4):635–639.
5. Middleton WD, Kneeland JB, Kellman GM, et al: MR imaging of the carpal tunnel: Normal anatomy and preliminary findings in the carpal tunnel syndrome. AJR Am J Roentgenol 1987; 148:307–316.

▪: FLEXOR RETINACULUM OF THE WRIST
▪ ACR Code: 43 (Wrist and Hand)

Technique ▪

Mesgarzadeh and colleagues performed axial MRI of the wrist with a 0.3-T Beta 300 unit (Fonar, Melville, NY), using 3-mm sections and T1 (500–700/28)-weighting.[1] Buchberger and colleagues did axial MRI of the wrist with a 1.5-T Magnetom machine (Siemens, Erlangen, Germany), using T1 (450–500/15)-weighting and 3- to 4-mm slice thickness.[2] Buchberger and group also performed axial real-time ultrasound of the wrist with 7.5-MHz linear probes, using a Picker LSC 9500 unit (Hitachi Medical Corp., Tokyo, Japan) and a stand-off pad.[2, 3]

Measurements ▪

Both groups of investigators drew a baseline (BL) between the hook of the hamate and the tubercle of the trapezium and a perpendicular line from the baseline to the apex (BA) of the flexor retinaculum.[1-3] Mesgarzadeh's group calculated a bowing ratio (BR) as follows: BR = BA/BR ×

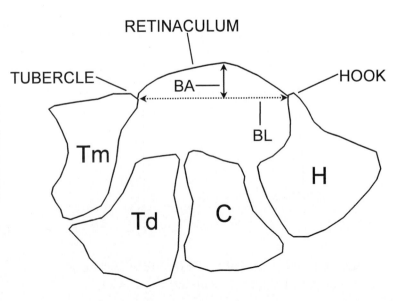

Figure 1 ▪ Measurement of palmar bowing of the flexor retinaculum at the level of the hook of the hamate with MRI and ultrasound. A baseline (BL) was drawn between the attachments of the retinaculum with the hamate (H) and the trapezium (Tm). The distance between BL and the apex of the retinaculum (BA) was measured in millimeters. To calculate the bowing ratio (BR), BA was divided by BL and multiplied by 100. The capitate (C) and trapezoid (Td) bones are also shown.

Table 1 ▪ Bowing of the Flexor Retinaculum of the Wrist

RESEARCHER	MODALITY	MEASUREMENT	SUBJECT CATEGORY	NO.	MEAN ± SD	RANGE
Mesgarzadeh	MRI	Bowing ratio (percent)	Normal	17	5.8±4.7%	0–15%
Buchberger	MRI	Baseline to apex (mm)	CTS	20	4.25±0.8	2.9–5.9
	U/S	Baseline to apex (mm)	Normal	28	2.1±0.8	0–3.1
	U/S	Baseline to apex (mm)	CTS	28	4.8±1.0	3.0–7.0
	U/S	Baseline to apex (mm)	CTS	20	3.7±1.1	2.0–6.0

SD = standard deviation. CTS = carpal tunnel syndrome.

100.[1] Buchberger's group simply recorded the length of BA in millimeters.[2,3] Figure 1 shows these measurements. Table 1 lists the measurements from all three papers.

Source ▪

Mesgarzadeh and colleagues studied 17 normal adult volunteers with no wrist problems.[1] Buchberger and colleagues evaluated 20 wrists in 18 adult patients with clinical carpal tunnel syndrome CTS with both ultrasound and MRI.[2] They also performed ultrasound only on 28 wrists from 25 adult patients (17 women, 8 men; mean age 61 years) affected with CTS and 28 wrists of 14 asymptomatic adult volunteers, of whom 9 were women and 5 were men.[3]

Comments ▪

Since neither paper reported the length of the baseline (BL), we cannot directly correlate the results from the two studies using MRI.[1,2] Furthermore, Buchberger and associates reported relatively poor correlation (r = .52) between MRI and ultrasound measurements of BA.[2] However, comparisons of the ultrasound BA measurement of both groups having CTS and normal subjects gave significant (p = .001) differences, with the retinaculum being more convex palmarly in patients with CTS.[2,3]

REFERENCES

1. Mesgarzadeh M, Schneck CD, Bonakdarpour A: Carpal tunnel: MR imaging. Part I. Normal anatomy. Radiology 1989; 171(3):743–748.
2. Buchberger W, Judmaier W, Birbamer G, et al: Carpal tunnel syndrome: Diagnosis with high-resolution sonography. AJR Am J Roentgenol 1992; 159(4):793–798.
3. Buchberger W, Schon G, Jungwirth W: High-resolution ultrasonography of the carpal tunnel. J Ultrasound Med 1991; 10(10):531–537.

▪: METACARPAL INDEX IN INFANTS
▪ ACR Code: 435 (Metacarpal)

Technique ▪

Central ray: Perpendicular to plane of film centered over palm.
Position: Posteroanterior.
Target-film distance: 30 inches.

Measurements (Figure 1 and Table 1) ▪

1. Axial length: Place a ruler along the center line of the shaft of the bone so that the shaft is divided into two equal part measurements (A).

2. Minimal width of shaft measurement (B).
3. Metacarpal index is calculated by measuring the second, third, fourth, and fifth metacarpals. The sum of lengths (A) is divided by the sum of widths (B).

Patients with Marfan syndrome had a metacarpal index of 7 or greater. In patients with Down syndrome, the metacarpal index is within normal limits.

Source ▪

Radiographs of both hands of 25 girls and 25 boys were taken at ages 6 months, 12 months, 18 months, and 24

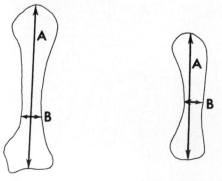

SECOND METACARPAL   FIFTH METACARPAL

Figure 1 ▪ Measurement of the metacarpal index.

Table 1 ▪ Metacarpal Index During First 2 Years

AGE (Mon)	GENDER	MEAN	SD
6	M	5.23	0.46
	F	5.60	0.37
12	M	5.30	0.41
	F	5.75	0.41
18	M	5.28	0.40
	F	5.82	0.45
24	M	5.40	0.43
	F	5.84	0.43

From Joseph MC, Meadow SR: Arch Dis Child 1969; 44:515. Used by permission.

months. The children were examined, were known to be healthy, and had been studied by Dr. Alice Stewart, Oxford University.

REFERENCE

1. Joseph MC, Meadow SR: The metacarpal index of infants. Arch Dis Child 1969; 44:515–516.

": METACARPAL INDEX IN ADULTS[1]
- ACR Code: 435 (Metacarpal)

Table 1 • Male Right Hand: Length, Width, and Relative Slenderness of Metacarpals, and Metacarpal Index

RIGHT METACARPAL		MEAN (mm)	RANGE (mm)	SD	COEFFICIENT OF VARIABILITY (%)*
1	Length	46.20	41–55	±2.9	6.3
	Width	10.98	8.5–13.0	±1.03	9.4
	Rel. slend.	4.25	3.6–5.2	±0.42	9.9
2	Length	68.60	57–79	±3.8	5.5
	Width	9.47	8.0–11.5	±0.76	8.0
	Rel. slend.	7.29	6.0–8.6	±0.61	8.4
3	Length	66.40	59–75	±3.2	4.8
	Width	9.31	8.0–10.5	±0.68	7.3
	Rel. slend.	7.16	6.3–8.1	±0.50	7.0
4	Length	59.40	51–65	±3.0	5.1
	Width	7.61	6.5–9.0	±0.58	7.6
	Rel. slend.	7.85	6.4–9.2	±0.63	8.0
5	Length	55.30	49–61	±2.7	4.9
	Width	9.01	7.5–10.5	±0.76	8.4
	Rel. slend.	6.18	5.0–7.7	±0.57	9.2
Index		6.86	5.9–8.1	±0.45	6.6

*Coefficient of variability = (SD/Mean) × 100.
From Parish JG: Br J Radiol 1966; 52–62. Used by permission.

Technique ■

Central ray: Perpendicular to plane of film centered over palm.
Position: Posteroanterior.
Target-film distance: 30 inches.

Measurements (Figure 1; Tables 1 through 4) ■

1. Axial length: Place a ruler along the center line of the shaft of the bone so that the shaft is divided into two equal parts (*A*).
2. Minimal width of shaft (*B*).
3. Relative slenderness of each bone = *A/B*.
4. Metacarpal index is calculated by averaging the relative slenderness of the second, third, fourth, and fifth metacarpals.

The metacarpal index is above the normal range in arachnodactyly and below normal in Morquio disease, Weill-Marchesani syndrome, and familial streptodactyly. Parish suggests for arachnodactyly a dividing line between normal and abnormal at the 3 SD level of 8.4 in men and 9.2 in women.

Source ■

Eighty-two female and 51 male patients between the ages of 21 and 45 years who were seen in the physical medicine department of Dryburn Hospital, Durham, England. Pa-

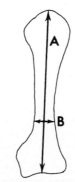
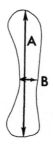

SECOND METACARPAL   FIFTH METACARPAL

Figure 1 • Measurement of the metacarpal index.

Table 2 • Male Left Hand: Length, Width, and Relative Slenderness of Metacarpals, and Metacarpal Index

LEFT METACARPAL		MEAN (mm)	RANGE (mm)	SD	COEFFICIENT OF VARIABILITY (%)*
1	Length	46.20	40–54	±3.1	6.7
	Width	10.93	9.5–13.0	±0.88	8.1
	Rel. slend.	4.24	3.5–5.1	±0.36	8.5
2	Length	68.60	63–78	±3.4	5.0
	Width	9.34	8.0–11.0	±0.77	8.2
	Rel. slend.	7.41	6.4–9.1	±0.59	8.0
3	Length	66.50	59–75	±3.2	4.8
	Width	9.22	7.5–10.5	±0.71	7.7
	Rel. slend.	7.25	6.3–9.1	±0.55	7.6
4	Length	59.40	55–66	±3.1	5.2
	Width	7.47	6.5–9.0	±0.56	7.5
	Rel. slend.	7.99	6.9–9.8	±0.60	7.5
5	Length	55.40	49–61	±2.7	4.9
	Width	8.68	7.5–10.0	±0.73	8.4
	Rel. slend.	6.42	5.4–7.7	±0.59	9.2
Index		7.02	6.0–85	±0.49	7.0

*Coefficient of variability = (SD/Mean) × 100.
From Parish JG: Br J Radiol 1966; 52–62. Used by permission.

Table 3 • Female Right Hand: Length, Width, and Relative Slenderness of Metacarpals, and Metacarpal Index

RIGHT METACARPAL		MEAN (mm)	RANGE (mm)	SD	COEFFICIENT OF VARIABILITY (%)*
1	Length	42.70	37–49	±2.3	5.4
	Width	9.04	7.5–11.0	±0.74	8.2
	Rel. slend.	4.74	3.8–6.1	±0.42	8.9
2	Length	64.40	58–74	±3.2	5.0
	Width	8.02	6.5–9.5	±0.62	7.7
	Rel. slend.	8.06	6.7–9.2	±0.63	7.8
3	Length	62.00	57–69	±3.1	5.0
	Width	8.03	6.5–9.5	±0.62	7.7
	Rel. slend.	7.76	6.4–9.1	±0.62	8.0
4	Length	55.60	50–61	±2.8	5.0
	Width	6.38	5.0–7.5	±0.55	8.6
	Rel. slend.	8.78	7.2–10.7	±0.83	9.5
5	Length	51.50	46–57	±2.5	4.9
	Width	7.35	6.0–9.0	±0.61	8.3
	Rel. slend.	7.05	5.4–8.8	±0.63	8.9
Index		7.60	6.3–8.9	±0.52	6.8

*Coefficient of variability = (SD/Mean) × 100.
From Parish JG: Br J Radiol 1966; 52–62. Used by permission.

Table 4 • Female Left Hand: Length, Width, and Relative Slenderness of Metacarpals, and Metacarpal Index

LEFT METACARPAL		MEAN (mm)	RANGE (mm)	SD	COEFFICIENT OF VARIABILITY (%)*
1	Length	42.40	37–49	±2.3	5.4
	Width	9.04	7.5–11.0	±0.71	7.9
	Rel. slend.	4.71	4.0–5.9	±0.42	8.9
2	Length	64.00	58–73	±3.1	4.8
	Width	7.90	6.5–9.0	±0.57	7.2
	Rel. slend.	8.13	6.9–9.7	±0.60	7.4
3	Length	61.70	56–70	±3.1	5.0
	Width	7.87	7.0–9.0	±0.53	6.7
	Rel. slend.	7.87	6.7–9.4	±0.53	6.7
4	Length	55.20	50–61	±2.8	5.1
	Width	6.13	5.0–7.0	±0.51	8.3
	Rel. slend.	9.05	7.6–10.9	±0.80	8.8
5	Length	51.10	46–57	±2.5	4.9
	Width	7.10	6.0–9.0	±0.65	9.2
	Rel. slend.	7.25	5.2–8.7	±0.67	9.2
Index		7.78	6.8–9.0	±0.49	6.3

*Coefficient of variability = (SD/Mean) × 100.
From Parish JG: Br J Radiol 1966; 52–62. Used by permission.

tients exhibiting bone or joint disease or congenital abnormalities of the skeletal system were excluded from the study.

REFERENCE

1. Parish JG: Radiographic measurements of the skeletal structure of the normal hand. Br J Radiol 1966; 39:52–62.

▪: METACARPOPHALANGEAL LENGTH IN THE EVALUATION OF SKELETAL MALFORMATION[1]

▪ ACR Code: 435 (Metacarpal)

Technique ▪

Central ray: Perpendicular to plane of film centered over palm.
Position: Posteroanterior.
Target-film distance: 36 inches.

Measurements (Figure 1) ▪

All measurements were total bone lengths, including epiphyses, and representing simple proximal-to-distal axial measurements, with the exception of the "hook" at the base of the third metacarpal, which is difficult to resolve. Measurements taken to the nearest 0.1 mm. The data are also applicable to the 39.37-inch (1-meter) focal film distance.

These dimensions are useful in the construction of metacarpophalangeal pattern profiles for the evaluation of skeletal malformations, as described by Poznanski and colleagues.[2]

Table 1 ▪ Standards for Metacarpal and Phalangeal Lengths and Variability (Age 2–10 Years)*

BONES		2 Mean	SD	3 Mean	SD	4 Mean	SD	5 Mean	SD	6 Mean	SD	7 Mean	SD	8 Mean	SD	9 Mean	SD	10 Mean	SD
MALES																			
Distal	5	8.8	—	8.4	0.6	9.0	0.7	9.9	0.6	10.7	0.6	11.4	0.8	12.2	0.9	12.6	1.0	13.5	0.9
	4	9.2	0.7	9.9	0.8	10.5	0.8	11.5	0.9	12.3	0.9	13.1	1.0	13.9	1.0	14.4	1.0	15.3	1.2
	3	8.7	0.9	9.5	0.8	10.2	0.8	11.1	0.8	11.8	0.9	12.7	1.0	13.4	1.0	14.0	1.0	14.8	1.2
	2	8.2	0.5	8.8	1.1	9.1	0.8	10.1	0.9	10.8	0.9	11.6	1.0	12.4	1.0	13.0	1.0	13.7	1.1
	1	11.1	0.6	12.3	0.8	13.2	1.0	14.4	0.9	15.4	0.9	16.5	1.0	17.4	1.0	17.9	1.2	19.0	1.2
Middle	5	8.8	0.9	9.8	0.8	10.6	1.0	11.2	1.0	12.0	1.0	12.7	1.1	13.5	1.1	14.3	1.2	15.0	1.2
	4	13.5	0.9	14.5	1.0	15.8	0.9	16.7	0.9	17.7	1.0	18.7	1.1	19.8	1.1	20.9	1.3	21.6	1.4
	3	14.1	0.8	15.1	1.1	16.5	1.0	17.6	1.0	18.7	1.1	19.8	1.2	20.9	1.2	22.0	1.4	22.9	1.4
	2	11.2	0.8	12.3	1.1	13.5	1.0	14.4	0.9	15.3	1.0	16.1	1.1	17.1	1.1	18.1	1.2	18.8	1.2
Proximal	5	16.1	0.7	17.8	0.9	19.2	1.0	20.6	1.0	21.8	1.0	23.0	1.1	24.2	1.3	25.2	1.5	26.4	1.5
	4	20.5	0.9	22.8	1.0	24.7	1.2	26.4	1.2	27.9	1.3	29.5	1.4	31.0	1.6	32.3	1.9	33.9	1.8
	3	21.8	1.0	24.2	1.1	26.3	1.4	28.1	1.4	29.8	1.4	31.5	1.6	33.2	1.8	34.7	2.2	36.1	1.9
	2	19.5	1.0	21.9	1.2	23.7	1.3	25.4	1.4	26.8	1.5	28.3	1.6	29.7	1.8	31.4	1.9	32.5	1.9
	1	15.2	—	15.9	1.1	17.2	1.1	18.3	1.2	19.6	1.2	20.8	1.3	21.8	1.3	23.1	1.5	24.2	1.4
Metacarpal	5	23.9	1.0	26.3	1.5	28.9	1.9	32.1	2.2	34.6	2.2	36.7	2.1	38.8	2.5	40.6	2.5	42.7	2.9
	4	25.5	1.1	28.9	1.5	31.7	2.1	35.0	2.5	37.9	2.7	40.1	2.5	42.2	3.1	44.1	2.8	46.5	3.5
	3	28.6	1.3	32.3	1.8	35.6	2.3	39.3	2.8	42.6	2.9	45.3	2.8	47.6	3.5	49.8	3.0	52.3	3.7
	2	30.6	1.5	34.5	1.7	37.9	2.3	41.6	2.7	44.9	2.9	47.7	2.8	50.2	3.4	52.6	3.0	55.0	3.9
	1	19.6	1.3	22.0	1.2	24.1	1.6	26.7	1.6	29.0	1.7	30.9	1.8	32.7	2.1	34.4	2.1	36.3	2.3
FEMALES																			
Distal	5	7.8	0.6	8.4	0.6	9.1	0.7	9.9	0.7	10.6	0.8	11.4	0.9	12.1	1.0	12.7	1.1	13.5	1.2
	4	9.1	0.7	9.9	0.7	10.6	0.8	11.5	0.9	12.4	1.0	13.2	1.1	14.0	1.1	14.4	1.2	15.5	1.4
	3	8.8	0.7	9.9	0.8	10.2	0.7	11.1	0.9	12.2	1.3	12.7	1.1	13.5	1.1	14.1	1.1	15.0	1.4
	2	8.0	0.8	8.6	0.7	9.4	0.7	10.1	0.8	10.9	0.9	11.7	1.0	12.3	1.1	13.1	1.1	13.8	1.4
	1	11.3	0.8	12.5	0.8	13.2	0.8	14.4	1.0	15.4	1.1	16.3	1.2	17.3	1.3	17.8	1.3	19.0	1.6
Middle	5	9.0	1.2	9.8	1.1	10.5	1.1	11.2	1.1	12.2	1.2	12.9	1.3	13.6	1.4	14.2	1.4	15.2	1.6
	4	13.5	0.9	14.9	1.0	15.8	1.1	16.9	1.2	18.1	1.3	19.1	1.4	20.1	1.4	20.9	1.5	22.2	1.7
	3	14.2	0.9	15.6	1.1	16.6	1.2	17.9	1.2	19.2	1.3	20.3	1.4	21.4	1.4	22.1	1.6	23.6	1.8
	2	11.6	0.9	12.8	1.0	13.6	1.1	14.8	1.1	16.0	1.2	16.8	1.3	17.8	1.4	18.1	1.5	19.6	1.7
Proximal	5	16.3	1.0	17.9	1.1	19.1	1.1	20.6	1.3	22.0	1.4	23.1	1.6	24.4	1.6	25.2	1.6	27.1	2.0
	4	20.7	1.1	22.9	1.3	24.6	1.3	26.3	1.5	28.2	1.7	29.7	1.9	31.2	2.0	32.4	2.0	34.5	2.4
	3	22.2	1.2	24.5	1.3	26.4	1.4	28.3	1.8	30.4	1.8	32.1	2.0	33.7	2.2	35.0	2.2	37.3	2.6
	2	20.1	1.2	22.3	1.3	24.0	1.8	25.8	1.7	27.7	1.7	29.2	1.9	30.7	2.0	31.5	2.4	34.0	2.4
	1	14.9	1.0	16.3	1.1	17.2	1.3	18.8	1.3	20.2	1.3	21.4	1.5	22.7	1.6	23.5	2.0	25.5	2.1
Metacarpal	5	23.7	1.5	26.9	2.1	29.4	1.8	32.6	2.0	35.1	2.1	37.2	2.4	39.4	2.5	40.8	2.5	43.8	2.8
	4	26.0	1.9	29.6	2.7	32.2	2.0	35.6	2.5	38.4	2.7	40.5	2.8	43.1	3.0	44.3	2.8	47.5	3.5
	3	29.4	2.1	33.4	2.9	36.3	2.2	40.3	2.7	43.3	3.1	45.8	3.1	48.7	3.2	49.9	3.2	53.6	3.8
	2	31.3	1.9	35.2	2.7	38.2	2.3	42.2	2.7	45.6	3.2	48.1	3.3	51.2	3.3	52.6	3.4	56.6	4.1
	1	19.9	1.6	22.7	1.6	24.8	1.7	27.3	1.8	29.6	1.9	31.5	2.0	33.5	2.1	34.8	2.4	37.4	2.6

*For each sex, n ≅ 150 at age 4 years, 124 at age 9 years, 78 in adulthood, and 30–85 at intermediate ages. All values are in millimeters.
From Garn SM, et al: Radiology 1972; 105:375–381. Used by permission.

Table 2 ▪ Standards for Metacarpal and Phalangeal Lengths and Variability (Age 11 Years–Adult)*

BONES		11 Mean	SD	12 Mean	SD	13 Mean	SD	14 Mean	SD	15 Mean	SD	16 Mean	SD	17 Mean	SD	18 Mean	SD	Adults Mean	SD
MALES																			
Distal	5	14.2	0.9	15.0	0.9	15.8	0.9	16.8	1.0	17.6	1.1	17.9	1.0	18.1	1.0	18.1	1.2	18.7	1.3
	4	16.1	1.2	17.0	1.3	17.8	1.4	18.8	1.3	19.6	1.4	20.0	1.3	20.3	1.3	20.0	1.3	20.5	1.2
	3	15.6	1.2	16.4	1.2	17.1	1.3	18.2	1.3	19.0	1.4	19.3	1.4	19.5	1.3	19.4	1.3	20.1	1.2
	2	14.3	1.1	15.0	1.0	15.7	1.4	16.7	1.2	17.5	1.2	17.8	1.3	18.2	1.3	18.1	1.3	18.8	1.4
	1	19.7	1.2	20.6	1.3	21.7	1.4	22.8	1.3	24.1	1.4	24.5	1.4	24.9	1.4	24.8	1.5	25.2	1.4
Middle	5	15.7	1.4	16.5	1.5	17.5	1.5	18.9	1.6	19.9	1.4	20.5	1.4	20.6	1.4	21.0	1.4	21.6	1.6
	4	22.6	1.5	23.6	1.5	24.8	1.7	26.5	1.6	27.7	1.5	28.4	1.5	28.7	1.4	29.1	1.5	29.6	1.6
	3	24.0	1.4	24.9	1.4	26.3	1.6	28.0	1.5	29.2	1.5	30.0	1.6	30.2	1.6	30.6	1.8	31.1	1.8
	2	19.8	1.8	20.4	1.3	21.6	1.6	23.2	1.5	24.3	1.5	25.0	1.5	25.3	1.4	25.6	1.7	26.1	1.6
Proximal	5	27.6	1.7	28.9	2.0	30.5	2.4	32.9	2.4	34.7	2.0	35.6	1.8	36.1	1.8	35.9	2.0	36.3	2.0
	4	35.3	2.0	37.0	2.4	38.8	2.8	41.6	2.8	43.7	2.6	44.9	2.3	45.4	2.2	45.2	2.5	45.5	2.3
	3	37.8	2.3	39.5	2.6	41.5	2.9	44.4	2.8	46.6	2.5	47.8	2.4	48.3	2.3	48.2	2.7	48.5	2.6
	2	33.9	2.1	35.5	2.4	37.2	2.6	39.8	2.6	41.8	2.2	42.8	2.0	43.3	2.1	43.4	2.4	43.7	2.2
	1	25.4	1.6	26.7	2.0	28.5	2.2	30.9	2.2	32.9	1.8	33.8	1.5	34.6	2.6	34.7	1.8	35.0	1.9
Metacarpal	5	44.6	2.8	47.7	3.2	49.1	4.0	52.2	3.9	55.4	3.6	57.1	2.8	57.9	2.5	57.5	2.9	58.0	3.0
	4	48.4	3.1	51.0	3.7	53.1	4.6	56.4	4.5	59.5	4.1	61.5	3.7	62.6	3.1	61.7	3.4	62.1	3.5
	3	54.6	3.4	57.3	4.0	59.5	5.1	63.1	4.9	66.7	4.4	68.7	4.1	69.7	3.3	69.0	3.7	69.0	3.8
	2	57.3	3.5	60.6	3.9	63.3	5.1	67.1	4.8	70.6	4.3	73.2	3.8	74.2	2.9	73.9	3.5	73.7	3.8
	1	38.2	2.4	40.2	2.7	42.5	3.0	45.1	2.8	47.6	2.6	48.8	2.3	49.5	2.1	49.4	2.7	49.6	2.9
FEMALES																			
Distal	5	14.2	1.3	15.0	1.3	15.4	1.3	15.6	1.3	15.9	1.4	15.9	1.4	16.2	1.3	16.0	1.2	16.2	1.2
	4	16.2	1.4	17.1	1.4	17.6	1.2	17.9	1.3	18.0	1.4	18.0	1.3	18.1	1.4	17.9	1.3	18.0	1.3
	3	15.8	1.3	16.6	1.4	17.1	1.4	17.3	1.3	17.6	1.5	17.5	1.4	17.6	1.4	17.4	1.3	17.7	1.3
	2	14.4	1.3	15.2	1.5	15.7	1.5	15.8	1.5	16.1	1.6	16.0	1.6	16.3	1.5	16.2	1.3	16.6	1.3
	1	20.0	1.7	20.9	1.7	21.4	1.6	21.7	1.6	22.0	1.7	22.0	1.7	22.1	1.8	22.0	1.6	22.1	1.6
Middle	5	16.2	1.7	17.2	1.7	17.9	1.8	18.1	1.6	18.4	1.7	18.5	1.7	18.5	1.9	18.6	1.7	18.7	1.7
	4	23.4	1.8	24.7	1.8	25.7	1.9	25.9	1.6	26.3	1.8	26.4	1.8	26.5	1.9	26.3	1.8	26.4	1.7
	3	24.9	1.9	26.2	1.9	27.2	2.0	27.5	1.7	28.1	1.8	28.0	1.9	28.0	1.8	27.8	1.8	27.9	1.7
	2	20.6	1.8	21.8	1.9	22.7	1.8	23.0	1.8	23.5	1.8	23.3	1.9	23.4	1.9	23.1	1.6	23.2	1.6
Proximal	5	28.7	2.1	30.5	2.2	31.9	2.2	32.3	2.1	32.9	2.2	32.8	2.3	32.8	2.3	32.5	2.0	32.5	1.9
	4	36.5	2.5	38.8	2.6	40.3	2.5	40.9	2.3	41.5	2.5	41.6	2.6	41.7	2.6	41.1	2.2	40.8	2.4
	3	39.5	2.7	41.7	2.8	43.5	2.8	44.1	2.4	44.8	2.6	44.8	2.7	44.8	2.5	44.2	2.4	44.0	2.3
	2	35.9	2.6	38.0	2.6	39.5	2.6	39.9	2.4	40.6	2.6	40.6	2.6	40.7	2.6	39.9	2.3	40.0	2.3
	1	27.2	2.3	29.2	2.4	30.6	2.2	31.1	1.9	31.8	2.0	31.7	2.1	31.9	2.2	31.3	1.9	31.4	2.0
Metacarpal	5	46.3	2.9	48.7	2.9	50.8	2.8	52.1	2.8	52.6	3.0	52.8	3.0	53.0	2.7	52.0	2.7	51.9	3.6
	4	50.2	3.8	52.8	3.7	55.1	3.6	56.2	3.6	56.9	3.6	57.2	3.9	57.2	3.5	56.1	2.9	56.0	3.5
	3	56.5	4.0	59.5	4.2	62.1	4.0	63.4	3.9	63.9	3.9	64.3	4.0	64.5	4.0	63.2	3.4	62.6	4.0
	2	59.9	4.3	63.2	4.4	66.2	4.2	67.4	3.9	68.1	4.2	68.6	4.3	68.9	4.1	67.5	3.4	66.9	4.3
	1	39.7	3.0	42.0	3.0	43.8	2.7	44.4	2.5	45.3	2.4	45.0	2.8	45.0	2.6	44.6	2.2	44.2	2.6

*For each sex, n ≅ 150 at age 4 years, 124 at age 9 years, 78 in adulthood, and 30–85 at intermediate ages. All values are in millimeters.
From Garn SM, et al: Radiology 1972; 105:375–381. Used by permission.

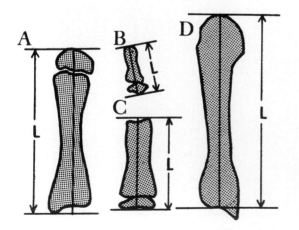

Figure 1 ▪ Length measurements of metacarpals (*A*), distals (*B*), and proximals (*C*), made at right angles to the long axis and including the epiphysis, when separate. The exception is the third metacarpal, excluding the styloid process as in *D*. (From Garn SM, et al: Radiology 1972; 105:375. Used by permission.)

Source ▪

Six hundred eighty-four metacarpal and phalangeal lengths were measured at the ages shown in Tables 1 and 2. All subjects were white and of European ancestry.

REFERENCES

1. Garn SM, Hertzog KP, Poznanski AK, Nagy JM: Metacarpophalangeal length in the evaluation of skeletal malformations. Radiology 1972; 105:375–381.
2. Poznanski AK, Garn SM, Nagy JM, Gale JC Jr: Metacarpophalangeal pattern profiles in the evaluation of skeletal malformations. Radiology 1972; 104:1–11.

▪: RELATIVE PROPORTIONS OF THE BONES OF THE THUMB[1]
▪ ACR Code: 438 (Thumb)

Table 1* ▪ Normal Metacarpal and Phalangeal Lengths

| | | MALES | | | | FEMALES | | | |
| | | Diaphysis and Epiphysis | | | Diaphysis | Diaphysis and Epiphysis | | | Diaphysis |
		Adult	9 Yr	4 Yr	1 Yr	Adult	9 Yr	4 Yr	1 Yr
Met 2/Met 1	Mean	1.49	1.53	1.57	1.64	1.52	1.52	1.55	1.60
	SD	0.05	0.05	0.06	0.06	0.07	0.06	0.07	0.09
Met 2/P 1	Mean	2.10	2.28	2.22	2.13	2.13	2.25	2.22	2.15
	SD	0.10	0.12	0.11	0.11	0.12	0.13	0.11	0.13
Met 2/D 1	Mean	2.93	2.93	2.88	2.85	3.02	2.96	2.90	2.89
	SD	0.16	0.15	0.16	0.18	0.20	0.16	0.14	0.19
Met 1/Met 2	Mean	0.67	0.66	0.64	0.61	0.66	0.66	0.65	0.63
	SD	0.02	0.02	0.02	0.02	0.04	0.03	0.03	0.04
Met 1/P 1	Mean	1.41	1.49	1.41	1.31	1.41	1.49	1.44	1.34
	SD	0.06	0.06	0.06	0.06	0.05	0.07	0.06	0.07
Met 1/D 1	Mean	1.97	1.92	1.82	1.74	1.99	1.95	1.88	1.81
	SD	0.12	0.10	0.10	0.10	0.12	0.11	0.11	0.14
P 1/Met 2	Mean	0.48	0.44	0.45	0.47	0.47	0.45	0.45	0.47
	SD	0.02	0.02	0.02	0.02	0.03	0.02	0.02	0.03
P 1/Met 1	Mean	0.71	0.67	0.71	0.77	0.71	0.67	0.70	0.75
	SD	0.03	0.03	0.03	0.04	0.03	0.03	0.03	0.04
P 1/D 1	Mean	1.40	1.29	1.30	1.34	1.42	1.32	1.31	1.35
	SD	0.08	0.07	0.07	0.08	0.09	0.08	0.07	0.09
D 1/Met 2	Mean	0.34	0.34	0.35	0.35	0.33	0.34	0.35	0.35
	SD	0.02	0.02	0.02	0.02	0.02	0.02	0.02	0.02
D 1/Met 1	Mean	0.51	0.52	0.55	0.58	0.50	0.51	0.53	0.56
	SD	0.03	0.03	0.03	0.03	0.03	0.03	0.03	0.04
D 1/P 1	Mean	0.72	0.78	0.77	0.75	0.71	0.76	0.77	0.75
	SD	0.04	0.04	0.04	0.04	0.04	0.05	0.04	0.05

*Met = metacarpal of the thumb; Met 2 = second metacarpal; P 1 = proximal phalanx of the thumb; D 1 = distal phalanx of the thumb.
From Poznanski AK, Garn SM, Holt JE: Radiology 1971, 100:115. Used by permission.

Technique ▪

Central ray: Perpendicular to plane of film projected over palm.
Position: Posteroanterior.
Target-film distance: Immaterial.

Measurements (See Figure 1 in Metacarpal Index in Adults and Table 1) ▪

Measurements are made along the axis of each bone, and the maximum length is used.

The ratio approach is more useful than comparisons with normal standards for length because it is not dependent on the size of the individual, and a relative disproportion in length of bones is more easily detected.

Source ▪

Measurements are from the studies of Garn at Fels Research Institute, Yellow Springs, Ohio.

REFERENCE

1. Poznanski AK, Garn SM, Holt JF: The thumb in the congenital malformation syndromes. Radiology 1971; 100:115–129.

CHAPTER 6

Pelvis and Hips

:: SYMPHYSIS PUBIS WIDTH
- ACR Code: 4414 (Symphysis Pubis)

Technique

Radiographs were performed of the pelvis or abdomen, using a focus-film distance of 1 meter.[1]

Measurements

The transverse width of the symphysis pubis was measured to the nearest millimeter. Using a phantom and by measuring the pubis from pelvic and abdominal films when both were done on the same subject, it was determined that there was no significant difference in symphysis width between centering at the iliac crests (abdominal films) or 5 cm above the pubis (pelvic films). Table 1 lists the symphysis width by age, with the mean and standard deviation (SD) given. Figure 1 is a plot of the mean and ± 2 SD for the same data.[1] An earlier study of adults (n = 400) yielded a mean ± SD for men of 5.9 ± 1.3 mm and for women of 4.9 ± 1.1 mm.[2] These numbers are included in Figure 1 as well.

Source

Subjects included 490 males and 398 females (total 888) whose ages ranged from newborn to 16 years. Patients with conditions known to be associated with widening of the symphysis were excluded.[1]

Comments

The logarithmic regression equations and r values for the mean symphysis pubis width and the +2 SD (95th percentile) value on age (from birth to 16 years) are given here and may be useful:

Table 1 ▪ Symphysis Pubis Width		
AGE	NO.	MEAN ± SD (mm)
0–6 mon	103	7.4 ± 1.3
7 mon–1 yr	66	7.1 ± 1.4
1–2 yr	89	6.9 ± 1.3
2–3 yr	91	6.3 ± 1.3
3–4 yr	88	6.5 ± 1.2
4–5 yr	65	6.1 ± 1.1
5–6 yr	57	6.2 ± 1.2
6–7 yr	42	5.8 ± 1.0
7–8 yr	50	6.0 ± 1.1
8–9 yr	42	5.8 ± 1.1
9–10 yr	38	5.9 ± 1.1
10–11 yr	40	6.1 ± 1.1
11–12 yr	32	6.2 ± 1.1
12–13 yr	32	5.8 ± 1.1
13–14 yr	25	5.9 ± 1.0
14–15 yr	14	5.9 ± 1.0
15–16 yr	14	5.4 ± 1.4
Adult male	—	5.9 ± 1.3
Adult female	—	4.9 ± 1.1

Values for children are from Patel[1] and for adults from Vix.[2] Measurements are in millimeters.
Modified from Patel K, Chapman S: Clin Radiol 1993; 47(1):56–57. Used by permission.

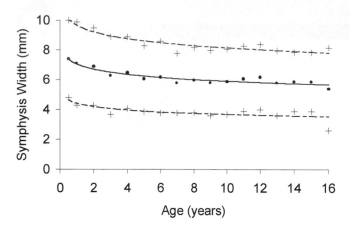

Figure 1 ▪ Symphysis pubis width by age. The mean (*circles*), ±2 standard deviations (*crosses*), and logarithmic regression lines (mean = *solid lines*, ±2 standard deviations = *dashed lines*) are shown. (From Patel K, Chapman S: Clin Radiol 1993; 47(1):56–57. Used by permission.)

Mean width in millimeters =

7.0513 − 0.4861 * ln (age in years), r = 0.93.

95th percentile width in millimeters = 9.6717 − 0.6511 * ln (age in years), r = 0.93.

REFERENCES

1. Patel K, Chapman S: Normal symphysis pubis width in children. Clin Radiol 1993; 47(1):56–57.
2. Vix VA, Ryu CY: The adult symphysis pubis: Normal and abnormal. AJR Am J Roentgenol 1971; 112(3):517–525.

⁘ THE ILIAC ANGLE AND THE ILIAC INDEX OF THE GROWING HIP[1]
▪ ACR Code: 442 (Hip Joint)

Technique ▪

Central ray: Perpendicular to plane of film centered to a point about 1 inch superior to the pubic symphysis.
Position: Anteroposterior.
Target-film distance: Immaterial.

Measurements (Figures 1 and 2; Table 1) ▪

The iliac angle is formed between a line drawn through the lower edges of the *Y* cartilages (the *Y-Y* line) and the oblique lines drawn through two points, the most lateral point of the iliac body below and the most lateral point on the iliac wing above (Figure 1).

The iliac index is a combination of the iliac angle and the acetabular angle (see next section) and may prove more useful than either single measurement. The iliac index is the sum of both acetabular angles and both iliac angles divided by 2. These measurements are useful in the diagnosis of Down syndrome, in which low values are obtained.

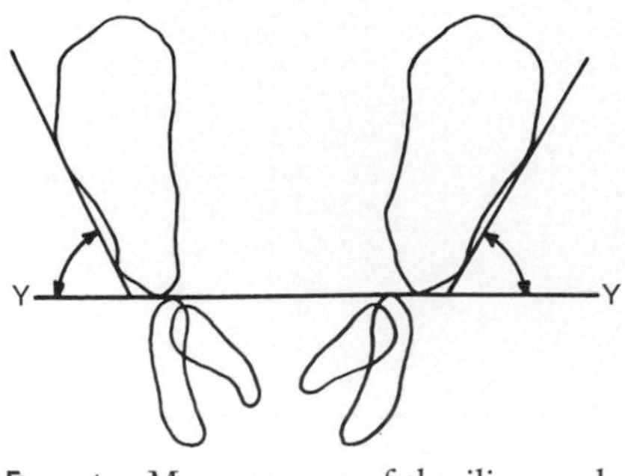

Astley states that if the iliac index is less than 60, Down syndrome is very possible.[2] If it is more than 78, the child is probably normal. If it lies in between, only a qualified report can be given. If the index is between 60 and 68, Down syndrome is probable, but a note must be added that 10% of normal subjects occur in this range. If the index is between 68 and 78, the child probably does not have Down syndrome, but a notation must be added that 6% of those with Down syndrome do occur in this range.

Source ▪

The data of Caffey and Ross are based on a study of 48 infants with Down syndrome, who varied in age from 2 days to 12 months, and on a previous study of 1500 unse-

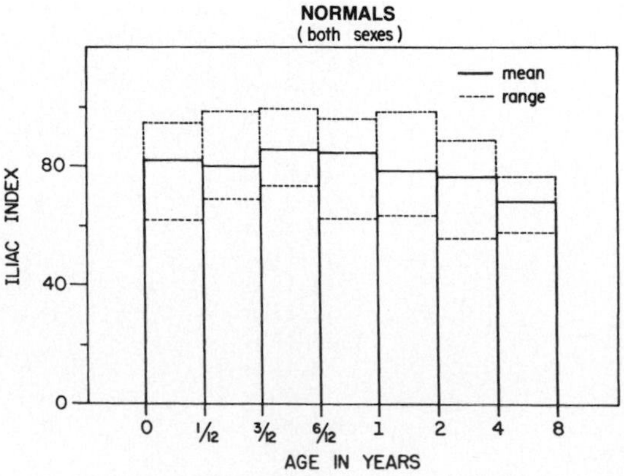

Figure 1 ▪ Measurement of the iliac angle.

Figure 2 ▪ Variation of the normal iliac index with age. (Adapted from Astley R: Br J Radiol 1963; 36:2.)

Table 1* ▪ Normal Iliac Angles and Indices

CATEGORY	MEAN	SD	2 SD RANGE	ACTUAL RANGE
Acetabular angles in degrees				
Younger with Down syndrome	16	4.5	25–7	29–9
Younger normal subjects	28	4.7	37–18	44–12
Older with Down syndrome	11	4.2	19–3	19–6
Older normal subjects	22	4.2	8–14	34–8
Iliac angles in degrees				
Younger with Down syndrome	44	6.5	56–30	58–35
Younger normal subjects	55	5.5	66–44	67–43
Older with Down syndrome	41	7.0	55–29	50–26
Older normal subjects	58	7.0	72–43	74–44
Iliac indices				
Younger with Down syndrome	60	9.9	80–49	87–48
Younger normal subjects	81	8.0	97–65	97–68
Older with Down syndrome	50	9.6	67–29	67–33
Older normal subjects	79	9.0	96–60	101–62

*Younger means younger than 3 months; older means 3–12 months of age.
From Caffey J, Ross S: AJR Am J Roentgenol 1958; 80:458. Used by permission.

lected newborn infants in whom the pelvis and hips were examined roentgenographically.[1]

Astley's study is based on 106 normal children from birth to 8 years and on 34 children in whom there was a clinical question of Down syndrome.[2]

REFERENCES

1. Caffey J, Ross S: AJR Am J Roentgenol 1958; 80:458.
2. Astley R: Br J Radiol 1963; 36:2

▪: THE ACETABULAR ANGLE OF THE GROWING HIP[1]
▪ ACR Code: 112 (Hip Joint)

Technique ▪

Central ray: Perpendicular to plane of film centered to a point about 1 inch superior to the pubic symphysis.
Position: Anteroposterior.
Target-film distance: Immaterial.

Measurements (Figure 1) ▪

The acetabular angle is formed between a transverse line drawn through the right and left *Y* cartilages in the ilia (the *Y-Y* line) and an oblique line connecting the medial and lateral ends of the bony edge behind and above the acetabular face.

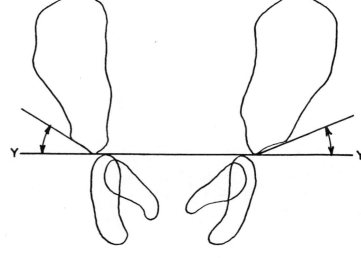

Figure 1 ▪ Measurement of the acetabular angle.

Table 1 ▪ Comparison of Acetabular Angles at Different Ages in All Categories

	MEAN VALUES (DEGREES)			2 SD RANGE (DEGREES)		
	Neonate	6 Mon	12 Mon	Neonate	6 Mon	12 Mon
White						
Male						
Right	25.8	19.4	19.1	34–17	26–12	26–12
Left	27.0	20.9	20.6	37–17	28–13	28–13
Female						
Right	28.3	22.1	20.5	38–18	30–14	28–13
Left	29.4	23.4	21.9	39–20	32–15	29–14
Black						
Male						
Right	24.8	21.4	20.5	34–15	31–12	29–12
Left	26.0	23.0	21.9	36–16	32–14	30–14
Female						
Right	27.7	23.9	22.5	38–18	32–16	30–15
Left	29.4	25.4	24.4	39–19	33–18	32–16

Adapted from Caffey J, et al: Pediatrics 1956; 17:632.

There are small differences in the left and right acetabular angles in all categories of patients (Table 1.) There is also a distinct difference in size of the angles on both sides in females and males.

Congenital dislocation of the hip is all but unknown in blacks.

Source ▪

The radiologic findings were derived from 627 newborn infants, of whom 551 were later reexamined at 6 months and 527 at 12 months. This study did not include premature infants, children with Down syndrome, children whose hips dislocated under observation, or children whose racial origins could not be determined accurately.

REFERENCE

1. Caffey J, et al: Pediatrics 1956; 17:632.

▪: EARLY DETECTION OF PERTHES DISEASE: THE TEARDROP DISTANCE
▪ ACR Code: 442 (Hip Joint)

Technique ▪

Central ray: Perpendicular to plane of film centered over midpelvis.
Position: Anteroposterior. Positioning does not alter the measurement, provided the femur is not rotated internally or externally more than 30°, flexed more than 30°, or abducted more than 15°.
Target-film distance: 40 inches.

Measurements (Figures 1 and 2) ▪

Measurement is made from the lateral margin of the pelvic teardrop to the medial border of the proximal femoral metaphysis. Measurements are independent of the age of the subject. The teardrop distance (*TDD*), when greater than 11 mm, or more than 2 mm greater than that of the opposite hip, is a sensitive indicator of hip joint disease.

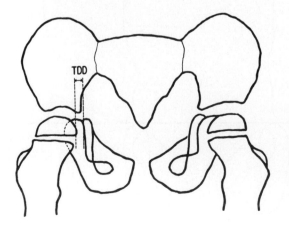

Figure 1 ▪ Measurement of the teardrop distance.

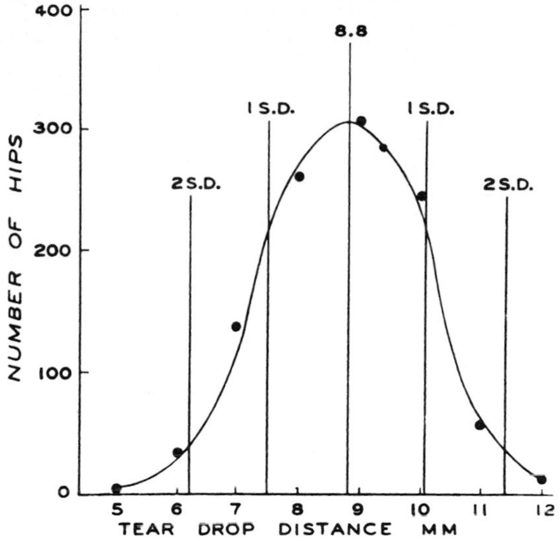

Figure 2 ▪ Frequency distribution of the teardrop distance in normal children. (From Eyring EJ, et al: AJR Am J Roentgenol 1965; 93:382. Used by permission.)

Source ▪

The data are based on a study of 1070 normal hips of children from 1 to 11 years and on 49 hips affected by Perthes disease.

REFERENCE

1. Eyring EJ, et al: AJR Am J Roentgenol 1965; 93:382.

▪▪ ULTRASOUND OF THE INFANT HIP (METHOD OF GRAF)
▪ ACR Code: 442 (Hip Joint)

Technique ▪

Linear transducers ranging in frequency from 5 to 7.5 MHz are used to perform real-time examination of the infant hip. A positioning device may be useful to help hold the infant in lateral decubitus position, with the hip to be examined up. Coronal images are made with the hip in neutral position so that the echogenic line of the ilium is parallel with the transducer, and the ossified proximal femur is imaged as an arcuate echogenic line. This basic view may be supplemented with coronal flexion, transverse neutral, and flexion, as well as stress views.

Measurements ▪

The single most important aspect of using Graf's technique for evaluation of infant hips is in producing a correctly aligned coronal image of the hip. Figure 1 shows such an image. A baseline is drawn paralleling the ilium bone and extending down into the femoral head. A line is drawn parallel to the bony acetabular roof between its lower edge and the promontory. The alpha angle is measured between this line and the baseline. A third line is drawn parallel to the cartilaginous roof between the promontory and the labrum. The beta angle is measured between this line and the baseline. Figure 2 shows these measurements. Table 1 lists the normal alpha and beta angles in infants from 0 to 6 months of age.[1] Table 2 shows the classification scheme as devised by Graf and refined by others.[2–8] Table 3 gives the median values of the alpha and beta angles for types I to IV.[9] Figure 3 shows the percentage of types I and IIB hips from 30 to 40 weeks (preterm infants) and from birth to 6 months in term infants. For this study, type I hips were divided into IA and IB (both having alpha angles of more than 60 degrees), with A having a sharp promontory and B having a slightly rounded promontory.[10]

Source ▪

Zieger and Schulz scanned 600 hips of normal infants ranging in age from 0 to 6 months.[1] Graf has examined many thousands of infant hips and developed a standardized classification scheme for hip dysplasia.[2–5] This scheme has been validated and refined by other investigators, each having extensive clinical experience with the technique.[6–8] Zieger and Schulz evaluated 334 hips of infants with varying degrees of dysplasia from completely normal (type I)

Table 1 ▪ Normal Values of the Alpha and Beta Angles in the Growing Hip

AGE (Mon)	ALPHA ANGLE	BETA ANGLE
0	61.1 ± 3.17	57.6 ± 4.90
1	62.2 ± 3.12	52.6 ± 5.04
2	62.8 ± 2.23	50.3 ± 3.61
3	64.6 ± 2.23	48.0 ± 3.84
4	65.0 ± 2.02	45.5 ± 3.08
5	65.5 ± 2.28	46.1 ± 4.28
6	65.2 ± 1.98	43.6 ± 3.21

Measurements are in degrees (mean ± standard deviation).
From Zieger M, Schulz RD: Pediatr Radiol 1987; 17:226–232. Used by permission.

Table 2 ▪ Classification of Infant Hips at Ultrasound

CLASS	SONOGRAPHIC TYPE	ACETABULAR MODELING	ACETABULAR PROMONTORY	CARTILAGE ROOF	α ANGLE (Degree)	β ANGLE (Degree)
I	Mature hip	Good	Sharp or slightly rounded	Narrow, extends far over femoral head	>60	<55
IIA	Immature hip, <3 months of age	Deficient (moderate)	Rounded	Broad, covers crown of head	50–60	55–77
IIB	Deficient, >3 months of age	Deficient (moderate)	Rounded	Broad, covers crown of head	50–60	55–77
IIC	Dysplasia (stable); also called critical zone	Deficient (moderate to severe)	Rounded	Broad, still covers femoral head	43–49	55–77
IID	Dysplasia (unstable); also called decentering	Deficient (severe)	Rounded or slightly flattened	Displaced upward	43–49	>77
III	Subluxed; also called eccentric	Poor	Flattened	Displaced, devoid of echoes or echogenic	<43	>77
IV	Dislocated	Poor	Deformed	Trapped between femoral head and ilium	Not measurable	>77

Modified from several researchers.[2–8]

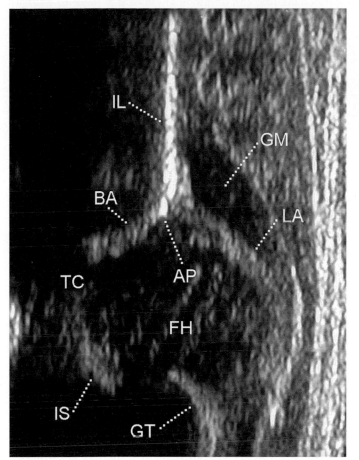

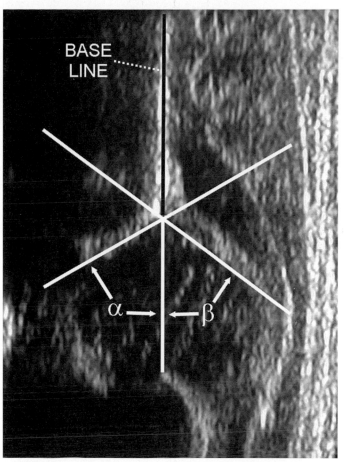

Figure 1 ▪ Coronal image of the infant hip in neutral position as required to measure the Graf angles. The image has been rotated so as to be anatomically correct. IL = ileum, BA = bony acetabulum, AP = acetabular promontory, GM = gluteal muscle, LA = labrum, TC = triradiate cartilage, FH = femoral head, IS = ischium, GT = greater trochanter.

Figure 2 ▪ Measurement of the alpha and beta angles from a coronal ultrasound of the hip in neutral position. The baseline, alpha angle, and beta angle are shown as described in the text.

Figure 3 ▪ Maturation of normal infant hips from 30 weeks through 6 months, expressed as percentages at each age. GA = gestational age, CA = chronologic age. Type IA (mature), *solid circles* and *solid line*. Type IB (transition form), *open circles* and *dashed line*. Type IIA (immature), *triangles* and *dotted line*. The lines represent an order 2 polynomial regression on age and percentage. (From Zieger M, Hilpert S: Pediatr Radiol 1987; 17:470–473. Used by permission.)

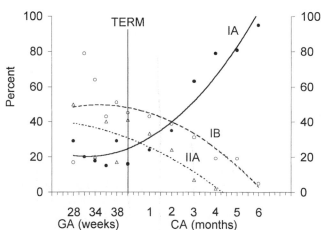

Table 3 ▪ Values of the Alpha and Beta Angles for Class I to IV Hips

Class	I	II	III	IV
Number	948	190	226	26
Alpha angle	66 ± 5.5	55 ± 5.0	48 ± 5.0	28 ± 9.5
Beta angle	33 ± 8	40 ± 8	47 ± 8	54 ± 8.5

Measurements are in degrees (median ± standard deviation).
From Zieger M: Pediatr Radiol 1986; 16(6):488–492. Used by permission.

to severely dysplastic (type IV). Each joint was scanned by two sonographers and the resulting hard copies were read by four individuals to derive mean values for each type.[9] In another study, Zieger and Hilpert scanned 200 normal hip joints in premature infants, ranging in gestational age from 28 to 38 weeks, within 10 weeks of birth, as well as 200 normal joints in term infants at various chronologic ages from birth to 6 months.[10] Using the Graf angles and morphologic features, the hips were classified in terms of maturity and the percentages tabulated.

Comments ▪

The alpha angle reflects the state of development of the acetabulum, and higher angles indicate better development and a deeper acetabulum. The beta angle reflects the amount of subluxation of the femoral head, with larger angles indicating greater degrees of subluxation/dislocation. In general, an alpha angle of greater than 60 degrees is normal at any age; between 50 and 59 degrees may be normal in infants less than 3 months old but is abnormal in older infants; and an alpha angle of less than 50 degrees is always abnormal. The measured angles are supplemented by observations about the morphology of the joint, as shown in Table 2. The acetabular morphology matures during the third trimester and the first several months of life, with type I hips comprising 93% of all normal subjects by 3 months of age, as shown in Figure 3.

REFERENCES

1. Zieger M, Schulz RD: Ultrasonography of the infant hip. Part III: Clinical application. Pediatr Radiol 1987; 17:226–232.
2. Graf R: The diagnosis of congenital hip-joint dislocation by the ultrasonic Comboung treatment. Arch Orthop Trauma Surg 1980; 97(2):117–133.
3. Graf R: New possibilities for the diagnosis of congenital hip joint dislocation by ultrasonography. J Pediatr Orthop 1983; 3(3):354–359.
4. Graf R: Classification of hip joint dysplasia by means of sonography. Arch Orthop Trauma Surg 1984; 102(4):248–255.
5. Graf R: Guide to Sonography of the Infant Hip. Thieme, New York, 1987.
6. Szoke N, Kuhl L, Heinrichs J: Ultrasound examination in the diagnosis of congenital hip dysplasia of newborns. J Pediatr Orthop 1988; 8(1):12–16.
7. Gerscovich EO: A radiologist's guide to the imaging in the diagnosis and treatment of developmental dysplasia of the hip. Skeletal Radiol 1997; 26:447–456.
8. DiPietro MA: Pediatric musculoskeletal and spinal sonography. In Holsbeeck MV, Introcaso JH (eds): Musculoskeletal Ultrasound. Mosby–Year Book, St. Louis, 1991, vol 1, pp 177–206.
9. Zieger M: Ultrasound of the infant hip. Part 2: Validity of the method. Pediatr Radiol 1986; 16(6):488–492.
10. Zieger M, Hilpert S: Ultrasonography of the infant hip. Part IV: Normal development in the newborn and preterm neonate. Pediatr Radiol 1987; 17:470–473.

▪▪ ACETABULAR COVERAGE OF THE FEMORAL HEAD
▪ ACR Code: 442 (Hip Joint)

Technique ▪

Morin and colleagues performed real-time ultrasound with 3.0- to 7.5-MHz linear transducers of infant hips with an MK100 machine (Advanced Technology Laboratories, Bellevue, WA).[1] Holen and colleagues used a 5-MHz transducer and a Picker 7000 machine (Picker International, Highland Heights, OH) for examination of infant hips.[2] Examinations were done in the coronal plane from the lateral position, in flexion[1] or semiflexion[2] positions.

Measurements ▪

Morin and colleagues drew a baseline parallel to the ilium down through the femoral head and two parallel lines through the joint capsule and acetabular floor. The percent of acetabular head coverage of the femoral head was calculated by dividing the distance between the ilial baseline and the acetabular floor line by the distance between the acetabular floor and joint capsule lines and multiplying by 100.[1] Holen and colleagues drew a line parallel to the transducer long axis through the acetabular apex and measured from that line to the acetabular floor, as well as the maximum width of the femoral head. Both measurements were perpendicular to the baseline of the scan, and the percentage was formed by dividing the covered portion by the width of the entire head and multiplying by 100.[2] Figure 1 shows the measurement technique. Table 1 lists the values obtained by patient group, including mean percent coverage, range, and standard deviation (when reported). There was no explanation in the text of Holen's paper for the discrepancy between the numbers of girls, boys, and total population.[2] Table 2 shows proposed cutoff values based on the study populations, as well as from a review of the subject by Millis and Share.[1–3]

Source ▪

Morin and colleagues evaluated 377 sonograms from 171 patients, ranging in age from 4 days to 28 months (mean 4

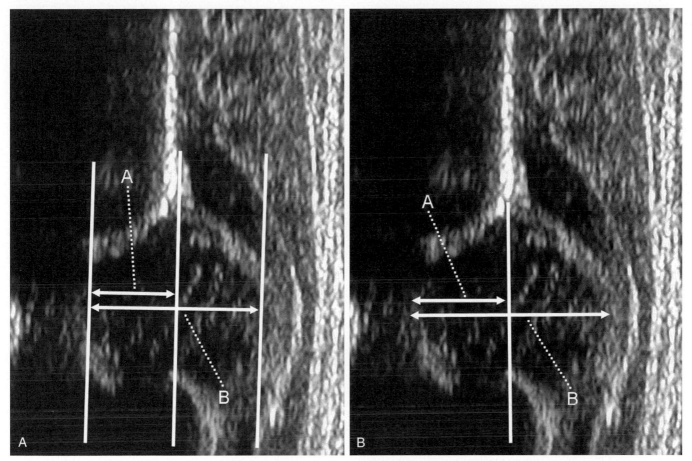

Figure 1 ▪ Measurement of acetabular coverage of the femoral head in infants. *A*, Method of Morin. Measurements are made between lines parallel to the ileal base line. *B*, Method of Holen. Measurements are made perpendicular to the transducer long axis. In both illustrations, *A* = distance between the acetabular apex and the floor; *B* = width of the femoral head. Percentage of coverage = A/B × 100.[1, 2]

Table 1 ▪ Coverage of the Femoral Head by the Acetabulum (%)[1, 2]

AUTHOR/ PATIENT GROUP	NO. IN GROUP	FEMORAL HEAD COVERAGE (%)		
		Mean	SD	Range
Morin et al				
Normal	236	59.3		37–89
Borderline	45	46.2		33–58
Abnormal	96	40.4		8–58
Holen et al				
Entire cohort	4459	54.8	5.2	21–76
Girls	2179	53.5	4.8	
Boys	2279	55.8	4.4	
Negative exam and negative U/S	4220	55.3	4.7	44–76
Abnormal exam and abnormal U/S	55	36.8	5.5	21–28
Equivocal exam and negative U/S	54	53.8	5.3	43–72
Negative exam and equivocal U/S	130	43.3	3.5	35–50

Table 2 ▪ Recommended Cut-Off Values for Femoral Head Coverage (%)

AUTHOR/PATIENT GROUP	FEMORAL HEAD COVERAGE (%)
Morin et al	
Normal	>58
Abnormal	≤58
Holen et al	
Normal	>50
Abnormal	≤50
Millis & Share	
Type I (mature)	>50
Type IIA (immature <3 months)	40–50
Type IIB (deficient >3 months)	40–50
Type IIC (dysplasia)	40–50
Type III (subluxation)	<40
Type IV (dislocation)	0

Morin and Holen from clinical studies, Millis from review article.[1–3]

months). There were 57 boys and 114 girls.[1] Holen and colleagues examined 4459 infants, almost all within 2 to 4 days after birth.[2] In both series, the patients were separated into groups based on physical examination, radiographic assessment, and standard ultrasound criteria for hip dysplasia or dislocation.

Comments ▪

The difference between the proposed cut-off values from the two studies can be attributed, in part, to slightly different techniques of obtaining the measurement.[1, 2] The method proposed by Holen and group seems to be somewhat easier to perform and the study population rather larger, which would militate for using 50% as the cut-off value.

REFERENCES

1. Morin C, Harcke HT, MacEwen GD: The infant hip: Real-time US assessment of acetabular development. Radiology 1985; 157:673–677.
2. Holen KJ, Terjesen T, Tegnander A, et al: Ultrasound screening for hip dysplasia in newborns. J Pediatr Orthop 1994; 14(5):667–673.
3. Millis MB, Share JC: Use of ultrasonography in dysplasia of the immature hip. Clin Orthop 1992; 274:160–171.

▪: OSSIFICATION OF THE FEMORAL HEAD
▪ ACR Code: 442 (Hip Joint)

Technique ▪

Anteroposterior (AP) radiographs of the abdomen.[1]

Measurements ▪

The presence or absence of the femoral head ossification center was noted and the cephalocaudal height measured directly from the film when visible.[1] Figure 1 shows the fraction of boys and girls with visible femoral head ossification at various ages from birth to 9 months. Figure 2 gives the height of the ossification center by age from birth to 1 year in boys and girls.

Source ▪

Subjects included 455 infants (241 boys and 214 girls) ranging in age from newborn to 1 year. Examinations were obtained for abdominal symptoms, urologic examination,

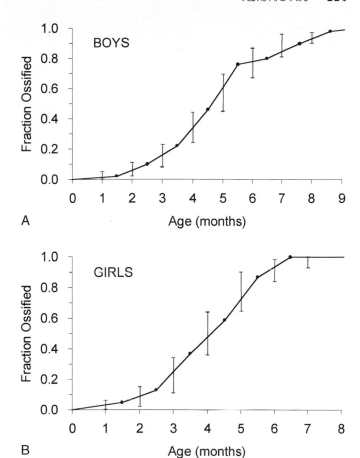

Figure 1 • Fraction of infants having radiographically visible femoral head ossification, from birth to 9 months in boys *(A)* and girls *(B)*. Observed values *(circles)* and 95% confidence intervals *(vertical lines)* are shown. (From Pettersson H, Theander G: Acta Radiol 1979; 20:170–179. Used by permission.)

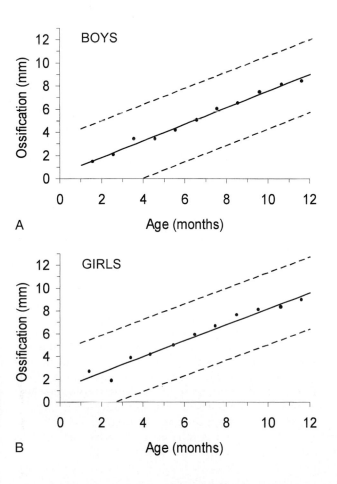

Figure 2 • Height of femoral head ossification center (in millimeters) from radiographs of boys *(A)* and girls *(B)*, from birth to 1 year. Shown are mean values *(circles)*, linear regression *(solid line)*, and 95% confidence intervals *(dashed lines)*. (From Pettersson H, Theander G: Acta Radiol 1979; 20:170–179. Used by permission.)

or swallowed foreign body. None of the infants had chronic, recurrent, or skeletal disease.[1]

Comments ▪

Ossification of the femoral head did not occur before 1 month and was always visible by 6 months in boys and 8 months in girls. Ossification was mostly seen bilaterally except in four boys aged 1 to 5 months and three girls aged 2 to 5 months.

REFERENCE

1. Pettersson H, Theander G: Ossification of femoral head in infancy. I. Normal standards. Acta Radiol 1979; 20:170–179.

▪: SIZE OF THE CARTILAGINOUS AND OSSIFIED FEMORAL HEAD
▪ ACR Code: 442 (Hip Joint)

Technique ▪

Zieger and associates performed ultrasound of the infant hip with linear transducers,[1, 2] and Harcke and colleagues used sector transducers.[3] The researchers used 7.5-MHz transducers until the infants were about 3 months of age and 5.0-MHz transducers for those between 3 and 7 months of age. Harcke and colleagues used 3.0-MHz transducers for children over 7 months of age.[3]

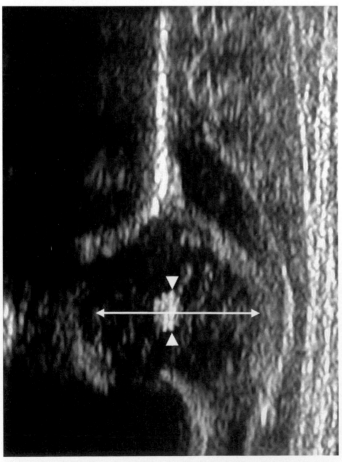

Figure 1 ▪ Measurement of the cartilaginous femoral head (*horizontal line with arrows*) and ossified nidus (*arrowheads*) from a longitudinal ultrasound of the infant hip.

Measurements ▪

Zieger and Hilpert measured the entire transverse diameter of the cartilaginous femoral head, as well as the cephalocaudal height of the ossified central nidus.[1] In the larger population of normal infants, Zieger and Schulz noted the presence or absence of an ossified central nidus in each femoral head.[2] Harcke and colleagues noted the presence or absence of central ossification in the femoral heads on ultrasound and radiographs and graded the size on a 4-point scale.[3] These measurements are depicted in Figure 1.

Figure 2 shows the size of the cartilaginous femoral head from 30 weeks' gestational age through 6 months and preterm and normal infants.[1] Figure 3 gives the percentage of ossified femoral heads from birth to 6 months.[2] This can be estimated by the following linear regression equation: Percent ossified = 20.5 × age in months − 10.5 (r = 0.97, p < .001). Figure 4 shows the size of the femoral ossification center from birth to 6 months.[1]

Harcke and group found agreement between radiographs and ultrasound in 689 of 742 hips (93%) in determining the presence or absence of ossification. Ultrasound showed ossification not seen on the radiograph in 52 of 742 (7%), and in one case ossification seen on the radiograph was not detected at ultrasound.[3] Further, in 150 cases in which ossification was seen in both hips on ultrasound and radiograph, 122 (81%) showed agreement between the two modalities in terms of symmetry of size. Sonography showed symmetric centers in 13 (9%) and asymmetry in 15 (10%), whereas the radiographs had opposite findings.[3]

Source ▪

Zieger and Hilpert scanned 200 normal hip joints in premature infants ranging in gestational age from 28 to 38 weeks within 10 weeks of birth, as well as 200 normal joints in term infants at various chronologic ages from birth to 6 months.[1] In another study, Zieger and Schulz scanned 1500 hips of normal infants ranging in age from 0 to 6 months.[2] Harcke and group reviewed 371 hip ultrasound studies done in 296 infants ranging in age from newborn to 1 year (total of 742 hips) and compared them with radiographs done within 1 week of the ultrasound.[3]

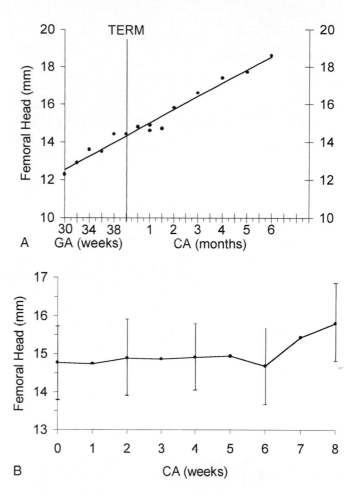

Figure 2 ▪ *A*, Size of the cartilaginous femoral head on ultrasound in 200 premature neonates and 200 normal infants up to age 6 months. Mean width *(circles)* and a linear regression are shown. *B*, Size of the cartilaginous femoral head in healthy infants during the first 2 months of life. The mean width = *circles and line*, 95% confidence intervals = *vertical lines*. CA = chronologic age, GA = gestational age. (From Zieger M, Hilpert S: Pediatr Radiol 1987; 17:470–473. Used by permission.)

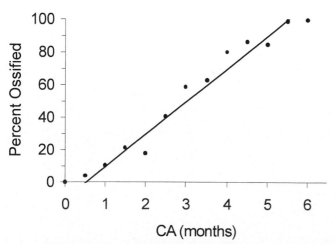

Figure 3 ▪ Development of femoral head ossification on ultrasound in 1500 normal hips by age fom birth to 6 months. Percentages at each age *(circles)* and a linear regression *(line)* are shown. (From Zieger M, Schulz RD: Pediatr Radiol 1987; 17:226–232. Used by permission.)

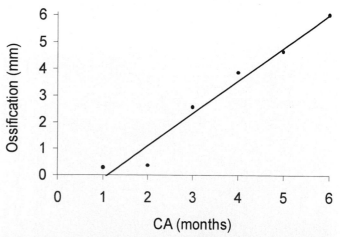

Figure 4 ▪ Height of femoral head ossification in 200 normal hip joints at ultrasound from birth to 6 months. The mean height in millimeters *(circles)* and linear regression *(line)* are shown. (From Zieger M, Hilpert S: Pediatr Radiol 1987; 17:470–473. Used by permission.)

REFERENCES

1. Zieger M, Hilpert S: Ultrasonography of the infant hip. Part IV: Normal development in the newborn and preterm neonate. Pediatr Radiol 1987; 17:470–473.

2. Zieger M, Schulz RD: Ultrasonography of the infant hip. Part III: Clinical application. Pediatr Radiol 1987; 17:226–232.

3. Harcke HT, Lee MS, Sinning L, et al: Ossification center of the infant hip: Sonographic and radiographic correlation. AJR Am J Roentgenol 1986; 147:317–321.

▪: ACETABULAR CARTILAGE THICKNESS
▪ ACR Code: 442 (Hip Joint)

Technique ▪

Real-time ultrasound of the infant hip was performed using various machines and 5.0 to 7.5-MHz transducers.[1]

Measurements ▪

Coronal neutral views of each hip (as used to calculate the Graf angles) were used. The ilial baseline and alpha angle were drawn first. The acetabular cartilage thickness was measured with electronic calipers between the apex of the alpha angle and the femoral head in a line parallel to the ilial baseline. Figure 1 shows this measurement. Conventional sonographic criteria, including Graf angles, morphologic evaluation, and dynamic examination, were listed at the same time to establish the presence of absence of dysplasia. Table 1 lists the cartilage thickness for controls, as well as study patients with and without dysplasia. The workers established a cut-off value of 3.4 mm; of the 22 initially normal hips exceeding this value in the study population, 16 developed dysplasia and/or subluxation on follow-up (6 weeks to 6 months). The test performance using 3.4 mm as a cut-off in detecting hip dysplasia (at the time of the test or developing later) is as follows: sensitivity 94%, specificity 97%, positive predictive value 91%, negative predictive value 98%.[1]

Source ▪

A control group consisted of 33 infants (66 hips) with no clinical suspicion for hip dysplasia who ranged in age from 1 day to 10 months of age (mean 42 days) and whose gestational age at birth ranged from 30.5 to 40 weeks (mean 39.5 weeks). The study group contained 110 infants (220 hips) referred for clinical findings or history suggesting hip dysplasia.[1] These patients ranged in age from 3 days to 8 months of age (mean 67 days), and the gestational age at birth ranged from 32 to 41 weeks (mean 39.5 weeks).

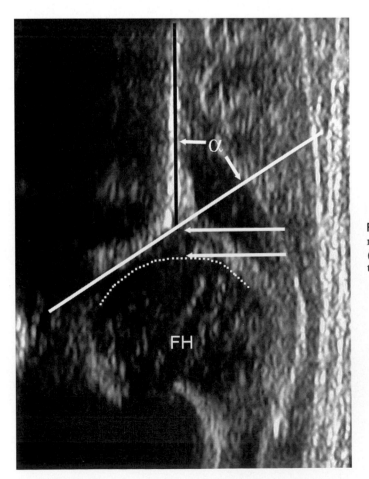

Figure 1 ▪ Measurement of acetabular cartilage thickness from coronal ultrasound of the hip. The ileal baseline (*black*) and alpha angle (*white*) lines are shown. The thickness (*arrows*) is measured between the acetabular apex and the femoral head (*dotted line*).

Table 1 ▪ Acetabular Cartilage Thickness in Infants at Ultrasound

GROUP	NO.	ACETABULAR CARTILAGE THICKNESS (mm)		
		Mean	Range	No. >3.4 mm
Controls	66	2.6	1.4–3.4	0
Study normal	170	3.0	1.2–6.4	22*
Study dysplastic	50	4.6	2.8–7.0	46

*16 of 22 infants with thickness >3.4 mm and initially normal ultrasound eventually developed dysplasia or instability.[1]

Comments ▪

This measurement is easy to perform at the time of standard examination of the infant hip and may add to the accuracy of the test, especially in terms of predicting subsequent development of dysplasia or instability.

REFERENCE

1. Soboleski DA, Babyn P: Sonographic diagnosis of developmental dysplasia of the hip: Importance of increased thickness of acetabular cartilage. AJR Am J Roentgenol 1993; 161(4):839–842.

▪: HIP JOINT SPACE
▪ ACR Code: 442 (Hip Joint)

Technique ▪

Well-centered anteroposterior (AP) pelvic radiographs with target-film distance of 100 cm (40 inches) were evaluated.[1, 3] Kaniklides and Dimopoulos used the ratio of diameters of the obturator foramen (RL = 0.56 to 1.8) to determine whether the films were truly AP,[1] and the other researchers utilized objective criteria to exclude rotated films.[2, 3]

Measurements ▪

Pogrund and Armbuster and associates measured the superior joint space from the uppermost point of the femoral head to the adjacent acetabulum in the vertical plane.[2, 3]

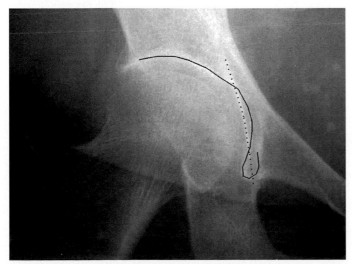

Figure 1 ▪ Landmarks for hip joint space measurement. The solid line depicts the acetabular margin ending inferiorly in the teardrop. The ilioischial line is shown by a dotted line. Depending on the obliquity of the radiograph, these lines may be in different orientations, and it is important to measure the joint space between the femoral head and the acetabular margin and not the ilioischial line.

Armbuster and colleagues measured the axial joint space just lateral to the acetabular fossa between the femoral head cortex to the acetabulum and the medial joint space along a horizontal line bisecting the femoral head.[3] Kaniklides and Dimopoulos measured the medial joint space between lines perpendicular to Hilgenreiner's horizontal (between the triradiate cartilages) that intersected the medial border of the femoral head and the lateral border of the teardrop.[1, 4] It is important not to confuse the ilioischial line and the floor of the acetabulum medially. This can be avoided by noting that the medial acetabular floor is in contiguity with the medial border of the teardrop. Figure 1 shows the ilioischial line, the acetabular margin, and the teardrop. Figure 2 shows the measurements described earlier. Table 1 presents measurements of the medial joint space in children and the superior joint space in adults.[1, 2] Table 2 lists all three positions in adults.[3]

Source ▪

Kaniklides and Dimopolous studied radiographs of 83 children (166 joints) ranging in age from 3 to 12 years. There were 51 boys and 32 girls.[1] Pogrund's subjects included 118 adult men and 122 adult women whose ages ranged between 45 and 84 years.[2] Armbuster and colleagues evaluated radiographs of 111 adult men and 39 adult women (300 hip joints): the ages were separated into those over 40 years (84%) and those 40 years of age or younger.[3] None of the subjects had clinical or radiologic evidence of hip disease at the time of the examination.[1–3]

Comments ▪

The superior and axial joint spaces will be abnormally decreased in adult osteoarthritis. The medial joint space may be increased in Legg-Calvé-Perthe disease. Eyring and group found that the upper limit of normal for the "teardrop distance" (medial joint space) was 11.0 mm, and Armbuster found 11.2 mm to be top normal.[3, 6] The joint spaces (especially medial) can be abnormally widened with hip

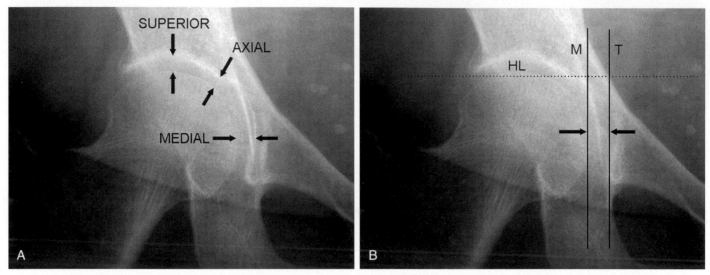

Figure 2 ▪ Measurement of the hip joint space on radiographs according to Armbuster and Pogrund and their colleagues *(A)* and Kaniklides et al *(B)*. The superior space is measured between the uppermost portion of the femoral head and the acetabulum. The axial space is measured just lateral to the acetabular fossa. *A,* The medial joint space is measured along a horizontal line through the middle of the femoral head or *B,* between lines *(arrows)* perpendicular to Hilgreiner's line *(HL)*, which are tangential to the medial femoral head *(M)* and the lateral margin of the teardrop *(T)*.

Table 1 ▪ Medial Joint Space in Children and Superior Joint Space in Adults[1, 2]

AGE RANGE (yr)	GENDER	NO.	KANIKLIDES: MEDIAL JOINT SPACE			
			Mean ± SD	Median	95th Percentile	98th Percentile
3–8	Male	68	8.5 ± 1.3	8.2	10.5	10.9
9–12	Male	34	7.2 ± 1.4	6.9	9.4	9.8
3–12	Male	102	8.1 ± 1.4	8.0	10.3	10.8
3–8	Female	40	7.1 ± 1.9	7.1	9.9	10.9
9–12	Female	24	6.0 ± 2.2	5.5	9.7	10.9
3–12	Female	64	6.7 ± 2.0	6.7	10.0	11.0
3–12	Both	166	7.5 ± 1.9	7.5	10.3	10.9

			POGRUND: SUPERIOR JOINT SPACE			
			Mean ± SD Right	Range Right	Mean ± SD Left	Range Left
45–54	Male	7	3.97 ± 0.76	3.2–5.0	3.83 ± 0.79	3.0–5.0
55–64	Male	18	3.91 ± 0.72	2.3–5.2	3.97 ± 0.69	2.5–5.6
65–74	Male	41	4.15 ± 0.71	2.8–5.5	4.15 ± 0.69	3.0–6.0
75–84	Male	52	3.81 ± 0.79	2.2–6.3	3.87 ± 0.77	2.8–6.2
45–84	Male	118	3.95	2.2–6.3	3.98	2.5–6.2
45–54	Female	16	3.73 ± 0.58	2.9–5.0	3.64 ± 0.53	2.6–4.5
55–64	Female	31	3.92 ± 0.79	2.5–5.4	3.79 ± 0.95	2.0–5.6
65–74	Female	34	4.06 ± 0.74	2.8–5.2	4.01 ± 0.78	1.7–5.2
75–84	Female	41	3.85 ± 1.09	2.4–4.7	3.78 ± 0.68	2.4–5.0
45–84	Female	122	3.91	2.5–5.4	3.83	1.7–5.6

Table 2 ▪ Medial, Superior, and Axial Hip Joint Space in Adults

GENDER	AGE (yr)	HIP JOINT SPACE (mm), MEAN (RANGE)		
		Medial	Superior	Axial
Both	≤40	8 (4–13)	4 (3–6)	4 (3–7)
	>40	8 (4–14)	4 (2–7)	4 (2–7)
Male	≤40	9 (6–13)	4 (3–7)	4 (3–7)
	>40	9 (4–14)	4 (2–7)	4 (2–7)
Female	≤40	8 (4–10)	4 (3–7)	4 (3–7)
	>40	8 (5–12)	4 (2–6)	4 (3–6)
Male	All	9 (4–14)	4 (2–7)	4 (2–7)
Female	All	8 (4–12)	4 (2–7)	4 (3–7)

From Armbuster TG, Guerra J Jr, Resnick D, et al: Radiology 1978; 128(1):1–10. Used by permission.

joint effusions in both children and adults, Sweeney and colleagues found that joint effusions caused the affected side to be 1 mm or more greater than the normal side in 10 patients with effusions documented by aspiration.[5]

REFERENCES

1. Kaniklides C, Dimopoulos P: Radiological measurement of femoral head position in Legg-Calvé-Perthes disease. Acta Radiol 1996; 36:863–869.
2. Pogrund H, Bloom R, Mogle P: The normal width of the adult hip joint: The relationship to age, sex and obesity. Skeletal Radiol 1983; 10:10–12.
3. Armbuster TG, Guerra J Jr, Resnick D, et al: The adult hip: An anatomic study. Part I: The bony landmarks. Radiology 1978; 128(1):1–10.
4. Hilgenreiner H: Zur Fruhdiagnose und Fruhbehandlung der angerborenen Huftgelenksverrenkung. Med Klin 1925; 21:1385.
5. Sweeney JP, Helms CA, Minagi H, Louie KW: The widened teardrop distance: A plain film indicator of hip joint effusion in adults. AJR Am J Roentgenol 1987; 149(1):117–119.
6. Eyring EJ, Bjornson DR, Peterson CA: Early diagnostic and prognostic signs in Legg-Calvé-Perthes disease. AJR Am J Roentgenol 1965; 93:382–386.

▪▪ ACETABULAR AND ARTICULAR CARTILAGE MEASUREMENTS IN PERTHES DISEASE BY MR[1]
▪ ACR Code: 442 (Hip Joint)

Technique ▪

1. 0.35-T superconductive magnet and a T1-weighted spin-echo sequence (700/30: repetition time [TR] msec/echo time [TE] msec).
2. 1.5-T magnet with a 600/20 pulse sequence.
3. Examinations performed with patients supine, with the hips in neutral position. 10-mm-thick coronal and axial sections obtained.

Measurements (Figure 1) ▪

The thickness of the femoral head cartilage was measured on the coronal image at four locations through the center of the femoral head. The superior and medial aspects of the acetabular cartilage were also measured.

The maximum thickness of the anterior and posterior aspects of the acetabular cartilage labrum was measured on the axial images.

The results of these measurements of both the normal and abnormal hips are given in Table 1.

The acetabulum-head index (AHI) and acetabulum-head quotient (AHQ) were used for evaluation of the degree of containment of the femoral head (Figure 2). Measurements were made from the cartilaginous surfaces of the femoral head and acetabulum.

Table 1 ▪ Femoral Head Cartilage Thickness and Acetabular Cartilage Thickness in 20 Patients with Legg-Calvé-Perthes Disease*

MEAN THICKNESS (mm)	FEMORAL HEAD CARTILAGE			
	Inferior	Medial	Superior	Lateral
Normal side	2.3 (18)	2.3 (18)	2.3 (17)	2.1 (18)
Abnormal side	5.2 (20)	5.9 (19)	4.2 (19)	5.0 (17)
Mean difference†	3.2 (18)	3.4 (17)	1.8 (16)	2.8 (15)

MEAN THICKNESS (mm)	ACETABULAR CARTILAGE			
	Medial	Superior	Anteroinferior	Posteroinferior
Normal side	2.4 (18)	2.9 (17)	2.2 (17)	4.0 (17)
Abnormal side	5.2 (19)	5.4 (20)	4.7 (18)	7.7 (19)
Mean difference†	2.9 (17)	2.9 (17)	2.4 (17)	3.9 (17)

*Measurements were made as shown in Figure 1. Numbers in parentheses are numbers of measurements available.
†Abnormal—normal.
From Rush BH, et al: Radiology 1988; 167:473–476. Used by permission.

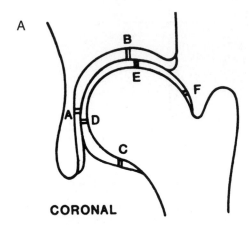

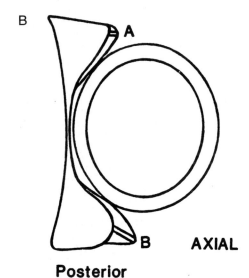

CORONAL

Anterior

Posterior

AXIAL

Figure 1 ▪ Measurement of articular and epiphyseal cartilage thickness. *A*, Coronal view. A = medial acetabulum; B = superior acetabulum; C = inferior femoral head; D = medial femoral head; E = superior femoral head; F = lateral femoral head. *B*, Axial view. A = anterior acetabular labrum; B = posterior acetabular labrum. (From Rush BH, et al: Radiology 1988; 167:473–476. Used by permission.)

Figure 2 ▪ Assessment of containment of femoral head within the acetabulum. (From Rush BH, et al: Radiology 1988; 167:473–476. Used by permission.)

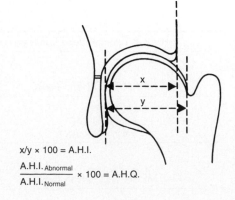

x/y × 100 = A.H.I.

$$\frac{\text{A.H.I.}_{\text{Abnormal}}}{\text{A.H.I.}_{\text{Normal}}} \times 100 = \text{A.H.Q.}$$

Table 2 • Degree of Containment of Femoral Head*

| | AHI | | |
CASE	Abnormal Side	Normal Side	AHQ
1	60.7	86.4	70.3
2	60.0	78.3	76.6
3	60.9	76.2	79.9
4	65.4	81.8	80.0
5	65.4	80.8	80.9
6	69.6	81.8	85.1
7	74.1	81.8	90.6
8	73.3	80.4†	91.2
9	74.1	80.0	92.6
10	75.0	76.2	98.4
11	80.8	80.44†	100.0
12	67.6	86.7	78.0
13	76.4	80.0	95.5
14	74.7	84.6	88.3
15	75.0	81.8	92.0
16	77.5	81.9	94.6
17	74.1	90.1	82.2
18	83.3	75.0	111.0
19	73.8	78.7	93.8
20	72.3	78.2	92.4

*Degree of containment was determined as shown in Figure 2. AHI = acetabulum-head index, AHQ = acetabulum-head quotient.
†Mean normal AHI used.
From Rush BH, et al: Radiology 1988; 167:473–476. Used by permission.

The AHI is a measure of the percent of the femoral head, with its cartilaginous rim, that is covered by superior acetabular cartilage. The results of these measurements are given in Table 2.

Source •

Data were derived from 20 patients with Perthes disease, ranging in age from 5 to 10 years, including 6 girls and 14 boys.

REFERENCE

1. Rush BH, Branson RT, Ogden JA: Legg-Calvé-Perthes disease: Detection of cartilaginous and synovial changes with MR imaging. Radiology 1988; 167:473–476.

⁚ THE CENTER EDGE ANGLE OF WIBERG
- ACR Code: 442 (Hip Joint)

Technique •

Anteroposterior (AP) radiographs of the pelvis (target-to-film distance not given) were evaluated. Rotated films (as evidenced by asymmetry of the obturator foramina) were excluded.[1, 2]

Measurements •

A horizontal line is drawn between the femoral head centers for reference, and a perpendicular vertical line is made through the center of the femoral head of the hip in question. A line between the center of the femoral head and the upper outer edge of the acetabulum is drawn, and the center edge angle is measured between it and the vertical.[1, 2] Figure 1 shows the measurement, and Table 1 lists the normal values.

Source •

Gusis and colleagues evaluated radiographs of 150 children (300 hips) ranging in age from 2 to 15 years.[1] Armbuster's subjects included 157 adults (314 hips). There were 116 males and 40 females; the age range was not given.[2] All subjects had radiographs for abdominal symptoms, gastrointestinal studies, or urographic examinations, and none had known disease affecting the hip joints.[1, 2]

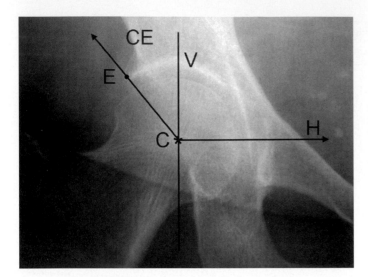

Figure 1 ▪ Measurement of the center edge *(CE)* angle from an AP radiograph of the hip. A horizontal line *(H)* is drawn between the centers of the femoral heads *(asterisk)*, and a perpendicular vertical *(V)* line is made through the center of the femoral head. A third line *(E)* is drawn from the center of the femoral head through the edge of the acetabulum, and the CE angle is measured between it and the vertical *(ECV)*.

Table 1 ▪ Center Edge (CE) Angle in Children and Adults

AUTHOR/ AGE (yr)	MALE		FEMALE		BOTH	
	No.	Mean	No.	Mean	No.	Mean
Gusis						
2	6	19.33	18	22.33	24	21.58
3	6	28.33	14	26.36	20	26.95
4	4	27.25	18	28.83	22	28.54
5	10	26.70	12	31.25	22	29.18
6	14	28.71	16	30.37	30	29.60
7	8	29.25	18	31.72	26	30.96
8	10	34.00	18	32.44	28	33.00
9	14	29.86	18	34.72	32	32.60
10	12	30.92	14	37.93	26	34.69
11	10	34.30	18	37.72	28	36.50
12	6	34.83	8	37.87	14	36.57
13	6	31.80	8	31.00	14	31.57
14	2	30.50	10	36.40	12	35.42
15	—	—	2	37.00	2	37.00
2–15	112	30.0±5.8	188	31.9±6.4	300	31.2±6.2
Armbuster						
≤40	36	37 (23–53)	24	38 (32–56)	60	38 (23–56)
>40	196	38 (25–59)	56	41 (24–59)	252	39 (24–59)
Adults	232	38 (23–59)	82	40 (24–59)	314	38.6 (23–59)

All measurements are in degrees. Mean values (± standard deviation for children 2 to 15 years and range for adults).[1, 2]

Comments ▪

Angles that are abnormally low may indicate dysplasia of the hip, and abnormally high values may be found in protrusio.[1-3] Gusis and Armbuster (see next section) both feel that the relationship between the medial acetabulum and the ilioischial line is a better indicator of protrusio.[1, 2]

REFERENCES

1. Gusis SE, Babini JC, Garay SM, et al: Evaluation of the measurement methods for protrusio acetabuli in normal children. Skeletal Radiol 1990; 19(4):279–282.
2. Armbuster TG, Guerra J Jr, Resnick D, et al: The adult hip: An anatomic study. Part I: The bony landmarks. Radiology 1978; 128(1): 1–10.
3. Wiberg G: Studies on dysplastic acetabula and congenital subluxation of the hip joint. Acta Chir Scand 1939; 58:5–135.

▪: RELATIONSHIP OF THE ACETABULAR AND ILIOISCHIAL LINES
▪ ACR Code: 442 (Hip Joint)

Technique ▪

Anteroposterior (AP) radiographs of the pelvis (target-to-film distance not given) were evaluated. Rotated films (as evidenced by asymmetry of the obturator foramina) were excluded.[1, 2]

Measurements ▪

The ilioischial line and medial acetabular rim were identified on each side. The acetabular rim can be recognized by virtue of the fact that its lower end is contiguous with the so-called "teardrop" just above and lateral to the upper outer portion of the obturator foramen. The distance between these two lines was measured where they cross a horizontal between the centers of the femoral heads. The measurement may be made at an angle of from 0 to 50 degrees with respect to the horizontal. If the acetabular margin was medial to the ilioichial line (called "reversed"), the maximum distance was recorded and given a negative

sign. When the situation was reversed (called "open"), the minimum distance was recorded and given a positive sign. When the lines coincide (called "crossed"), a value of zero was given. Figure 1 shows these measurements, and Table 1 lists normal values by age and gender.[1, 2]

Source ▪

Gusis and colleagues evaluated radiographs of 150 children (300 hips) ranging in age from 2 to 15 years.[1] Armbuster's subjects included 157 adults (314 hips). There were 116 males and 40 females, and the age range was not given.[2] All subjects had radiographs for abdominal symptoms, gastrointestinal studies, or urographic examinations, and none had known disease affecting the hip joints.[1, 2]

Comments ▪

These relationships are useful in diagnosing protrusio of the hip in rheumatoid arthritis and trauma.[1, 2] This method

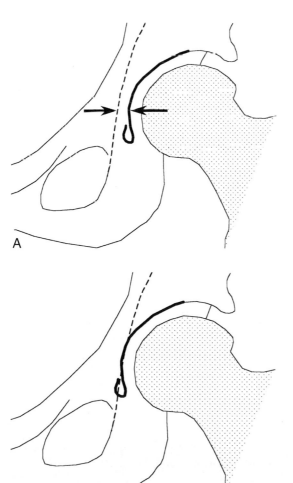
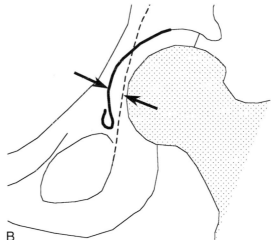

Figure 1 ▪ The distance between the acetabular and ilioischial lines. Measurements are made at the level of a horizontal line through the centers of the femoral heads and may be from 0 to 50 degrees with respect to it. When the acetabular margin (*heavy solid line*) is lateral to the ilioischial (*dotted*) line as in *A*, the minimum distance (millimeters) is measured (*arrows*) and given a positive sign. When the acetabular line is medial to the ilioischial line as in *B*, the maximum distance (millimeters) is measured (*arrows*) and given a negative sign. The measurement is zero when the lines cross, as in *C*.

Table 1 • Acetabular to Ilioischial Line Distances in Children and Adults

AUTHOR/ AGE (yr)	MALE		FEMALE		BOTH	
	No.	Mean	No.	Mean	No.	Mean
Gusis						
2	6	2.92	18	3.11	24	3.06
3	6	4.29	14	1.78	20	2.35
4	4	2.12	18	1.32	22	1.46
5	10	2.35	12	1.46	22	1.86
6	14	2.36	16	2.05	30	2.19
7	8	1.94	18	1.42	26	1.57
8	10	2.55	18	1.53	28	1.89
9	14	2.93	18	0.33	32	1.47
10	12	2.17	14	0.96	26	1.52
11	10	2.50	18	1.14	28	1.62
12	6	1.33	8	−0.81	14	0.11
13	6	3.20	8	−0.50	14	2.14
14	2	3.00	10	0.45	12	0.87
15	—	—	2	0	2	0
2–15	112	2.6 ± 1.7	188	1.3 ± 2.0	300	1.8 ± 2.0
Armbuster						
≤ 40	36	1 (−4 to 7)	24	−2 (−5 to 5)	60	0 (−5 to 7)
> 40	196	2 (−4 to 8)	56	−1 (−8 to 6)	252	1 (−8 to 8)
Adults	232	2 (−4 to 8)	82	−1 (−8 to 6)	314	0.8 (−8 to 8)

All measurements are in millimeters. Mean values (± standard deviation for children 2 to 15 years and range for adults).[1,2]

was felt to be superior to visual inspection of the "teardrop" in relationship to the ilioischial line, as the latter is more prone to error from rotation due to differences in anterior to posterior position of the anatomic structures responsible for the radiographic features. Gusis and colleagues suggest a cut-off of −0.8 mm for boys and −2.7 mm for girls (mean = 2 × SD), and Armbuster and group cited cut-off values of −3 mm for men and −6 mm for women.[1,2]

REFERENCES

1. Gusis SE, Babini JC, Garay SM, et al: Evaluation of the measurement methods for protrusio acetabuli in normal children. Skeletal Radiol 1990; 19(4):279–282.
2. Armbuster TG, Guerra J Jr, Resnick D, et al: The adult hip: An anatomic study. Part I: The bony landmarks. Radiology 1978; 128(1): 1–10.

∷ MEASUREMENT OF ACETABULAR DEPTH[1]
- ACR Code: 442 (Hip Joint)

Technique •

Central ray: Perpendicular to plane of film.
Position: Anteroposterior supine.
Target-film distance: 120 cm.

Measurements (Figure 1) •

A line is drawn between the edge of the articular surface of the acetabulum and the upper corner of the symphysis pubis on the same side.

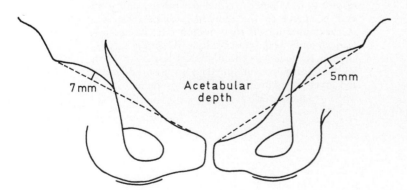

Figure 1 • Measurement of acetabular depth. (Adapted from Murray RO: Br J Radiol 1965; 38:809.)

The average depth of the acetabulum in females was 12 mm, ranging from a maximum of 18 mm to a minimum of 9 mm. In males, the average was 13 mm, ranging from a maximum of 18 mm to a minimum of 7 mm. The mean figure was 12 mm. Murray believes that an acetabular depth of less than 9 mm is considered an imperfectly formed acetabulum, which may lead to osteoarthritis of the hip.[1]

Source ▪

Based on a study at 25 males and 25 females, making a total at 100 hips.

REFERENCE

1. Murray RO: The aetiology of primary osteo-arthritis of the hip. Br J Radiol 1965; 38:810–824.

▪: MEASUREMENT OF PROTRUSIO ACETABULI[1]
- ▪ ACR Code: 442 (Hip Joint)

Technique ▪

Central ray: Perpendicular to plane of film centered over midpelvis.
Position: Anteroposterior.
Target-film distance: Immaterial.

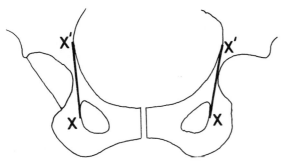

Figure 1 ▪ Köhler's line. Adapted from Hubbard MJS: AJR Am J Roentgenol 1969; 106:506.)

Measurements (Figure 1) ▪

The outline of the dome of the acetabulum meets Köhler's line X′X. This line is drawn from the pelvic border of the ilium to the medial border of the body of the ischium.

If the outline of the acetabular dome passes medial to line X′X, a protrusion exists.

This method is applicable to serial roentgenograms of an individual patient but is not suitable for comparing patients.

Source ▪

The data are from 242 patients with a diagnosis of degenerative arthritis of the hip.

REFERENCE

1. Hubbard MJS: The measurement of progression in protrusio acetabuli. AJR Am J Roentgenol 1969; 106:506–508.

▪: ACETABULAR ANTEVERSION AND SECTOR ANGLES
- ▪ ACR Code: 442 (Hip Joint)

Technique ▪

An anteroposterior (AP) scout view of the pelvis is obtained. Axial CT slices with the gantry unangled were then made through the centers of the femoral heads.

Measurements ▪

On the axial slice best depicting the centers of both femoral heads, a horizontal line is drawn between them (H or C1C2 by Anda). To measure the acetabular anteversion (AcAV), a line is drawn perpendicular to the H line through the posterior acetabular margin (P), and a second line is drawn connecting P and the anterior acetabular margin (A). The angle between them is the AcAV. To measure the horizontal, anterior, and posterior acetabular sector angles (HASA, AASA, and PASA), the line between the centers of the femoral heads (H or C1C2) is again used. Lines are then drawn connecting the center of the femoral head (C) with the anterior (A) and posterior (P) margins. The HASA is measured between the anterior and posterior margins, the AASA is measured between the anterior margin and horizontal, and the PASA is measured between the posterior margin and horizontal.[1, 2]

Figure 1 depicts the acetabular sector angle (AcSA) measurement; Figure 2 shows the technique for determining HASA, AASA, and PASA. Table 1 gives the results in normal adults.

Table 1 ▪ Acetabular Anteversion and Sector Angles in Adults

	MEN	WOMEN
Number	42	40
AcAV	18.5 ± 4.5	21.5 ± 5
HASA	167 ± 11	169 ± 10
AASA	64 ± 6	63 ± 6
PASA	102 ± 8	105 ± 8

All measurements are in degrees (mean ± standard deviation).
AcAV = acetabular anteversion, HASA = horizontal acetabular sector angle, AASA = anterior acetabular sector angle, PASA = posterior acetabular sector angle.[1–3]

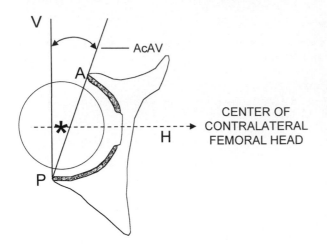

Figure 1 ▪ Measurement of acetabular anteversion (*AcAV*) from an axial CT slice through the femoral heads. The *asterisk* indicates the center of the femoral head.

H = horizontal line connecting femoral head centers
P = posterior margin of acetabulum
A = anterior margin of acetabulum
V = line perpendicular to line H through point P
AcAV = angle VPA.[3]

Figure 2 ▪ Measurement of acetabular sector angles (*horizontal = HASA, anterior = AASA, posterior = PASA*) from an axial CT slice through the femoral heads. The *asterisk* indicates the center of the femoral head.

H = horizontal line connecting femoral head centers
C = center of femoral head
P = posterior margin of acetabulum
A = anterior margin of acetabulum
HASA = angle ACP
AASA = angle ACH
HASA = angle HCP.[3]

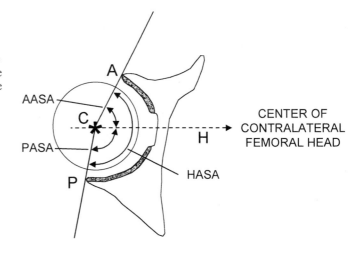

Source ▪

Normal adults (21 men, 20 women); both hips were measured in each subject.

Comments ▪

Sector angles below the normal range indicate dysplasia of the acetabulum.[1, 2]

REFERENCES

1. Anda S, Terjesen T, Kvistad KA, Svenningsen S: Acetabular angles and femoral anteversion in dysplastic hips in adults: C T investigation. J Comput Assist Tomogr 1991; 15:115–120.
2. Anda S, Terjesen T, Kvistad KA: Computed tomograph measurements of the acetabulum in adult dysplastic hips: Which level is appropriate? Skeletal Radiol 1991; 20:267–271.
3. Anda S: Personal communication, 1992.

▪▪ MEASUREMENTS OF ADULT HIPS FOR DYSPLASIA
▪ ACR Code: 442 (Hip Joint)

Technique ▪

Delaunay and colleagues performed a review of the medical literature concerning various measurements of adult hips on radiographs and CT scans to detect and quantify dysplasia.[1]

Measurements ▪

Most of the measurements described here are made from anteroposterior (AP) radiographs of the hip joint or pelvis and utilize several landmarks that are shown in Figure 1. The center edge (CE) angle of Wiberg (Figure 2) is of primary importance in describing the superior and lateral coverage of the femoral head by the acetabulum.[2] The "horizontal toit externe" (HTE) angle (Figure 3) is used to assess the orientation of the acetabular roof as well as femoral head coverage.[3] The acetabular index of depth to width (Figure 4) describes the depth of the acetabulum.[4] The percentage of femoral head coverage by the acetabulum (Figure 5) quantifies the congruity of the head in the acetabulum, which, if inadequate, can lead to early degenerative changes.[5] When acetabular dysplasia is identified on an AP view, it is useful to perform a standing false-profile view (Figure 6) of the joint to determine the anterior coverage of the head by the acetabulum.[6] The vertical-center-anterior (VCA) angle (Figure 7) quantifies these relationships.[3, 6, 7]

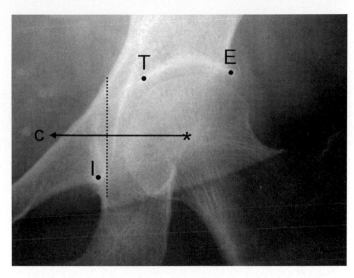

Figure 1 • Landmarks for hip measurements. The asterisk indicates the center of the femoral head of the hip in question. A line drawn from there through the opposite femoral head (*C*) serves as a horizontal reference. The medial limit of the acetabulum is indicated by a vertical dotted line. The E point is the lateral border of the edge of the acetabulum, and the T point is the medial limit of the weight-bearing portion of the acetabular roof. The weight-bearing acetabular portion is sclerotic and wedge arched (between the E and T points). The inferiormost point of the acetabulum (*I*) is the bottom of the teardrop.[1]

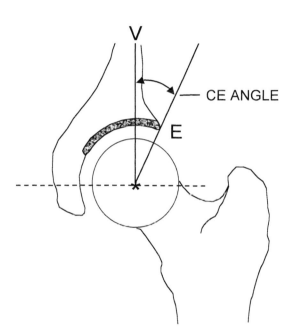

Figure 2 • Center edge (CE) angle of Wiberg. A vertical line (*V*) is drawn though the center of the femoral head (*asterisk*) perpendicular to the horizontal (*dashed*) line, and a second line (*E*) is drawn from the center of the femoral head contacting the E point. The CE angle is formed by VE and should be greater than 25 degrees in normal subjects. (From Delaunay S, Dussault RG, Kaplan PA, Alford BA: Skeletal Radiol 1996; 26:75–81. Used by permission.)

Figure 3 • HTE angle. A line is drawn parallel to the horizontal (*dashed*) line through the T point. A second line is drawn from the T point through the E point. The angle between them is the HTE angle and is less than or equal to 10 degrees in normal subjects. (From Delaunay S, Dussault RG, Kaplan PA, Alford BA: Skeletal Radiol 1996; 26:75–81. Used by permission.)

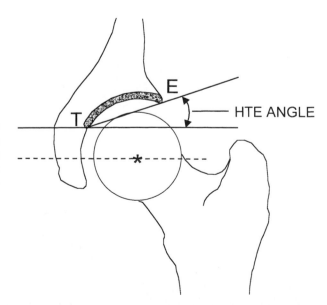

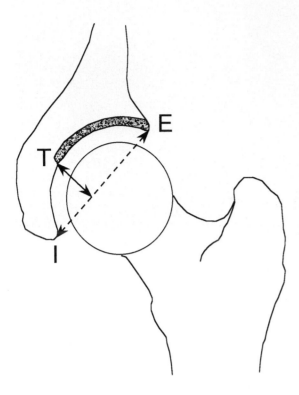

Figure 4 ▪ Acetabular index. The width *(dotted)* line is measured between the inferior acetabular margin *(I)* and the E point. The depth *(solid area)* is measured between the T point and the width line. The acetabular index is calculated by depth/width × 100 and should be greater than 38 degrees in normal subjects, with an average value of around 60 degrees. (From Delaunay S, Dussault RG, Kaplan PA, Alford BA: Skeletal Radiol 1996; 26:75–81. Used by permission.)

Figure 5 ▪ Femoral head coverage percentage. Lines are drawn (perpendicular to the horizontal) through the medialmost aspect of the joint space *(1)*, through the E point *(2)*, and through the lateral margin of the femoral head *(3)*. Two measurements are made between these lines: A = 1–2 and B = 1–3. Percentage coverage is calculated as follows: (A/B) × 100. This should normally be greater than or equal to 75%. (From Delaunay S, Dussault RG, Kaplan PA, Alford BA: Skeletal Radiol 1996; 26:75–81. Used by permission.)

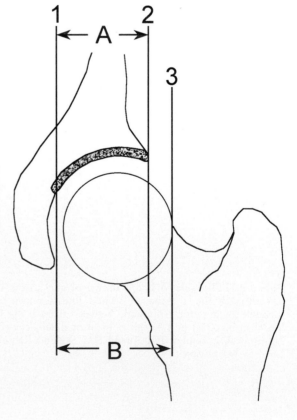

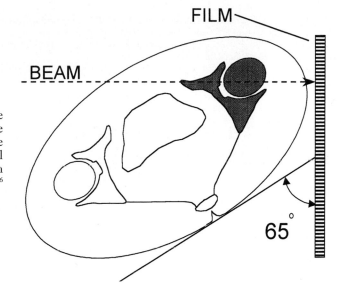

Figure 6 ▪ Technique for standing false profile radiograph. The feet are parallel to the film plane while the pelvis is rotated 65 degrees relative to the film, with the side to be examined *(shaded)* positioned against the cassette. The exposure is made with the beam centered on the femoral head, and the radiograph is deemed adequate if the distance between femoral heads is approximately equal to the size of one femoral head.[1, 6]

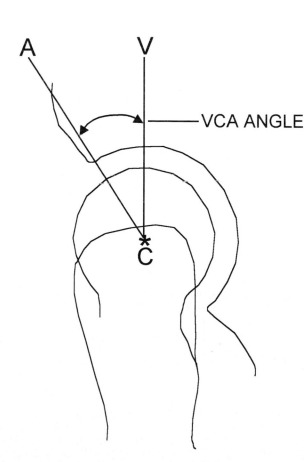

Figure 7 ▪ VCA angle as measured from the false profile view. A line *(V)* is drawn vertically through the center of the femoral head *(C)*, and a second line is drawn from the center of the femoral head through the anterior border of the acetabulum *(A)*. The VCA angle is measured between the two and is greater than 25 degrees in normal subjects. (From Delaunay S, Dussault RG, Kaplan PA, Alford BA: Skeletal Radiol 1996; 26:75–81. Used by permission.)

Source ▪

See references.

REFERENCES

1. Delaunay S, Dussault RG, Kaplan PA, Alford BA: Radiographic measurements of dysplastic adult hips. Skeletal Radiol 1996; 26:75–81.
2. Wiberg G: Studies on dysplastic acetabula and congenital subluxation of the hip joint. Acta Chir Scand 1939; 58:5–135.
3. Lequesne M: Coxometrie. Mesure des angles fondamentaux de la hanche radiographique de l'adulte par un rapporteur combine. Rev Rhum 1963; 30:479–485.
4. Murphy SB, Ganz R, Muller ME: The prognosis in untreated dysplasia of the hip: A study of radiographic factors that predict the outcome. J Bone Joint Surg Am 1995; 77(7):985–989.
5. Cooperman DR, Wallensten R, Stulberg SD: Acetabular dysplasia in the adult. Clin Orthop 1983; 175:79–85.
6. Lequesne M, de Seze S: Le faux-profi du bassin. Rev Rhum 1961; 28:643–652.
7. Lequesne M, Lemoine A, Massare C: Le "complet" radiographique coxo-femoral. Depistage et bilan pre-operatoire des vices architecturaux de la hanche. J Radiol Electrol 1964; 1–2:27–44.

▪: AXIAL RELATIONSHIPS OF THE HIP JOINT[1]
▪ ACR Code: 443 (Proximal Femur)

Technique ▪

Central ray: Passes through a point 1 inch below the center of the inguinal ligament perpendicular to the plane of the film.
Position: Anteroposterior. The patient is placed flat on the back with the toe of the foot pointing somewhat to the median plane.
Target-film distance: Immaterial.

Measurements (Figure 1) ▪

AB = Line along midaxis of femoral shaft.
CD = Line along midaxis of femoral head and neck.

Angle *FA* = Angle of the femoral neck at the intersection of *AB* and *CD*.

Source ▪

The data are based on a study of 50 normal adult subjects, equally divided between men and women, ranging in age from 19 to 76 years.

REFERENCE

1. Keats TE, Teeslink R, Diamond AE, Williams JH: Normal axial relationships of the major joints. Radiology 1966; 87:904–907.

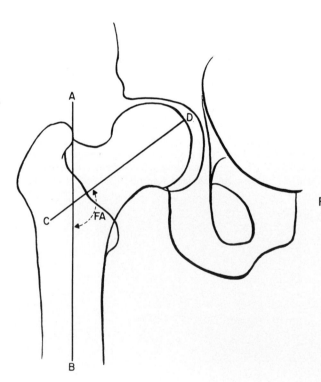

Figure 1 ▪ Femoral angle (FA): men, 128 degrees; women, 127 degrees.

⁚ CRITERIA FOR DETECTION OF SLIPPED CAPITAL FEMORAL EPIPHYSIS[1]
▪ ACR Code: 443 (Proximal Femur)

Technique ▪

Central ray: Perpendicular, center at level of hips.
Position: Anteroposterior supine, toes may be slightly pointed toward median.
Target-film distance: Immaterial.

Measurement (Figure 1) ▪

AB = Line intersecting a superior lateral segment of the femoral head.
AC = Line tangential to the arc of the femoral head. When slipping occurs (*dotted line*), the head descends and the neck rides upward. Line *AC* therefore disappears, to overlie line *AB*, which is now a tangential line on the femoral head rather than an intersecting line.
1 and *2* = *Arrows* indicating the usual concavoconvexity at the superior epiphyseal junction.

Source ▪

These measurements were derived from the work of many investigators. The reader will find an extensive bibliography to these sources in the article by Martin.

REFERENCE

1. Martin HE. Radiology 1951; 56:842.

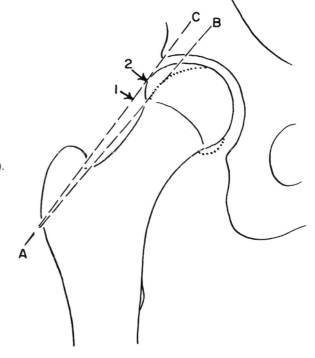

Figure 1 ▪ Measurements for slipped femoral epiphysis (see text for details). (Adapted from Martin HE: Radiology 1951; 56:842.)

⁚ GRADING OF AVASCULAR NECROSIS OF THE HIP
▪ ACR Code: 443 (Proximal End of Femur)

Technique ▪

Anteroposterior radiographs of hips, MRI of hips, and technetium bone scans were performed. Occasionally, CT and/or radiographic tomograms of the hip were done to assess the extent of collapse of the femoral head.[1]

Measurements ▪

The new staging system is detailed in Table 1 and shown in Figure 1. In Table 1, the grades from the previously most commonly used system are shown as well. The major difference is that Steinberg's new system divides the standard stages III and IV into four stages. This is to reflect the clinical importance of the distinction between subchondral collapse (Steinberg stage III) and flattening of the femoral head (Steinberg stage IV), which were previously both given a stage of III. Also, the finding of joint narrowing and minimal-to-mild acetabular changes (Steinberg stage V) is separated from frank degenerative change in the joint (Steinberg stage VI), whereas in the prior system these groups were joined into stage IV.[1]

The other significant difference in Steinberg's new system is the addition of a lettered system for grading changes in a quantitative system. For clinical use, stages I through V are divided into three lettered grades (A, B, and C). The quantitative grading system is listed in Table 2 and depicted in Figure 2. In stages I and II, the grade depends on the percentage of area involved with sclerosis and/or cyst

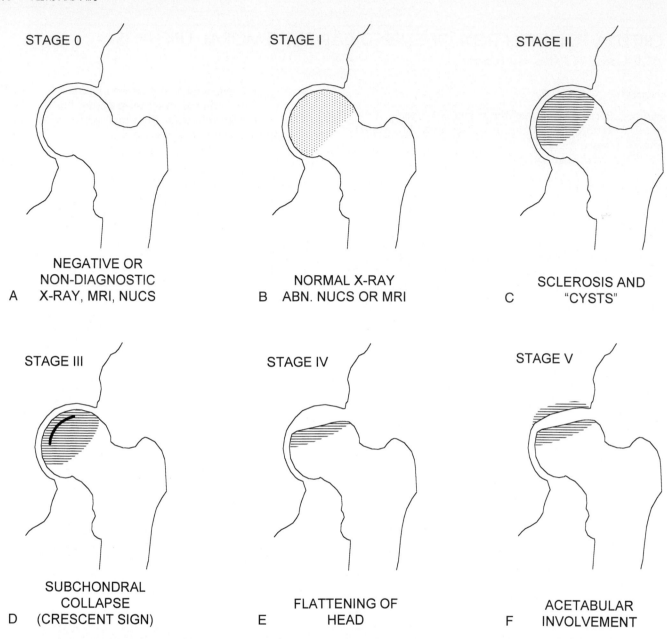

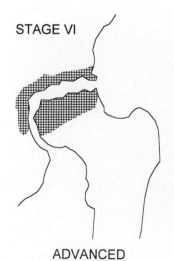

Figure 1 ▪ Staging of avascular necrosis (AVN) of the hip. Figure parts A through G depict stages 0 through VI, respectively. Staging can be done on either MRI or radiographs, although x-ray alone is probably sufficient, once the diagnosis has been established, and for higher stages. (From Steinberg ME, Hayken GD, Steinberg DR: J Bone Joint Surg Br 1995; 77(1):34–41. Used by permission.)

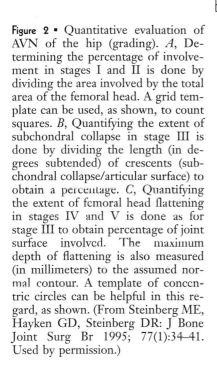

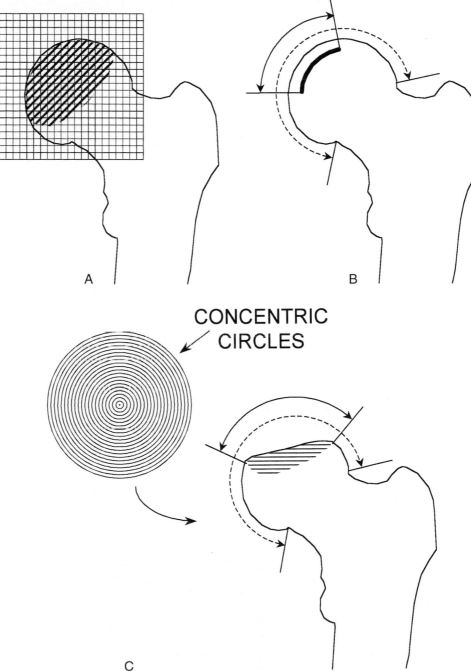

Figure 2 · Quantitative evaluation of AVN of the hip (grading). *A*, Determining the percentage of involvement in stages I and II is done by dividing the area involved by the total area of the femoral head. A grid template can be used, as shown, to count squares. *B*, Quantifying the extent of subchondral collapse in stage III is done by dividing the length (in degrees subtended) of crescents (subchondral collapse/articular surface) to obtain a percentage. *C*, Quantifying the extent of femoral head flattening in stages IV and V is done as for stage III to obtain percentage of joint surface involved. The maximum depth of flattening is also measured (in millimeters) to the assumed normal contour. A template of concentric circles can be helpful in this regard, as shown. (From Steinberg ME, Hayken GD, Steinberg DR: J Bone Joint Surg Br 1995; 77(1):34–41. Used by permission.)

CONCENTRIC CIRCLES

A

B

C

Table 1 ▪ Staging System for Avascular Necrosis of the Hip

STAGE (Steinberg)	STAGE (Standard)	DESCRIPTION
0	0	Normal radiograph, normal or nondiagnostic MRI and bone scan
I	I	Normal radiograph, abnormal MRI or bone scan
II	II	Mottled sclerotic and "cystic" changes in the femoral head
III	III	Subchondral collapse, producing a "crescent" sign
IV	III	Flattening of the femoral head
V	IV	Joint narrowing, variable acetabular changes
VI	IV	Advanced degenerative changes

The proposed stages (Steinberg) are shown alongside a commonly used system (Standard).
From Steinberg ME, Hayken GD, Steinberg DR: J Bone Joint Surg Br 1995; 77(1):34–41. Used by permission.

Table 2 ▪ Quantitative Grading of Avascular Necrosis of the Hip

STAGE	GRADE	DESCRIPTION
I and II	A, mild	<15% of head involvement as seen on radiograph or MRI
	B, moderate	15% to 30%
	C, severe	>30%
III	A, mild	Subchondral collapse (crescent) beneath <15% of articular surface
	B, moderate	Crescent beneath 15% to 30%
	C, severe	Crescent beneath >30%
IV	A, mild	<15% of surface has collapsed and depression is <2 mm
	B, moderate	15% to 30% collapsed or 2 to 4 mm depression
	C, severe	>30% collapsed or >4 mm depression
V	A, B, or C	Average of femoral head involvement, as determined in stage IV, and estimated acetabular involvement

Each stage from I through V is qualified with a lettered grade as shown.
From Steinberg ME, Hayken GD, Steinberg DR: J Bone Joint Surg Br 1995; 77(1):34–41. Used by permission.

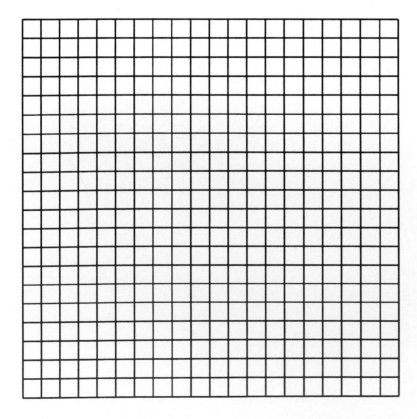

Figure 3 ▪ Template of 5-millimeter squares to help in quantifying area involved.

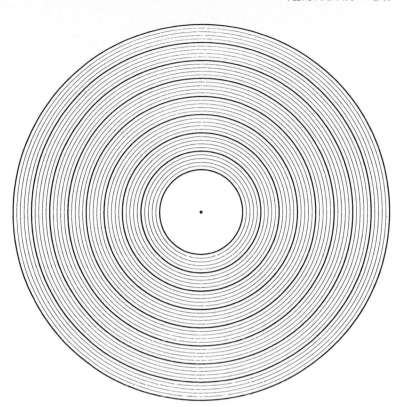

Figure 4 ▪ Template of 1-millimeter concentric circles *(heavy lines every 5 mm)* to help in quantifying subchondral collapse.

formation on radiographs or MRI. In stages III to V, the grade depends on the percentage of the femoral head joint surface affected by subchondral collapse or flattening and the measured amount of maximal flattening. Templates are provided in Figures 3 and 4 that may be copied onto transparency stock and used as shown in Figure 2.

Source ▪

Over 1000 hips suspected or affected with avascular necrosis (AVN) of the hip were evaluated and graded with a proposed 7-level quantitative system.[1] A subset of 115 hips was graded according to a previously described system with 5 levels.[2–4] Another subset of 73 hips was evaluated to determine whether quantitative determination of lesion size correlated with outcome after core decompression and bone grafting in stages I and II.[1, 5]

Comments ▪

The lettered grading system is adequate for clinical evaluation. If desired, the percentages of involvement and mea-sured flattening can be directly recorded for use in research purposes. The investigators found radiographic progression by using the new stage/grade system in 74% of 115 hips, whereas the standard stage system showed progression only in 50%. Further, in 73 early-stage hips evaluated with the new system prior to therapy, the lesion size (grade) pre-dicted radiologic and clinical outcome much better than stage alone.[1, 5]

REFERENCES

1. Steinberg ME, Hayken GD, Steinberg DR: A quantitative system for staging avascular necrosis. J Bone Joint Surg Br 1995; 77(1):34–41.
2. Berquist TH: Pelvis, hips, and thigh. In Berquist TH (ed): MRI of the Musculoskeletal System, 3rd ed. Lippincott-Raven, Philadelphia, 1996, pp 197–284.
3. Ficat RP, Arlet J: Necrosis of the femoral head. In Hungerford DS (ed): Ischemia and Necrosis of Bone. Williams & Wilkins, Baltimore, 1980, pp 171–182.
4. Ficat RP: Idiopathic bone necrosis of the femoral head: Early diagnosis and treatment. J Bone Joint Surg Br 1985; 67:3–9.
5. Steinberg ME, Bands RE, Parry S, et al: Does lesion size affect outcome in avascular necrosis? Orthop Trans 1992–1993; 16:706–707.

CHAPTER 7

Lower Extremity

·: MEASUREMENT OF FEMORAL TORSION WITH BIPLANE RADIOGRAPHS

- ACR Code: 44 (Femur)

Technique ·

The films required for Magilligan's method[1] include a standard anteroposterior (AP) radiograph and a horizontal lateral (HL) radiograph of the same side. The leg should be extended and in the neutral position as far as rotation is concerned. The AP radiograph is made with the beam centered over the hip of the side in question The HL view is done by having the opposite leg flexed at the hip and knee and positioning the tube so as to direct the beam through the hip in question from medial to lateral. The cassette is placed against the flank on the side to be examined, parallel to the table top and to the long axis of the femoral neck (looking at the AP view is helpful in this regard). The leg to be examined may be abducted/adducted to achieve correct position for the HL view but must not be rotated after the AP view. Figure 1 shows the HL view geometry.

For the method of Ogata,[2] an AP view is also done, with the only difference being that the knees are flexed to 90 degrees over the end of the table. A tabletop lateral (TL) view of the proximal femur is done with the hip and knee flexed to 90 degrees and the lateral aspect of the leg contacting the tabletop. Figure 2 shows the TL view geometry.

Measurements ·

From the AP view, the projected cervicofemoral (alpha) angle is measured as shown in Figure 3. From the HL or TL view, the projected anteversion angle (Hbeta or Tbeta) is measured as shown in Figure 4. Based on geometric calculations by Magilligan, the true anteversion (TA) angle may be obtained by: $\tan(TA) = \tan(Hbeta)/\sin(alpha)$. Note that as the alpha angle approaches 90 degrees, its sine is very nearly equal to 1.0, so that between alpha = 80 to 100 degrees, TA = beta.[1] Similar analysis by Ogata and Goldsand resulted in the following relationship for calculating true anteversion: $\tan(TA) = \tan(Tbeta)/\tan(alpha)$. With this geometry, when alpha = 45 degrees, TA = beta.[2]

Tables 1 and 2 list TA angles for various combinations of alpha and beta as calculated from Magilligan's and Ogata's formulas.[1, 2]

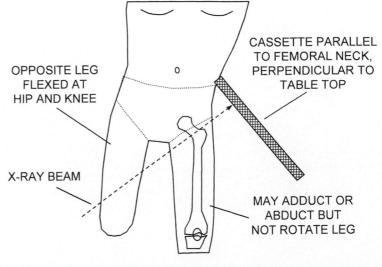

Figure 1 · Positioning for horizontal lateral view of the left hip.

OPPOSITE LEG FLEXED AT HIP AND KNEE

CASSETTE PARALLEL TO FEMORAL NECK, PERPENDICULAR TO TABLE TOP

X-RAY BEAM

MAY ADDUCT OR ABDUCT BUT NOT ROTATE LEG

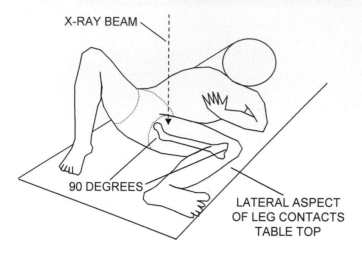

Figure 2 ▪ Positioning for tabletop lateral view of the hip.

X-RAY BEAM

90 DEGREES

LATERAL ASPECT
OF LEG CONTACTS
TABLE TOP

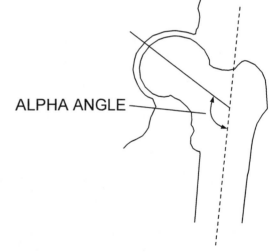

ALPHA ANGLE

Figure 3 ▪ Measurement of the projected cervicofemoral (alpha) angle from an AP radiograph. The long axis of the femoral shaft (*dotted line*) and the axis of the femoral neck (*solid line*) form the angle.

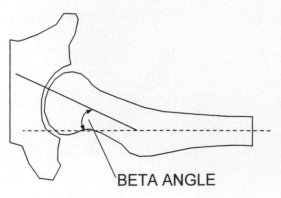

BETA ANGLE

Figure 4 ▪ Measurement of the projected anteversion angle (beta) from the lateral radiograph. The long axis of the femoral shaft (*dotted line*) and the axis of the femoral neck (*solid line*) form the angle. This is done in the same fashion from horizontal (Hbeta) or tabletop (Tbeta) views. However, because of the different geometry, the formulas for true anteversion using these angles are different (see text).

Table 1 ▪ Obtaining True Anteversion Angle from Measured Alpha and Beta Angles (Horizontal Lateral View)

BETA	ALPHA												
	5	10	15	20	25	30	35	40	45	50	60	70	80–100
5	45	27	19	14	12	10	9	8	7	7	6	5	5
10	64	45	34	27	23	19	17	15	14	13	12	11	10
15	72	57	46	38	32	28	25	23	21	19	17	16	15
20	77	64	55	47	41	36	32	30	27	25	23	21	20
25	79	70	61	54	48	43	39	36	33	31	28	26	25
30	81	73	66	59	54	49	45	42	39	37	34	32	30
35	83	76	70	64	59	54	51	47	45	42	39	37	35
40	84	78	73	68	63	59	56	53	50	48	44	42	40
45	85	80	75	71	67	63	60	57	55	53	49	47	45
50	86	82	78	74	70	67	64	62	59	57	54	52	50
55	87	83	80	77	74	71	68	66	64	62	59	57	55
60	87	84	82	79	76	74	72	70	68	66	63	62	60
65	88	85	83	81	79	77	75	73	72	70	68	66	65
70	88	86	85	83	81	80	78	77	76	74	73	71	70
75	89	87	86	85	84	82	81	80	79	78	77	76	75
80	89	88	87	87	86	85	84	84	83	82	81	81	80
85	90	89	89	88	88	87	87	87	86	86	86	85	85

To use, apply measured alpha to the first row and beta to the first column and read the true anteversion angle from the appropriate cell.[1]

Table 2 ▪ Obtaining True Anteversion Angle from Measured Alpha and Beta Angles (Tabletop Lateral View)

BETA	ALPHA																
	5	10	15	20	25	30	35	40	45	50	55	60	65	70	75	80	85
5	45	26	18	14	11	9	7	6	5	4	4	3	2	2	1	1	0
10	64	45	33	26	21	17	14	12	10	8	7	6	5	4	3	2	1
15	72	57	45	36	30	25	21	18	15	13	11	9	7	6	4	3	1
20	76	64	54	45	38	32	27	23	20	17	14	12	10	8	6	4	2
25	79	69	60	52	45	39	34	29	25	21	18	15	12	10	7	5	2
30	81	73	65	58	51	45	40	35	30	26	22	18	15	12	9	6	3
35	83	76	69	63	56	50	45	40	35	30	26	22	18	14	11	7	4
40	84	78	72	67	61	55	50	45	40	35	30	26	21	17	13	8	4
45	85	80	75	70	65	60	55	50	45	40	35	30	25	20	15	10	5
50	86	82	77	73	69	64	60	55	50	45	40	35	29	23	18	12	6
55	86	83	79	76	72	68	64	60	55	50	45	40	34	27	21	14	7
60	87	84	81	78	75	72	68	64	60	55	50	45	39	32	25	17	9
65	88	85	83	80	78	75	72	69	65	61	56	51	45	38	30	21	11
70	88	86	84	82	80	78	76	73	70	67	63	58	52	45	36	26	14
75	89	87	86	84	83	81	79	77	75	72	69	65	60	54	45	33	18
80	89	88	87	86	85	84	83	82	80	78	76	73	69	64	57	45	26
85	90	89	89	88	88	87	86	86	85	84	83	81	79	76	72	64	45

Source ▪

The methods were worked out with dried specimens and applied clinically.[1, 2]

Comments ▪

There are several biplane radiographic methods for measuring femoral torsion.[3–6] Many of these require special positioning devices, and the method of Hermann and Egund[6] requires three radiographs. The two techniques described herein seem to offer a compromise between simplicity and accuracy.

REFERENCES

1. Magilligan DJ: Calculation of the angle of anteversion by means of horizontal lateral roentgenography. J Bone Joint Surg Am 1956; 38A: 1231–1246.
2. Ogata K, Goldsand E: A simple biplanar method of measuring femoral anteversion and neck-shaft angle. J Bone Joint Surg Am 1979; 61:846–850.
3. Dunn DM: Anteversion of the neck of the femur: A method of measurement. J Bone Joint Surg Br 1952; 34B:181–186.
4. Ryder CT, Crane L: Measuring femoral anteversion: The problem and a method. J Bone Joint Surg Am 1953; 35A:321–328.
5. Dunlap K, Shands A, Hollister L, et al: A new method for determination of torsion of the femur. J Bone Joint Surg Am 1953; 35A:289–311.
6. Hermann KL, Egund N: Measuring femoral anteversion in the femoral neck from routine radiographs. Acta Radiol 1998; 39:410–415.

▪▪ MEASUREMENT OF FEMORAL TORSION BY FLUOROSCOPY
▪ ACR Code: 44 (Femur)

Technique ▪

The patient is placed prone on the fluoroscopic table, and the image intensifier is centered over the femoral neck of the side in question. The patient's knee is flexed to 90 degrees (the hip stays extended). Under fluoroscopic guidance the lower leg is moved so as to rotate the femur (usually externally—foot across the opposite leg) until the femoral neck lies directly in line with the femoral shaft. Once this geometry has been achieved, the angle between the limb and the plane of the table is the anteversion angle. This is shown in Figures 1 and 2. If the femur must be internally rotated (foot lateral) to achieve the proper geometry, retroversion is present.[1, 2]

Measurements ▪

A goniometer with a long pointer (as shown in Figure 1) is helpful. The angle of anteversion is read directly from the instrument with reference to the plane of the tabletop as 0 degrees.[1, 2] In Ruby's study with a dried femur at anteversion angles of from 0 to 90 degrees, the Rogers fluoroscopic method[2] had a mean error of +1.4 degrees and a range of error of −4 to +7 degrees. This compared favorably with the Ryder-Crane biplane radiographic method,[3] which had a mean error of +2.7 degrees and a range of error of −5 to +8 degrees. In 28 normal limbs, the fluoroscopic method gave mean ± SD of 35 ± 11 degrees, compared with 32 ± 12 degrees for the Ryder-Crane method.[1]

Source ▪

Ruby and colleagues used a dried femur that was cut at the intertrochanteric level to allow simulating different torsion angles. Clinical material consisted of 32 patients (64 hips), of whom 14 had normal lower extremities and 18 had rotational abnormalities.[1]

Comments ▪

Ruby and colleagues calculated radiation dosage from the Ryder-Crane method at 0.12 rad and with fluoroscopy, 1.0 rad. For this reason, they favor the use of the former but note that it does require special equipment.[1] With more modern equipment, the dosages at fluoroscopy are probably lower.

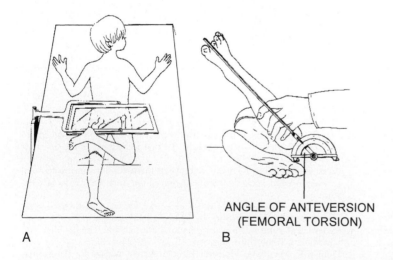

ANGLE OF ANTEVERSION
(FEMORAL TORSION)

A   B

Figure 1 ▪ Fluoroscopic method of determining femoral torsion. *A*, Patient position to examine the right leg. *B*, Measurement of the angle after leg positioning under fluoroscopy. (From Ruby L, Mital MA, O'Conner J, Patel U: J Bone Joint Surg Am 1979; 61:46–51. Used by permission.)

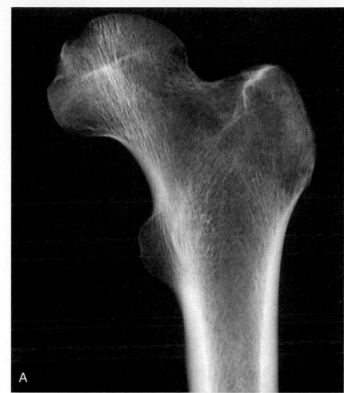

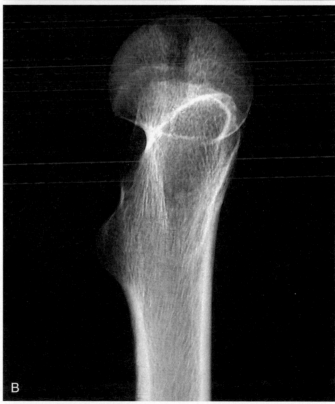

Figure 2 ▪ Appearance of the proximal femur (dried specimen). *A*, In neutral rotation and *B*, after rotation so that the femoral neck and shaft are aligned.

REFERENCES

1. Ruby L, Mital MA, O'Conner J, Patel U: Anteversion of the femoral neck: Comparison of methods of measurements in patients. J Bone Joint Surg Am 1979; 61:46–51.

2. Rogers SP: A method for determining the angle of torsion of the neck of the femur. J Bone Joint Surg 1934; 13:821–824.

3. Ryder CT, Crane L: Measuring femoral anteversion: The problem and a method. J Bone Joint Surg Am 1953; 35A:321–328.

˙: MEASUREMENT OF FEMORAL TORSION WITH COMPUTED TOMOGRAPHY AND MRI
- ▪ ACR Code: 44 (Femur)

Technique ▪

Computed tomography (CT) is performed with the patient supine and with the long axis of the femur to be examined parallel to the long axis (Z) of the gantry. It is helpful to have the femoral neck and condyles at the same vertical (Y) level, as this minimizes geometric distortions. After a localizer scan in the anteroposterior (AP) plane, slices are made through the femoral head/neck and the distal femur just above the joint. Section thickness and technical parameters are not critical and may be selected to minimize dose while maintaining adequate images showing the bony contours.[1-3] The same positioning requirements hold for MRI as for CT. Using the machine's body coil allows scanning the proximal and distal femur without moving the patient, and fine detail (as would be obtained with surface coils) is not critical. Any rapid sequence that displays bony detail well may be used (T1, FLASH, or others).

Measurements ▪

The condylar axis is measured from an axial slice through the distal femur where the condyles are the widest (Figure 1A) and may be determined by several methods (Figure 1B–D). The axis of the femoral neck is measured from axial slices through the femoral head and neck at one of four possible levels (Figure 2A). The axis may be measured from single sections that include both the head and neck or the neck alone (Figure 2B), or from a pair of sections through the center of the head and the base of the neck (Figure 2C). The angle of anteversion is the angle between the condylar axis and the axis of the neck.[1-3]

Murphy's experiments with CT of 12 cadaveric femora showed that those made using two sections (Figure 2C, method II) for the axis of the femoral neck were considerably more accurate and precise than those made from only one slice (Figure 2B, method I). When compared with

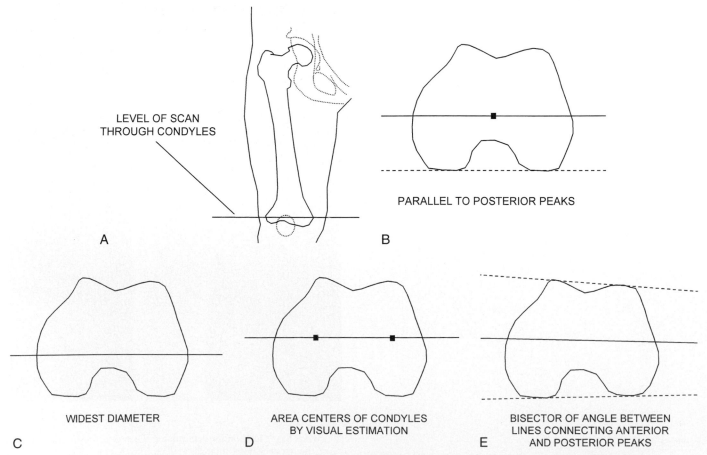

LEVEL OF SCAN
THROUGH CONDYLES

PARALLEL TO POSTERIOR PEAKS

A

B

WIDEST DIAMETER

AREA CENTERS OF CONDYLES
BY VISUAL ESTIMATION

BISECTOR OF ANGLE BETWEEN
LINES CONNECTING ANTERIOR
AND POSTERIOR PEAKS

C

D

E

Figure 1 ▪ Determination of the condylar axis of the femur. *A*, Scan plane through distal femur. *B*, Parallel to line through the posterior peaks. *C*, Through the widest diameter of the condyles. *D*, Through the area center of each condyle. *E*, Bisector of lines through anterior and posterior peaks. (From Murphy SB, Simon SR, Kijewski PK, et al: J Bone Joint Surg Am 1987; 69:1169–1176. Used by permission.)

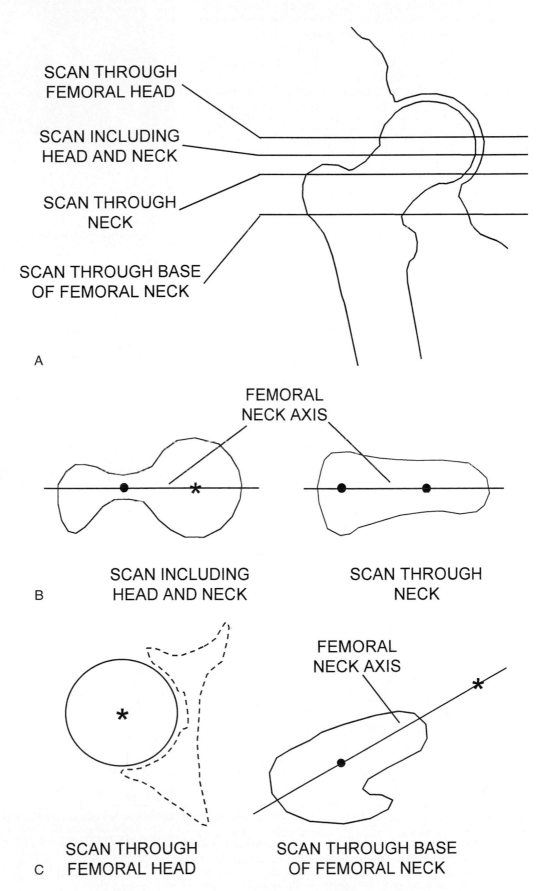

SCAN THROUGH
FEMORAL HEAD

SCAN INCLUDING
HEAD AND NECK

SCAN THROUGH
NECK

SCAN THROUGH BASE
OF FEMORAL NECK

A

FEMORAL
NECK AXIS

SCAN INCLUDING
HEAD AND NECK

SCAN THROUGH
NECK

B

FEMORAL
NECK AXIS

SCAN THROUGH
FEMORAL HEAD

SCAN THROUGH BASE
OF FEMORAL NECK

C

Figure 2 ▪ Determination of the axis of the femoral neck. *A,* possible section levels. *B,* Axis of the femoral neck measured from a single level through either the head and neck or the neck alone. *C,* Axis of the femoral neck measured from scans through the head and the base of the neck. The center of the femoral head *(asterisk)* and middle of the neck *(circles)* are shown. (From Murphy SB, Simon SR, Kijewski PK, et al: J Bone Joint Surg Am 1987; 69:1169–1176. Used by permission.)

direct measurements according to Billing's definitions,[4] method II overestimated true anteversion by 0.32 degree and had a variance of 0.4 ± 0.6 degree, compared with underestimation of 9 degrees and variance of 13 ± 3.6 degrees for method I. As for methods of determining the condylar axis, the methods using the posterior condylar peaks (Figure 1B) and area centers (Figure 1D) were least influenced by changing the level of the slice through the distal femur. These differences were smaller than those found in the proximal measurements. Figure 3 shows the recommended measurement procedure with the three pertinent slices superimposed.[1]

Considerations for measurements from axial MRI images through the proximal and distal femur are identical to those just described. MRI has the advantage of multiplanar imaging, and oblique images parallel to the femoral neck can be made.[5–8] Figure 4 shows this modification. Tomczak found MRI-derived anteversion angles to be about 10 degrees less than those obtained with CT in children. Anteversion with CT averaged 34 degrees, with a range of 5 to 82, and MRI-measured anteversion averaged 23 degrees, with a range of 0 to 65.[5, 6] Schneider and colleagues found that as the proximal slice orientation became more steeply inclined, the measured anteversion was 11.2 ± 5.4 degrees with transverse orientation, 12.1 ± 6.0 degrees with slightly inclined orientation, and 16.7 ± 6.3 degrees at steep angulation. Measurements from angled scans were felt to be more accurate, as this approximates Murphy's method.[8]

Source ▪

Adult femora (n = 20) were embedded in plaster and sectioned for direct measurements or scanned with CT (n = 12) to determine optimal section levels and measurement landmarks for femoral torsion.[1] Guenther and associates measured femoral torsion with CT and MRI in 37 hips of 19 children (7 boys, 12 girls, mean age 11 years; age range 3.5 to 17.5 years). Of these, four had cerebral palsy, six had developmental dysplasia, and five had Legg-

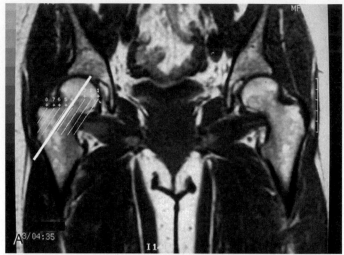

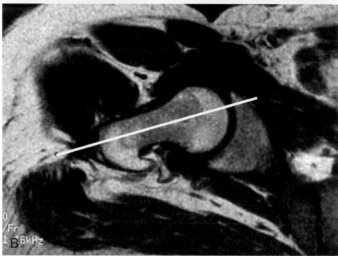

Figure 4 ▪ Modification of proximal femoral scan plane for MRI. *A,* Coronal localizer scout view with femoral neck scan plane shown. *B,* Oblique image through femoral neck, with axis drawn. Measurements of the distal femur from axial images are done in the same manner as for CT.

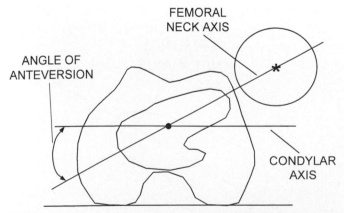

Figure 3 ▪ Recommended method for measuring femoral torsion from axial scans (either CT or MRI) through the femoral head, the base of the neck, and the condyles. These are shown superimposed, with the femoral neck axis drawn between the center of the head *(asterisk)* and the center of the base of the neck *(circle)*. The condylar axis is taken to be parallel to the posterior peaks. (From Murphy SB, Simon SR, Kijewski PK, et al: J Bone Joint Surg Am 1987; 69:1169–1176. Used by permission.)

Calvé-Perthes disease.[6] Schneider performed MRI of 98 femurs in healthy adult volunteers whose mean age was 42 years.[8]

Comments ▪

Exactly how to mark the landmarks and measure the angles depends on software available at the operator's console of the CT or MRI machine or in offline processing equipment. If it is possible to superimpose multiple slices on the display or on hard copy without obscuring anatomy, the task is much easier.

REFERENCES

1. Murphy SB, Simon SR, Kijewski PK, et al: Femoral anteversion. J Bone Joint Surg Am 1987; 69:1169–1176.
2. Hernandez RJ, Tachdjian MO, Poznanski AK, Dias LS: CT determination of femoral torsion. AJR Am J Roentgenol 1981; 137:97–101.
3. Weiner DS, Cook AJ, Hoyt WA Jr, Oravec CE: Computed tomography in the measurement of femoral anteversion. Orthopedics 1978; 1:299–306.
4. Billing L: Roentgen examination of the proximal femur end in children and adolescents. Acta Radiol 1954; Suppl 110.

5. Tomczak R, Gunther K. Pfeifer T, et al: [The measurement of the femoral torsion angle in children by NMR tomography compared to CT and ultrasound] [German]. Fortschr Röntgenstr 1995; 162:224–228.
6. Guenther KP, Tomczak R, Kessler S, et al: Measurement of femoral anteversion by magnetic resonance imaging: Evaluation of a new technique in children and adolescents. Eur J Radiol 1995; 21:47–52.
7. Schneider B, Laubenberger J, Wildner M, et al: [NMR tomographic measurement of femoral ante-torsion and tibial torsion] [German]. Fortschr Röntgenstr 1995; 162:229–231.
8. Schneider B, Laubenberger J, Jemlich S, et al: Measurement of femoral antetorsion and tibial torsion by magnetic resonance imaging. Br J Radiol 1997; 70:575–579.

▪: FEMORAL TORSION ANGLES IN CHILDREN AND ADULTS
▪ ACR Code: 44 (Femur)

Technique ▪

Numerous techniques exist for measuring femoral torsion clinically, from cadavers or dried specimens, and with imaging. Several imaging methods are described in this text.

Measurements ▪

When the axis of the femoral neck is anteriorly inclined with respect to the transcondylar axis, anteversion is said to be present (the normal situation), and these angles are given a positive sign by convention. When the femoral neck axis is posteriorly inclined, the term *retroversion* is used, and the angles have a negative sign by convention. Table 1 lists reported values in children and Table 2 lists reported values in adults.[1–12] Figure 1 is a graphic depiction of femoral anteversion (antetorsion) based on cadaveric measurements and anatomic investigations compiled by Weiner.[13]

Table 1 ▪ Values of Femoral Anteversion in Children

AGE	FABRY	SHANDS	DUNLAP	BUDIN
1	31.1 ± 8.9	39	31 (20–41)	(30–50)
2	30.0 ± 8.5	31	24 (13–38)	30
3	26.7 ± 7.3	29	20 (12–32)	
4	26.2 ± 7.8			25
5	26.7 ± 7.4	27	20 (11–36)	
6	26.6 ± 7.2			
7	23.2 ± 7.0	26	19 (7–32)	
8	24.4 ± 6.5			
9	21.3 ± 5.5	24	18 (10–27)	20
10	20.9 ± 6.6			
11	20.6 ± 7.5	24	17 (5–28)	
12	19.9 ± 6.4			
13	20.0 ± 6.1	21	14 (3–24)	
14	14.5 ± 8.6			17
15	15.4 ± 8.0	16	10 (5–26)	
16	15.4 ± 7.6			
16–20				11

All measurements are in degrees. Fabry's results are given as mean ± standard deviation. Reported ranges are in parentheses.[1–4]

Table 2 ▪ Values of Femoral Anteversion in Adults

AUTHOR	METHOD	NUMBER	MEAN ± SD	RANGE
Dunlap	Radiographic	200	10	5–26
	Meta-analysis	1524	11.2	−20–50
Budin	Literature review	—		8–15
Brouwer	Radiographic	100	10.9	−9–38
Hermann	Radiographic	18	19	−5–29
	CT	18	23	−1–32
Hoiseth	Radiographic	19	12.3 ± 7.4	
	CT	19	11.4 ± 11.2	
Jend	CT	32	15.3 ± 11.9	
Strecker	CT	505	24.1 ± 17.4	
Anda	CT	20	21.6 ± 5.1	10–31
Tomczak	MRI	25	22.2	0–37
	CT	25	15.7	3–48
Schneider	MRI	98	10.4 ± 6.2	
Axial	MRI	42	11.2 ± 5.4	
Moderate	MRI	42	12.1 ± 6.0	
Steep	MRI	42	16.7 ± 6.3	

All measurements are in degrees. Standard deviations are listed when reported. The subgroups under Schneider refer to various angulations of the scan through the femoral neck.[3–12]

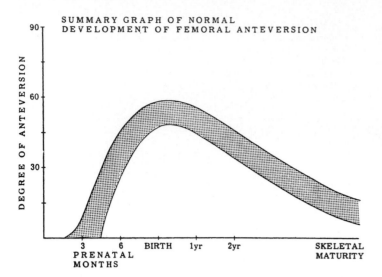

SUMMARY GRAPH OF NORMAL
DEVELOPMENT OF FEMORAL ANTEVERSION

Figure 1 ▪ Femoral anteversion angle in the fetus, infant, and during childhood until skeletal maturity. (From Weiner DS, Cook AJ, Hoyt WA Jr, Oravec CE: Orthopedics 1978; 1:299–306. Used by permission.)

Source ▪

See references.

REFERENCES

1. Fabry G, MacEwen GD, Shands AR: Torsion of the femur: A follow-up study in normal and abnormal conditions. J Bone Joint Surg Am 1973; 55:1726–1738.
2. Shands A, Steele M: Torsion of the femur: A follow-up report on the use of the Dunlap method for its determination. J Bone Joint Surg Am 1958; 40:803–816.
3. Dunlap K, Shands A, Hollister L, et al: A new method for determination of torsion of the femur. J Bone Joint Surg Am 1953; 35A:289–311.
4. Budin E, Chandler E: Measurement of femoral neck anteversion by a direct method. Radiology 1957; 69:209–213.
5. Brouwer KJ, Molenaar JC, van Linge B: Rotational deformities after femoral shaft fractures in childhood: A retrospective study. Acta Orthop Scand 1981; 52:81–89.
6. Hermann KL, Egund N: CT measurement of anteversion in the femoral neck. The influence of femur positioning. Acta Radiol 1997; 38(4 Pt 1):527–532.
7. Hoiseth A, Reikeras O, Fonstelien E: Evaluation of three methods for measurement of femoral neck anteversion. Acta Radiol Diagn 1989; 30:69–73.
8. Jend HH: [Computed tomographic determination of the anteversion angle. Premises and possibilities] [German]. Fortschr Röntgenstr 1986; 144:447–452.
9. Strecker W, Keppler P, Gebhard F, Kinzl L: Length and torsion of the lower limb. J Bone Joint Surg Br 1997; 79:1019–1023.
10. Anda S, Terjesen I, Kvistad KA, Svenningsen S: Acetabular angles and femoral anteversion in dysplastic hips in adults: CT investigation. J Comput Assist Tomogr 1991; 15:115–120.
11. Tomczak RJ, Guenther KP, Rieber A, et al: MR imaging measurement of the femoral antetorsional angle as a new technique: Comparison with CT in children and adults. AJR Am J Roentgenol 1997; 168:791–794.
12. Schneider B, Laubenberger J, Jemlich S, et al: Measurement of femoral antetorsion and tibial torsion by magnetic resonance imaging. Br J Radiol 1997; 70:575–579.
13. Weiner DS, Cook AJ, Hoyt WA Jr, Oravec CE: Computed tomography in the measurement of femoral anteversion. Orthopedics 1978; 1:299–306.

▪▪ MUSCLE AND FAT THICKNESS IN THE THIGH
▪ ACR Code: 449 (Soft Tissues of the Thigh)

Technique ▪

Ultrasound of the anterior thigh was done with 5-MHz linear transducers, using a SAL 20A machine (Toshiba, Tokyo, Japan). The subjects were seated with the knee extended and relaxed. Scanning was done midway between the greater trochanter and the knee joint in the transverse plane (Figure 1*A*). Prior to obtaining measurements, the transducer orientation was changed to get the brightest echo from the femur bone so as to be perpendicular to the long axis of the thigh. The authors stress that transducer pressure must be kept at a minimum to avoid distortion of the anatomy.[1]

Measurements ▪

Using frozen images and electronic calipers, the thickness of the subcutaneous fat (SQFT) from skin to outer muscular fascia, and the thickness of the quadriceps muscle complex thickness (QMT) from outer fascia to the femur were measured in millimeters. Figure 1*B* shows these measurements. Table 1 lists QMT for girls and boys and Figure 2 gives the same information in graphic form (combined sexes). Figure 3 depicts SQFT for girls and boys.[1]

Source ▪

One leg of 276 children ranging from infants to 12 years of age was examined. The age and gender distribution are listed in Table 1. Subjects were inpatients without neuromuscular disease, children attending a local school, and newborn babies in the nursery.[1]

Comments ▪

There were no significant differences in QMT between genders, whereas the SQFT was greater in girls than in boys after infancy. Multiple regression analyses failed to

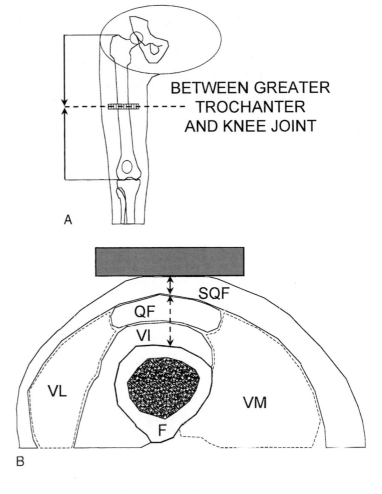

Figure 1 ▪ Measurement of quadriceps muscle complex thickness (QMT) and subcutaneous fat (SQF) in the thigh. *A,* The scanning position is midway between the greater trochanter and the knee joint *(arrows and dotted line). B,* Measurements are made from transverse images between the skin surface and the outer muscular fascia *(solid line with arrowheads)* for SQF and between the outer fascia and the femur *(dashed line with arrowheads)* for QMT. QF = quadriceps femoris, F = femur, VL = vastus lateralis, VI = vastus intermedialis, VM = vastus medialis.

Table 1 ▪ **Quadriceps Muscle Thickness in Children**

AGE	BOYS		GIRLS	
	No.	Mean ± SD	No.	Mean ± SD
0–1	16	16.5 ± 2.6	8	16.3 ± 3.3
1–2	5	22.0 ± 3.5	9	21.2 ± 3.1
2–3	9	23.3 ± 3.5	11	22.7 ± 4.2
3–4	12	21.6 ± 3.5	11	24.6 ± 4.5
4–5	15	26.0 ± 4.0	7	24.7 ± 3.3
5–6	12	26.8 ± 4.0	12	25.8 ± 3.4
6–7	12	25.5 ± 4.7	17	25.7 ± 4.0
7–8	8	26.5 ± 3.2	13	26.5 ± 3.7
8–9	11	28.5 ± 5.0	9	31.0 ± 4.8
9–10	14	28.6 ± 5.4	11	30.5 ± 6.0
10–11	12	32.0 ± 5.7	21	29.1 ± 6.2
11–12	10	31.7 ± 3.8	9	27.6 ± 5.3

All measurements are in millimeters. SD = standard deviation.
From Heckmatt JZ, Pier N, Dubowitz V: J Clin Ultrasound 1988; 16:171–176. Used by permission.

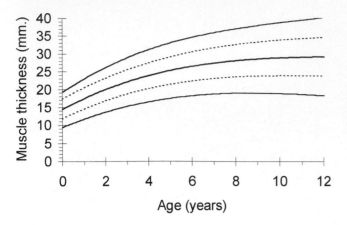

Figure 2 ▪ Quadriceps muscle thickness in children. Mean *(solid line)*, ± 1 standard deviation *(dotted lines)*, and ± 2 standard deviations *(solid lines)* are shown. Girls and boys are combined. (From Heckmatt JZ, Pier N, Dubowitz V: J Clin Ultrasound 1988; 16:171–176. Used by permission.)

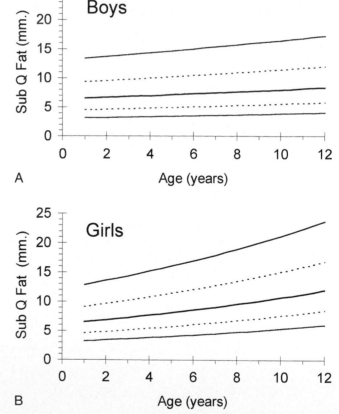

Figure 3 ▪ Subcutaneous fat thickness in boys *(A)* and girls *(B)*. Mean *(solid line)*, ± 1 standard deviation *(dotted lines)*, ± 2 standard deviations *(solid lines)* are shown. (From Heckmatt JZ, Pier N, Dubowitz V: J Clin Ultrasound 1988; 16:171–176. Used by permission.)

yield a model for QMT, whereas logarithmic equations were found to predict SQFT from age and sex as follows:

$$SQFT \text{ (boys)} = 10^{[0.802 + 0.0099 \text{ Age (years)}]}$$
$$\text{Standard deviation} = 0.1578$$

$$SQFT \text{ (girls)} = 10^{[0.788 + 0.0241 \text{ Age (years)}]}$$
$$\text{Standard deviation} = 0.1489$$

These measurements are useful in assessing muscle atrophy or hypertrophy in neuromuscular disease.[1]

REFERENCE

1. Heckmatt JZ, Pier N, Dubowitz V: Measurement of quadriceps muscle thickness and subcutaneous tissue thickness in normal children by real-time ultrasound imaging. J Clin Ultrasound 1988; 16:171–176.

▪: SAGITTAL PLANE RELATION OF FEMORAL CONDYLES TO THE LONG AXIS OF THE FEMUR[1]

▪ ACR Code: 451 (Distal End of Femur)

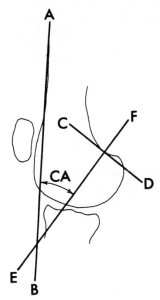

Figure 1 ▪ (Adapted from Lindahl O, Movin A: Acta Radiol Diagn 1970; 10:108. Used by permission.)

Technique ▪

Central ray: Projected through the knee joint space, perpendicular to the plane of the film.
Position: True lateral.
Target-film distance: Immaterial (Lindahl used 100 cm).

Measurements (Figure 1) ▪

AB = Line drawn along the anterior cortical demarcation of the shaft of the femur.
CD = Plane for the floor of the intercondylar fossa (the intercondylar plane).
EF = Perpendicular to line *CD* intersecting line *AB*.

CA = Angle formed by roof of intercondylar fossa and long axis of femur.

Mean value, 34.0° ± 0.5°; range, 26° to 44°. Right and left sides in the same patient showed differences of 0.2° ± 0.2°.

Source ▪

Two hundred normal knee joints of 100 patients without knee complaints.

REFERENCE

1. Lindahl O, Movin A: Roentgenologic angulation measurement in supracondylar fractures of the femur. Acta Radiol Diagn 1970; 10:108–112.

▪: PROXIMAL TROCHLEAR GROOVE

▪ ACR Code: 451 (Distal End of Femur)

Technique ▪

Lateral radiographs of the knee were performed on a remote control examination table (other data not given). Correlative radiographs were done in other projections, including 30-degree (flexion) axial views with external ankle rotation to assess for lateral patellar subluxation.[1, 2]

Measurements ▪

On the lateral view, the distance between the trochlear groove to the lateral and medial anterior femoral condyles was measured (in millimiters) and the average computed.

This was done 1 cm below the upper limit of the trochlear groove (proximal) and in the middle of the cephalocaudal extent of the groove (medial). Figure 1 shows these measurements. Table 1 lists the measurements for each population group as well as combined figures for knees with stable and subluxing patellas.[1]

Source ▪

Asymptomatic subjects (10 women, 10 men, mean age 28 years) had radiographs of both knees. Unselected patients with various complaints (39 women, 30 men, mean age 35 years) had radiographs of one or both knees. Patients with

Table 1 ▪ Depth of the Trochlear Groove from Lateral Radiographs

CLINICAL STATUS	NO. OF KNEES	LATERAL SUBLUXATION ON 30° VIEW: POSITIVE/ EXAMINED (%)	PROXIMAL (Mean ± SD)	MEDIAL (Mean ± SD)
Asymptomatic	40	0/40 (0)	5.94 ± 1.74	7.77 ± 1.78
Various symptoms (stable)	96	0/96 (0)	5.84 ± 1.53	6.83 ± 1.30
Various symptoms (subluxing)	11	11/11 (100)	5.05 ± 1.37	6.27 ± 0.68
Patellar instability (treated knee)	40	27/27 (100)	3.83 ± 1.06	5.55 ± 1.04
Patellar instability (untreated knee)	22	11/13 (85)	2.74 ± 1.35	5.65 ± 1.34
Asymptomatic and various (stable)	136	0/136 (0)	5.87 ± 1.59*	7.11 ± 1.46*
Various (subluxing) and patellar instability	73	71/73 (97)	3.69 ± 1.20*	5.69 ± 1.10*

*Calculated from the reported data.[1]
All measurements are in mm. SD = standard deviation.

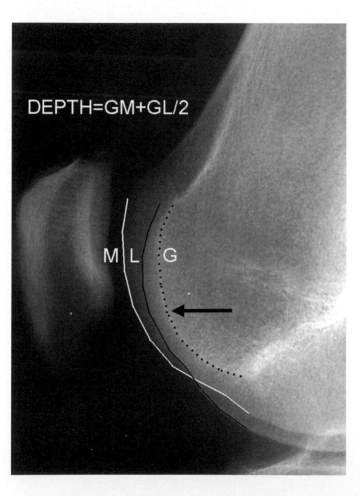

Figure 1 ▪ Measurement of trochlear depth. The trochlear groove (*dotted, G*) as well as the anterior margins of the medial (*white, M*) and lateral (*black, M*) condyles have been outlined. Proximal measurements are made 1 cm below the upper margin of the trochlear groove. The depth is calculated by GM + GL/2. If the upper trochlear groove margin is not well seen, the physis may be used as a landmark. The same measurements may be made in the midpoint (called medial by Malghem and Maldague) of the groove, as shown by the arrow.[1]

a history of lateral patellar subluxation (21 women, 13 men, mean age 21 years) were also included. Radiographs of 40 knees that had received corrective surgery and 22 contralateral knees were included.[1] Of the 209 knees evaluated with lateral radiographs, 187 had the 30-degree axial views of the externally rotated ankle available.[1]

Comments ▪

A mixed subset of 50 subject radiographs was measured by the researchers in both papers to determine inter- and intraobserver variability, these values were calculated at 0.8 and 0.5 mm, respectively. Modestly rotated radiographs produce variances in the measurement of up to 15%. Proximal measurements were significantly lower in subjects with subluxing patellas (p < 0.001), as were the medial measurements, though to a lesser degree (p = 0.1–0.001). The researchers state that a proximal measurement of the trochlear depth of less than 5.0 mm greatly increases the risk of patellar instability.[1]

REFERENCES

1. Malghem J, Maldague B: Depth insufficiency of the proximal trochlear groove on lateral radiographs of the knee: Relation to patellar dislocation. Radiology 1989; 170:507–510.
2. Malghem J, Maldague B: Patellofemoral joint: 30 degree axial radiograph with lateral rotation of the leg. Radiology 1989; 170:566–567.

▪: DEPTH OF THE LATERAL FEMORAL SULCUS
▪ ACR Code: 451 (Distal End of Femur)

Technique ▪

Standard lateral radiographs of the knee were performed following knee injury.[1-3] The source-to-film distance was specified in one paper at 100 cm.[3] Clinical correlation to confirm the presence or absence of anterior cruciate ligament (ACL) tear was performed with various combinations of physical examination (anterior drawer, pivot-shift, and Lachman tests), arthrometer studies, MRI examinations, arthroscopy, or surgery.[1-3]

Measurements ▪

The lateral femoral sulcus may form an arcuate depression in the contour of the lateral femoral condyle on true lateral radiographs and is seen midway between the patellar and tibial articular surfaces. Measurement of the depth of the sulcus was performed in all three studies by the method initially described by Warren and colleagues.[1] Figure 1 shows the sulcus on a normal radiograph, and Figure 2 depicts the measurement of its depth on a tracing of the same radiograph. Table 1 lists the measured depths from the three cited studies in terms of mean, standard deviation, and range, as well as percent above two cut-off depths (1.5 and 2.0 mm) for knees with intact and torn ACL.[1-3]

Source ▪

Warren and colleagues studied radiographs of 47 adults (age and gender not given) with intact ACL, 52 with acute ACL tear, and 101 with chronic ACL tear.[1] Cobby's subjects included 62 people with intact ACL (48 men, 14 women, mean age 42 years; age range 15 to 70 years) and 41 with ACL tears (27 men, 14 women, mean age 32 years; age range 17 to 58 years).[2] Yu and colleagues evaluated 26 patients with intact ACL (20 men, 6 women, mean age 27 years; age range 12–43 years) and 124 having tears of the ACL (88 men, 36 women, mean age 27 years; age range 13 to 52 years).[3]

Comments ▪

A sizable fraction (50% with intact ACL, 30% with acutely torn ACL, and 40% with chronic ACL tear) of radiographs will not display the sulcus at all.[3] An impaction fracture in the lateral femoral condyle directly over the anterior horn of the meniscus is felt to be responsible for the widening of the notch in ACL tear.[2] Warren and Yu and their associates state that a depth of greater than 2.0 mm is indicative of a torn ACL.[1,3] Yu and associates calculated test statistics from their series: sensitivity 3.2%, specificity 100%, positive predictive value 100%.[3] Cobby and colleagues cited a cut-off depth of greater than 1.5 mm, which was 3 standard deviations above their mean.[2]

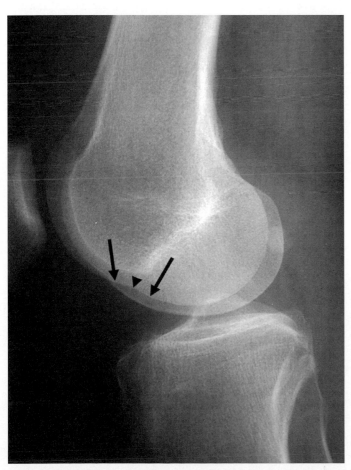

Figure 1 ▪ Lateral femoral sulcus in a normal lateral radiograph of the knee. The anterior and posterior borders of the notch are indicated (*arrows*), as well as its base (*arrowhead*).

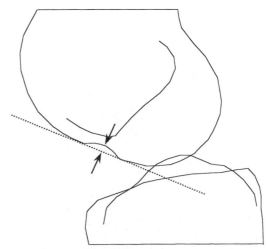

Figure 2 ▪ Measurement of the depth of the lateral femoral sulcus. A line (*dotted*) is drawn tangential to the junctions of the sulcal depression with the lateral condylar margin. The depth is measured between the line and the base of the sulcus (*arrows*).

Table 1 ▪ Lateral Femoral Sulcus Depth[1-3]

RESEARCHER	PATIENT CATEGORY	NO.	DEPTH			
			≥1.5 mm (%)	≥2.0 mm (%)	Mean ± SD	Range
Warren et al	Neg. tear	47	1 (2)	0	—	—
	Pos. tear (acute)	52	2 (4)	0	—	—
	Pos. tear (chronic)	101	13 (13)	8 (8)	—	—
Cobby et al	Neg. tear	62	0	—	0.45	0.0–1.2
	Pos. tear	41	5 (12)	—	0.89	0.0–5.0
Yu et al	Neg. tear	26	3 (12)	0	0.31 ± 0.35	0.0–1.0
	Pos. tear	124	11 (9)	4 (3.2)	0.57 ± 0.57	0.0–3.3

REFERENCES

1. Warren RF, Kaplan N, Bach BR: The lateral notch sign of anterior cruciate ligament insufficiency. Am J Knee Surg 1988; 1:119–124.
2. Cobby MJ, Schweitzer ME, Resnick D: The deep lateral femoral notch: An indirect sign of a torn anterior cruciate ligament. Radiology 1992; 184(3):855–858.
3. Yu JS, Bosch E, Pathria MN, et al: Deep lateral femoral sulcus: Study of 124 patients with anterior cruciate ligament tear. Emerg Radiol 1995; 2:129–134.

▪: AXIAL RELATIONSHIPS OF THE KNEE JOINT[1]
▪ ACR Code: 452 (Knee Joint)

Technique ▪

Central ray: Passes through a point about 0.5 inch below the tip of the patella, so that it will pass directly through the knee joint space, perpendicular to the plane of the film.
Position: Anteroposterior.
Target-film distance: Immaterial.

Measurements (Figure 1; Table 1) ▪

AB = Line drawn along the midaxis of the femoral shaft.
CD = Line drawn along the midaxis of the tibial shaft.
EF = Line tangent to the articular surfaces of the condyles.
GH = Line tangent to the lateral and medial extremities of the tibial plateau.

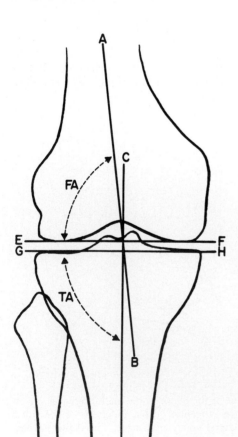

Figure 1 ▪ Measurement of the axial knee joint angles (see text for details).

Table 1 ▪ Normal Axial Angles of the Knee	FA	TA
Male	75°–85°	85°–100°
Female	75°–85°	87°–98°
Average	81°	93°

FA = Femoral angle; TA = tibial angle.
From Keats TE, et al: Radiology 1966; 87:904–907. Used by permission.

FA = Femoral angle at intersection of *AB* and *EF*.
TA = Tibial angle at intersection of *CD* and *GH*.

Source ▪

The data were based on a study of 50 normal adult subjects, equally divided between males and females and ranging in age from 18 to 66 years.

REFERENCE

1. Keats TE, Teeslink R, Diamond AE, Williams JH: Normal axial relationships of the major joints. Radiology 1966; 87:904–907.

▪: KNEE JOINT SPACE HEIGHT
- ACR Code: 452 (Knee Joint)

Technique ▪

Non–weight-bearing posteroanterior (PA) radiographs were taken of the knee, using 12.5 mA, 63 kV, and a focus-film distance of 110 cm.[1] Weight-bearing films were done with similar technique but with the subject standing.

Measurements ▪

The height of the medial and lateral joint spaces in millimeters was measured using a digital analysis system.[2] Figure 1 shows these measurements. Table 1 lists the mean values and ranges for males, females, all patients, with and without weight bearing.[1]

		MEDIAL JOINT SPACE HEIGHT		LATERAL JOINT SPACE HEIGHT	
SUBJECT GROUP	**NO.**	**Mean**	**Range**	**Mean**	**Range**
All subjects	669	6.43	5.58–7.15	7.00	6.30–7.58
Male	315	7.03	6.91–7.15	7.44	7.30–7.58
Female	370	5.73	5.58–5.88	6.44	6.30–6.58
Non–weight bearing	30	5.31	4.89–5.73	6.12	5.64–6.60
Weight bearing	30	5.15	4.85–5.45	5.90	5.60–6.18

Table 1 ▪ Knee Joint Space Height

Measurements are in millimeters.[1]

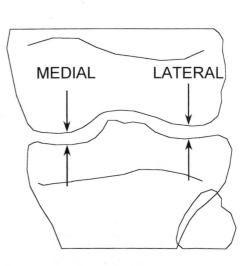

MEDIAL   LATERAL

Figure 1 ▪ Measurement of knee joint space. The distances between the lateral and medial articular margins of the femur and tibia were measured in millimeters as shown (*arrows*).[1]

Source ▪

Patients evaluated in the casualty radiology department for knee pain (n = 302, male 47, female 155, median age 35.1 years, age range 12 to 85 years) or acute injury (n = 369, male 232, female 137, median age 34.9, age range 10 to 86 years). None of the patients had clinical or radiographic evidence of significant injury or arthritis at the time of the study. Data on height and weight were obtained from 213 of the patients. A separate population of 30 normal female volunteers had weight-bearing films, and these were compared with age-matched members of the patient group.[1]

Comments ▪

The lateral compartment was wider than the medial (p < .001); males had larger measurements in both compartments (p < .001); and weight bearing caused a 4% decrease in height of both compartments. There was no significant correlation between height, weight, or calculated body mass index and joint space height.[1]

REFERENCES

1. Dacre JE, Scott JA, Da Silva P, et al: Joint space in the radiologically normal knee. Br J Rheumatol 1991; 30:426–428.
2. Dacre JE, Huskisson EC: The automatic assessment of knee radiographs in osteoarthritis using digital image analysis. Br J Rheumatol 1989; 28:506–510.

▪: SIZE OF THE QUADRICEPS TENDON, PATELLAR TENDON, AND SUPRAPATELLAR BURSA
- ACR Code: 452 (Knee Joint)

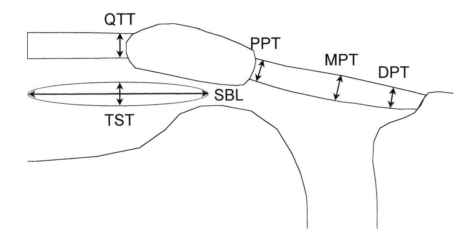

Figure 1 ▪ Ultrasound measurements about the anterior knee. The following structures were measured (abbreviations also used in the table of normal values):

QTT = quadriceps tendon thickness
PPT = proximal patellar tendon thickness
MPT = midpatellar tendon thickness
DPT = distal patellar tendon thickness
TST = total synovial thickness of suprapatellar bursa
SBL = suprapatellar bursal length

(From van Holsbeeck MV, Introcaso JH: Mosby–Year Book, St. Louis, 1991, vol 1, pp 315–319. Used by permission.)

Table 1 ▪ Normal Measurements of Anterior Knee Joint Structures

MEASUREMENT	SEDENTARY MALES (n = 24)	SEDENTARY FEMALES (n = 21)	MALE ATHLETES (n = 52)	FEMALE ATHLETES (n = 43)
Right QTT	5.1 ± 0.6	4.9 ± 0.6	4.9 ± 0.8	5.1 ± 0.7
Left QTT	5.2 ± 0.8	4.8 ± 0.5	5.2 ± 0.9	5.1 ± 0.6
Right PPT	3.0 ± 0.4	2.6 ± 0.4	3.4 ± 0.9	3.3 ± 0.8
Left PPT	3.1 ± 0.3	2.7 ± 0.4	3.5 ± 0.7	3.1 ± 0.4
Right MPT	3.1 ± 0.4	2.9 ± 0.5	3.6 ± 0.7	3.3 ± 0.8
Left MPT	3.2 ± 0.4	2.9 ± 0.3	3.5 ± 0.6	3.1 ± 0.4
Right DPT	3.1 ± 0.4	2.6 ± 0.4	3.4 ± 0.9	3.3 ± 0.8
Left DPT	3.1 ± 0.4	2.7 ± 0.4	3.5 ± 0.7	3.1 ± 0.4
Right TST	2.5 ± 0.5	2.3 ± 0.5	2.5 ± 0.7	2.3 ± 0.6
Left TST	2.5 ± 0.4	2.3 ± 0.5	2.6 ± 0.6	2.2 ± 0.6
Right SBL	22.3 ± 3.8	21.2 ± 4.3	21.2 ± 4.2	19.5 ± 5.0
Left SBL	21.8 ± 4.2	20.6 ± 5.3	23.9 ± 4.8	20.8 ± 4.9

All measurements in millimeters (mean ± standard deviation). Structure abbreviations are listed in Figure 1.
From van Holsbeeck MV, Introcaso JH: Mosby–Year Book, St. Louis, 1991, vol 1, pp 315–319. Used by permission.

Technique ▪

Ultrasound of the knee was done with high-frequency linear transducers over the anterior knee.[1]

Measurements ▪

Frozen images were used to measure the thickness of the quadriceps tendon above the patella, the patellar tendon in three locations, and the thickness and length of the suprapatellar bursa in normal subjects.[1] Figure 1 shows the locations of measurements and lists abbreviations used in the table of normal values (Table 1).

Source ▪

The study population consisted of 96 adults divided according to lifestyle (sedentary or athletic) and gender.[1]

REFERENCE

1. van Holsbeeck MV, Introcaso JH: Appendix: Table of Normal Values. In van Holsbeeck MV, Introcaso JH (eds): Musculoskeletal Ultrasound. Mosby–Year Book, St. Louis, 1991, vol 1, pp 315–319.

▪: THICKNESS OF THE PATELLAR TENDON
▪ ACR Code: 4528 (Patellar Tendon)

Technique ▪

El-Khoury and colleagues used a 1.5-T Signa unit (GE Medical Systems, Milwaukee, WI) and Reiff and colleagues used a 1.5-T Magnetom machine (Siemens Medical Systems, Iselin, NJ) to perform MRI of the knee. Both groups used dedicated surface coils, and all sequences were performed in the sagittal plane with minimal obliquity (15 to 20 degrees) and 3-mm section thickness.[1, 2] El-Khoury and colleagues obtained spin-echo sequences with T1 (350–567/15)-, Proton density (2000–2150/17–20)-, and T2 (2000–2150/80)-weighting.[1] Reiff and colleagues performed gradient echo (GRE) sequences (12/30/40 degrees) on their subjects.[2]

Measurements ▪

Measurements of the patellar tendon (PT) thickness were made from the most central image of the tendon at the inferior pole of the patella (proximal), at the middle, and at the tibial insertion (distal) site.[1, 2] Measurements were made perpendicular to the long axis of the tendon.[2] Figure 1 shows the measurement sites and Table 1 gives the results from both studies.

Source ▪

El-Khoury and colleagues studied 10 healthy volunteers and 50 patients (40 men, 20 women, mean age 29 years, age range 16 to 72 years) without complaints or imaging findings to suggest PT abnormality. They also studied 13 knees from 11 patients (8 men, 3 women, mean age 21 years, age range 16 to 34 years) with clinical patellar tendinitis.[1] Reiff's subjects were 60 patients (38 males, 22 females, mean age 32 years, age range 14 to 60 years) with routine studies of the knee that had no anterior compartment symptomatology.[2]

Comments ▪

El-Khoury and group performed oblique and straight images in four subjects and found less than 1.0 mm difference in the PT measurements. The proximal PT thickness was significantly greater in patients with patellar tendinits than in normal subjects (p < .0001). Though the numbers were not given, El-Khoury and group state that in severe patellar tendinitis the middle PT thickness was also increased. An upper limit of 7.0 mm was proposed for the proximal measurement.[1]

Figure 1 ▪ Measurement of patellar tendon thickness from midsagittal MRI. The thickness is measured perpendicular to the long axis of the tendon at the patellar origin *(PROX)*, at the midpoint *(MIDDLE)*, and at the tibial insertion *(DISTAL)*.

Table 1 ▪ Patellar Tendon Thickness from Sagittal MRI

AUTHOR/GROUP	SEQUENCE	NO.	PROXIMAL		MIDDLE		DISTAL	
			Mean ± SD	Range	Mean ± SD	Range	Mean ± SD	Range
El-Khoury et al	T1, PD, T2							
Normal		60	3.7 ± 1.2	2.0–6.0	4.3 ± 1.1	—	5.6 ± 1.1	—
Patellar tendinitis		13	10.9 ± 2.3	8.0–15.0	—	—	—	—
Reiff et al	GRE							
Males (normal)		38	5.5 ± 1.5	2.9–8.8	3.9 ± 0.9	2.5–5.9	5.0 ± 1.4	2.5–8.8
Females (normal)		22	5.6 ± 2.1	1.5–10.3	4.0 ± 1.1	1.5–6.6	4.9 ± 1.4	1.5–7.4

All measurements are in millimeters. SD = standard deviation, PD = proton density, GRE = gradient echo.[1, 2]

REFERENCES

1. El-Khoury GY, Wira RL, Berbaum KS, et al. MR imaging of patellar tendinitis. Radiology 1992; 184(3):849–854.

2. Reiff DB, Heenan SD, Heron CW: MRI appearances of the asymptomatic patellar tendon on gradient echo imaging. Skeletal Radiol 1995; 24(2):123–126.

▪: MEASUREMENT FOR ASSESSING THE HEIGHT OF THE PATELLA[1]
▪ ACR Code: 453 (Patella)

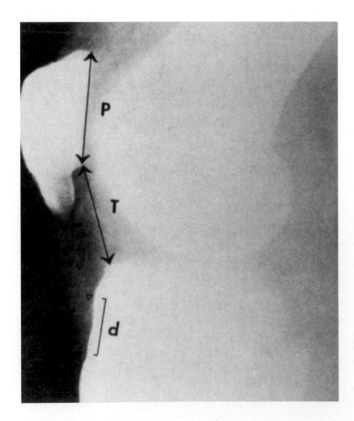

Figure 1 ▪ Low kv exposure radiograph illustrating an example of measurement of the distance (P) between the upper and lower limits of the articular surface of the patella, and the shortest distance (T) between this same lower limit and the tibial plateau. (From de Carvalho A, Andersen AH, Topp S, et al: Int Orthop 1985; 9:195–197. Used by permission.)

Table 1 ▪ Limits of Confidence of the T/P Ratio									
	LOWER LIMITS (PATELLA INFERA)					UPPER LIMITS (PATELLA ALTA)			
Levels of significance									
Two-sided	0.01	0.02	0.05	0.10	0.20	0.20	0.10	0.05	0.02	0.01
One-sided	0.005	0.01	0.025	0.05	0.10	0.10	0.05	0.025	0.01	0.005
T/P ratio	0.56	0.59	0.64	0.68	0.72	1.06	1.11	1.15	1.20	1.23

From de Carvalho A, et al: Int Orthop 1985; 9:195–197. Used by permission.

This technique may be used in place of the preceding entry in those cases in which there is lack of definition of the posterior surface of the patellar tendon and loss of sharpness of the notch on the tibia, or in cases in which the lower limit of the tendon does not coincide with the notch of the tibial tubercle.

Technique ▪

Central ray: Perpendicular to plane of film.
Position: Lateral with 30% flexion of the knee.
Target-film distance: Immaterial.

Measurement (Figure 1) ▪

The ratio of T/P (see Figure 1) is calculated, and the cutoffs at various levels of confidence for patella infera and patella alta are shown in Table 1.

Source ▪

Data were derived from a study of 150 subjects without knee complaints, ages 20 to 60 years.

REFERENCE

1. de Carvalho A, Holst Andersen A, Topp S, Jurik AG: A method for assessing the height of the patella. Int Orthop 1985; 9:195–197.

▪: PATELLAR POSITION ON LATERAL RADIOGRAPHS
▪ ACR Code: 453 (Patella)

Technique ▪

Lateral radiographs of the knee in semiflexion (30 degrees) were performed, with the central ray perpendicular to the film and centered on the joint.[1–3]

Measurements ▪

Kannus, and Insall and Salvati, measured the length of the patellar tendon *(LT)* from the lower patellar margin to its insertion on the tibia, as well as the maximum cephalocaudal length of the patella *(LP)*, and formed a ratio between the two.[1, 2] De Carvalho and colleagues measured the distance between the lower articular margin of the patella and the anterior tibial plateau *(PTD)*, as well as the length of the articular surface of the patella *(ASL)*, and formed a ratio between them.[3] Figure 1 shows these measurements, and Table 1 lists the results as reported.[1–3]

Source ▪

Kannus studied 45 adults (21 men, 24 women, age range 61 to 48 years, mean age 27 years) with unilateral patellar pain syndrome. This was defined by at least 2 months of pain and crepitus, with flexion in the affected joint (right 26, left 19), and accompanying characteristic physical findings. The contralateral joint was normal and there was no clinical or radiographic evidence of fracture, ligamentous injury or inflammation, or arthritis.[1] Insall and Salvati evaluated radiographs of 114 knees without patellar disease.[2] De Carvalho and colleagues studied radiographs of 150 adults without knee complaints who were aged from 20 to 60 years.[3]

Comments ▪

When the patellar tendon or its insertion notch on the tibia can be clearly seen, the method of Insall and Salvati (LT/LP) may be used.[2] When these landmarks are invisible, the alternative method (PTD/ASL) is useful.[3] Kannus

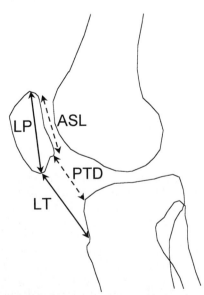

Figure 1 ▪ Measurements of patellar position from lateral knee radiographs. The length of the patellar tendon *(LT)* and the cephalocaudal length of the patella *(LP)* are used to form a ratio *(LT/LP)*. Alternatively, the distance between the lower articular margin of the patella and the anterior tibial plateau *(PTD)* and the length of the patellar articular surface *(ASL)* can be used to form a ratio *(PTD/ASL)*.[1, 3]

Table 1 ▪ Patellar Height Ratios

AUTHOR/POPULATION	PARAMETER	LT/LP RATIO	PTD/ASL RATIO
Kannus Normal (n = 45)	Mean ± SD	1.17±0.16	0.97±0.23
	Range	0.85–1.47	0.47–1.38
Kannus Pain synd. (n = 45)	Mean ± SD	1.30±0.17	1.17±0.27
	Range	1.08–1.76	0.80–2.13
Insall and Salvati Normal (n = 114)	Median	1.00	
	Range	0.8–1.2	
de Carvalho et al Normal (n = 150)	Mean ± SD		0.89±0.13
	Range		0.47–1.28

Measurements are unitless. Pain Synd. = patellar pain syndrome, SD = standard deviation. Other abbreviations as in Figure 1 and the text.

found significant differences in the LT/LP ratio between the normal knees and the knees affected by patellar pain syndrome (p < 0.01). This was caused by lengthening of the LT measurement (p < 0.01) with no difference in LP.[1] Frank rupture of the patellar tendon will also cause both ratios to be abnormally high (patella alta). When the patella is low riding (patella infra), the calculated ratios will fall below normal limits.

REFERENCES

1. Kannus PA: Long patellar tendon: Radiographic sign of patellofemoral pain syndrome—a prospective study. Radiology 1992; 185:859–863.
2. Insall J, Salvati E: Patella position in the normal knee joint. Radiology 1971; 101(1): 101–104.
3. de Carvalho A, Holst Andersen A, Topp S, Jurik AG: A method for assessing the height of the patella. Int Orthop 1985; 9(3): 195–197.

▪: PATELLAR CARTILAGE THICKNESS
▪ ACR Code: 453 (Patella)

Technique ▪

Fresh cadaver patellas were placed in "supine" position in a plastic box and scanned with a 1.5-T Signa machine (GE Medical Systems, Milwaukee, WI). Axial images were performed with several sequences: T1 (500/20), proton density (1800/20), T2 (1800/80), fast spin echo (3600/84/echo train = 16), gradient echo (47/12/flip angle = 20 degrees). Fat suppression was used for the proton density, T2, and fast spin echo sequences. The gradient echo images were obtained with 1.2-mm section thickness and the rest with 4-mm thickness and 1-mm gap.[1] For direct measurements (after MRI scanning), the patellas were frozen and sectioned at 5-mm intervals, fixed, decalcified, sliced to 6 μm, and stained with hematoxylin and eosin.

Measurements ▪

Measurements of cartilage thickness were made from four images from each MRI sequence, with a scaled loupe with 7× magnification to the nearest 0.1 mm. A CUE-2 (Olympus) semiautomated morphometry system with a 4-power lens was used to measure the patellar cartilage thickness from anatomic sections corresponding to the MRI images. Measurements were made in three locations on each MRI image and anatomic section: opposite the apex of the patella, 30 degrees medial, and 30 degrees lateral from the apical line. A total of 180 measurements was available for each sequence, 300 for each position, and 60 from each patella. A subset of 20 randomly selected positions from all MRI sequences (total = 100) was measured 4 weeks after the initial determination by the same experimenter, as well as by a second observer to assess inter- and intraobserver variability.[1] Figure 1 shows the measurement positions, and Table 1 gives the results by sequence and measurement position.

Source ▪

Fresh cadaveric patellas from three women and five men (total patellas 15), whose ages at the time of death ranged from 30 to 77 years.[1]

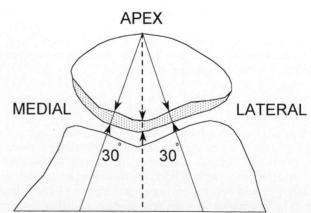

Figure 1 ▪ Measurement of patellar cartilage thickness. A line (dotted) was drawn from the apex of the patella through the cartilage and its thickness measured there (arrows). Medial and lateral measurements (arrows) were made 30 degrees on either side of the middle (solid lines).[1]

Table 1 ▪ Patellar Cartilage Thickness

SEQUENCE	MEASUREMENT POSITION	NO. OF MEASUREMENTS	THICKNESS	DIFFERENCE FROM DIRECT MEASUREMENT (Mean ± SD)	CORRELATION MRI–DIRECT r VALUE
T1 weighted	Combined	180	3.19	0.25 ± 0.59	0.85
T2 weighted	Combined	180	3.46	0.46 ± 0.71	0.79
Proton density	Combined	180	3.26	0.33 ± 0.62	0.82
Fast spin echo	Combined	180	3.41	0.47 ± 0.79	0.79
Gradient echo	Combined	180	3.50	0.49 ± 0.74	0.78
Combined	30° Medial	300	3.2 (1.1–6.6)	—	—
Combined	At apex	300	3.0 (1.3–6.5)	—	—
Combined	30° Lateral	300	3.1 (1.3–6.6)	—	—

All measurements are in millimeters. SD = standard deviation. For the combined sequence thickness at each position, the range is given in parentheses.[1]

Comments ▪

The intraobserver variability was −0.09 to 0.05 mm, with correlation coefficients of 0.867 to 0.920, whereas the interobserver variability had a range of −0.04 to 0.11 and correlation coefficients of 0.850 to 0.983. Differences between MRI and direct measurements of more than 1.0 mm were felt to be related to focal surface defects seen as subtle signal intensity changes on MRI leading to overestimation of the thickness. The measurements made from T1 and proton density sequences were determined to be closest to the direct measurements.

Reference

1. van Leersum MD, Schweitzer ME, Gannon F, et al: Thickness of patellofemoral articular cartilage as measured on MR imaging: Sequence comparison of accuracy, reproducibility, and interobserver variation. Skeletal Radiol 1995; 24(6):431–435.

▪: MEASUREMENTS OF RELATIONSHIPS OF THE PATELLOFEMORAL JOINT[1]

▪ ACR Code: 453 (Patella)

Technique (Figure 1) ▪

Central ray: Directed parallel to the anterior border of the tibia and the patellofemoral space perpendicular to the film.
Position: Patient seated with knees in 20 degrees of flexion. The feet are plantar flexed.
Target-film distance: Immaterial.

Measurements ▪

1. The lateral patellofemoral angle (Figure 2). The drawing is that of a left knee, and the left side of the drawing is the lateral side of the knee. Line *AA* joins the summits of the femoral condyles. Line *BB* joins the limits of the lateral patellar facet. The angle lies above line *AA* and, when normal, is always open laterally. In instances of patellar tilt with subluxation *(below)*, the lateral patellofemoral angle is open medially or the lines are parallel.
2. The patellofemoral index (Figure 3). The index corresponds to the ratio of the thickness of the medial patellofemoral interspace *(a)* over the lateral patellofemoral interspaces *(b)*. In normal individuals, this ratio is 1.6, because the medial patellofemoral interspace is equal to or slightly greater than the lateral patellofemoral interspace. In patients with chondromalacia patellae, there is tilt of the patella with an increase in the medial interspace, and the patellofemoral index will be more than 1.6.

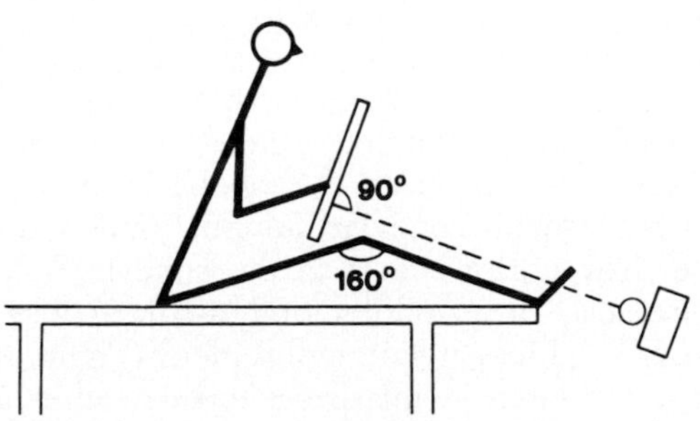

Figure 1 ▪ Roentgen technique. (From Laurin CA, et al: Clin Orthop 1979; 144:16. Used by permission.)

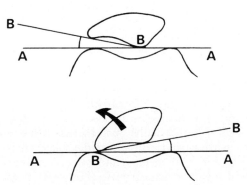

Figure 2 ▪ The lateral patellofemoral angle. (From Laurin CA, et al: Clin Orthop 1979; 144:16. Used by permission.)

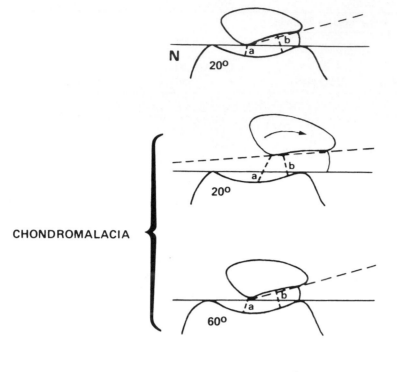

Figure 3 ▪ The patellofemoral index. (From Laurin CA, et al: Clin Orthop 1979; 144:16. Used by permission.)

Source ▪

Normal measurements determined from 100 normal patients and 100 patients with chondromalacia patellae and 30 patients with patellar subluxation.

REFERENCE

1. Laurin CA, Dussault R, Levesque HP: The tangential x-ray investigation of the patello-femoral joint: X-ray technique, diagnostic criteria, and their interpretation. Clin Orthop Rel Res 1979; 144:16–26.

▪▪ PATELLOFEMORAL RELATIONSHIPS ON TANGENTIAL VIEWS
▪ ACR Code: 453 (Patella)

Technique ▪

Several radiographic techniques for tangential evaluation of the patellofemoral joint are available. Three of the more commonly used were described by Ficat, Merchant, and Laurin and their colleagues.[1–3] These are shown in Figure 1. Ficat and Hungerford suggest a series of views, including 30, 60, and 90 degrees of knee flexion.[1] The measurements below are typically described as being done on 20- to 30-degree views, as patellar displacements may be reduced with greater degrees of knee flexion.[4]

Measurements ▪

Wiberg described patellar morphology as having three common types, and these are shown in Figure 2.[5] Type II (medial facet slightly smaller than lateral) is the most common, and with type III (small medial facet) there may be hypoplasia of the medial trochlear facet of the femur.[6, 7] The lateral-medial trochlear ratio (Figure 3) measures dysplasia of the medial aspect of the trochlea and is considered abnormal when greater than 1.7.[7, 8] The sulcus angle (Figure 4) quantifies the depth of the trochlear groove, and when greater than 142 to 145 degrees may be related to recurrent patellar dislocation.[1, 2, 4, 6, 7] The congruence angle (Figure 5) relates the patellar position with the apex of the trochlear groove and normally is slightly negative (medial). Positive (lateral) angles of 16 or more degrees are abnormal—patients with recurrent dislocation average +23 degrees.[2, 4, 6–8]

The lateral patellofemoral angle (Figure 6) relates the lateral articular facet of the patella with the femoral condyles. It is open laterally in most normal subjects (90%) and parallel or open medially with subluxation.[3, 4, 6, 7, 10] Patellar displacement (Figure 7) may be assessed by measuring the distance between the medial border of the patella and the medial condylar summit. When the patella lies more than 1 mm lateral to the condyle, subluxation, chondromalacia, or patellofemoral cartilage loss may be considered.[3, 4, 6] The patellofemoral index (Figure 8) relates the medial and lateral joint spaces to each other. In chondromalacia it is greater than 1.6 (medial space larger), though this may reduce at higher degrees of knee flexion.[3, 6]

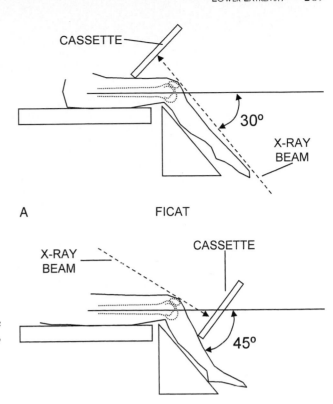

A   FICAT

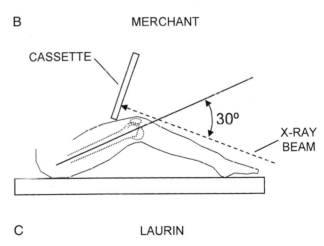

B   MERCHANT

Figure 1 ▪ Different methods of performing tangential radiographs of the patellofemoral joint, as described by *A*, Ficat; *B*, Merchant; and *C*, Laurin.[1-3]

C   LAURIN

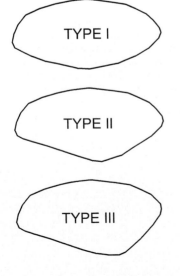

Figure 2 ▪ Classification of patellar shape by Wiberg. Type I has equal lengths of medial and lateral facets. Type II (most normal subjects) has a slightly shorter medial facet. Type III has a rather short medial facet with a steep angle.[5]

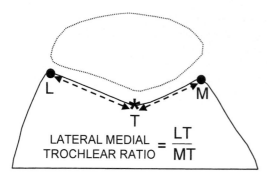

Figure 3 ▪ The lateral medial trochlear ratio formed by dividing the distance from the lowest point of the intercondylar sulcus *(T)* to the medial condylar summit *(M)* by the distance between T and the lateral condylar summit *(L)*. Normally it is less than 1.7 mm.[7, 8]

Figure 4 ▪ The sulcus (or trochlear) angle is formed between lines joining the summits of the condyles (circles) and the lowest point of the intercondylar sulcus *(asterisk)*. Normal values are reported as 141, 142, 137, 124–145, and 136 ± 6 degrees. The latter seems to be frequently cited.[1, 2, 4, 6, 7]

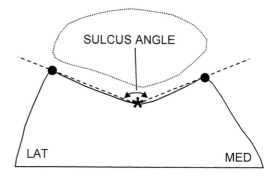

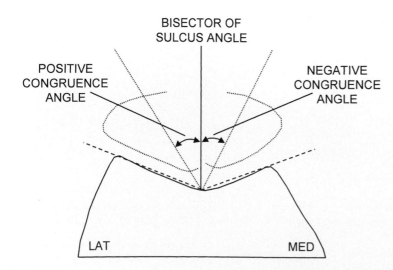

Figure 5 ▪ The congruence angle is formed between a line *(solid)* bisecting the sulcus angle and a line *(dotted)* from the lowest point of the intercondylar sulcus through the apex of the patella. The angle is given a positive sign if lateral and a negative sign if medial. The normal value is reported as −6 or −8, with a standard deviation of 6 degrees.[2, 4, 6–8]

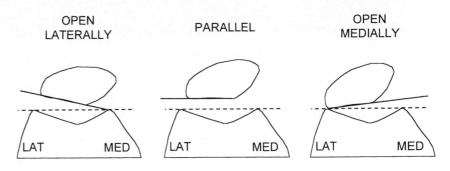

OPEN LATERALLY   PARALLEL   OPEN MEDIALLY

Figure 6 ▪ The lateral patellofemoral angle is formed between a line *(dashed)* joining the condylar summits and a line *(solid)* through the lateral patellar facet joint surface. The angle may be open laterally (most normal subjects), parallel, or open medially.[3, 4, 6, 7, 10]

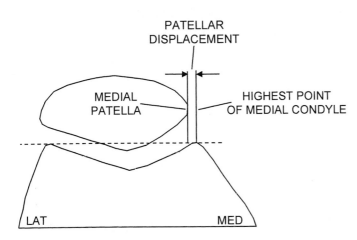

PATELLAR DISPLACEMENT

MEDIAL PATELLA

HIGHEST POINT OF MEDIAL CONDYLE

LAT   MED

Figure 7 ▪ Patellar displacement may be measured by drawing lines *(solid)* parallel to a line *(dashed)* through the condylar summits that intersect the medial edge of the patella and the medial condylar summit. In 97% of normal subjects, the medial edge of the patella lies medial to the condylar summit, and in 3% it lies lateral (as shown), but the distance is less than 1 mm.[3, 4, 6]

Figure 8 ▪ The patellofemoral index is formed by dividing the shortest distance between the lateral limit of the medial facet of the patella and the condyle *(MPFD)* by the shortest distance between the lateral patellar facet and the lateral condyle *(LPFD)*. It is normally 1.6 mm or less.[3, 6]

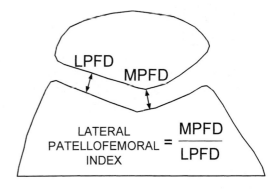

LPFD   MPFD

$$\text{LATERAL PATELLOFEMORAL INDEX} = \frac{\text{MPFD}}{\text{LPFD}}$$

Source ▪

The material here was abstracted from review articles and book chapters describing radiologic assessment of patellofemoral relationships.[1–10]

REFERENCES

1. Ficat RP, Hungerford DS: Disorders of the Patellofemoral Joint. Williams & Wilkins, Baltimore, 1977.
2. Merchant AC, Mercer RL, Jacobsen RH, Cool CR: Roentgenographic analysis of patellofemoral congruence. J Bone Joint Surg Am 1974; 56:1391–1396.
3. Laurin CA, Dussault R, Levesque HP: The tangential x-ray investigation of the patello-femoral joint: X-ray technique, diagnostic criteria, and their interpretation. Clin Orthop 1979; 144:16–26.
4. Weissman, BN, Sledge CB: The knee. In Weissman BN, Sledge CB (eds): Orthopedic Radiology. WB Saunders, Philadelphia, 1986, pp 500–517.
5. Wiberg G: Roentgenographic and anatomic studies on the femoropatellar joint. With special reference to chondromalacia patellae. Acta Orthop Scand 1941; 12:319–411.
6. Rand JA, Berquist TH: The knee. In Berquist TH (ed): Imaging of Orthopedic Trauma and Surgery. WB Saunders, Philadelphia; 1986, pp 307–319.
7. Beaconsfield T, Pintore E, Maffulli N, Petri GJ: Radiological measurements in patellofemoral disorders. A review. Clin Orthop 1994; 308:18–28.
8. Walch G, Dejour H: La radiologie dans la pathologie femoro-patellaire. In Dejour H, Walch G (eds): La Pathologie Femoro-patellaire. Sixiemes Journees Lyonnaises de Chirugie du Genou, Lyon, France, 1987, pp 25–33.
9. Aglietti P, Insall JN, Cerulli G: Patellar pain and incongruence. I: Measurements of incongruence. Clin Orthop 1983; 176:217–223.
10. Laurin CA, Levesque HP, Dussault R, et al: The abnormal lateral patello-femoral angle: A diagnostic roentgenographic sign of recurrent patellar subluxation. J Bone Joint Surg Am 1978; 60: 55–60.

▪: SECONDARY SIGNS OF ANTERIOR CRUCIATE TEAR
▪ ACR Code: 4526 (Cruciate Ligament)

Technique ▪

The following data are from studies of indirect signs of anterior cruciate ligament (ACL) tear.[1-10] Several of the papers include evaluation of two or more such signs,[1-5, 10] and the rest describe one of the signs.[6-9] Sagittal MRI of the knee was done on various machines, with field strength ranging from 0.5 to 1.5 T, usually with the knee laterally rotated about 15 degrees and/or oblique scanning to parallel the plane of the ACL. Images were done with T1 and T2 weighting using various techniques, sometimes including fat suppression for T2. Proton density as well as gradient echo sequences were sometimes included as well.

Measurements ▪

A torn ACL alters the relationships of the tibia and distal femur in the sagittal plane, often resulting in visible manifestations relating to the posterior cruciate ligament (PCL). The main abnormality is posterior displacement of the tibia with respect to the distal femur, which causes shortening of the distance between the PCL attachments, manifested in alterations of the PCL line (Figure 1), contour (Figure 2), index of curvature (Figure 3), and angle (Figure 4). The orientation of the torn ACL itself is also changed as it tends to assume a horizontal position, as seen in its angle with respect to the femur (Figure 5) and tibial plateau (Figure 6). Anterior tibial displacement may be assessed by noting the relationship of its posterior margin with the lateral meniscus and the distal femur (Figure 7). When the ACL is torn, the posterior rim of the tibial plateau has an impact on the distal lateral femur, deepening the normally occurring notch (Figure 8).

Table 1 lists these signs and gives normal and abnormal criteria or measurement values. Tables 2 and 3 give the observed sensitivity and specificity of each sign as reported in the literature cited.

Source ▪

All the papers included a subset of subjects (volunteers or patients) with no clinical or imaging evidence of ACL injury, as well as a group with documented ACL tear (by surgery, imaging, and/or convincing clinical evidence). The patients with ACL tear were often divided into acute versus chronic or complete versus incomplete types. When possible, the measurement values and test performance data given herein are for all tears as compared with normal knees.[1-10]

Comments ▪

In a recent study, Brandser and colleagues sought to separate the secondary signs and measurements described previously from primary signs (discontinuity, irregularity, and signal abnormalities of the ACL), using receiver operating characteristics (ROC) analysis of the performance of three observers in diagnosing ACL tear. They found areas under the ROC curve for secondary signs alone of 0.73 to 0.84, for primary signs alone of 0.95 to 0.99, and for both together of 0.94 to 0.98.[10] Gentili states that the ACL

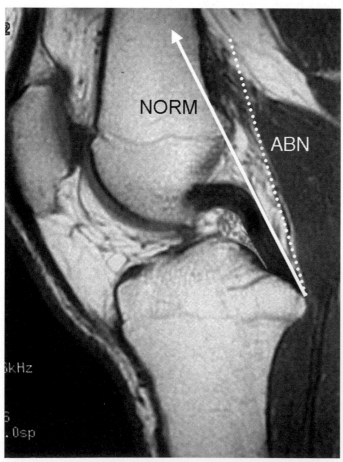

Figure 1 ▪ The posterior cruciate ligament (PCL) line. This is measured from the slice best depicting the PCL. A line (*solid white with arrow*) is drawn through the posterior margin of the PCL and extended toward the femur. Normally, this line should cross the cortex and enter the medullary cavity within 5 mm of the distal posterior femur. An abnormal PCL line (*dotted white*) will fail to intersect with the femur or do so higher along the posterior margin.

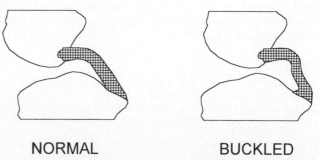

NORMAL   BUCKLED

Figure 2 ▪ The PCL contour. This is determined from the slice best showing the PCL. The normal PCL is concave anterior-inferiorly. A buckled PCL has at least one portion that is concave posteriorly.

Text continued on page 277

Figure 3 ▪ The PCL index. This is measured on the slice best depicting the PCL. A line *(FT)* is drawn between the anterior portions of the femoral *(F)* and tibial *(T)* attachments of the PCL. The maximum distance *(CA)* between line FT and the apex *(A)* of the PCL is measured perpendicularly to line *FT.*

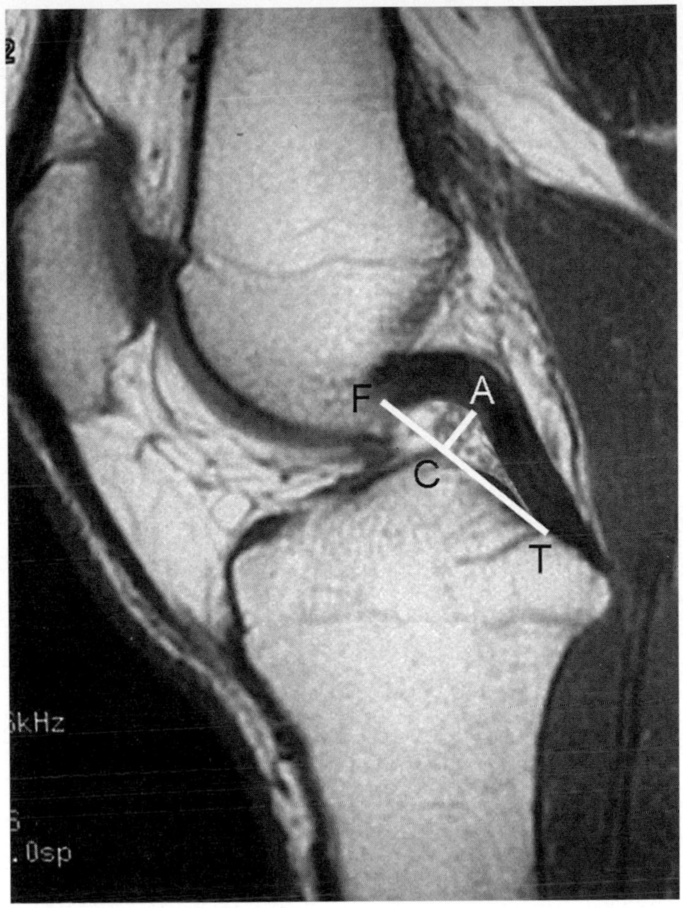

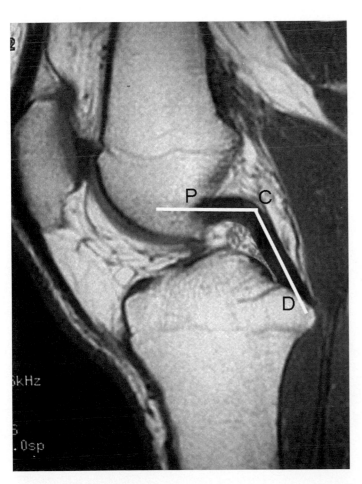

Figure 4 ▪ The PCL angle. This is measured on the slice best depicting the PCL. A line *(PC)* is drawn through the proximal portion of the PCL. A second line *(DC)* is drawn through the distal portion of the PCL. The angle (PCD) is measured.

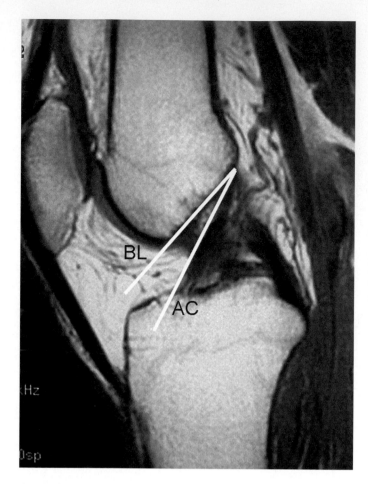

Figure 5 ▪ The anterior cruciate ligament (ACL) angle in relation to the femur. This is measured on the slice best depicting the ACL. A line (Blumenstaat = *BL*) is drawn through the posterior surface of the femur. A second line *(AC)* is drawn through the anterior margin of the ACL. The angle between the two lines is measured. If the apex of the angle is posterior (as shown), the angle is given a negative sign. When the apex is anterior (as in torn and displaced ACL), the sign is positive.

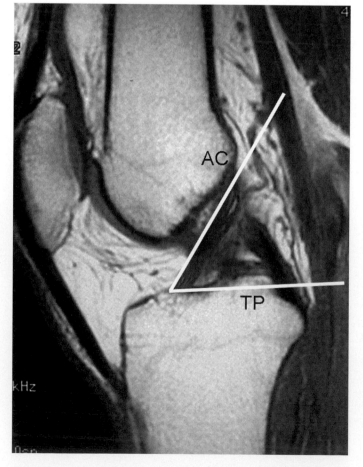

Figure 6 ▪ The ACL angle in relation to the tibial plateau. This is measured on the slice best depicting the ACL. A line *(TP)* is drawn through the tibial plateau. A second line *(AC)* is drawn through the anterior margin of the ACL. The angle between the two lines is measured.

Figure 7 ▪ Lateral meniscal uncovering. This is measured on the slice midway between the tibial insertion of the PCL and the lateralmost part of the tibial condyle. A line is drawn through the posterior tibial plateau parallel to the tibial long axis *(PT)*. The distance from this line to the posterior margin of the lateral meniscus *(M)* is measured. Here it would be given a negative value. If the meniscus touches the PT line, the value is 0, and if posterior it is positive.

Tibial translation is measured on the same slice with the same reference line *(PT)*. The distance between line PT and the posteriormost cortex of the lateral femoral condyle *(F)* is given a negative sign if anterior, 0 if they coincide, and positive numbers when the condyle is posterior to PT.

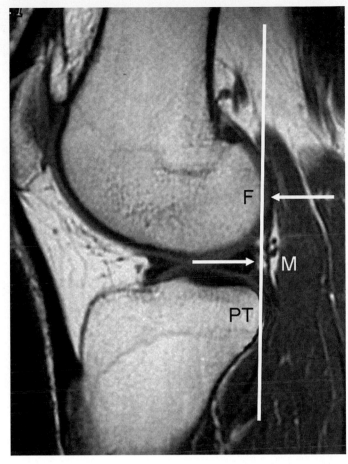

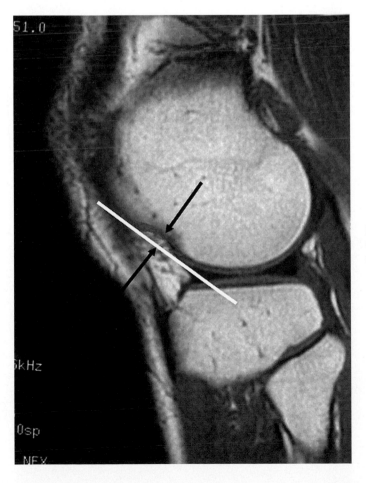

Figure 8 ▪ Lateral femoral notch. This is measured on the lateral slice that best depicts the notch. A line *(white)* is drawn across the roof of the notch and the maximum depth measured *(black arrows)*.

Table 1 ▪ Definition of Secondary Signs and Measurements for ACL Tear on Sagittal MRI

MEASUREMENT	FIGURE NO.	REFERENCES	HOW REPORTED	NORMAL CRITERIA/ MEASUREMENT	ABNORMAL CRITERIA
PCL line	1	1, 2, 9, 10	Abnormal-normal	Intersects medullary cavity of femur within 5 mm of the distal cortex	Fails to intersect within 5 mm; often entirely posterior to femur
PCL shape	2	1–3, 6, 10	Buckled-normal	Concave anteriorly-inferiorly	Wavy contour, concave posteriorly
PCL index	3	1, 3, 5, 8, 10	ratio	0.19	>0.20–>0.39
PCL angle	4	1, 4	Degrees	114–123	<100–<107
ACL angle WRT BL	5	1, 2	Degrees	−1.6	>9–>15
ACL angle WRT TP	6	1, 3	Degrees	56	<45–<50
Lateral meniscus uncovering	7	1, 3–5, 10	Millimeters	0.54	≥0–>5.0
Tibial translation	7	1, 2, 6, 7, 10	Millimeters	2.17	>5–>7
Lateral femoral notch	8	1, 2, 10	Millimeters	0.35	>1–>1.5

ACL = anterior cruciate ligament, PCL = posterior cruciate ligament, WRT = with respect to, BL = Blumenstaat line, TP = tibial plateau.

Table 2 ▪ Performance of Secondary Signs (Involving the ACL and PCL) of ACL Tear on Sagittal MRI

MEASUREMENT	POSITIVE CRITERION	REFERENCE	TEAR POSITIVE (No.)	TEAR NEGATIVE (No.)	SENSITIVITY (%)	SPECIFICITY (%)
PCL line	Posterior to femur	2	43	60	66	86
PCL line	Posterior to femur	9	22	59	86	94
PCL line	Posterior to femur	1	54	35	51	91
PCL shape	Concave posteriorly	2	43	60	38	90
PCL shape	Concave posteriorly	6	60	29	17	100
PCL shape	Concave posteriorly	3	52	36	71	—
PCL index	>0.20	8	31	31	87	84
PCL index	>0.34	3	52	36	50	—
PCL index	>0.39	5	50	53	44	96
PCL index	>0.39	1	54	35	34	100
PCL angle	<100	1	54	35	37	100
PCL angle	<105	4	39	29	73	83
PCL angle	<107	1	54	35	52	94
ACL angle WRT BL	Not parallel	2	43	60	79	86
ACL angle WRT BL	>9	1	54	35	91	86
ACL angle WRT BL	>15	1	54	35	89	100
ACL angle WRT TP	<45	1	54	35	91	97
ACL angle WRT TP	<40	1	54	35	89	100
ACL angle WRT TP	<50	3	52	36	50	—

ACL = anterior cruciate ligament, PCL = posterior cruciate ligament, WRT = with respect to, BL = Blumenstaat line, TP = tibial plateau.

Table 3 ▪ Performance of Secondary Signs (Involving the Femur, Tibia, and Lateral Meniscus) of ACL Tear on Sagittal MRI

MEASUREMENT	POSITIVE CRITERION	REFERENCE	TEAR POSITIVE (No.)	TEAR NEGATIVE (No.)	SENSITIVITY (%)	SPECIFICITY (%)
Lateral meniscus	≥0	3	52	36	31	—
Lateral meniscus	≥0	4	39	29	56	99
Lateral meniscus	≥0	5	50	53	44	96
Lateral meniscus	>3.5	1	54	35	44	94
Lateral meniscus	>5	1	54	35	20	100
Tibial translation	>5	1	54	35	63	80
Tibial translation	>5	2	43	60	60	88
Tibial translation	>5	6	60	29	58	93
Tibial translation	>5	7	21	91	86	99
Tibial translation	>7	6	60	29	38	100
Tibial translation	>7	1	54	35	41	91
Lateral femoral notch	>1	1	54	35	30	94
Lateral femoral notch	>1.5	1	54	35	19	100
Lateral femoral notch	>1.5	2	43	60	32	99

angles with respect to the femur (Blumenstaat line) and the tibial plateau were the most accurate, which is a reflection of the fact that they represent quantification of abnormalities of the ACL itself.[1]

Note: The MRI images have been enhanced to show the measured structures to better advantage.

REFERENCES

1. Gentili A, Seeger LL, Yao L, Do HM: Anterior cruciate ligament tear: Indirect signs at MR imaging. Radiology 1994; 193(3):835–840.
2. Robertson PL, Schweitzer ME, Bartolozzi AR, Ugoni A: Anterior cruciate ligament tears: Evaluation of multiple signs with MR imaging. Radiology 1994; 193:829–834.
3. Yao L, Gentili A, Petrus L, Lee JK: Partial ACL rupture: An MR diagnosis?. Skeletal Radiol 1995; 24(4):247–251.
4. McCauley TR, Moses M, Kier R, et al: MR diagnosis of tears of anterior cruciate ligament of the knee: Importance of ancillary findings. AJR Am J Roentgenol 1994; 162(1):115–119.
5. Tung GA, Davis LM, Wiggins ME, Fadale PD: Tears of the anterior cruciate ligament: Primary and secondary signs at MR imaging. Radiology 1993; 188:661–667.
6. Vahey TN, Hunt JE, Shelbourne KD: Anterior translocation of the tibia at MR imaging: A secondary sign of anterior cruciate ligament tear. Radiology 1993; 187(3):817–819.
7. Chan WP, Peterfy C, Fritz RC, Genant HK: MR diagnosis of complete tears of the anterior cruciate ligament of the knee: Importance of anterior subluxation of the tibia. AJR Am J Roentgenol 1994; 162(2):355–360.
8. Liu SH, Osti L, Dorey F, Yao L: Anterior cruciate ligament tear. A new diagnostic index on magnetic resonance imaging. Clin Orthop 1994; (302): 147–150.
9. Schweitzer ME, Cervilla V, Kursunoglu-Brahme S, Resnick D: The PCL line: An indirect sign of anterior cruciate ligament injury. Clin Imag 1992; 16(1):43–48.
10. Brandser EA, Riley MA, Berbaum KS, et al: MR imaging of anterior cruciate ligament injury: Independent value of primary and secondary signs. AJR Am J Roentgenol 1996; 167(1):121–126.

▪▪ MEDIAL COLLATERAL LIGAMENT THICKNESS
▪ ACR Code: 4527 (Collateral Ligament)

Technique ▪

Coronal T1 (500/30) or gradient echo (500-650/20-35, 25-30 degree flip angle) images were made using a surface coil on a 0.5-T machine (Philips Medical Systems, Eindoven, Netherlands). Section thickness was 5 to 5.2 mm, with 0.5 to 0.52-mm gap; field of view was 20 cm and four excitations were averaged.[1] Ultrasound of the knee was done with high-frequency linear transducers in the coronal plane over the medial knee.[2]

Measurements ▪

From the coronal MRI image through its midportion, Staron and colleagues measured the transverse thickness of the medial collateral ligament (MCL) directly from the films, using the scale printed on the film for calibration. This was done at the femoral attachment, in the midpoint, and just proximal to where it became indistinguishable with the tibial cortex. These three distances were averaged in each subject, and the intraligamentous thickness variance (thickest—thinnest) was computed. Differences between normal and injured knees were compared using the Fisher exact test.[1] The MCL thickness was measured from frozen ultrasound images proximally and distally.[2] Figure 1 shows the sites of measurement of the MCL, Table 1 lists the MRI results, and Table 2 lists the ultrasound thicknesses.

Source ▪

Staron's study group consisted of 16 patients (19 scans) with arthroscopic proof of anterior cruciate ligament (ACL) and medial meniscal tears. There were 13 men and 3 women whose age ranged from 19 to 56 years (mean age 34.8 years), and they were examined between 1 day and 2 years (mean 6 months) from the injury. For comparison, scans of 19 patients (10 men, 9 women, age range 19 to 55 years, mean age 35.5 years) with no history or imaging findings of knee pathology were evaluated.[1] Van Holsbeeck performed ultrasound of the MCL on 96 adults separated by lifestyle (sedentary or athletic) and gender.[2]

Comments ▪

In addition to significantly thicker measurements of the MCL, the variation in thickness was greater in the injured knees at MRI. There was also fluid superficial to the MCL in 15 (79%) of the injured knees up to 2 years after injury. The increased thickness of the MCL was attributed to edema and hemorrhage, inflammatory reaction, or scarring, depending on the acuity. Adjacent fluid may persist because of abnormal mechanics due to instability.[1]

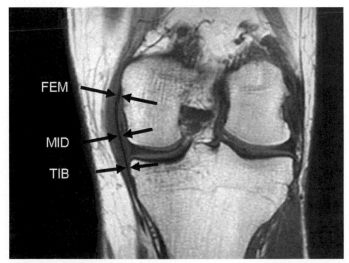

Figure 1 ▪ Measurement of the thickness of the medial collateral ligament (MCL) from coronal MR images. The scan through the middle of the anteroposterior extent of the MCL is chosen, and the thickness is measured just below the femoral attachment *(FEM)*, in the midportion *(MID)*, and proximal to the tibial attachment *(TIB)*. Ultrasound measurements were made proximally *(FEM)* and distally *(TIB)*.[1,2]

Table 1 • Thickness of the Medial Collateral Ligament on MRI

LOCATION	INJURED KNEES (n = 19)		NORMAL KNEES (n = 19)		P VALUE
	Mean ± SD	Range	Mean ± SD	Range	
Femoral end	2.5 ± 1.1	0.7–3.8	1.7 ± 0.5	0.9–2.6	.011
Midpoint	2.1 ± 0.7	1.3–3.5	1.5 ± 0.2	1.3–2.0	.002
Tibial end	1.5 ± 0.6	0.7–3.0	1.3 ± 0.3	0.9–1.7	.171
Average	2.0 ± 0.6	0.9–3.3	1.5 ± 0.2	1.2–2.0	.001
Thickest—thinnest	1.3 ± 0.9	0.0–2.9	0.6 ± 0.5	0.0–1.7	.006

All measurements are in millimeters. SD = standard deviation.
From Staron RB, Haramati N, Feldman F, et al: Skeletal Radiol 1994; 23(8):633–636. Used by permission.

Table 2 • Thickness of the Medial Collateral Ligament on Ultrasound

SUBJECTS	NUMBER	PROXIMAL (MEAN ± SD)		DISTAL (MEAN ± SD)	
		Right	Left	Right	Left
Sedentary men	22	3.8 ± 0.5	3.7 ± 0.6	2.3 ± 0.3	2.3 ± 0.4
Male athletes	24	3.8 ± 0.5	3.8 ± 0.5	2.0 ± 0.4	2.0 ± 0.4
Sedentary women	21	3.6 ± 0.7	3.3 ± 0.7	2.3 ± 0.4	2.3 ± 0.3
Female athletes	19	3.8 ± 0.5	3.6 ± 0.5	2.1 ± 0.3	2.1 ± 0.3

All measurements are in millimeters. SD = standard deviation.
From van Holsbeeck MV, Introcaso JH: Mosby–Year Book, St. Louis, 1991, vol 1, pp 315–319. Used by permission.

REFERENCES

1. Staron RB, Haramati N, Feldman F, et al: O'Donoghue's triad: Magnetic resonance imaging evidence. Skeletal Radiol 1994; 23(8):633–636.

2. van Holsbeeck MV, Introcaso JH: Appendix: Table of Normal Values In van Holsbeeck MV, Introcaso JH (eds): Musculoskeletal Ultrasound. Mosby–Year Book, St. Louis, 1991, vol 1, pp 315–319.

∷ MEASUREMENT OF THE METAPHYSEAL-DIAPHYSEAL ANGLE FOR THE DIFFERENTIATION OF PHYSIOLOGIC BOWING OF THE KNEES AND TIBIA VARA[1]

• ACR Code: 454 (Proximal End of Tibia)

Technique •

Central ray: Centered over knees.
Position: Anteroposterior standing.
Target-film distance: Immaterial.

Measurement (Figure 1 and Table 1) •

A line is drawn perpendicular to the longitudinal axis of the tibia, and another is drawn through the two beaks of the metaphysis to determine the transverse axis of the tibial metaphysis. The metaphyseal-diaphyseal angle is bisected by those two lines.

The data of Levine and Drennan[1] show that in 29 of 30 affected extremities with an initial metaphyseal-diaphyseal angle of more than 11.0 degrees, radiographic changes of tibia vara developed. However, only 3 of 58 extremities with a metaphyseal-diaphyseal angle of 11.0 degrees or less later had any of the diagnostic changes. This measurement allows accurate early diagnosis of bowleg deformity.

Table 1 • Results

	METAPHYSEAL-DIAPHYSEAL ANGLE (DEGREES)	
	Average	Range
Physiologic bowing (age)		
11–20 mon	5.1 ± 2.8	0–11
21–30 mon	3.7 ± 3.1	0–10
Tibia vara (age)		
11–20 mon	16.4 ± 4.3	8–22
21–30 mon	13.7 ± 4.3	7–22

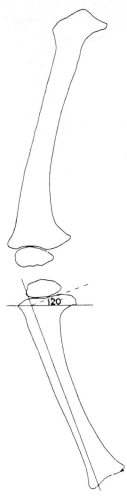

Figure 1 ▪ Tibia vara, the metaphyseal angle. (From Levine AM, Drennan JC: J Bone Joint Surg 1982; 64A:1158. Used by permission.)

Source ▪

Data based on 52 limbs of children with physiologic bowing and 32 limbs of children with tibia vara (Blount disease).

REFERENCE

1. Levine AM, Drennan JC: Physiological bowing and tibia vara. The metaphyseal-diaphyseal angle in the measurement of bowleg deformities. J Bone Joint Surg Am 1982; 64:1158–1163.

▪ MEASUREMENT OF THE TIBIAL PLATEAU ANGLE FOR DETERMINATION OF DEPRESSION DUE TO FRACTURE[1]
▪ ACR Code: 454 (Proximal End of Tibia)

Technique ▪

Central ray: Perpendicular to plane of film centered over joint.
Position: Lateral.
Target-film distance: Immaterial.

Measurements (Figure 1) ▪

The angle of the tibial plateau is defined by a line drawn tangential to the tibial crest, a second line tangential to the proximal tibial articular surfaces, and a third line perpendicular to the tibial crest line. The

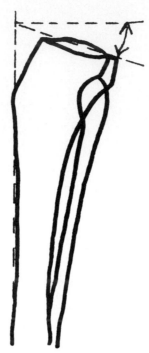

Figure 1 ▪ Method of measuring plateau angle. (Adapted from Moore TM, et al: J Bone Joint Surg 1974; 56A:155. Used by permission.)

interval found between the second and third lines defines the angle.

The normal angles range from 7 degrees to 22 degrees with a mean of 14 degrees and a standard deviation of ± 3.6 degrees. This angle is useful in determining the degree of depression of the tibial plateau due to fracture.

Source ▪

Data were based on a study of 50 true lateral roentgenograms of normal knees.

REFERENCE

1. Moore TM, Harvey JP Jr: Roentgenographic measurement of tibial-plateau depression due to fracture. J Bone Joint Surg Am 1974; 56:155–160.

▪: MEASUREMENT OF TIBIAL TORSION BY FLUOROSCOPY
▪ ACR Code: 458 (Tibia and Fibula)

Technique ▪

Clementz and Magnusson used a BV 21 portable C-arm fluoroscopy device (Phillips, Best, The Netherlands) to visualize the knee joint in the lateral (LAT) projection and then the ankle joint in anteroposterior (AP) projection. Subjects were supine, with the leg to be examined extended and the contralateral leg flexed so as to allow an unimpeded view of the side of interest. Between visualization of the two joints, the leg was kept stationary.[1, 2]

Measurements ▪

During LAT fluoroscopy of the knee joint, the leg was rotated so that the posterior margins of the femoral condyles were superimposed, as shown in Figure 1. The C-arm was repositioned over the ankle joint and rotated during fluoroscopy until the anterior and posterior margins of the medial malleolus were superimposed. The difference in angulation (as read from the C-arm protractor) was taken to be the angle of tibial torsion. Figure 2 shows the second step. Lastly, a second check of the knee joint was done to make sure the condyles were still superimposed. If there was any change, the procedure was repeated.[1, 2]

An additional fluoroscopic landmark (anterior talus in the LAT view) and an anatomic landmark (axis of the sole of the foot) were tried but were more error prone.[1] The standard error for a single tibial torsion determination was found to be 0.74 degree with the aforementioned method.[1] When fluoroscopy was compared with cryosection and direct measurement in excised cadaveric lower legs, the absolute error was 1.01 degrees and the standard error was 0.98 degree.[2] In the same study, CT determinations had an absolute error of 1.1 degrees and a standard error of 1.07 degrees compared with direct measurements, and between

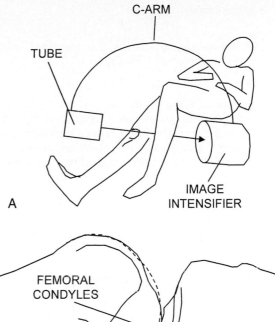

A

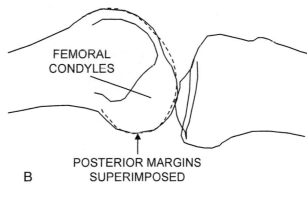

B

Figure 1 ▪ First step in measurement of tibial torsion. *A*, The knee joint was imaged in the lateral projection with the leg extended. *B*, Under fluoroscopy, the leg was rotated until the posterior femoral condyles superimposed.[1]

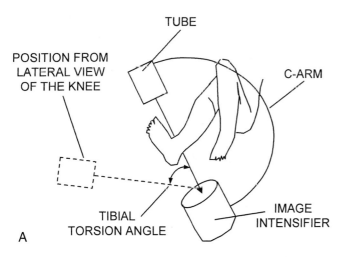

A

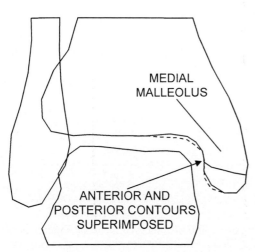

B

Figure 2 ▪ Second step in measurement of tibial torsion. *A*, The ankle joint was imaged in the anteroposterior plane. *B*, The C-arm was rotated during fluoroscopy until the anterior and posterior margins of the inner border of the medial condyle superimposed. Tibial torsion was recorded as the difference in angles from the two views.[1]

CT and fluoroscopy the absolute error was 1.37 degrees with a standard error of 1.22 degrees.[2]

Source •

Measurement of tibial torsion was performed in 100 adult volunteers (40 men, 60 women, mean age 31 years, age range 18 to 61 years) with no reported history of knee or leg problems.[1] Ten human necropsy specimens were used to compare CT, fluoroscopic, and direct measurement of tibial torsion.[2]

Comments •

Tibial torsion refers to the twist of the distal relative to the proximal articular axes of the tibia in the transverse plane.[1, 2]

This relationship is important in treatment of tibial fracture, and the C-arm technique is ideally suited to use in an operating room during reduction.[1] The method can also be performed in the radiology department on appropriate equipment.

REFERENCES

1. Clementz BG, Magnusson A: Fluoroscopic measurement of tibial torsion in adults: A comparison of three methods. Arch Orthop Trauma Surg 1988; 108:150–153.
2. Clementz BG: Assessment of tibial torsion and rotational deformity with a new fluoroscopic technique. Clin Orthop 1989; 245: 199–209.

▪▪ MEASUREMENT OF TIBIAL TORSION WITH CT AND MRI
▪ ACR Code: 458 (Tibia and Fibula)

Technique •

The most important technical consideration with either computed tomographic (CT) or magnetic resonance (MRI) determination of tibial torsion is that the leg be positioned on the scanning couch parallel to the long axis (Z) of the machine. Other imaging parameters are less important as long as bony detail is displayed well and the scans are performed in the axial plane (unangled). Rapid MRI sequences or CT protocols help minimize the possibility of movement of the limb during the evaluation. For MRI, surface coils are problematic unless separate coils can be placed at the knee and ankle, since moving a single coil during the examination likely would alter the position of the leg. Regardless of machine type, axial images just below the knee and just above the ankle joint are required for these measurements.[1–4]

Measurements •

Tibial torsion (TT) was measured by drawing reference lines through the proximal tibia and the distal tibia and fibula. The proximal line of reference (PLR) was measured from a slice just above the fibular head and defined by a line joining the dorsal ridges[2, 4] or by visual estimation of the transverse axis of the midtibia.[1, 3] This is shown in Figure 1. The distal line of reference (DLR) was determined from a slice just above the ankle joint. Jend and Schneider and colleagues superimposed a circle over the tibial pilon (including the fibular notch and excluding the medial malleolus). The DLR was drawn between the center of this circle and a point midway between the margins of the fibular notch.[2, 4] Laasonen and colleagues formed the DLR between the centers of the tibia and fibula or between the tibial center and the middle of the fibular notch.[3] These methods are shown in Figure 2. The TT angle was calculated by the difference between PLR and DLR, as shown in Figure 3.[1–14] Jakob and group used the tibial and fibular centers for DLR endpoints.[1]

Laasonen and colleagues found significant variation (25 to 38 degrees) in TT measured by different combinations of methods. They found either PLR method combined with DLR drawn through the tibial and fibular centers to

be the most consistent and accurate, with differences in repeated measurements of 4.35 to 4.50 degrees.[3] Jend and colleagues found errors of repeated measurements to be 1.1 degrees for PLR and 1.5 degrees for DLR.[2] Jakob and colleagues calculated interobserver error of 5 degrees for TT measurements.[1]

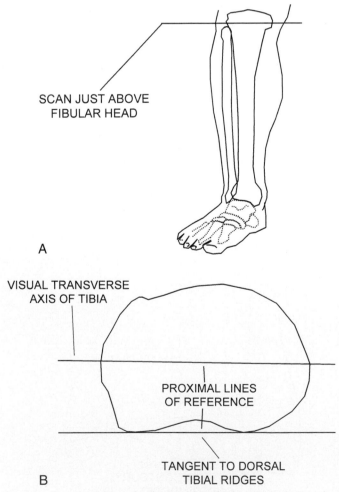

SCAN JUST ABOVE
FIBULAR HEAD

A

VISUAL TRANSVERSE
AXIS OF TIBIA

PROXIMAL LINES
OF REFERENCE

TANGENT TO DORSAL
TIBIAL RIDGES

B

Figure 1 • Proximal line of reference for tibial torsion. *A,* Level of axial scan. *B,* Two methods for drawing the reference line.

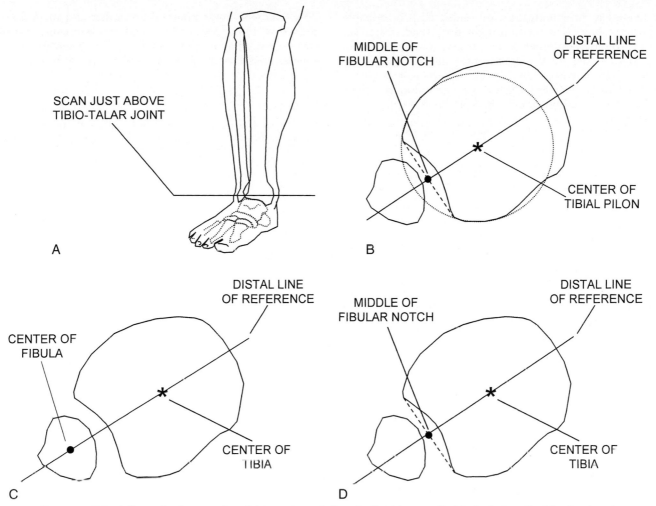

Figure 2 • Distal line of reference for tibial torsion. *A,* Level of axial scan. *B,* Method described by Jend and associates, with the center of the tibial pilon *(asterisk and dotted circle)* and midpoint of fibular notch *(circle)* forming the endpoints. *C,* Through centers of the tibia *(asterisk)* and fibula *(circle)*. *D,* Through the center of the fibula *(asterisk)* and midpoint of fibular notch *(circle)*.[2, 3]

Figure 3 • Tibial torsion is measured as the angle between proximal *(dashed)* and distal *(solid)* lines of reference.

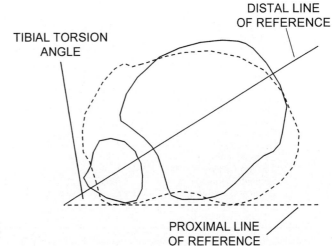

The choice of methods for determining PLR is probably not critical. The DLR method defined by Jend and group (circle through pilon) gives larger measurements (40 to 42 degrees) than the tibial/fibular center method (25 to 31 degrees). The normal value for TT in adults from direct measurement in cadavers, clinical measurement, and fluoroscopic determination ranges up to about 30 degrees (see next section).

Source ▪

Jakob and colleagues performed CT of 45 cadaveric tibia.[1] Jend and colleagues examined (with CT) 61 adult patients of both sexes, with 68 limbs having a history of fracture and 70 being normal.[2] Laasonen and colleagues studied (with CT) 11 patients (6 men, 5 women, age range 49 to 72 years) who had unilateral gonarthrosis and underwent tibial osteotomy. All were scanned preoperatively and eight were scanned after the procedure.[3] Schneider and colleagues performed MRI of 98 legs from healthy adult volunteers with a mean age of 45 years.[4]

REFERENCES

1. Jakob RP, Haertel M, Stussi E: Tibial torsion calculated by computerized tomography and compared to other methods of measurement. J Bone Joint Surg Br 1980; 62:238–242.
2. Jend HH, Heller M, Dallek M, Schoettle H: Measurement of tibial torsion by computed tomography. Acta Radiol 1981; 22(3A):271–276.
3. Laasonen EM, Jokio P, Lindholm TS: Tibial torsion measured by computed tomography. Acta Radiol 1984; 25:325–329.
4. Schneider B, Laubenberger J, Jemlich S, et al: Measurement of femoral antetorsion and tibial torsion by magnetic resonance imaging. Br J Radiol 1997; 70:575–579.

▪▪ TIBIAL TORSION ANGLES IN CHILDREN AND ADULTS
▪ ACR Code: 458 TF (Tibia and Fibula)

Technique ▪

Numerous techniques exist for measuring tibial torsion clinically, from cadavers or dried specimens, and with imaging. Several imaging methods are described in this text.

Measurements ▪

Tibial torsion refers to the twist of the tibia on its longitudinal axis. When the distal tibia is twisted laterally with respect to the proximal, the term *external torsion* is applied and measured angles are by convention given a positive sign. When the distal tibia is turned medially with respect to the proximal, the term *internal torsion* is used and measured angles are given a negative by convention. Many measurements use the distal fibula and the medial malleolus as the distal reference line, and the measurement is probably more properly called tibiofibular torsion though the terms are often used interchangeably. Table 1 lists reported normal values from several sources and methods in children and adults.[1-12] Figure 1 shows the distribution of tibial torsion angles in 61 adults as determined by Jend and colleagues with CT.[8]

Hutter and Scott have stated that the normal range of

Table 1 ▪ Tibial Torsion in Children and Adults

AUTHOR (AGE GROUP)	METHOD	NUMBER	TORSION (Degrees)	R/L DIFFERENCE (Degrees)
Ritter (children)	Clinical			
Birth		1000	4±5	
6 mon		302	6±2	
1 yr		154	10±2	
2 yr		105	11±3	
Staheli (children)	Clinical	160		
Birth–1 yr			4–7	
2–8 yr			9–11	
9–13 yr			12–14	
Staheli (adults)	Clinical	20	14±4.5	
Hutter (adults)	Direct from cadavers	40	20 (0–40)	
Wynne-Davies (adults)	Clinical		20	
Turner (adults)	Clinical	137	19±4.8	
Jakob (adults)	CT	45	30	
Elgeti (adults)	CT	10	28.8±6.7	
Jend (adults)	CT	70	40±9	5±2
Laasonen (adults)	CT	11	28–38	
Strecker (adults)	CT	504	34.9±15.9	4.9
Schneider (adults)	MRI	98	41.7±8.8	6.1±4.5
Clementz (adults)	C-arm			
Right		100	30.7±7.8	
Left		100	28.6±7.6	2.1±5.2

Measurements are listed as mean ± standard deviation when reported. From Staheli, ranges of mean values for each age group are shown. From Hutter, the mean and range are given. From Laasonen, a range of values obtained with different reference lines is given.[1-12]

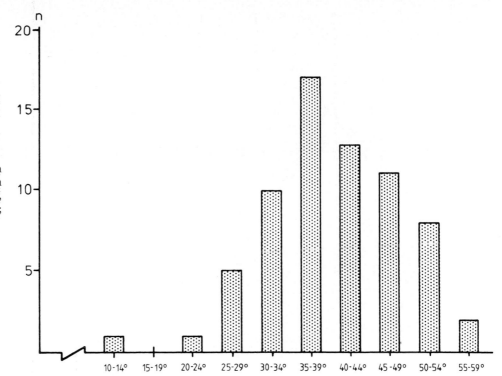

Figure 1 ▪ Distribution of tibial torsion by CT in 61 normal adult legs. (From Jend HH, Heller M, Dallek M, Schoettle H: Acta Radiol 1981; 22(3A):271–276. Used by permission.)

tibial torsion is 0 to 40 degrees, with internal torsion (negative angles) and severe external torsion (greater than 40 degrees) being abnormal.[3] Jend and colleagues found an average difference between sides of 5 ± 2 degrees, with upper limits of normal being 8 degrees.[8]

Source ▪

See references.

REFERENCES

1. Ritter MA, DeRosa GP, Babcock JL: Tibial torsion? Clin Orthop 1976; 120:159–163.
2. Staheli LT, Engel GM: Tibial torsion: A method of assessment and a survey of normal children. Clin Orthop 1972; 86:183–186.
3. Hutter CG, Scott W: Tibial torsion. J Bone Joint Surg Am 1949; 31:511–518.
4. Wynne-Davies R: Talipes equinovarus: A review of eighty-four cases after completion of treatment. J Bone Joint Surg Br 1964; 46:464–476.
5. Turner MS, Smillie IS: The effect of tibial torsion on the pathology of the knee. J Bone Joint Surg Br 1981; 63:396–398.
6. Jakob RP, Haertel M, Stussi E: Tibial torsion calculated by computerized tomography and compared to other methods of measurement. J Bone Joint Surg Br 1980; 62:238–242.
7. Elgeti H, Grote R, Giebel G: [Measurement of tibial torsion by axial computerized tomography] [German]. Unfallheikunde 1980; 83:14–19.
8. Jend HH, Heller M, Dallek M, Schoettle H: Measurement of tibial torsion by computed tomography. Acta Radiol 1981; 22(3A):271–276.
9. Laasonen EM, Jokio P, Lindholm TS: Tibial torsion measured by computed tomography. Acta Radiol 1984; 25:325–329.
10. Strecker W, Keppler P, Gebhard F, Kinzl L: Length and torsion of the lower limb. J Bone Joint Surg Br 1997; 79:1019–1023.
11. Schneider B, Laubenberger J, Jemlich S, et al: Measurement of femoral antetorsion and tibial torsion by magnetic resonance imaging. Br J Radiol 1997; 70:575–579.
12. Clementz BG: Tibial torsion measured in normal adults. Acta Orthop Scand 1988; 59:441–442.

▪▪ MEASUREMENT OF THE AXIAL ANGLES OF THE ANKLE[1]
- ACR Code: 463 (Ankle Joint)

Technique ▪

Central ray: Perpendicular to plane of film projected through the center of the talotibial joint.
Position: Anteroposterior, with great toe pointing slightly medially.
Target-film distance: Immaterial.

Measurements ▪ (Figure 1 and Table 1)

AB = The axis of the shaft of the tibia. This line is perpendicular to the horizontal plane of the ankle joint and is continuous with the vertical axis of the talus.
CD = Line tangent to the articular surface of the medial malleolus.

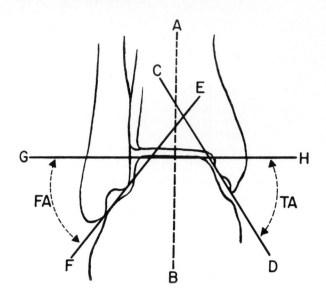

Figure 1 • Measurement of the axial angles of the ankle (see text for details).

Table 1 • Normal Axial Angles of the Ankle			
	MEN	WOMEN	AVERAGE
FA	45°–63°	43°–62°	52°
TA	45°–61°	49°–65°	53°

FA = fibular angle; TA = tibial angle.
From Keats TW, et al: Radiology 1966; 87:904. Used by permission.

EF = Line tangent to the articular surface of the lateral malleolus.
GH = Line tangent to the articular surface of the talus.
A = Fibular angle at the intersection of EF and GH.
TA = Tibial angle at the intersection of CD and GH.

Source •

The data were based on a study of 50 normal adult subjects, equally divided between men and women, ranging in age from 18 to 85 years.

REFERENCE

1. Keats TE, Teeslink R, Diamond AE, Williams JH: Normal axial relationships of the major joints. Radiology 1966; 87:904–907.

▪: MEASUREMENT OF THE WIDTH OF THE ANKLE JOINT[1]
▪ ACR Code: 463 (Ankle Joint)

Technique •

Central ray: Perpendicular to plane of film centered over the ankle joint.
Position: Anteroposterior, with patient sitting or supine, and lateral.
Target-film distance: 120 cm.

Measurements • (Figure 1)

The six measurements were averaged. Figure 2 shows the average joint space in each measuring point.

Figure 3 shows the average joint space related to age. The average joint space in men was 3.4 mm ± 0.4 mm and in women 2.9 mm ± 0.4 mm. The joint space is wider in the medial part in the AP view.

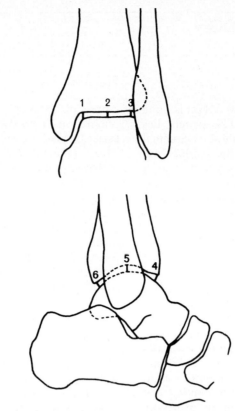

Figure 1 ▪ Measuring points of the ankle. (From Jonsson K, et al: Acta Radiol Diagn 1984; 25:147–149. Used by permission.)

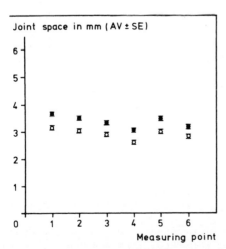

Figure 2 ▪ Average joint space in each measuring point. Men = *closed circles*; women = *open circles*. (From Jonsson K, et al: Acta Radiol Diagn 1984; 25:147–149. Used by permission.)

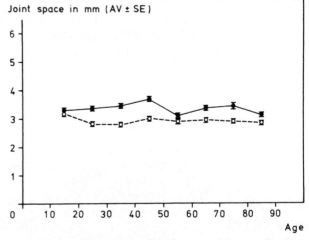

Figure 3 ▪ Average joint space related to age. Men = *closed circles*; women = *open circles*. (From Jonsson K, et al: Acta Radiol Diagn 1984; 25:147–149. Used by permission.)

Source ▪

Data are based on a study of 160 normal adults, 80 men and 80 women.

REFERENCE

1. Jonsson K, Fredin HO, Cederlund CG, Bauer M: Width of the normal ankle joint. Acta Radiol Diagn 1984; 25:147–149.

▪: SIZE OF THE ACHILLES TENDON
▪ ACR Code: 469 (Achilles Tendon)

Technique ▪

Ultrasound with linear transducers (5 to 10 MHz) is done over the dorsal aspect of the ankle.[1–10] The patient lies prone with the feet over the end of the table. Longitudinal scanning best depicts the morphology of the tendon, and measurements of tendon dimensions are typically done in the transverse plane. In one study, MRI of the ankle was done in the axial plane using a 0.5-T Gyroscan machine (Phillips Medical Systems, Irvine, CA), T1 (550/30) weighting, and 10-mm section thickness.[9]

Measurements ▪

Transverse scanning at the level of the medial malleolus was done to make measurements of the tendon thickness in the anteroposterior (AP) dimension and (sometimes) width in the transverse (TRV) dimension.[1–10] This is typically done with electronic calipers from frozen images and recorded in millimeters. It is important to keep the transducer perpendicular to the long axis of the tendon to avoid error (especially in the AP measurement). A standoff pad may be helpful for acoustic coupling and to place the tendon in the middle of the field of view. In the one study using MRI for measurement, the AP and TRV dimensions were taken 2 cm from the calcaneal insertion.[9]

Figure 1 shows the method of measurement. Table 1 lists normal width and thickness measurements by age, gender, and activity. Table 2 lists thickness measurements from clinical studies of injured tendons and of hypercholesterolemia patients with associated normal controls (as cited).

Source ▪

Three of the studies cited here were of purely normal populations, with the age ranges, gender, and other characteristics (sedentary/athletic) given in the data tables.[1–3] Measurements of the tendon thickness have been made in patients with tendinitis, rupture, and after surgery for rupture.[4, 5] The diagnosis in these patients was confirmed by clinical findings, imaging morphology, follow-up, or surgery. Patients with familial hypercholesterolemia (mostly type IIa) confirmed by family history and lipid profile analysis have also been studied.[6–10] These include populations with visible Achilles tendon xanthomas,[6] normal Achilles tendons on physical examination,[7] and unselected patients.[8, 9] Many of these clinical studies included normal control groups,[4–8] and these are shown.

Comments ▪

Steinmetz's normative data for thickness have been cited frequently for hypercholesterolemia studies. The cut-off is 7.1 mm, which is 2 standard deviations above the mean.[8] Bureau applied this cut-off to a population of 94 hypercholesterolemic patients and found thickness greater than 7.1 mm in 57 of 62 (92%) of those with palpable xanthomas and 2 of 32 (6%) of those with negative physical examination. Further, 100% of 62 patients with palpable xanthomas and 26 of 32 (81%) of those with negative examination had focal hypoechoic defects representing xanthomas.[10] This was confirmed by Bude's study of clinically negative tendons in hypercholesterolemic patients in which 36 of 46 (78%) of tendons and 19 of 23 (83%) of individuals had

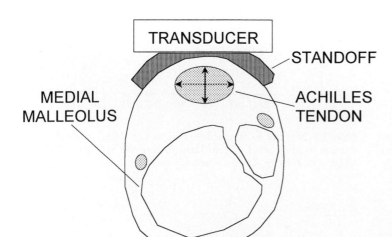

Figure 1 ▪ Measurement of Achilles tendon dimensions from transverse ultrasound. Measurements are taken at the level of the medial malleolus. Anteroposterior (AP) thickness (*solid line, arrows*) and transverse width (*dotted line, arrows*) can be measured.

Table 1 ▪ Normal Achilles Tendon Measurements

AUTHOR/GROUP DESCRIPTION	GENDER	AGES	NO.	AP (mm) Mean ± SD	TRV (mm) Mean ± SD
Koivunen-Niemela					
Normal	Male	0–9	12	4.5 ± 0.8	
		10–17	22	6.3 ± 0.9	
		18–29	224	6.3 ± 0.5	
		30–80	84	7.1 ± 1.2	
Normal	Female	0–9	18	4.6 ± 0.8	
		10–17	32	5.9 ± 0.7	
		18–29	40	6.1 ± 0.4	
		30–80	102	6.7 ± 0.8	
van Holsbeeck					
Sedentary right	Male	Adult	24	6.2 ± 0.8	9.0 ± 1.0
Sedentary left			24	6.1 ± 0.8	8.8 ± 0.8
Athlete right	Male	Adult	52	5.7 ± 0.8	13.0 ± 2.8
Athlete left			52	5.9 ± 1.0	12.8 ± 2.4
Sedentary right	Female	Adult	21	5.5 ± 0.7	9.2 ± 0.9
Sedentary left			21	5.7 ± 1.1	8.7 ± 1.0
Athlete right	Female	Adult	43	5.4 ± 0.7	12.3 ± 1.4
Athlete left			43	5.5 ± 0.7	12.3 ± 1.5
Kallinen					
Sedentary	Male	70–81	11	6.1 ± 0.9	12.0 ± 2.2
Athletes	Male	70–81	18	6.2 ± 0.9	13.9 ± 1.8

All measurements made with ultrasound. SD = standard deviation.[1–3]

Table 2 ▪ Achilles Tendon Thickness (AP) in Injured and Hypercholesterolemic Patient Groups

AUTHOR/GROUP DESCRIPTION	AGES (yr)	NO. (tendons)	AP THICKNESS (mm) Mean ± SD	Range
Mathieson				
Controls	13–60	10	6.1	
Tendinitis		13	6.1 ± 1.4	4–8
Rupture		3		13–15
Fornage				
Normal	12–78	23	5.3	4–6
Tendinitis (chronic)		28	10	7–16
Postoperative		7	15.5	11–20
Steinmetz				
Normal	Adults	32	5.7 ± 0.7	5–8
Hypercholesterolemia, unselected		38	13.4 ± 5.9	6–20
Bude				
Hypercholesterolemia, unselected	18–76	44	8.9 ± 2.8	5.0–16.6
Bude				
Hypercholesterolemia, no palpable tendon thickening	16–69	46	5.3 ± 0.8	4.0–8.2
Liem				
Controls	22–60	12	6.2 ± 1.2	4–9
Controls (MRI)			5.6 ± 1.1	4–7
Hypercholesterolemia, visible xanthomas	26–60	14	12.3 ± 3.7	8–18
Hypercholesterolemia (MRI), visible xanthomas			11.9 ± 3.8	8–18

All measurements with ultrasound except where noted (MRI). SD = standard deviation.[4–9]

hypoechoic defects. All but one of these tendons were less than 7.1 mm in thickness.[7]

REFERENCES

1. Koivunen-Niemela T, Parkkola K: Anatomy of the Achilles tendon (tendo calcaneus) with respect to tendon thickness measurements. Surg Radiol Anat 1995; 17(3):263–268.
2. van Holsbeeck MV, Introcaso JH: Appendix: Table of Normal Values. In van Holsbeeck MV, Introcaso JH (eds): Musculoskeletal Ultrasound. Mosby–Year Book, St. Louis, 1991, vol 1, pp 315–319.
3. Kallinen M, Suominen H: Ultrasonographic measurements of the Achilles tendon in elderly athletes and sedentary men. Acta Radiol 1994; 35(6):560–563.
4. Mathieson JR, Connell DG, Cooperberg PL, Lloyd-Smith DR: Sonography of the Achilles tendon and adjacent bursae. AJR Am J Roentgenol 1988; 151:127–131.
5. Fornage BD: Achilles tendon: US examination. Radiology 1986; 159:759–764.
6. Steinmetz A, Schmidt W, Schuler P, et al: Ultrasonography of achilles tendons in primary hypercholesterolemia: Comparison with computed tomography. Atherosclerosis 1988; 74:231–239.
7. Bude RO, Alder RS, Bassett DR, et al: Heterozygous familial hypercholesterolemia: Detection of xanthomas in the achilles tendon with US. Radiology 1993; 188:567–571.
8. Bude RO, Nesbitt SD, Adler RS, Rubenfire M: Sonographic detection of xanthomas in normal-sized achilles tendons of individuals with heterozygous familial hypercholesterolemia. AJR Am J Roentgenol 1998; 170:621–625.
9. Liem MS, Leuven JA, Bloem JL, Schipper J: Magnetic resonance imaging of Achilles tendon xanthomas in familial hypercholesterolemia. Skeletal Radiol 1992; 21(7):453–457.
10. Bureau NJ, Roederer G: Sonography of achilles tendon xanthomas in patients with heterozygous familial hypercholesterolemia. AJR Am J Roentgenol 1998; 171:645–749.

⠂⠒ BOEHLER ANGLE OF THE CALCANEUS
▪ ACR Code: 4642 (Calcaneus)

Technique ▪

Ankle radiographs were made in the mediolateral projection, with the central ray centered over the malleoli. Correct positioning is confirmed when the two malleoli are projected over one another.[1–3]

Measurements ▪

A line is drawn between the posterior tuberosity to the apex of the posterior facet. A second line is drawn between the apices of the posterior facet and the anterior process. The angle between them is the Boehler angle. This is shown in Figure 1. The normal values and suggested lower limits are given in Table 1.

Source ▪

Boehler studied approximately 1900 patients who were treated for fracture of the calcaneus. In each case, both the normal and injured sides were radiographed.[1] Hauser and Kroeker evaluated 120 bilateral radiographs from 61 patients.[2] Chen and colleagues studied 120 patients (63 men, 57 women, age range 16 to 81 years, mean age 34 years) who had radiographs of the foot or ankle for reasons other than trauma.[3] Steel and colleagues evaluated 82 radiographs of 41 women volunteers (age range 40 to 60 years).[4]

Comments ▪

Normal side-to-side variation in Boehler's angle ranges up to 3.6 degrees.[2–4] Comparison with the uninjured side may be useful in borderline cases. In Chen's subjects, 37 of 120 (31%) had an angle that would be abnormally low using the commonly cited cut-off of 28 degrees, and they suggest using 18 degrees instead. This was based on their mean minus 2 standard deviations and resulted in only one case falling below the cut-off.[2]

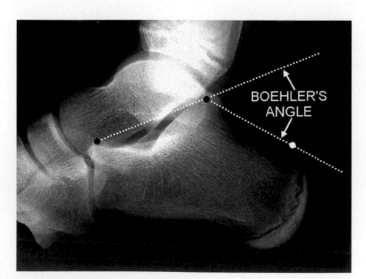

Figure 1 ▪ Measurement of Boehler's angle from a lateral ankle radiograph. The angle is measured between lines passing through the apices of the anterior process and posterior facet (*black circles*) and a line passing through the posterior facet and the posterior tuberosity (*white circle*).

Table 1 ▪ Boehler Angle Normative Values

AUTHOR	GROUP	NUMBER	MEAN ± SD	RANGE	LOWER LIMIT
Boehler	Adults	1900	30–35*	28–40	28
Hauser	Adults	122	32±6	20–44	20
Chen	Men	63	30±6	—	
Chen	Women	57	29±6	—	
Chen	Adults	120	30±6	14–50	18
Steel	Females	82	35±8	22–48	

*Boehler gave a "range" for the mean.
All measurements are in degrees. SD = standard deviation.

REFERENCES

1. Boehler L: Diagnosis, pathology and treatment of fractures of the os calcis. J Bone Joint Surg 1931; 13:75–89.
2. Hauser ML, Kroeker RO: Boehler's angle: A review and study. J Am Podiatr Med Assoc 1975; 65:517–521.
3. Chen MY, Bohrer SP, Kelley TF: Boehler's angle: A reappraisal. Ann Emerg Med 1991; 20(2): 122–124.
4. Steel MW, Johnson KA, DeWitz MA, Ilstrup DM: Radiographic measurements of the normal adult foot. Foot Ankle 1980; 1:151–158.

⁛ AXIAL RELATIONSHIPS OF THE FOOT AND CRITERIA FOR DETERMINATION OF CONGENITAL ABNORMALITIES
▪ ACR Code: 464 (Tarsal Bones) 465 (Metatarsals)

Technique ▪

Central ray: Perpendicular to plane of film, over midportion of foot in both projections.

Position: Anteroposterior (AP) and lateral.[1] Technique must be carefully standardized. Slight variations in rotation in either projection can markedly alter the relationship of the bones shown on the film. For the anteroposterior view, the knees must be held together and must fall in a plane that is perpendicular to the film (Figure 1A). The tendency of the technologist to "correct" the abnormality by placing the foot normally on the cassette must be discouraged. From the lateral projection (Figure 1B), the technique for lateral ankle view is the correct one. Templeton and coworkers exert pressure against the foot with a plastic board in both projections to simulate weight bearing.

Target-film distance: Immaterial.

Measurements ▪

Figure 2: Normal foot. Recorded angles with weight bearing.[2, 3]

Figure 3: Clubfoot.

Figure 4: "Rocket" deformity.[3]

Figure 5: Flatfoot.[3]

Figure 6: Metatarsus varus.[3]

Figure 7: Pes cavus.[3]

Figures 8–9: Diagrammatic representation of hindfoot and forefoot relationships.[4]

Source ▪

The angles of the normal foot reported by Templeton are based on AP and lateral weight-bearing radiographs of 160 normal children, ages 12 days to 12 years.[2]

Davis and Hatt's diagrams are not based on any statistically valid sample. They are arranged as a guide for the radiologist in describing certain abnormalities. No particular numbers are assigned to the ankles, and the context should be interpreted in a manner similar to that for any other descriptive radiologic finding.[3]

A standard text of pediatric orthopedic radiology provides an additional set of diagrams (Figures 8–9) that is also very helpful in visualizing the relationships of the hindfoot and forefoot in normal patients as well as those with varus or valgus.[4]

Text continued on page 299

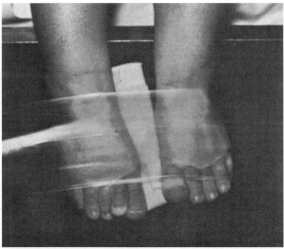
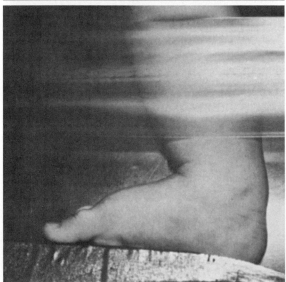

Figure 1 ▪ Proper positioning of a child's foot for AP and lateral radiographs. A wooden wedge is used on the lateral film to dorsiflex the foot as much as possible and to show the presence or absence of equinus. The position of the bones is not affected by holding the foot in the restrictive plastic strap to procure the anteroposterior view. (From Keim HA: Clin Orthop 1970; 70:133. Used by permission.)

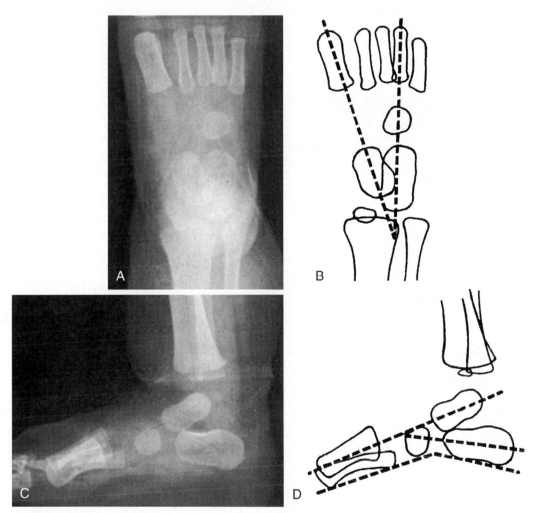

Figure 2 ▪ Normal foot. *A* and *B*, AP projection. The angle between the talus and calcaneus varies with age. In infants and young children, the angle is between 30 degrees and 50 degrees (weight bearing). In children older than 5 years, the talocalcaneal angle varies from 15 degrees to 30 degrees (weight bearing). The line through the midtalus points to the head of the first metatarsal. The line through the midcalcaneus points to the head of the fourth metatarsal. The midtalar and midcalcaneal lines generally coincide with midshaft lines of the first and fourth metatarsals, respectively. Lines of metatarsal shafts are very nearly parallel.

C and *D*, Lateral projection. The midtalar line and the line through the shaft of the first metatarsal coincide in children over 5 years of age on weight bearing, but in infants and young children the talus is positioned more vertically, and the midtalar line passes inferiorly to the shaft of the first metatarsal. An obtuse angle is formed by the line through the inferior cortex of the fifth metatarsal, ranging from 150 degrees to 175 degrees (weight bearing). The midtalar line and midcalcaneal line form an acute angle that varies normally from 25 degrees to 50 degrees (weight bearing).

(A and C from Templeton AW: AJR Am J Roentgenol 1965; 93:374. Drawings from Davis LA, Hatt WS: Radiology 1955; 64:818. Used by permission.)

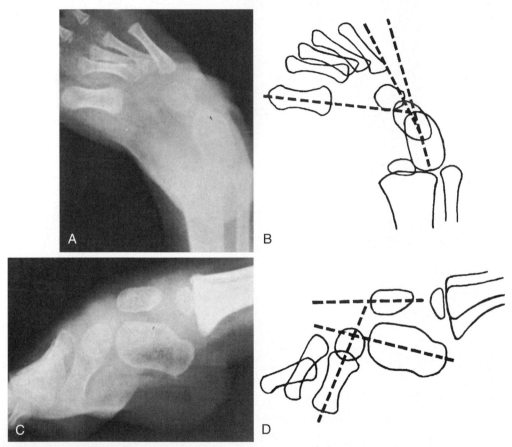

Figure 3 ▪ Clubfoot. *A* and *B*, AP projection. The talocalcaneal angle approaches 0 degrees or is even reversed. The midtalar line points lateral to normal position. The midcalcaneal line points lateral to normal position. The midtalar line and the line through the shaft of the first metatarsal now form an angle. There is a loss of parallelism of metatarsals with convergence posteriorly. *C* and *D*, Lateral projection. The midtalar line and the line through the shaft of the first metatarsal form an obtuse angle. Midtalar and midcalcaneal lines approach parallelism. (From Davis LA, Hatt WS: Radiology 1955; 64:818. Used by permission.)

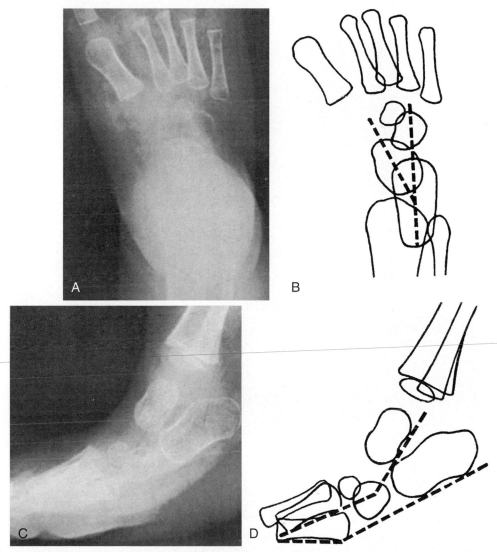

Figure 4 ▪ "Rocker" deformity (overcorrected clubfoot). *A* and *B*, AP projection. The angle between the calcaneus and talus is less than average. The forefoot may or may not be normal. *C* and *D*, Lateral projection. Reverse angle between inferior cortex of calcaneus and fifth metatarsal. Reverse angle between inferior cortex of talus and first metatarsal in severe cases. (From Davis LA, Hatt WS: Radiology 1955; 64:81. Used by permission.)

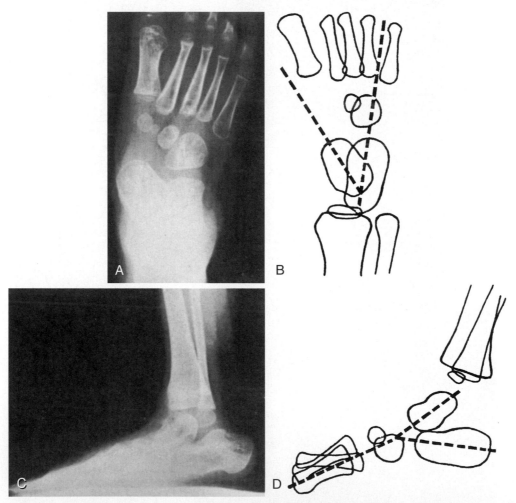

Figure 5 ▪ Flatfoot. *A* and *B*, AP projection. Increased talocalcaneal angle. *C* and *D*, Lateral projection. The line of the first metatarsal makes an angle instead of coinciding with the midtalar line. Frequently there is an increased talocalcaneal angle. (From Davis LA, Hatt WS: Radiology 1955; 64:81. Used by permission.)

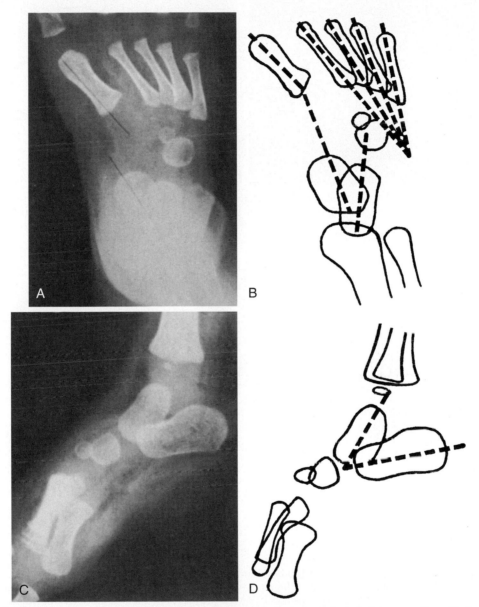

Figure 6 ▪ Metatarsus varus. *A* and *B*, AP projection. There is an increased angle between the midtalar line and the line of the shaft of the first metatarsal. The lines of the metatarsals converge posteriorly. The midcalcaneal line runs lateral to the normal position. *C* and *D*, Lateral projection. The angle between the midcalcaneal and midtalar lines may increase. (From Davis LA, Hatt WS: Radiology 1955; 64:81. Used by permission.)

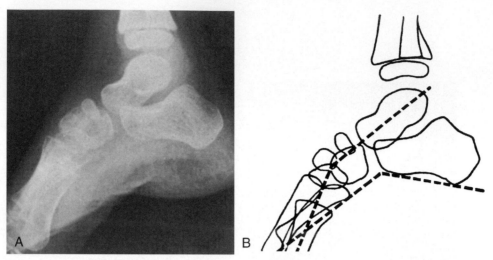

Figure 7 ▪ Pes cavus. The AP projection is unchanged from the normal. *A* and *B*, Lateral projection. Increased angle between the line through the inferior cortex of the calcaneus and inferior cortex of the fifth metatarsal. There is now an angle between the midtalar line and the line through the shaft of the first metatarsal. (From Davis LA, Hatt WS: Radiology 1955; 64:81. Used by permission.)

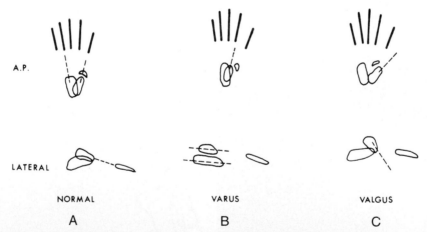

Figure 8 ▪ Diagrammatic representation of hindfoot and forefoot relationships. *A,* Normal hindfoot. The talar axial line intersects or points slightly medial to the first metatarsal base. The navicular is situated directly opposite the head of the talus. The calcaneus points toward the fourth metatarsal base, making a definable angle with the talus. On the lateral projection, the anterior portion of the talus is slightly plantarflexed, the calcaneus slightly dorsiflexed. The talar axial line points down the shaft of the first metatarsal.

B, Hindfoot varus. The talocalcaneal angle is decreased, with these two bones more nearly parallel to each other or actually superimposed. The navicular is medially displaced, and the axial talar line points lateral to the first metatarsal base. On the lateral projection, the calcaneus and talus are both more nearly horizontal and parallel to each other. *C,* Hindfoot valgus. The talocalcaneal angle is increased, with navicular and other midfoot bones displaced lateral to the talus. The talar axial line will pass medial to the first metatarsal base. On the lateral projection, the talus is more nearly vertical than normal.

(From Ozonoff MB: Philadelphia, WB Saunders Co, 1979, pp 288–289. Used by permission.)

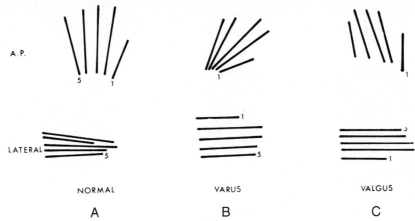

Figure 9 ▪ *A*, Normal forefoot. The metatarsals converge proximally, with overlap at the bases. On the lateral projection, the fifth metatarsal is most plantar, with the other metatarsals being superimposed. *B*, Forefoot varus. The forefoot is narrowed, with increased convergence at the bases and more than normal superimposition. On the lateral projection, a ladder-like arrangement is seen, with the first metatarsal highest. *C*, Forefoot valgus. The forefoot is broadened, with the metatarsals more nearly parallel than normal and with decreased overlap at the bases. On the lateral projection, a ladder-like arrangement is rarely seen, because the degree of eversion is rarely enough to show this finding. If it is present, however, the first metatarsal will be most plantar. (From Ozonoff MB: WB Saunders Co, Philadelphia, 1979, pp 288–289. Used by permission.)

REFERENCES

1. Keim HA, Ritchie GW: Weight-bearing roentgenograms in the evaluation of foot deformities. Clin Orthop 1970; 70:133–136.
2. Templeton AW, McAlister WH, Zim ID: Standardization of terminology and evaluation of osseous relationships in congenitally abnormal feet. AJR Am J Roentgenol 1965; 93:374–381.
3. Davis LA, Hatt WS: Congenital abnormalities of the feet. Radiology 1955; 64:818–825.
4. Ozonoff MB: Pediatric Orthopedic Radiology. WB Saunders, Philadelphia, 1979, pp 288–289.

⁚ MEASUREMENT OF THE FEET OF NORMAL INFANTS AND CHILDREN[1]
▪ ACR Code: 464 (Tarsal Bones) 465 (Metatarsals)

Technique ▪

Central ray: Perpendicular to plane of film.
Position: Standing. For the AP projection, the knee was flexed and the beam directed at the head of the talus. For the true lateral and maximum dorsiflexion lateral radiographs, the ankle was held in neutral or maximally dorsiflexed, the beam directed at the talus.
Target-film distance: Immaterial.

Measurements ▪ (Figure 1, A through K)

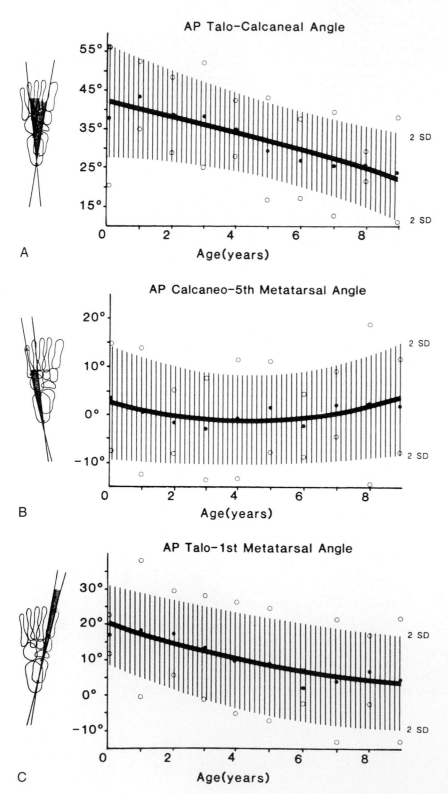

Figure 1 ▪ *A–K*, The mean and standard deviations for each of the 10 angles and the calculated talocalcaneal index were plotted for each of the ten age groups. *Solid lines* show the mean changes with age, *shaded areas*, the normal ranges; *solid circles*, the mean measurements for each age group; *open circles*, 2 standard deviations for each age group. (From Vanderwilde R, et al: J Bone Joint Surg 1988; 70A: 407–414.)

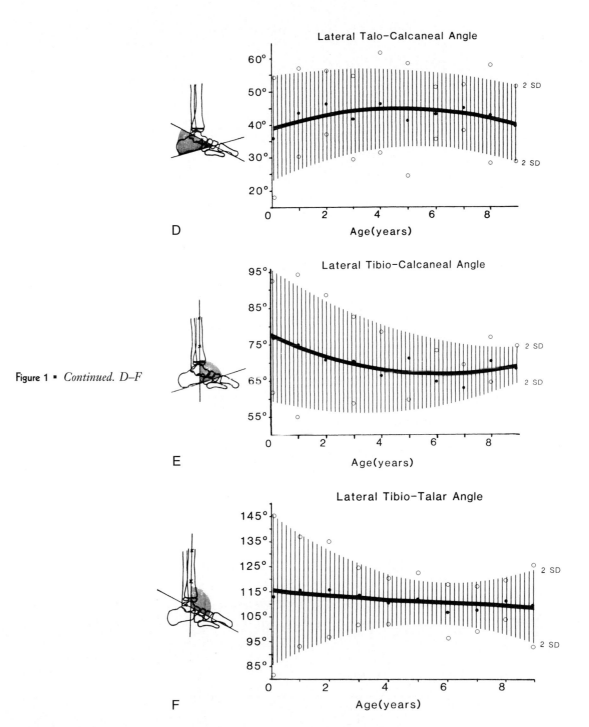

Figure 1 ▪ *Continued. D–F*

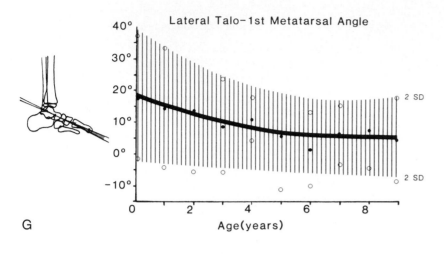

G

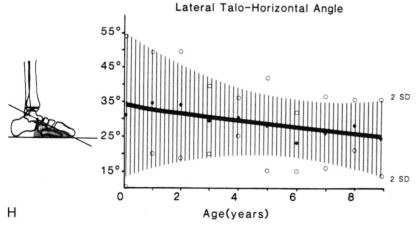

H

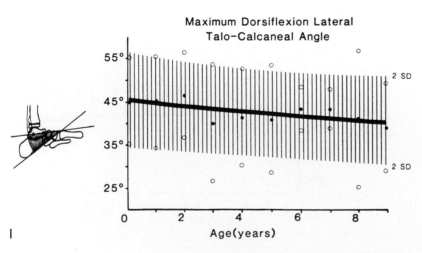

I

Figure 1 ▪ *Continued. G–I*

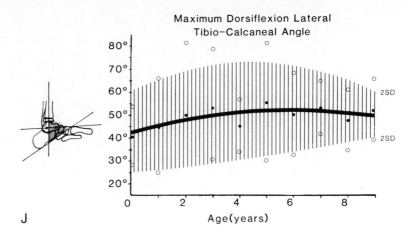

J

Figure 1 • *Continued. J–K*

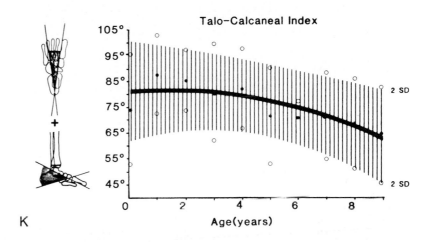

K

Source •

Data were based on radiographs of 74 normal infants and children ranging in age from 6 to 127 months, including 39 boys and 35 girls.

REFERENCE

1. Vanderwilde R, Staheli LT, Chew DE, Malagon V: Measurements on radiographs of the foot in normal infants and children. J Bone Joint Surg Am 1988; 70:407–415.

⁚ LENGTH PATTERN OF METATARSAL BONES[1]
- ACR Code: 465 (Metatarsals)

Technique •

Central ray: Perpendicular to plane of film, over midportion of foot.
Position: Anteroposterior.
Target-film distance: Immaterial.

Measurements • (Figure 1)

Total joint line angle is 142.5 degrees mean. First metatarsal is shorter than second. Second metatarsal is longest. Third metatarsal is shorter than second. Fourth metatarsal is shorter than third. Fifth metatarsal is shorter than fourth.

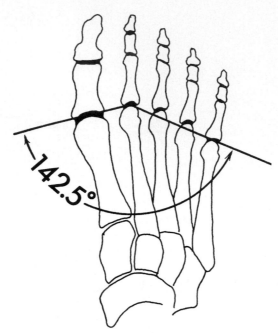

Figure 1 ▪ Angle formed by distal metatarsal bones. (Adapted from Gamble FO, Yale I: Williams & Wilkins Co., Baltimore, 1966, p 158. Used by permission.)

Source ▪

Gamble and Yale used 279 foot roentgenograms.

REFERENCE

1. Gamble FO, Yale I: Clinical Foot Roentgenology. Williams & Wilkins Co., Baltimore, 1966, p 158.

▪: MEASUREMENTS PERTAINING TO HALLUX VALGUS
▪ ACR Code: 468 (Metatarsals and Phalanges)

Technique ▪

Radiographs for these measurements are made with the patient standing and are exposed in the anteroposterior (AP) projection (also called dorsoplantar). The central ray is directed 15 degrees toward the heel and centered on the midfoot. A source-to-film distance of at least 40 inches (102 cm) is used.[1] Richardson and colleagues made radiographs of amputated first rays by placing them in a device to simulate a standing radiograph and using a similar radiographic technique.[2]

Measurements ▪

Four angles of the first ray may be measured from radiographs of the foot. These help describe the severity and location of any valgus deformity and are important for surgical planning. Figure 1 shows angle measurements of the first ray, with the cut-offs for abnormal angles listed.[1, 3-5] The relative length of the first metatarsal with respect to the second (Figure 2), congruency of the first metatarsal phalangeal joint (Figure 3), and the position of the tibial sesamoid with respect to the first metatarsal (Figure 4) are also important to foot surgeons.[1]

The distal metatarsal articular angle (DMAA) can be helpful in assessing the need for osteotomy to correct excessive valgus tilt of the articular surface in addition to soft tissue repair.[2] A method for measurement of DMAA in congruous and subluxed joints is shown in Figure 5. The normal mean in Richardson's postmortem study was 6.1 degrees, and the range was −3 to 26 degrees, with positive numbers indicating valgus tilt.[2]

Source ▪

Karasick and Wapner reviewed the medical literature and applied clinical experience to write an overview of pertinent measurements and observations from AP radiographs in assessment of hallux valgus.[1] Richardson and colleagues radiographed 100 first rays amputated at the cuneiform articulation. The age at time of death and gender of these 74 cadavers and 26 fresh specimens were not given, and none had been operated on for hallux valgus.[2]

Comments ▪

Richardson and colleagues did not provide a cut-off for normal or the standard deviation in their paper about the DMAA. The standard deviation was estimated by us from a bar graph of frequency distributions at 5.5 mm. Therefore, an angle of 19 degrees would be just above the 99th percentile, and a value of 20 degrees for abnormal would be reasonable.

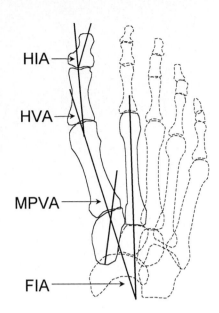

Figure 1 ▪ Angle measurements of the first ray of the foot from standing AP radiographs. HIA = Hallux interphalangeus angle, between the long axes of the phalanges. Normally less than 8 degrees. HVA = Hallux valgus angle, between the long axes of the metatarsal and the proximal phalanx. Normally less than 15 degrees. MPVA = Metatarsus primus varus angle, between the long axes of the medial cuneiform and the metatarsal. Normally less than 25 degrees. FIA = First intermetatarsal angle, between the long axes of the first and second metatarsals. Normally less than 10 degrees.[1, 3–5]

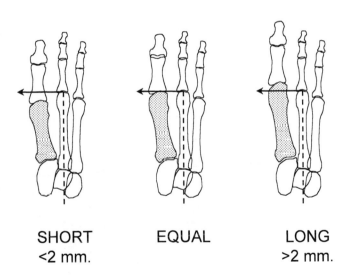

SHORT
<2 mm.

EQUAL

LONG
>2 mm.

Figure 2 ▪ Relative lengths of the first and second metatarsals. A line (arrow) perpendicular to the long axis of the second metatarsal (dashed line) is projected from its distal end toward the first metatarsal. If the line falls within 2 mm of the end of the first metatarsal, the bones are considered to be of equal length. If the line crosses the first metatarsal, the metatarsal is considered to be long, and if it crosses the proximal phalanx, the metatarsal is short.[1]

Figure 3 ▪ First metatarsal phalangeal joint congruence. Lines are drawn through the medial and lateral ends of the articular surfaces of the distal metatarsal and proximal phalanx. In a congruent joint, the lines are parallel. If the joint is deviated, the lines intersect medial to the joint, whereas in a subluxed joint, the lines intersect within the joint.[1]

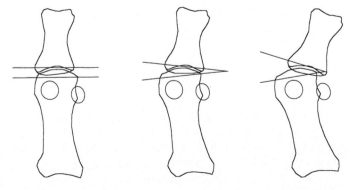

CONGRUENT   DEVIATED   SUBLUXED

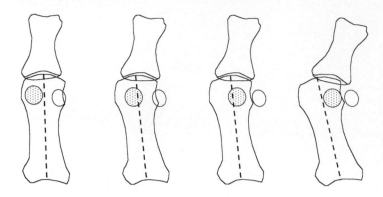

GRADE 0   GRADE 1   GRADE 2   GRADE 3

Figure 4 ▪ Tibial sesamoid position. A line *(dashed)* is drawn through the middle of the first metatarsal long axis. If the tibial sesamoid *(shaded)* falls medial to the line, a grade of 0 is assigned. If more than 50% of the sesamoid is medial, the grade is 1, and if more than 50% is lateral, the grade is 2. A grade of 3 is assigned when the tibial sesamoid lies entirely lateral to the line. As shown, increasing lateral deviation is associated with deviation/subluxation.[1]

Figure 5 ▪ Distal metatarsal articular angle (DMAA). In congruous joints, a line is drawn between medial and lateral distal articular margins of the metatarsal. A second line is drawn to intersect the first, which is perpendicular to the long axis of the metatarsal *(dashed)*. The angle between them (apex lateral) is the DMAA. If the joint is subluxed, the medial joint margin may be identified by the sagittal groove. The lateral margin is located by measuring the distance *(arrows)* between the sagittal groove and the medial edge of the phalanx. The same distance *(arrows)* is subtracted from the lateral edge of the phalanx and projected to the metatarsal. This method assumes that the joint surfaces of the two bones are the same width.[2]

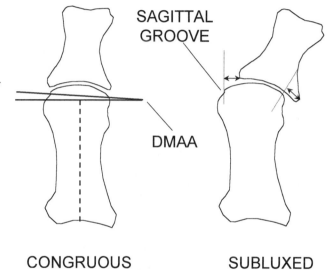

CONGRUOUS   **SUBLUXED**

REFERENCES

1. Karasick D, Wapner KL: Hallux valgus deformity: Preoperative radiologic assessment. AJR Am J Roentgenol 1990; 155(1):119–123.
2. Richardson EG, Graves SC, McClure JT, Boone RT: First metatarsal head-shaft angle: A method of determination. Foot Ankle 1993; 14(4):181–185.
3. LaPorta G, Melillo T, Olinsky D: X-ray evaluation of hallux abducto valgus deformity. J Am Podiatr Med Assoc 1974; 64:544–566.
4. Spinner SM, Lipsman S, Spector F: Radiographic criteria in the assessment of hallux abductus deformities. J Foot Surg 1984; 23:25–30.
5. Smith RW, Reynolds JC, Stewart MJ: Hallux valgus assessment: Report of research committee of American Orthopaedic Foot and Ankle Society. Foot Ankle 1984; 5:92–102.

▪▪ MEASUREMENTS PERTAINING TO BUNIONETTE DEFORMITY
▪ ACR Code: 468 (Metatarsals and Phalanges)

Technique ▪

Radiographs for these measurements are made with the patient standing and are exposed in the anteroposterior (AP) projection (also called dorsoplantar). The central ray is directed 15 degrees toward the heel and centered on the midfoot. A source-to-film distance of at least 40 inches (102 cm) is used.[1]

Measurements ▪

Four measurements are combined in the evaluation of the painful fifth ray.[1–3] The metatarsophalangeal angle (MPA) helps define the bunionette deformity. The fifth intermeta-

tarsal angle (FIA) quantifies the divergence of the fifth metatarsal, which may result in a symptomatic lesion. The shape of the fifth metatarsal itself is also important in prognosis and treatment planning and is described by the lateral divergence angle (LDA) and the width of the head.[1] These measurements and the cut-off values for abnormality are shown in Figure 1.

Source ▪

Karasick reviewed the medical literature and applied clinical experience to write an overview of pertinent measurements and observations from AP radiographs is assessment of hallux valgus (1).

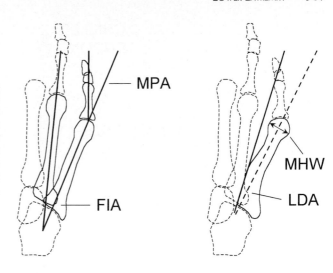

Figure 1 ▪ Measurements of the fifth ray for bunionette deformity. MPA = Metatarsalphalangeal angle, between the long axes of the metatarsal and proximal phalanx. Normally less than 10 degrees. FIA = Fifth intermetatarsal angle, between the long axes of the fourth and fifth metatarsals. Normally less than 8 degrees. LDA = Lateral deviation angle, between the long axis of the distal metatarsal (*dashed line*) and a line parallel to the proximal medial cortex (*solid*). Normally less than 3 degrees. MHW = Metatarsal head width. The greatest width of the metatarsal head (*arrows*) perpendicular to the long axis (*dashed line*). Normally less than 13 mm.[1-3]

Comments ▪

Three anatomic variations leading to symptomatic bunionette are recognized. Type 1 (27% of cases) is characterized by a large metatarsal head of 13 mm or more. Type 2 (23% of cases) is associated with lateral bowing where the LDA is 3 degrees or more. Type 3 (50% of cases) is characterized by a large FIA measuring 8 degrees or more.[1, 4] When the type 3 deformity is combined with an abnormally large first intermetatarsal angle (10 degrees or more), the resulting combination is termed splayfoot.[1]

References

1. Karasick D: Preoperative assessment of symptomatic bunionette deformity: Radiologic findings. AJR Am J Roentgenol 1995; 164(1): 147–149.
2. Nestor BJ, Kitaoka HB, Ilstrup DM, et al: Radiologic anatomy of the painful bunionette. Foot Ankle 1990; 11:6–11.
3. Fallat LM, Bucholz J: Analysis of the tailor's bunion by radiographic and anatomic display. J Am Podiatr Med Assoc 1980; 70:597–603.
4. Coughlin MJ: Treatment of bunionette deformity with longitudinal diaphyseal osteotomy with distal soft tissue repair. Foot Ankle 1991; 11:195–203.

▪: PLANTAR FASCIA
▪ ACR Code: 469 (Plantar Fascia)

Technique ▪

Cardinal and colleagues and Gibbon performed longitudinal ultrasound over the dorsum of the foot posteriorly to visualize the plantar aponeurosis with 7- to 7.5-MHz linear transducers. The patients were scanned prone, with the feet hanging from the examination table.[1-3] Berkowitz and colleagues used a 1.5-T Signa MRI machine (GE Medical Systems, Milwaukee, WI) to produce sagittal T1 (400-600/20) and coronal PD/T2 (1700-2200/20-30, 80) images. An extremity coil was used, and the section thickness was 3 mm with 0- to 1.5-mm gap.[4]

Measurements ▪

The normal plantar fascia appears as a striated hyperechoic structure on ultrasound and as a band of decreased signal on MRI. On both ultrasound and sagittal MRI, the maximum thickness of the plantar fascia was measured at the proximal end near the calcaneal insertion.[1-4] With coronal MRI images, the slice showing the proximal plantar fascia at its thickest point and to best advantage was used to measure the thickness.[4] Figure 1 shows the technique of measurement and Table 1 lists the results.

Source ▪

Cardinal and colleagues studied 15 patients (9 women, 6 men, age range 30 to 74 years, mean age 45 years) with typical symptoms and physical findings of plantar fasciitis (19 symptomatic feet, 11 asymptomatic feet). None had been operated on.[1] A control group (age/gender not given) of 15 asymptomatic volunteers (30 feet) was also scanned.[1] Gibbon has evaluated 190 patients with plantar fasciitis (297 feet) and 48 asymptomatic volunteers (96 feet). The ages and gender distribution were not given.[2, 3] Berkowitz and colleagues studied 8 patients (7 women, 1 man, age range 28 to 73, mean age 43 years) and obtained scans of 10 symptomatic feet. Controls consisted of nine feet from five asymptomatic women (age range 32 to 46 years, mean age 41 years) and six nonpainful feet from five men whose ages ranged from 29 to 33 years.[4]

Comments ▪

In addition to thickening of the fascia, ultrasound may show loss of normal striations and hypoechogenicity in cases of fasciitis. This was demonstrated in 84% by Berkowitz and group and in 74% by Gibbon and Long[1, 3] on MRI areas of increased signal within the tendons of 90% of patients with fasciitis.

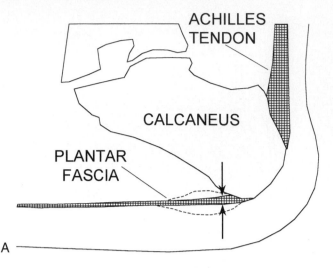

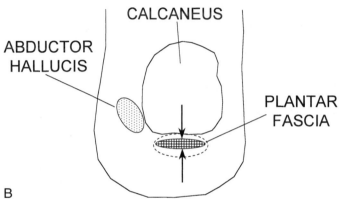

Figure 1 ▪ Measurement of the plantar fascia thickness may be done in the sagittal (*A*, ultrasound or MRI) or coronal plane (*B*, MRI). The thickness of the normal fascia *(arrows)* is measured proximally near the calcaneal insertion at its maximum. Typically, fasciitis produces proximal swelling *(dashed lines)*.

AUTHOR (MODALITY)/ GROUP DESCRIPTION	NO. OF FEET	THICKNESS (mm)	
		Mean ± SD	Range
Cardinal (U/S)			
Control	30	2.6 ± 0.48	1.6–3.8
Asymptomatic heel	11	2.9 ± 0.7	2.0–4.0
Fasciitis	15	5.2 ± 1.13	3.2–6.8
Gibbon (U/S)			
Control	96	3.3 ± 0.38	2.4–4.3
Fasciitis	297	5.9 ± 0.97	4.1–9.1
Berkowitz (MRI sagittal T1)			
Male control	6	3.0 ± 0.8	
Female control	9	3.22 ± 0.44	
Fasciitis	10	7.4 ± 1.17	
Berkowitz (MRI coronal T2)			
Male control	6	3.0 ± 0.0	
Female control	9	3.44 ± 0.53	
Fasciitis	10	7.56 ± 1.01	

Table 1 ▪ Plantar Fascia Thickness[1, 3, 4]

REFERENCES

1. Cardinal E, Chhem RK, Beauregard CG, et al: Plantar fasciitis: Sonographic evaluation. Radiology 1996; 201:257–259
2. Gibbon WW: Plantar fasciitis: US imaging (letter). Radiology 1992; 182:285.
3. Gibbon W, Long G: Plantar fasciitis: US evaluation (letter). Radiology 1997; 203:290.
4. Berkowitz JF, Kier R, Rudicel S: Plantar fasciitis: MR imaging. Radiology 1991; 179:665–667.

CHAPTER 8

Skeletal Maturation, Body Surface Area

■■
■

■: CALCULATION OF BODY SURFACE AREA

Measurements ■

The calculation of body surface area (BSA) is often done using the formula of Du Bois and Du Bois, which is based on direct measurements of nine individuals, one of whom was a child.[1] However, two more recent papers written by Gehan and George and by Haycock and colleagues were based on larger samples (401 and 81, respectively).[2,3] These investigators produced equations of the same form as Du Bois and Du Bois but with different constants and exponents. Bailey and Briars have stated that since Gehan's formula was developed with least squares analysis and from the largest population, it should be the medical standard.[4] Mosteller has proposed a simplified formula by assuming that the two exponents are equal to 0.5.[5] This easy-to-remember equation accounts for 98% of the total variation in the 401 observations reported by Gehan and George.

Table 1 lists the various formulas for calculating BSA from weight and height. When the calculated BSA values from these tables are compared with those derived using Haycock's formula, the percentage difference is 1.5 ± 0.93 (mean $\pm$ SD over the usable range of weight and height). Tables 2 and 3 contain BSA as calculated by the formula of Gehan and George based on height and weight. Figures 1 and 2 are nomograms for determining BSA in children and adults from known height and weight,[7] which are based on the Du Bois relationship.[1]

As a rough approximation, the BSA of 9, 10, and 12 to 13 year old children is 1.07, 1.14, and 1.33 meters squared, respectively. Adult male BSA is approximately 1.9 meters squared, and adult females have a BSA of about 1.6 meters squared.[6]

Source ■

See references.

Table 1 ■ Formulas for Calculating Body Surface Area When Weight and Height Are Known

RESEARCHER	NO.	FORMULA
Du Bois and Du Bois[1]	9	$BSA\ (m^2) = Wt(kg)^{0.425} \times Ht(cm)^{0.725} \times 0.007184$
Gehan and George[2]	401	$BSA\ (m^2) = Wt(kg)^{0.51456} \times Ht(cm)^{0.42246} \times 0.02350$
Haycock et al[3]	81	$BSA\ (m^2) = Wt(kg)^{0.5378} \times Ht(cm)^{0.3964} \times 0.024265$
Mosteller[5]	—	$BSA\ (m^2) = \sqrt{\dfrac{Wt(kg) \times Ht(cm)}{3600}}$
		$BSA\ (m^2) = \sqrt{\dfrac{Wt(lb) \times Ht(in)}{3131}}$

Table 2 ▪ Body Surface Area Versus Height (from 50–150 cm) and Weight (from 5–95 kg)

HEIGHT (cm)	WEIGHT (kg)																		
	5	10	15	20	25	30	35	40	45	50	55	60	65	70	75	80	85	90	95
50	0.28	0.40	0.49	0.57	0.64	0.71	0.76	0.82	0.87	0.92	0.96	1.01	1.05	1.09	1.13	1.17	1.21	1.24	1.28
55	0.29	0.42	0.51	0.60	0.67	0.73	0.80	0.85	0.91	0.96	1.00	1.05	1.09	1.14	1.18	1.22	1.26	1.29	1.33
60	0.30	0.43	0.53	0.62	0.69	0.76	0.83	0.88	0.94	0.99	1.04	1.09	1.13	1.18	1.22	1.26	1.30	1.34	1.38
65	0.31	0.45	0.55	0.64	0.72	0.79	0.85	0.91	0.97	1.03	1.08	1.13	1.18	1.22	1.26	1.31	1.35	1.39	1.43
70	0.32	0.46	0.57	0.66	0.74	0.81	0.88	0.94	1.00	1.06	1.11	1.16	1.21	1.26	1.30	1.35	1.39	1.43	1.47
75	0.33	0.48	0.59	0.68	0.76	0.84	0.91	0.97	1.03	1.09	1.14	1.20	1.25	1.30	1.34	1.39	1.43	1.47	1.52
80	0.34	0.49	0.60	0.70	0.78	0.86	0.93	1.00	1.06	1.12	1.18	1.23	1.28	1.33	1.38	1.43	1.47	1.52	1.56
85	0.35	0.50	0.62	0.72	0.80	0.88	0.96	1.02	1.09	1.15	1.21	1.26	1.31	1.37	1.42	1.46	1.51	1.55	1.60
90	0.36	0.51	0.63	0.73	0.82	0.90	0.98	1.05	1.11	1.18	1.24	1.29	1.35	1.40	1.45	1.50	1.55	1.59	1.64
95	0.37	0.53	0.65	0.75	0.84	0.93	1.00	1.07	1.14	1.20	1.26	1.32	1.38	1.43	1.48	1.53	1.58	1.63	1.68
100	0.38	0.54	0.66	0.77	0.86	0.95	1.02	1.10	1.17	1.23	1.29	1.35	1.41	1.46	1.52	1.57	1.62	1.66	1.71
105	0.38	0.55	0.68	0.78	0.88	0.97	1.04	1.12	1.19	1.26	1.32	1.38	1.44	1.49	1.55	1.60	1.65	1.70	1.75
110	0.39	0.56	0.69	0.80	0.90	0.98	1.07	1.14	1.21	1.28	1.34	1.41	1.47	1.52	1.58	1.63	1.68	1.73	1.78
115	0.40	0.57	0.70	0.81	0.91	1.00	1.09	1.16	1.24	1.30	1.37	1.43	1.49	1.55	1.61	1.66	1.71	1.77	1.82
120	0.41	0.58	0.71	0.83	0.93	1.02	1.11	1.18	1.26	1.33	1.40	1.46	1.52	1.58	1.64	1.69	1.75	1.80	1.85
125	0.41	0.59	0.73	0.84	0.95	1.04	1.12	1.20	1.28	1.35	1.42	1.48	1.55	1.61	1.67	1.72	1.78	1.83	1.88
130	0.42	0.60	0.74	0.86	0.96	1.06	1.14	1.22	1.30	1.37	1.44	1.51	1.57	1.63	1.69	1.75	1.81	1.86	1.91
135	0.43	0.61	0.75	0.87	0.98	1.07	1.16	1.24	1.32	1.40	1.47	1.53	1.60	1.66	1.72	1.78	1.83	1.89	1.94
140	0.43	0.62	0.76	0.88	0.99	1.09	1.18	1.26	1.34	1.42	1.49	1.56	1.62	1.69	1.75	1.81	1.86	1.92	1.97
145	0.44	0.63	0.77	0.90	1.01	1.11	1.20	1.28	1.36	1.44	1.51	1.58	1.65	1.71	1.77	1.83	1.89	1.95	2.00
150	0.45	0.64	0.79	0.91	1.02	1.12	1.21	1.30	1.38	1.46	1.53	1.60	1.67	1.74	1.80	1.86	1.92	1.98	2.03

Calculated from the formula by Gehan and George.[2]

Table 3 ▪ Body Surface Area Versus Height (from 150–225 cm) and Weight (from 30–130 kg)

HEIGHT (cm)	WEIGHT (kg)																		
	30	35	40	45	50	55	60	65	70	75	80	85	90	95	100	105	110	115	120
150	1.12	1.21	1.30	1.38	1.46	1.53	1.60	1.67	1.74	1.80	1.86	1.92	1.98	2.03	2.09	2.14	2.19	2.24	2.29
155	1.14	1.23	1.32	1.40	1.48	1.55	1.63	1.69	1.76	1.82	1.89	1.95	2.00	2.06	2.11	2.17	2.22	2.27	2.32
160	1.15	1.25	1.34	1.42	1.50	1.58	1.65	1.72	1.78	1.85	1.91	1.97	2.03	2.09	2.14	2.20	2.25	2.30	2.35
165	1.17	1.26	1.35	1.44	1.52	1.60	1.67	1.74	1.81	1.87	1.94	2.00	2.06	2.11	2.17	2.23	2.28	2.33	2.39
170	1.18	1.28	1.37	1.46	1.54	1.62	1.69	1.76	1.83	1.90	1.96	2.02	2.08	2.14	2.20	2.25	2.31	2.36	2.42
175	1.20	1.30	1.39	1.48	1.56	1.64	1.71	1.78	1.85	1.92	1.98	2.05	2.11	2.17	2.23	2.28	2.34	2.39	2.45
180	1.21	1.31	1.41	1.49	1.58	1.66	1.73	1.80	1.87	1.94	2.01	2.07	2.13	2.19	2.25	2.31	2.37	2.42	2.47
185	1.23	1.33	1.42	1.51	1.59	1.67	1.75	1.83	1.90	1.97	2.03	2.10	2.16	2.22	2.28	2.34	2.39	2.45	2.50

HEIGHT (cm)	WEIGHT (kg)																		
	40	45	50	55	60	65	70	75	80	85	90	95	100	105	110	115	120	125	130
185	1.42	1.51	1.59	1.67	1.75	1.83	1.90	1.97	2.03	2.10	2.16	2.22	2.28	2.34	2.39	2.45	2.50	2.56	2.61
190	1.44	1.53	1.61	1.69	1.77	1.85	1.92	1.99	2.05	2.12	2.18	2.24	2.30	2.36	2.42	2.48	2.53	2.59	2.64
195	1.45	1.54	1.63	1.71	1.79	1.87	1.94	2.01	2.08	2.14	2.21	2.27	2.33	2.39	2.45	2.50	2.56	2.61	2.67
200	1.47	1.56	1.65	1.73	1.81	1.89	1.96	2.03	2.10	2.17	2.23	2.29	2.36	2.41	2.47	2.53	2.59	2.64	2.70
205	1.48	1.58	1.67	1.75	1.83	1.91	1.98	2.05	2.12	2.19	2.25	2.32	2.38	2.44	2.50	2.56	2.61	2.67	2.72
210	1.50	1.59	1.68	1.77	1.85	1.93	2.00	2.07	2.14	2.21	2.28	2.34	2.40	2.47	2.52	2.58	2.64	2.70	2.75
215	1.51	1.61	1.70	1.78	1.87	1.94	2.02	2.09	2.16	2.23	2.30	2.36	2.43	2.49	2.55	2.61	2.67	2.72	2.78
220	1.53	1.63	1.72	1.80	1.88	1.96	2.04	2.11	2.19	2.25	2.32	2.39	2.45	2.51	2.58	2.63	2.69	2.75	2.81
225	1.54	1.64	1.73	1.82	1.90	1.98	2.06	2.13	2.21	2.28	2.34	2.41	2.48	2.54	2.60	2.66	2.72	2.78	2.83

Calculated from the formula by Gehan and George.[2]

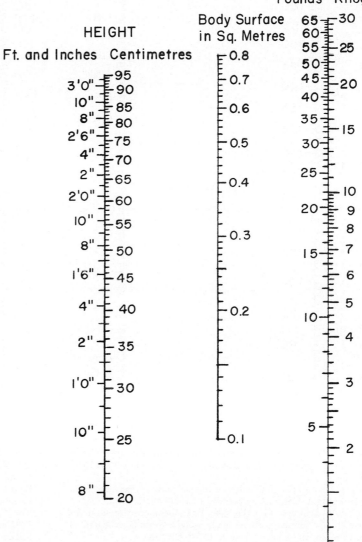

Figure 1 ▪ Nomogram for determination of body surface area in children when height and weight are known. (From Geigy: Scientific Tables, ed 6. Basel, Switzerland, 1962. Used by permission.)

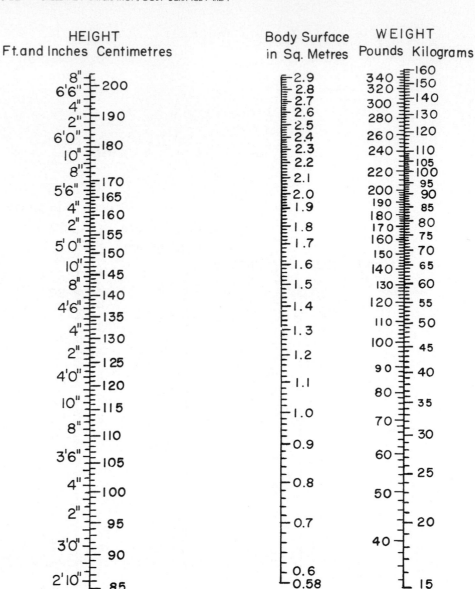

HEIGHT
Ft.and Inches Centimetres

Body Surface
in Sq. Metres

WEIGHT
Pounds Kilograms

Figure 2 ▪ Nomogram for determination of body surface area in adults when height and weight are known. (From Geigy: Scientific Tables, ed 6. Basel, Switzerland, 1962. Used by permission.)

REFERENCES

1. Du Bois D, Du Bois EF: A formula to estimate the approximate surface area if height and weight be known. Arch Intern Med 1916; 17:863–871.
2. Gehan EA, George SL: Estimation of human body surface area from height and weight. Cancer Chemother Res 1970; 54:225–235.
3. Haycock GB, Schwartz GJ, Wisotsky DH: Geometric method for measuring body surface area: A height-weight formula validated in infants, children, and adults. J Pediatr 1978; 93:62–66.
4. Bailey BJ, Briars GL: Estimating the surface area of the human body. Stat Med 1996; 15:1325–1332.
5. Mosteller RD: More on simplified calculation of body-surface area. N Engl J Med 1988; 318:1130.
6. Chapman RM: Gonadal toxicity and teratogenicity. In Perry MC (ed): The Chemotherapy Source Book. Williams & Wilkins, Baltimore, 1992, p 711.
7. Scientific Tables. Ciba-Geigy, Basel, Switzerland, 1962.

▪▪ ASSESSMENT OF GESTATIONAL AGE FROM LUMBAR SPINE DIMENSIONS
- ▪ ACR Code: 33.127 (Bone Age Determination, Spine)

Technique ▪

Portable anteroposterior (AP) radiographs of the chest and upper abdomen (details not given) were made.[1]

Measurements ▪

The width of the L1 vertebral body *(W)* and the distance from the top of L1 to the bottom of L2 *(H)* were measured with needle-pointed calipers applied to the film and then to a ruler. Measurement was made to the nearest 0.1 mm.[1] These are shown in Figure 1. Stepwise multiple regression was performed (including measurement of the distance between the L1 pedicles) to determine the best predictors of gestational age (GA) and the best model for fit. A linear function of W and H gave the best predictions:

$$GA = 11.89 + (0.77 \times W) + (0.93 \times H).$$

The standard error (SE) of the predicted GA can be calculated by the following:

$$SE = \sqrt{2.93 \times 0.00907W^2 + 0.00764H^2 - 0.195W - 0.22H + 2.64}$$

The 95% prediction interval for the estimate is approximated by:

$$GA \pm 2SE.$$

Williamson and Edwards developed a nomogram for estimating GA from W and H, which is shown in Figure 2.

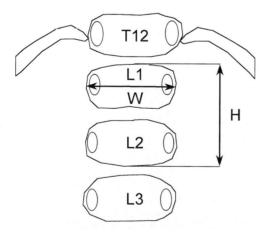

Figure 1 ▪ Measurements of the upper lumbar spine from supine radiographs for prediction of gestational age. The width of L1 (W) is measured between the lateral margins of the vertebral body. The combined height (H) of L1 and L2 is measured from the superior endplate of L1 to the inferior endplate of L2.

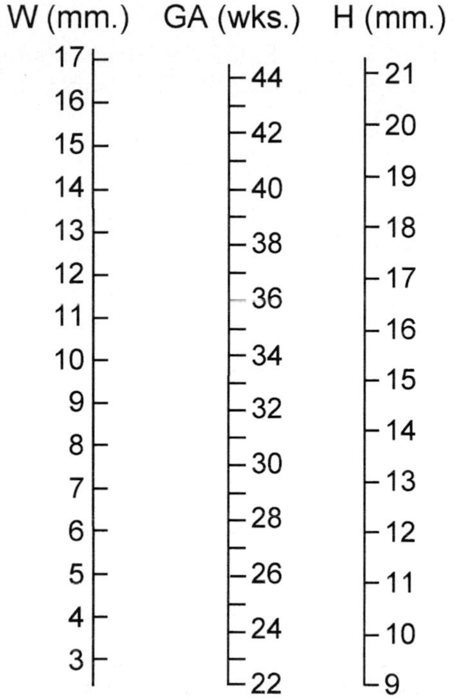

W (mm.)	GA (wks.)	H (mm.)
17		21
16	44	20
15	42	
14	40	19
13	38	18
12	36	17
11		16
10	34	15
9	32	
8	30	14
7	28	13
6		12
5	26	11
4	24	10
3	22	9

Figure 2 ▪ Nomogram for predicting gestational age (GA) from L1 width (W) and combined height (H) of L1 and L2. A straight line connecting the measured values of W and H will intersect the central line at the predicted GA. (From Williamson MR, Edwards DK: Pediatr Radiol 1980; 9(4):229–231. Used by permission.)

Source ▪

A total of 183 white infants was studied. The gestational age was determined by the Dubowitz method.[2] All infants had appropriate birth weight for gestational age.[1]

Comments ▪

The error (95% prediction interval as described above) of the estimate of GA increases as the values of W and H deviate from the mean values obtained in the study. For example, for W = 11 mm and H = 14 mm (near the respective means), the estimated GA would be 33.4 ± 0.34 weeks; with W = 10.8 mm and H = 14.4 mm, the estimated GA would be 33.6 ± 2.9 weeks. Nearly all age estimates will be within ± 3.0 weeks.[1]

References

1. Williamson MR, Edwards DK: Prediction of gestational age of infants from the abdominal radiograph. Pediatr Radiol 1980; 9(4):229–231.
2. Dubowitz LMS, Dubowitz V, Goldberg C: Clinical assessment of gestational age in the newborn infant. J Pediatr 1970; 77:1–10.

▪: MRI APPEARANCE OF MARROW DEVELOPMENT IN THE THORAX, PELVIS, AND EXTREMITIES
- ACR Code: 4 (Skeletal Marrow Development)

Technique ▪

MRI was done with an Esatom 5000 machine (manufacturer not given) using T1 (500/20)-weighted spin-echo sequences in three planes.[1]

Measurements ▪

A visual grading system (Table 1) was devised for describing marrow signal intensity and applied to each defined anatomic region. Results were grouped by age and gender. The data were presented as absolute numbers of examinations having a particular grade at each anatomic site. We have calculated percentages (even though some are for small numbers) as this seemed to be somewhat easier to apply clinically. Tables 2, 3, and 4 list the results (as percentages) for the thorax and shoulder, pelvis, and proximal femur. Table 5 lists results in the upper and lower extremities by segment.[1]

Table 1 ▪ MRI Signal Intensity Grading System

GRADE	SIGNAL INTENSITY
1	≤Muscle
2	>Muscle>,<<Fat
3	>Muscle<Fat
4	=Fat

From Taccone A, Oddone M, Dell'Acqua AD, et al: Pediatr Radiol 1995; 25(8):596–606. Used by permission.

Table 2 ▪ Thoracic Wall and Shoulder Bone Marrow of 122 Patients According to Signal Intensity, Gender, and Age

		AGE (yr)										
		0–1		1–3		4–6		7–10		11–15		16–24	
	GRADE	M	F	M	F	M	F	M	F	M	F	M	F
Chest wall:													
Sternal manubrium	1	93	100	17	50			60	75	45	50	100	
	2	7		83	50	100	100	40	25	35	50	0	100
	3												
	4												
Ribs	1	93	80	30									
	2	7	20	50	100	100	100	50	71	33			
	3			20				50	29	67	100	100	100
	4												
Scapular body	1	57	80	14									
	2	36	20	57	57	33	50	44	40	33			
	3	7		29	43	67	50	56	60	67	100	100	
	4												
Proximal humerus:													
Epiphysis	1	50	75										
	2	29		13									
	3	21	25	75	100	86	50	50	20	43		33	
	4			13			14	50	80	57	100	67	100
Metaphysis	1	92	100	17	29		25	18					
	2	8		83	71	100	75	36	86	43			
	3							45	14	57	100	100	100
	4												
Proximal diaphysis	1	42	75	14	100	100	50	55	33	43			
	2	33	25	86			50	45	67	57	100	100	100
	3												
	4												
Total patients		14	5	7	9	4		14	12	23	14	17	3

All numbers except bottom row are percentages for each age and gender group within each structure.
From Taccone A, Oddone M, Dell'Acqua AD, et al: Pediatr Radiol 1995; 25(8):596–606. Used by permission.

Table 3 ▪ Pelvic Marrow of 121 Patients According to Signal Intensity, Gender, and Age

| | | AGE (yr) | | | | | | | | | | | |
| | | 0–1 | | 1–3 | | 4–6 | | 7–10 | | 11–15 | | 16–24 | |
	GRADE	M	F	M	F	M	F	M	F	M	F	M	F
Pelvis:													
Posterior ilium	1												
	2	100	100	63	71	11		13	21			25	18
	3			38	29	89	100	87	79	100	100	75	82
	4												
Anterior ilium	1												
	2	89	89										
	3	11	11	88	86	78	100	53	50	27	50	50	73
	4			13	14	22		47	50	73	50	50	27
Acetabulum	1	44	33										
	2	44	56	13	43								
	3	11	11	50	43	78	100	73	79	82	92	88	91
	4			38	14	22		27	21	18	8	13	9
Ischium	1	22	22										
	2	78	78	63	64	11		13	14				
	3			38	36	89	100	87	86	91	92	75	82
	4									9	8	25	18
Pubis	1	11	22										
	2	89	78	63	71	22	100	20	29	0	0	13	9
	3			38	29	78		80	71	82	83	63	64
	4									18	17	25	27
Sacrum	1												
	2	100	100	25	57			13	14			13	27
	3			75	43	100	100	87	86	100	100	88	73
	4												
Total patients		9	9	8	14	9	1	15	14	11	12	8	11

All numbers except bottom row are percentages for each age and gender group within each structure.
From Taccone A, Oddone M, Dell'Acqua AD, et al: Pediatr Radiol 1995; 25(8):596–606. Used by permission.

Table 4 ▪ Proximal Femoral Marrow of 121 Patients According to Signal Intensity, Gender, and Age

| | | AGE (yr) | | | | | | | | | | | |
| | | 0–1 | | 1–3 | | 4–6 | | 7–10 | | 11–15 | | 16–24 | |
	GRADE	M	F	M	F	M	F	M	F	M	F	M	F
Proximal femur:													
Epiphysis	1	75	44										
	2		22										
	3	25	33	25	29								
	4			75	71	100	100	100	100	100	100	100	100
Metaphysis	1	100	100	25	21								
	2			75	79	100	100	100	100	55	50	33	55
	3									45	50	56	45
	4											11	0
Proximal diaphysis	1												
	2	100	100	63	57	33	100						
	3			38	43	67	0	100	100	73	83	100	100
	4									27	17		
Greater trochanter	1												
	2	100	100	100	100								
	3												
	4					100	100	100	100	100	100	100	100
Total patients		9	9	8	14	9	1	15	14	11	12	8	11

All numbers except bottom row are percentages for each age and gender group within each structure.[1]
From Taccone A, Oddone M, Dell'Acqua AD, et al: Pediatr Radiol 1995; 25(8):596–606. Used by permission.

Table 5 ▪ Upper and Lower Extremity Marrow According to Signal Intensity, Gender, and Age

AGE GROUP	0–12 MON				2– YR				6–10 YR			11–15 YR			16–24 YR		
GRADE	1	2	3	4	1	2	3	4	1&2	3	4	1&2	3	4	1&2	3	4
Epiphyses:																	
Humeral capitellum			50	50				100			100			100			100
Olecranon			25	75				100			100			100			100
Distal radius							50	50			100			100			100
Metacarpophalangeal							25	75			100			100			100
Distal femur	33	8	25	33				100			100			100			100
Proximal tibia	33	8	25	33				100			100			100			100
Distal tibia			100					100			100			100			100
Metatarsophalangeal								100			100			100			
Metaphyses:																	
Distal humerus	75	25			100					100			50	50			100
Proximal radius	100				17	67	17				100			100			100
Distal radius						75	25				100			100			
Metacarpophalangeal								100			100			100			100
Distal femur	75	25			13	69	19		26	74			44	56		13	87
Proximal tibia	75	25			13	75	13			79	21		11	89			100
Distal tibia	100					100					100			100			
Metatarsophalangeal			100					100			100			100			
Diaphyses:																	
Humerus		50	50			33	67				100			100			100
Radius			100			22	78			20	80			100			100
Metacarpophalangeal								100			100			100			100
Femur		33	67			19	81			16	84			100			100
Tibia		31	62	8		16	63	21		5	95			100			100
Metatarsophalangeal			100					100			100			100			100
Round bones:																	
Capitate								100			100			100			100
Talus			38	63				100			100			100			100
Calcaneus			38	63				100			100			100			100
Patella					15	8	15	62		11	89			100			100

All numbers are percentages for each age and gender group within each structure.
From Taccone A, Oddone M, Dell'Acqua AD, et al: Pediatr Radiol 1995; 25(8):596–606. Used by permission.

Source ▪

A retrospective study of 122 MRI examinations of the thoracic wall and shoulder, 131 pelvic and proximal femur examinations, and 128 studies of the upper and lower extremities. Patient age ranged from 7 days to 25 years. None of the subjects had any history or findings of disease processes that would alter the normal marrow development.[1]

Comments ▪

These "road maps" provide a good overview of the age-related change from red to yellow marrow in the appendicular skeleton.

Reference

1. Taccone A, Oddone M, Dell'Acqua AD, et al: MRI "road-map" of normal age-related bone marrow. II. Thorax, pelvis and extremities. Pediatr Radiol 1995; 25(8):596–606.

⠐⠂ SKELETAL MATURATION: METHOD OF SONTAG, SNELL, AND ANDERSON[1]

■ ACR Code: 4 (Skeletal Maturation)

Technique ■

Roentgenograms are taken of the following areas of the left side of the body: shoulder, elbow, wrist and hand, hip, knee (anteroposterior; lateral after 24 months), ankle and foot (anteroposterior; lateral after 48 months).

Measurements (Tables 1 and 2) ■

The total number of ossification centers in the left half of the body is counted. A center is counted as soon as it casts a small shadow on the roentgenogram.

Source ■

These data have been taken from roentgenograms made at regular intervals of all the bones and joints of the left upper and lower extremities of 149 normal children during their first 5 years of life. The children came from the rural and metropolitan area near Yellow Springs, Ohio. There were 75 boys and 74 girls, and they represented a fair economic cross-section. Three black children (1 boy and 2 girls) were included.

REFERENCE

1. Sontag LW, Snell D, Anderson M: Am J Dis Child 1939; 58:949.

Table 1 ■ List of Centers (Total, 67)

Shoulder
 Coracoid process
Humerus
 Proximal medial epiphysis
 Proximal lateral epiphysis
 Capitellum
 Medial epicondyle
Radius
 Proximal epiphysis
 Distal epiphysis
Hand
 Capitatum
 Hamatum
 Triquetrum
 Lunate
 Navicular
 Greater multangular bone
 Lesser multangular bone
 5 distal phalangeal epiphyses
 4 middle phalangeal epiphyses
 5 proximal phalangeal epiphyses
 5 metacarpal epiphyses

Femur
 Proximal epiphysis
 Greater trochanter
 Distal epiphysis
Knee
 Patella
Tibia
 Proximal epiphysis
 Distal epiphysis
Fibula
 Proximal epiphysis
 Distal epiphysis
Foot
 Cuboid
 First cuneiform
 Second cuneiform
 Third cuneiform
 Navicular
 Epiphysis of calcaneus
 5 distal phalangeal epiphyses
 4 middle phalangeal epiphyses
 5 proximal phalangeal epiphyses
 5 metatarsal epiphyses

Table 2 ■ Mean Total Number of Centers on the Left Side of Body Ossified at Given Age Levels

AGE (IN MON)	BOYS		GIRLS	
	Mean No.	SD	Mean No.	SD
1	4.11	1.41	4.58	1.76
3	6.63	1.86	7.78	2.16
6	9.61	1.95	11.44	2.53
9	11.88	2.66	15.36	4.92
12	13.96	3.96	22.40	6.93
18	19.27	6.61	34.10	8.44
24	29.21	8.10	43.44	6.65
30	37.59	7.40	48.91	6.50
36	43.42	5.34	52.73	5.48
42	47.06	5.26	56.61	3.98
48	51.24	4.59	57.94	3.91
54	53.94	4.35	59.89	3.36
60	56.24	4.07	61.52	2.69

⁚ SKELETAL MATURATION: METHOD OF GIRDANY AND GOLDEN[1]
▪ ACR Code: 4 (Skeletal Maturation)

Technique ▪

Conventional technique for each body part.

Measurements ▪

The numbers on Figures 1 and 2 indicate the range from the 10th to the 90th percentile in appearance time of centers of ossification, obtained from the studies on bone growth available in 1950. Statistically significant studies of the time of appearance of ossification centers have been made of relatively few portions of the skeleton after the 6th year of life. Figures followed by *m* mean months; otherwise all numbers indicate years. Where two sets of numbers are given for one center of ossification, the upper figures refer to males and the lower figures refer to females. A single set of figures applies to both sexes. *AB* indicates that the ossification center is visible at birth. Figures in parentheses give approximate time of fusion.

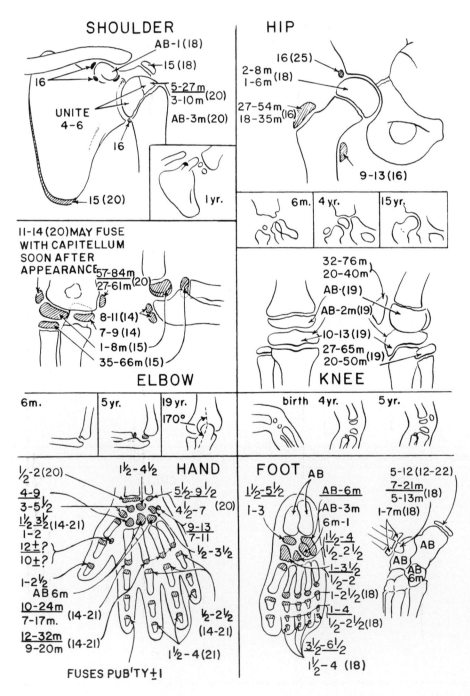

Figure 1 ▪ (From Girdany BR, Golden R: AJR Am J Roentgenol 1952; 68:922. Used by permission.)

VERTEBRA

OSSIFY FROM 3 PRIMARY CENTERS AND 9 SECONDARY CENTERS – ANY OF THESE SECONDARY CENTERS, EXCEPT FOR ANNULAR EPIPHYSES, MAY FAIL TO FUSE.

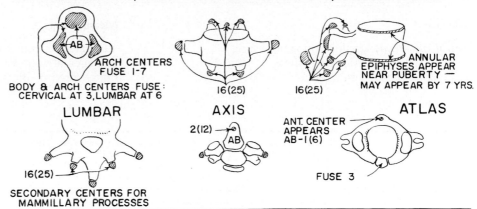

ARCH CENTERS FUSE 1-7

BODY & ARCH CENTERS FUSE: CERVICAL AT 3, LUMBAR AT 6

16(25)

16(25)

ANNULAR EPIPHYSES APPEAR NEAR PUBERTY – MAY APPEAR BY 7 YRS.

LUMBAR

AXIS

ATLAS

2(12)

ANT. CENTER APPEARS AB-1(6)

16(25)

SECONDARY CENTERS FOR MAMMILLARY PROCESSES

FUSE 3

SACRUM & COCCYX

LOWER SACRAL BODIES FUSE AT 18 ··· ALL FUSE BY 30

INNOMINATE

Figure 2 ▪ (From Girdany BR, Golden R: AJR Am J Roentgenol 1952; 68:922. Used by permission.)

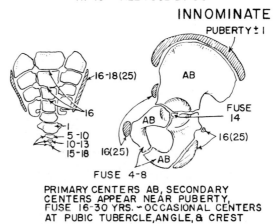

PUBERTY ± 1

AB

16-18(25)

16

1
5-10
10-13
15-18

AB

AB

FUSE 14

16(25)

16(25)

AB

FUSE 4-8

PRIMARY CENTERS AB, SECONDARY CENTERS APPEAR NEAR PUBERTY, FUSE 16-30 YRS. – OCCASIONAL CENTERS AT PUBIC TUBERCLE, ANGLE, & CREST

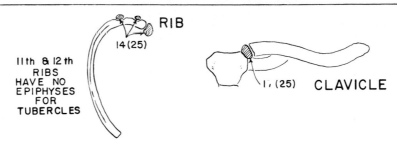

RIB

14(25)

11th & 12th RIBS HAVE NO EPIPHYSES FOR TUBERCLES

17 (25)

CLAVICLE

Source ▪

The figures giving the range of time of appearance of the most important ossification centers have been adapted from multiple sources, including

Scammon RE, in (Schaeffer JP (ed): Morris' Human Anatomy, ed 11. Blakiston Company, Philadelphia, 1953, p 11.

Vogt EC, Vickers VS: Radiology 1938; 31:441.

Milman DH, Bakwin H: J Pediatr 1950; 36:617.

Buehl CC, Pyle SI: J Pediatr 1942; 21:331.

Ruckensteiner E: Die normale Entwicklung des Knochensystems im Roentgenbilg. Georg Thieme, Leipzig, 1931.

Bailey W: AJR Am J Roentgenol 1939; 42:85.

REFERENCE

1. Girdany BR, Golden R: AJR Am J Roentgenol 1952; 68:922.

▪⫶ SKELETAL MATURATION: METHOD OF GRAHAM[1]

▪ ACR Code: 4 (Skeletal Maturation)

Technique ▪

Central ray: Perpendicular to plane of film.
Position: Anteroposterior and lateral.
Target-film distance: Immaterial.

Measurements ▪

The selected examinations that yield the most data at various ages are shown in Figure 1. The age-at-appearances for selected ossification centers is shown in Table 1. This

Table 1 ▪ Age-at-Appearance (years, months) Percentiles for Selected Ossification Centers*

CENTERS	BOYS			GIRLS		
	5th	50th	95th	5th	50th	95th
Humerus, head	—	0–0	0–4	—	0–0	0–4
Tibia, proximal	—	0–0	0–1	—	0–0	0–0
Coracoid process of scapula	—	0–0	0–4	—	0–0	0–5
Cuboid	—	0–1	0–4	—	0–1	0–2
Capitate	—	**0–3**	**0–7**	—	**0–2**	**0–7**
Hamate	**0–0**	**0–4**	**0–10**	—	**0–2**	**0–7**
Capitellum of humerus	**0–1**	**0–4**	**1–1**	**0–1**	**0–3**	**0–9**
Femur, head	**0–1**	**0–4**	**0–8**	**0–0**	**0–4**	**0–7**
Cuneiform 3	**0–1**	**0–6**	**1–7**	—	**0–3**	**1–3**
Humerus, greater tuberosity	**0–3**	**0–10**	**2–4**	**0–2**	**0–6**	**1–2**
Toe phalanx 5M	—	1–0	3–10	—	0–9	2–1
Radius, distal	0–6	1–1	2–4	0–5	0–10	1–8
Toe phalanx 1 D	0–9	1–3	2–1	0–5	0–9	1–8
Toe phalanx 4 M	0–5	1–3	2–11	0–5	0–11	3–0
Finger phalanx 3 P	0–9	1–4	2–2	0–5	0–10	1–7
Toe phalanx 3 M	0–5	1–5	4–3	0–3	1–0	2–6
Finger phalanx 2 P	0–9	1–5	2–2	0–5	0–10	1–8
Finger phalanx 4 P	0–10	1–6	2–5	0–5	0–11	1–8
Finger phalanx 1 D	0–9	1–6	2–8	0–5	1–0	1–9
Toe phalanx 3 P	0–11	1–7	2–6	0–6	1–1	1–11
Metacarpal 2	0–11	1–7	2–10	0–8	1–1	1–8
Toe phalanx 4 P	0–11	1–8	2–8	0–7	1–3	2–1
Toe phalanx 2 P	1–0	1–9	2–8	0–8	1–2	2–1
Metacarpal 3	0–11	1–9	3–0	0–8	1–2	1–11
Finger phalanx 5 P	1–0	1–10	2–10	0–8	1–2	2–1
Finger phalanx 3 M	1–0	2–0	3–4	0–8	1–3	2–4
Metacarpal 4	1–1	2–0	3–7	0–9	1–3	2–2
Toe phalanx 2 M	0–11	2–0	4–1	0–6	1–2	2–3
Finger phalanx 4 M	1–0	2–1	3–3	0–8	1–3	2–5
Metacarpal 5	1–3	2–2	3–10	0–10	1–4	2–4
Cuneiform 1	**0–11**	**2–2**	**3–9**	**0–6**	**1–5**	**2–10**
Metatarsal 1	1–5	2–2	3–1	1–0	1–7	2–3
Finger phalanx 2 M	1–4	2–2	3–4	0–8	1–4	2–6
Toe phalanx 1 P	1–5	2–4	3–4	0–11	1–7	2–6
Finger phalanx 3 D	1–4	2–5	3–9	0–9	1–6	2–8
Triquetrum	0–6	2–5	5–6	0–3	1–8	3–9
Finger phalanx 4 D	1–4	2–5	3–9	0–9	1–6	2–10
Toe phalanx 5 P	1–6	2–5	3–8	1–0	1–9	2–8
Metacarpal 1	1–5	2–7	4–4	0–11	1–7	2–8
Cuneiform 2	**1–2**	**2–8**	**4–3**	**0–10**	**1–10**	**3–0**
Metatarsal 2	1–11	2–10	4–4	1–3	2–2	3–5
Femur, greater trochanter	1–11	3–0	4–4	1–0	1–10	3–0
Finger phalanx 1 P	1–10	3–0	4–7	0–11	1–9	2–10
Navicular of foot	**1–1**	**3–0**	**5–5**	**0–9**	**1–11**	**3–7**
Finger phalanx 2 D	1–10	3–2	5–0	1–1	2–6	3–3
Finger phalanx 5 D	2–1	3–3	5–0	1–0	2–0	3–5
Finger phalanx 5 M	1–11	3–5	5–10	0–11	2–0	3–6
Fibula, proximal	**1–10**	**3–6**	**5–3**	**1–4**	**2–7**	**3–11**
Metatarsal 3	2–4	3–6	5–0	1–5	2–6	3–8
Toe phalanx 5 D	2–4	3–11	6–4	1–2	2–4	4–1
Patella	**2–7**	**4–0**	**6–0**	**1–6**	**2–6**	**4–0**
Metatarsal 4	2–11	4–0	5–9	1–9	2–10	4–1
Lunate	1–6	4–1	6–9	1–1	2–7	5–8
Toe phalanx 3 D	3–0	4–4	6–2	1–4	2–9	4–1

Table 1 ■ Age-at-Appearance (years, months) Percentiles for Selected Ossification Centers* *Continued*

	BOYS			GIRLS		
CENTERS	5th	50th	95th	5th	50th	95th
Metatarsal 5	3–1	4–4	6–4	2–1	3–3	4–11
Toe phalanx 4 D	2–11	4–5	6–5	1–4	2–7	4–1
Toe phalanx 2 D	3–3	4–8	6–9	1–6	2–11	4–6
Radius, head	**3–0**	**5–3**	**8–0**	**2–3**	**3–10**	**6–3**
Navicular of wrist	3–7	5–8	7–10	2–4	4–1	6–0
Greater multangular	3–6	5–10	9–0	1–11	4–1	6–4
Lesser multangular	3–1	6–3	8–6	2–5	4–2	6–0
Medial epicondyle of humerus	**4–3**	**6–3**	**8–5**	**2–1**	**3–5**	**5–1**
Ulna, distal	5–3	7–1	9–1	3–3	5–4	7–8
Calcaneal apophysis	**5–2**	**7–7**	**9–7**	**3–6**	**5–4**	**7–4**
Olecranon of ulna	**7–9**	**9–8**	**11–11**	**5–7**	**8–0**	**9–11**
Lateral epicondyle of humerus	**9–3**	**11–3**	**13–8**	**7–2**	**9–3**	**11–3**
Tibial tubercle	**9–11**	**11–10**	**13–5**	**7–11**	**10–3**	**11–10**
Adductor sesamoid of thumb	11–0	12–9	14–7	8–8	10–9	12–8
Os acetabulum	11–11	13–6	15–4	9–7	11–6	13–5
Acromion	**12–2**	**13–9**	**15–6**	**10–4**	**11–11**	**13–9**
Iliac crest	**12–0**	**14–0**	**15–11**	**10–10**	**12–9**	**15–4**
Coracoid apophysis	**12–9**	**14–4**	**16–4**	**10–4**	**12–3**	**14–4**
Ischial tuberosity	**13–7**	**15–3**	**17–1**	**11–9**	**13–11**	**16–0**

*P = proximal, M = middle, D = distal.
Adapted from Garn SM, et al: Med Radiogr Photogr 1967; 43:45–66.

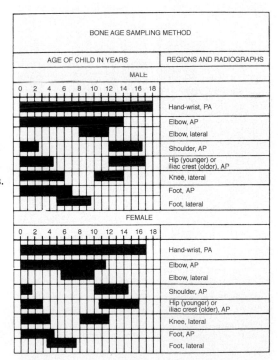

Figure 1 ■ Suggested films for determination of osseous maturation at various ages. (From Graham CB: Radiol Clin North Am 1972; 10:185. Used by permission.)

table is derived from Garn and colleagues[2] and modified to be more useful. Important "happenings" at various age levels are boldfaced. These data are based on a white population. American black and Hong Kong Chinese infants are relatively slightly advanced.

Source ■

Data derived by Garn and colleagues in the Fels Research Institute Program of Human Development were based on a study of 143 healthy, middle-class Ohio-born children of Northwestern European ancestry.

References

1. Graham CB: Assessment of bone maturation—methods and pitfalls. Radiol Clin North Am 1972; 10:185–202.
2. Garn SM, Rohmann CG, Silverman FN: Radiographic standards for postnatal ossification and tooth calcification. Med Radiogr Photogr 1967; 43:45–66.

˙: STANDARDS FOR LIMB BONE LENGTH RATIOS IN CHILDREN
▪ ACR Code: 4 (Skeletal Maturation)

Technique ▪

Central ray: Perpendicular to plane of film centered over midlimb.
Position: Anteroposterior or posteroanterior.
Target-film distance: 7½ feet (228.6.cm) to eliminate magnification.

Measurement (Figure 1) ▪

From age 0 to 2 months to 12 years, the length of the limbs was measured parallel to the long axis of the most proximal edge to the most distal edge of the diaphysis. From 10 years through adolescence, length measurements were made from the most proximal edge of the epiphysis

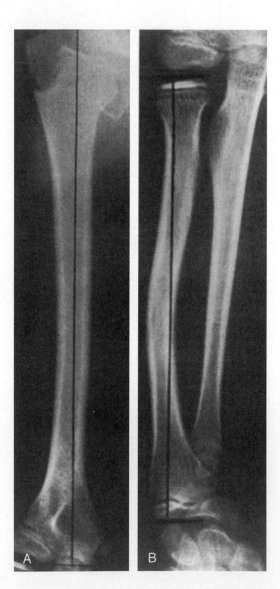

Figure 1 ▪ Guidelines for measuring total bone lengths in humerus *(A)* and radius *(B)*. (From Robinow M, Chumlea WC: Radiology 1982; 143:433. Used by permission.)

Table 1 ▪ Diaphyseal Bone Length Ratios

BONE RATIO	AGE (yr)	NO.	MEAN	SD	PERCENTILE				
					5	10	50	90	95
Radius / Humerus	0.2–0.49	134	0.82	0.04	0.77	0.78	0.82	0.87	0.89
	0.5–0.99	132	0.79	0.03	0.74	0.75	0.78	0.83	0.85
	1.0–1.49	45	0.77	0.03	0.73	0.74	0.77	0.81	0.82
	1.5–1.99	123	0.76	0.02	0.72	0.73	0.76	0.79	0.80
	2.0–9.99	218	0.75	0.02	0.71	0.72	0.74	0.77	0.78
	10.0–15.0	170	0.75	0.02	0.71	0.72	0.75	0.78	0.78
Tibia / Femur	0.2–0.49	133	0.81	0.04	0.75	0.77	0.82	0.86	0.87
	0.5–0.99	132	0.81	0.03	0.76	0.77	0.81	0.84	0.85
	1.0–1.49	45	0.81	0.02	0.78	0.78	0.81	0.83	0.83
	1.5–1.99	124	0.81	0.02	0.78	0.78	0.81	0.84	0.84
	2.0–9.99	218	0.81	0.02	0.78	0.78	0.81	0.84	0.85
	10.0–15.0	170	0.82	0.02	0.78	0.79	0.82	0.85	0.86
Humerus / Femur	0.2–0.49	133	0.83	0.05	0.75	0.76	0.83	0.90	0.92
	0.5–0.99	132	0.79	0.03	0.73	0.74	0.79	0.82	0.83
	1.0–1.49	45	0.77	0.02	0.73	0.74	0.77	0.80	0.80
	1.5–1.99	124	0.76	0.02	0.73	0.73	0.76	0.79	0.80
	2.0–9.99	218	0.71	0.03	0.67	0.68	0.71	0.75	0.75
	10.0–15.0	170	0.69	0.02	0.65	0.66	0.69	0.71	0.72
Radius / Tibia	0.2–0.49	134	0.84	0.05	0.77	0.78	0.83	0.90	0.94
	0.5–0.99	132	0.77	0.03	0.72	0.73	0.77	0.81	0.82
	1.0–1.49	45	0.74	0.02	0.69	0.70	0.74	0.77	0.78
	1.5–1.99	123	0.71	0.03	0.67	0.68	0.71	0.75	0.76
	2.0–9.99	218	0.65	0.03	0.61	0.62	0.65	0.69	0.70
	10.0–15.0	170	0.63	0.02	0.59	0.60	0.62	0.65	0.66

From Robinow M, Chumlea WC: Radiology 1982; 143:433. Used by permission.

Table 2 ▪ Total Bone Length Ratios

BONE RATIO	AGE (yr)	NO.	MEAN	SD	PERCENTILE				
					5	10	50	90	95
Radius / Humerus	10.0–15.0	174	0.75	0.02	0.72	0.72	0.74	0.77	0.78
Tibia / Femur	10.0–15.0	174	0.84	0.02	0.80	0.81	0.84	0.87	0.88
Humerus / Femur	10.0–15.0	174	0.67	0.02	0.64	0.65	0.67	0.69	0.70
Radius / Tibia	10.0–15.0	174	0.59	0.02	0.57	0.57	0.60	0.62	0.62

From Robinow M, Chumlea WC: Radiology 1982; 143:433. Used by permission.

at the opposite end. From 10 through 12 years there are, therefore, two sets of measurements.

Tables 1 and 2 show the means and standard deviations for each ratio and respective percentiles. These data are useful in evaluating disproportional limb growth in various types of short-limb dwarfing.

Source ▪

Radiographs made at regular intervals from 2 months to 18 years of all children enrolled in the Child Research Council study, Denver, between 1935 and 1967. All children were white. See Tables 1 and 2 for breakdown of numbers and ages.

REFERENCE

1. Robinow M, Chumlea WC: Standards for limb bone length ratios in children. Radiology 1982; 143:433.

": SKELETAL MATURATION: METHOD OF GREULICH AND PYLE
- ACR Code: 4.127 (Bone Age Determination)

Technique •

Central ray: Perpendicular to plane of film and centered halfway between tips of fingers and distal end of radius.
Position: Posteroanterior.
Target-film distance. Immaterial.

Measurements (Figure 1) •

The patient's film is compared with the standard of the same gender and nearest chronologic age. It is next com-pared with adjacent standards, both older and younger than the one that is of the next chronologic age. For a more detailed comparison, select the standard that superficially appears to resemble the patient's film most closely.

Source •

Each of the standards was selected from 100 films of chil-dren of the same gender and age. The film chosen was selected as the most representative of the central tendency

Text continued on page 329

MALE

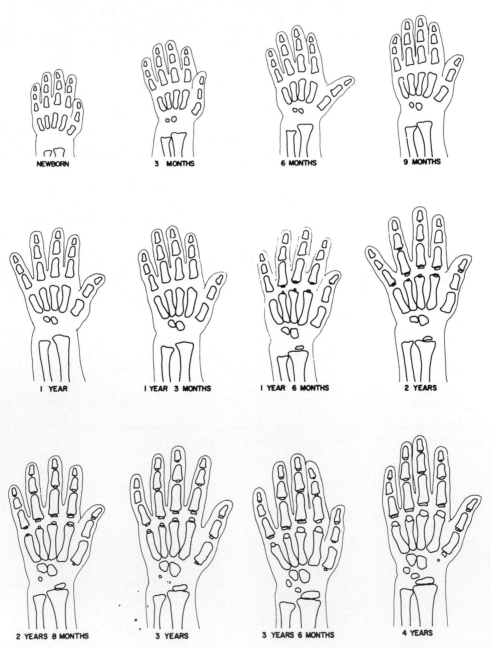

Figure 1 • (Adapted from Greulich WW, Pyle SI: Stanford, CA, Stanford University Press, 1959.)

MALE (continued)

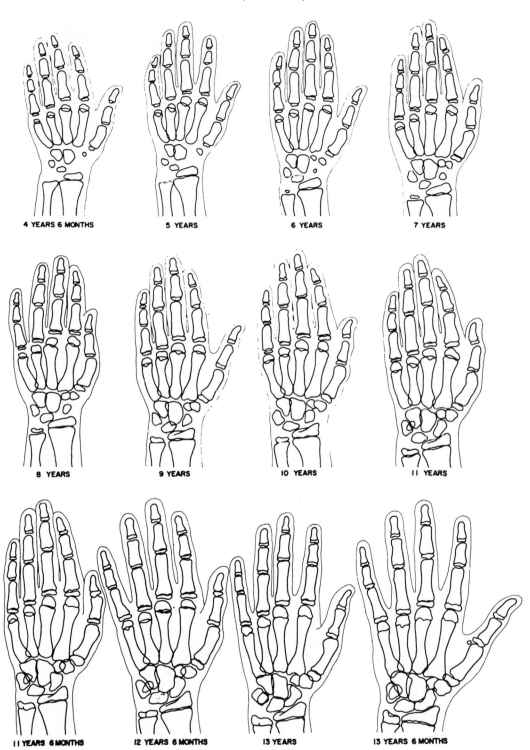

4 YEARS 6 MONTHS **5 YEARS** **6 YEARS** **7 YEARS**

8 YEARS **9 YEARS** **10 YEARS** **11 YEARS**

11 YEARS 6 MONTHS **12 YEARS 6 MONTHS** **13 YEARS** **13 YEARS 6 MONTHS**

Figure 1 ▪ *Continued.*

Illustration continued on following page

MALE (continued)

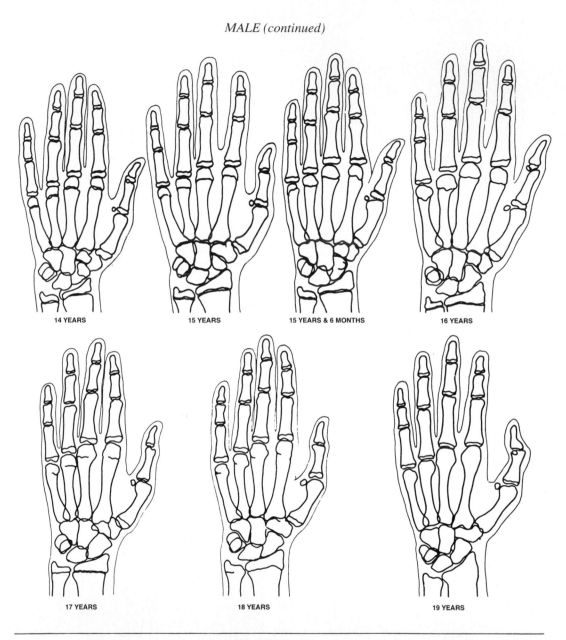

14 YEARS 15 YEARS 15 YEARS & 6 MONTHS 16 YEARS

17 YEARS 18 YEARS 19 YEARS

FEMALE

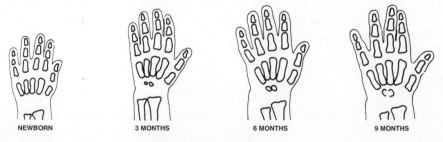

NEWBORN 3 MONTHS 6 MONTHS 9 MONTHS

Figure 1 ▪ *Continued.*

FEMALE (continued)

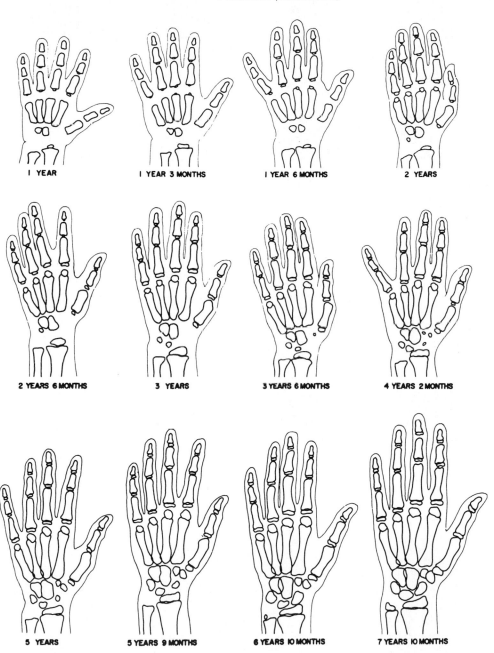

Figure 1 ▪ *Continued.*

Illustration continued on following page

FEMALE *(continued)*

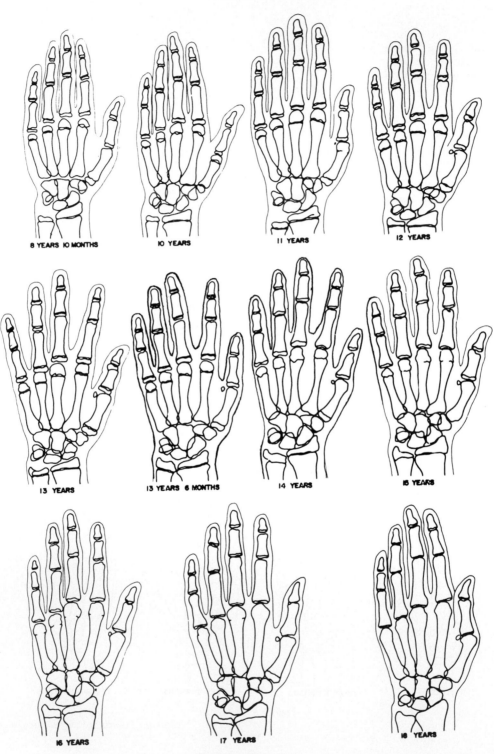

Figure 1 ▪ *Continued.*

of the group. All children were white; all were born in the United States; almost all were of North European ancestry. The entire group included 1000 children.

Note: Pyle, Waterhouse, and Greulich[1] published in 1971 a radiographic reference standard for the assessment of skeletal age from hand-wrist films of children and youths. The reference standard is based in part on the 1959 Greulich and Pyle Atlas that contains one series of reference films for males and another series for females. The new reference standard uses a single series of reference films. The osseous features indicating one and the same skeletal maturity level of each hand-wrist bone appear in the male and female at different chronologic ages. The films in the single film series are calibrated to show the natural chronologic differences between the appearance of the osseous features in males and females.

Studies of skeletal age assessments by research workers using left hand-wrist films and the bone-specific Greulich and Pyle method showed intraobserver differences ranging from 0.25 to 0.47 year. Observer training improves reliability of assessments.[2, 3]

REFERENCES

1. Pyle SI, Waterhouse AM, Greulich WW: A Radiographic Standard of Reference for the Growing Hand and Wrist. The Press of Case Western Reserve University, Cleveland, 1971.
2. Roche AF, Rohmann CG, French NY, Davila GH: Effect of training on replicability of assessments of skeletal maturity (Greulich-Pyle). AJR Am J Roentgenol 1970; 108:511–515.
3. Johnson GF, Dorst JP, Kuhn JP, et al: Reliability of skeletal age assessments. AJR Am J Roentgenol 1973; 118:320–327.

▪: APPLICABILITY OF THE GREULICH AND PYLE BONE AGE STANDARDS
- ACR Code: 4.127 (Bone Age Determination)

Technique ▪

Hand radiographs were obtained in standard fashion.[1]

Measurements ▪

Two experienced observers, blinded to patient age, gender, and ethnicity, compared the radiographs of children under study with the bone age (BA) standards of Greulich and Pyle.[2] The resulting BA determinations were grouped by age (Table 1), gender, and ethnicity and compared with the chronologic age (CA) of the child. The results of these comparisons (mean ± SD of BA–CA) and of paired t tests (p values) are listed in Table 2.

Source ▪

The study group included 294 girls and 471 boys who had hand radiographs for minor trauma and were otherwise healthy. Hand radiographs obtained for other illnesses or to determine bone age were excluded.[1]

Comments ▪

The mean difference of BA determinations between the two observers (47 readings) was 26 days, the correlation was excellent (r = 0.99), and paired t tests yielded p = .4298. Ontell and colleagues concluded that when determining BA using the Greulich and Pyle standards, the age, gender, and ethnicity of the patient should be taken into account. BA determinations were particularly error prone in African-American and Hispanic adolescent girls and Asian and Hispanic adolescent boys.[1] In a previous similarly designed study, Loder and colleagues found that the Greulich and Pyle standards were not applicable to white boys after early childhood, African-American girls of any age, or African-American adolescents.[3]

Table 1 ▪ Age Group Definitions[1]		
GENDER/ AGE GROUP	START AGE (yr/mon)	END AGE (yr/mon)
Boys		
Early childhood	birth	3/9
Middle childhood	3/10	7/6
Late childhood	7/7	13/3
Adolescence	13/4	18
Girls		
Early childhood	birth	3/10
Middle childhood	3/11	8/4
Late childhood	8/5	13/3
Adolescence	13/4	18

Table 2 ▪ Differences Between Chronologic Age and Bone Age Grouped by Gender, Ethnicity, and Age

ETHNICITY/ AGE GROUP	GIRLS			BOYS		
	No.	Difference (Yr) Mean ± SD	p Value	No.	Difference (Yr) Mean ± SD	p Value
White						
Early childhood	15	−0.039 ± 0.406	0.7184	16	−0.317 ± 0.432	0.0101*
Middle childhood	25	−0.037 ± 1.190	0.8788	25	−0.533 ± 0.749	0.0016*
Late childhood	42	0.084 ± 1.127	0.6332	81	−0.669 ± 1.285	<0.0001*
Adolescence	48	0.330 ± 0.974	0.0231	86	0.152 ± 1.201	0.2448
African-American						
Early childhood	18	0.397 ± 0.363	0.0002*	11	0.055 ± 0.527	0.7383
Middle childhood	12	0.000 ± 1.428	0.9999	10	−0.341 ± 0.766	0.1925
Late childhood	15	0.846 ± 1.313	0.0258*	27	0.374 ± 1.181	0.1120
Adolescence	20	0.800 ± 0.963	0.0015*	47	0.413 ± 1.311	0.0359*
Asian						
Early childhood	8	0.143 ± 0.299	0.2183	10	−0.347 ± 0.535	0.0707
Middle childhood	5	−0.074 ± 0.606	0.7993	10	−1.233 ± 1.034	0.0044*
Late childhood	8	0.334 ± 1.061	0.4033	16	−0.397 ± 1.995	0.4386
Adolescence	9	0.520 ± 1.270	0.2541	27	0.788 ± 1.418	0.0078*
Hispanic						
Early childhood	20	−0.144 ± 0.466	0.1826	13	−0.339 ± 0.303	0.0016*
Middle childhood	13	0.482 ± 0.956	0.0941	11	−0.497 ± 0.992	0.1276
Late childhood	19	0.570 ± 1.415	0.0960	32	−0.229 ± 1.312	0.3313
Adolescence	17	0.739 ± 0.926	0.0046*	49	0.956 ± 0.985	<0.0001*

Positive differences indicate that bone age exceeds chronologic age. Negative differences indicate that bone age trails chronologic age. Asterisks (*) next to p values indicate groups to which the Greulich and Pyle standard do not apply well.

From Ontell FK, Ivanovic M, Ablin DS, Barlow TW: AJR Am J Roentgenol 1996; 167:1395–1398. Used by permission.

REFERENCES

1. Ontell FK, Ivanovic M, Ablin DS, Barlow TW: Bone age in children of diverse ethnicity. AJR Am J Roentgenol 1996; 167:1395–1398.
2. Greulich WW, Pyle SL: Radiographic Atlas of Skeletal Development of the Hand and Wrist, 2nd ed. Stanford University Press, Stanford, CA, 1959, pp 61–183.
3. Loder RT, Estle DT, Morrison K, et al: Applicability of the Greulich and Pyle skeletal age standards to black and white children of today. Am J Dis Child 1993; 147:1329–1333.

▪: DETERMINATION OF NEONATAL MATURATION BY TOOTH APPEARANCE ON THE CHEST RADIOGRAPH[1]

▪ ACR Code: 25 (Teeth, Maturation)

Technique ▪

Central ray: Perpendicular to plane of film centered over midchest.
Position: Anteroposterior and lateral.
Target-film distance: Immaterial.

Measurements (Figures 1 and 2) ▪

No second deciduous molar appeared prior to 36 to 37 weeks of gestational age. No first deciduous molar was visibly mineralized before 33 to 34 weeks of gestational age. Tooth age appears to correlate more closely with gestational age than with bone age.

Source ▪

Based on study of 51 white infants of both sexes. All films were taken within 2 days of birth. No difference in tooth development exists between races.

REFERENCE

1. Kuhns LR, Sherman MP, Poznanski AK: Determination of neonatal maturation on the chest radiograph. Radiology 1972; 102:597–603.

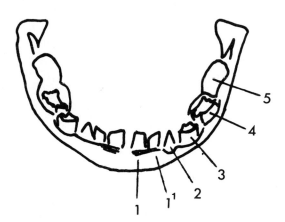

Figure 1 ▪ Tracing of an anteroposterior view of the mandible of a hypothyroid newborn infant. Deciduous teeth are labeled: *1* = central incisors, *1'* = lateral incisor, *2* = lateral incisor (canine), *3* = first molar, *4* = second molar, *5* = follicle of the first permanent molar, the enamel of which is not yet visibly mineralized. (From Kuhns LR, Sherman MP, Poznanski AK: Radiology 1972; 102:597. Used by permission.)

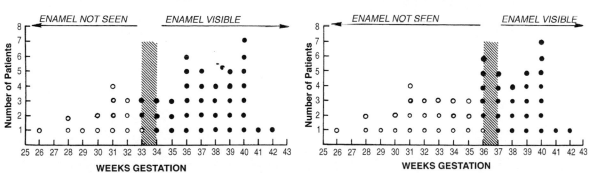

Figure 2 ▪ Summary of first and second deciduous molar mineralization. (From Kuhns LR, Sherman MP, Poznanski AK: Radiology 1972; 102:597. Used by permission.)

": DEVELOPMENT OF THE TEETH
- ACR Code: 25 (Teeth, Maturation)

See Figure 1[1] and Table 1.[2]

REFERENCES

1. Schour I, Poncher H: Publication copyright 1940 and 1945 by Mead Johnson & Company.

2. Pendergrass EP, Schaeffer JP, Hodes P: The Head and Neck in Roentgen Diagnosis. Charles C Thomas, Springfield, IL, 1956, vol 1, p 442.

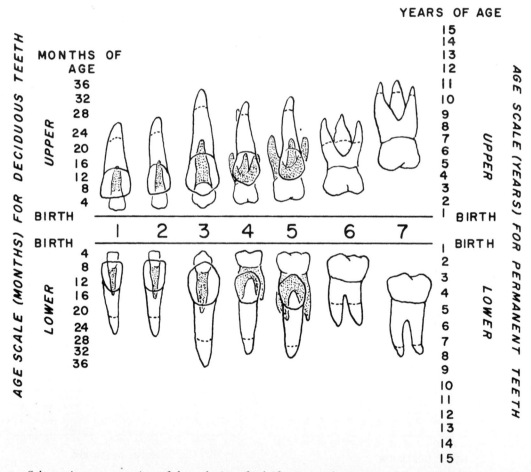

Figure 1 • Schematic representation of the velocity of calcification and eruption of the teeth. The position of the biting edge of the crowns in the age scale indicates the age at which calcification of each tooth begins. Dotted lines on the roots signify the age at which each tooth erupts and its approximate size at that time. The position of the ends of the roots on the age scale measures the age at which calcification of each tooth is completed. The third permanent molar is not shown because of its great normal developmental variation. It usually begins to calcify between ages 7 and 10, erupts between ages 17 and 21, and completes calcification between ages 18 and 25. Deciduous teeth are *shaded*; permanent teeth are *unshaded*. (Adapted from Schour I, Poncher H: Publication copyright 1940 and 1945 by Mead Johnson & Company.)

Table 1 • Approximate Periods of Eruption

DECIDUOUS TEETH	ERUPTION OCCURS	SHEDDING BEGINS
Medial incisors	6–8 mon	7th yr
Lateral incisors	7–12 mon	8th yr
First molars	14–15 mon	10th yr
Canines	18–19 mon	10th yr
Second molars	20–24 mon	11th–12th yr

PERMANENT TEETH	YEAR ERUPTION OCCURS	
	Girls	Boys
First molars	6.0	6.5
Medial incisors	6.5	7.0
Lateral incisors	8.0	8.5
First premolars	9.0	10.0
Second premolars	10.0	11.0
Canines	11.0	11.5
Second molars	11.5	12.0
Third molars	17–25	17–25

From Pendergrass EP, Schaeffer JP, Hodes P: Charles C Thomas, Publisher, Springfield, IL, 1956, vol 1, p 442. Used by permission.

∴ HAND MEASUREMENTS FOR DETECTION OF GONADAL DYSGENESIS
■ ACR Code: 43 (Hand, Maturation)

Metacarpal Sign[1] ■

The Carpal Sign[2] ■

Phalangeal Sign[3] ■

Technique

Central ray: Perpendicular to plane of film centered over palm.
Projection: Posteroanterior.
Target-film distance: Immaterial.

Measurements

Metacarpal sign (Figure 1): A line drawn tangentially to the distal end of the heads of the fifth and fourth metacarpals extends distally to the head of the third metacarpal. A positive sign is present when the line passes through the head of the third metacarpal. When the line is tangential to the head of the third metacarpal, the sign is considered borderline. A positive metacarpal sign, while not diagnostic in itself, is an accessory sign of gonadal dysgenesis to be correlated with other radiographic and clinical findings. It has no significance when detectable in more than one generation.

The *carpal sign* (Figure 2): Two tangents are drawn, the first touching the proximal contour of the navicular and lunate bones and the second touching the triangular and lunate bones. In normal subjects, a value of 131.5° is obtained. In patients with gonadal dysgenesis, the carpal angle is 117° or less.

The *phalangeal sign* (Figure 3): Comparison of the length of the fourth metacarpal with the total length of the distal plus proximal phalanges of the fourth finger in normal subjects indicates equal dimensions of these bones; the differences do not exceed 2 mm. In some cases of gonadal aplasia, the total height of the distal and proximal phalanges

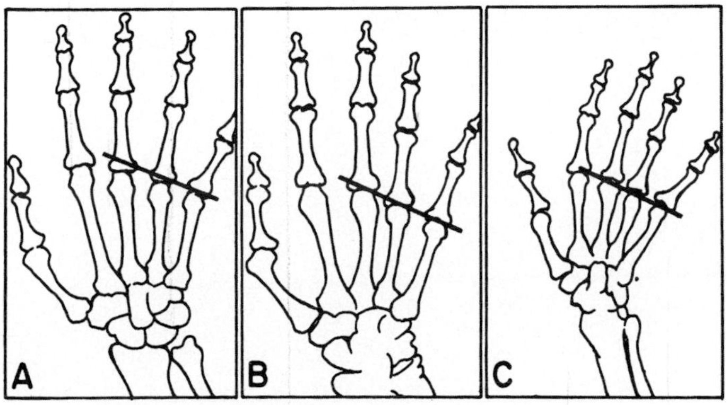

The Carpal Sign†

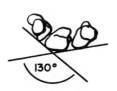

NORMAL   **TURNER'S SYNDROME**

Figure 2 • Carpal sign. See text for details.[2]

Figure 1 • Metacarpal sign. See text for details.[1]

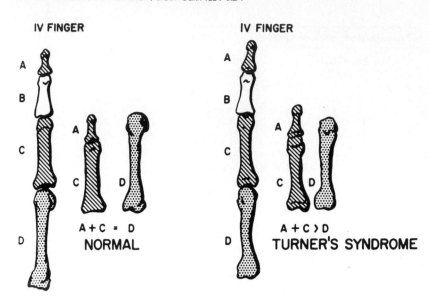

IV FINGER

A + C = D
NORMAL

IV FINGER

A + C ⟩ D
TURNER'S SYNDROME

Figure 3 ▪ Phalangeal sign. See text for details.[3]

exceeds by 3 mm or more the height of the fourth metacarpal.

Source

The metacarpal sign is based on a study of 2594 unselected patients. The carpal and phalangeal signs of Kosowicz are based on measurements of 466 normal subjects.

References

1. Archibald RM, et al: J Clin Endocrinol 1959; 19:1312.
2. Kosowicz J: J Clin Endocrinol 1962; 22:949.
3. Kosowicz J: AJR Am J Roentgenol 1965; 93:354.
4. Keats TE, Burns TW: Radial Clin North Am 1964; 2:297.

⠶ OSSIFICATION AND FUSION OF THE STERNUM
▪ ACR Code: 472 (Sternum, Maturation)

See Figure 1.

Reference

1. Currarino G, Silverman FN: Radiology 1958; 70:532.

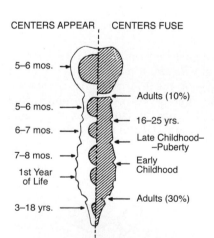

CENTERS APPEAR   CENTERS FUSE

5–6 mos.

5–6 mos.   Adults (10%)

6–7 mos.   16–25 yrs.

                              Late Childhood–
                              –Puberty
7–8 mos.
                              Early
1st Year   Childhood
of Life
                              Adults (30%)
3–18 yrs.

Figure 1 ▪ Sequence of ossification and fusion of the sternum.[1]

CHAPTER 9

Heart and Great Vessels

▪: DISTRIBUTION OF CARDIAC OUTPUT BY VIDEO DILUTION
▪ ACR Code: 5 (Heart and Great Vessels)

Technique ▪

Measurements were carried out at the time of contrast arteriography of the cerebral circulation, upper extremities, lower extremities, or visceral arteries. An initial (reference) injection of 20 to 30 ml of contrast was made into the ascending or upper abdominal aorta via a pigtail catheter. Video fluoroscopy was recorded onto video tape during the injections. For evaluation of flow in branch arteries, injection of 1 to 2 ml of contrast was done via selective catheters in the proximal portion of the vessel under study, and video fluoroscopy was again recorded on video tape during injection.[1]

Measurements ▪

A video densitometer was used to obtain time-density curves over a selected portion of the vessel under study from the video tape made during injection of contrast. The time-density curve was recorded on a strip chart, and the area (A) under the curve was measured with a planimeter. The flow (Q) was calculated by $Q = M/Ak$, where $M =$ the amount of contrast injected and $k =$ the calibration factor. Fractional flow in each vessel was calculated by dividing the flow in each vessel by the flow in the aorta (ascending for head and upper extremity, proximal abdominal for abdominal and iliac branches) obtained from the reference injection. Even though the calibration factor (k) and therefore absolute flows were not determined, the fractional flows were accurate since k cancels out. In a subset of 10 patients, injections were made into both ascending and distal descending aorta and the fractional flow in the descending aorta thus calculated at 0.605. The abdominal and iliac fractional flows were multiplied by this number to normalize them to represent fraction of cardiac output. No attempt was made to quantify coronary flow.[1] Table 1 lists the values obtained as percent of cardiac output.

Source ▪

Subjects included 70 patients with presumed normal regional flow distribution who were examined during the course of routine angiography. Patients were all supine, fasting, and awake. Demerol (50 mg IM) was given prior to the study in those having cerebral angiography.[1]

Comments ▪

The method has been validated in a hydrodynamic flow model and with 389 video dilution measurements made in 20 dogs by correlation with an electromagnetic flowmeter. The correlation between measurements in both studies was quite good, with r = 0.99.[2, 3]

Table 1 ▪ Regional Distribution of Cardiac Output by Video Densitometry		
ARTERY	NUMBER	% CO (Mean ± SD)
Above hemidiaphragms		
Common carotid	40	8.5 ± 0.9
Internal carotid	24	5.3 ± 1.0
External carotid	24	3.2 ± 0.4
Subclavian	9	8.1 ± 0.8
Vertebral	5	1.9 ± 0.5
Axillary	7	6.2 ± 0.9
Descending aorta	10	60.5 ± 4.6
Below hemidiaphragms		
Celiac	12	15.7
Hepatic	14	8.8 ± 3.0
Splenic	12	6.9 ± 1.5
Superior mesenteric	15	15.4 ± 2.8
Inferior mesenteric	1	2.0
Renal	26	8.6 ± 0.9
Common iliac	8	6.0 ± 1.3

CO = cardiac output, SD = standard deviation.
From Lantz BMT, Foerster JM, Link DP, Holcroft JW: AJR Am J Roentgenol 1981; 137:903–907. Used by permission.

REFERENCES

1. Lantz BMT, Foerster JM, Link DP, Holcroft JW: Regional distribution of cardiac output: Normal values in man determined by video dilution technique. AJR Am J Roentgenol 1981; 137:903–907.
2. Lantz BMT: Relative flow measured by roentgen videodensitometry in hydrodynamic model. Acta Radiol 1975; 16:503–519.
3. Holcroft JW, Lantz BMT, Link DP, Foerster JM: Video dilution technique accurately measures blood flow. Surg Forum 1980; 31:324–325.

▪: MEASUREMENT OF THE HEART IN CHILDREN (CARDIOTHORACIC INDEX)[1-3]

▪ ACR Code: 51 (Heart)

Technique ▪

Central ray: Perpendicular to plane of film centered over midpoint of chest.

Positions:
1. Bakwin and Bakwin: Anteroposterior erect. No timing according to phase of respiration.
2. Maresh and Washburn: Infants, posteroanterior supine; from age 3 or 3½ years, posteroanterior erect.
3. Lincoln and Spillman: Posteroanterior erect. Moderately deep inspiration.

Target-film distances:
1. Bakwin and Bakwin: 2 meters.
2. Maresh and Washburn: Infants, 1.5 meters (5 feet); from 3 or 3½ years, 2.1 meters (7 feet).
3. Lincoln and Spillman: 6 feet.

Measurements (Fig. 1; Tables 1 through 3) ▪

MRD = Maximum transverse diameter of the right side of the heart, which is a line drawn from the midline of the spine to the most distant point on the right cardiac margin.

MLD = Maximum transverse diameter on the left side of the heart.

ID = Internal diameter of the thorax drawn parallel to the transverse cardiac diameters through the tip of the dome of the right side of the diaphragm. It extends from the right to the left pleural surface.

The total transverse cardiac diameter is the sum of *MRD* and *MLD*. The cardiothoracic index is obtained by dividing the sum of *MRD* and *MLD* by *ID*. Originally, the heart was considered pathologically enlarged when the ratio exceeded 0.50. Experience has demonstrated that there is a consider-

Table 1 ▪ First Year of Life			
AGE RANGE (wk)	NO. OF CASES	MEAN CARDIO-THORACIC INDEX	RANGE (Within 1 SD)
0–3	52	0.55	0.60–0.50
4–7	36	0.58	0.64–0.52
8–15	71	0.57	0.62–0.51
16–23	42	0.57	0.62–0.51
24–31	27	0.56	0.61–0.50
32–39	35	0.56	0.61–0.51
40–47	19	0.54	0.60–0.49
48–55	22	0.53	0.57–0.49

Data from Bakwin H, Bakwin RM: Am J Dis Child 1935; 49:861.

Table 2 ▪ First 6 Years of Life			
AGE (yr)	NO. OF CASES	MEAN CARDIO-THORACIC INDEX	ACTUAL TOTAL RANGE
0–1	357	0.49	0.65–0.39
1–2	211	0.49	0.60–0.39
2–3	183	0.45	0.50–0.39
3–4	152	0.45	0.52–0.40
4–5	87	0.45	0.52–0.40
5–6	33	0.45	0.50–0.40

Data from Maresh MM, Washburn AH: Am J Dis Child 1938; 56:33.

Table 3 ▪ 7 to 12 Years				
AGE (yr)	NO. OF CASES	TOTAL TRANSVERSE DIAMETER OF HEART (cm)	INTERNAL DIAMETER OF THORAX (cm)	NORMAL RANGE
Boys				
7	35	9.2	19.7	0.49–0.43
8	32	9.4	20.5	0.49–0.42
9	35	9.5	21.1	0.49–0.41
10	21	9.8	21.5	0.49–0.43
11	21	9.9	22.0	0.49–0.43
12	19	10.1	23.0	0.46–0.40
Girls				
7	36	9.1	19.3	0.50–0.44
8	32	9.3	20.0	0.50–0.44
9	28	9.5	20.6	0.49–0.43
10	22	9.7	20.9	0.49–0.43
11	24	9.9	22.0	0.49–0.41
12	21	10.4	22.9	0.49–0.41

cm = centimeters.
Data from Lincoln EM, Spillman R: Am J Dis Child 1928; 35:791.

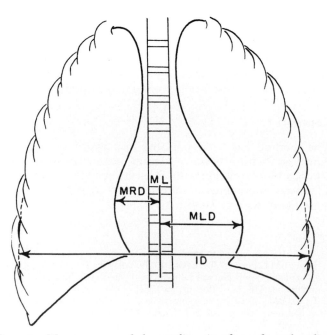

Figure 1 ▪ Measurement of the cardiac size from frontal radiographs in children. See text for details.

able range for the normal values of the cardiothoracic index, the range being widest during the first year of life.

Source ▪

Bakwin and Bakwin:[1] Data based on study of 165 infant boys and 146 infant girls born in Bellevue Hospital. Only infants of white antecedents were studied.

Maresh and Washburn:[2] Data based on study of 38 normal boys and 29 normal girls examined by the Child Research Council every 3 months since birth. One thousand twenty-six roentgenograms were measured.

Lincoln and Spillman:[3] Study made over a period of 7 school years and based on yearly roentgenograms of 246 normal school children.

References

1. Bakwin H, Bakwin RM: Am J Dis Child 1935; 49:861.
2. Maresh MM, Washburn AH: Am J Dis Child 1938; 56:33.
3. Lincoln EM, Spillman R: Am J Dis Child 1928; 35:791.

▪: MEASUREMENT OF THE HEART IN ADULTS (CARDIOTHORACIC RATIO)[1]

▪ ACR Code: 51 (Heart)

Technique ▪

Central ray: Perpendicular to plane of film centered over midportion of chest.
Position: Posteroanterior erect. Breathing suspended in midrespiration.
Target-film distance: 6 feet.

Measurements (Figure 1) ▪

MRD = Maximum transverse diameter of the right side of the heart, which is a line drawn from the midline of the spine to the most distant point on the right cardiac margin.
ML = Midline of the spine.
MLD = Maximum transverse diameter on the left side of the heart.

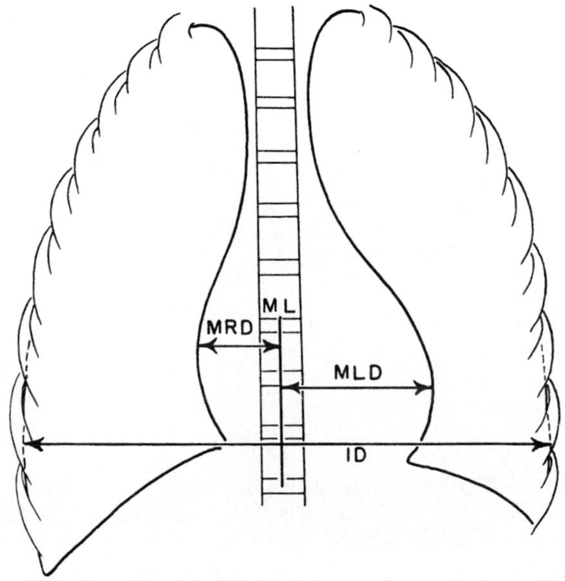

Figure 1 ▪ Measurement of the cardiac size from frontal radiographs in adults. See text for details.

ID = Greatest internal diameter of the thorax, which is usually at the level of the apex or one space lower, measuring the inner borders of the ribs.

The transverse diameter (TD) of the heart = MRD + MLD.

$$\frac{\text{Maximum transverse diameter heart } (TD)}{\text{Maximum transverse diameter thorax } (ID)}$$

The normal heart is usually less than half the greatest diameter of the thorax. The normal cardiothoracic ratio varies between 39% and 50%, with an average of about 45%. Because of variations due to cardiac filling and phase of respiration, a margin of safety of 2% above the upper limit is claimed.

Source ▪

The method was tested on approximately 500 patients. In Danzer's opinion, the results of this test warrant its practicability and usefulness in the estimation of cardiac size, particularly in cases of moderate or early enlargement.

Cardiac Measurements in Systole and Diastole
(Table 1)[2] ▪

1. Two chest films obtained on each of 359 patients.
2. Films taken during systole and diastole.
3. Summary of size changes in the widest transverse measurements of the heart.

Table 1 ▪ Cardiac Size Differences Between Systole and Diastole

DIFFERENCES IN HEART SIZE	NO. OF PATIENTS	PERCENT OF PATIENTS
0.0–0.3 cm	169	52
0.4–0.9 cm	113	41
1.0–1.7 cm	22	7

Cardiac Measurement in the Anteroposterior Projection[3] ▪

A study of the cardiothoracic ratio in erect anteroposterior projection has shown an upper limit of cardiothoracic ratio of 55% and of heart diameter of 165 mm in males and 150 mm in females. These measurements have been shown to provide useful discrimination between normal and abnormal heart size.

REFERENCES

1. Danzer CS: Am J Med Sci 1919; 157:313.
2. Gammill SL, Krebs C, Meyers P, et al: Cardiac measurements in systole and diastole. Radiology 1970; 94:115–120.
3. Kabala JE, Wilde P: The measurement of heart size in the anteroposterior chest radiograph. Br J Radiol 1987; 60:981–986.

▪: MEASUREMENT OF CARDIAC VOLUME
▪ ACR Code: 51 (Heart)

Technique ▪

Central ray: Perpendicular to plane of film centered over midchest.
Position: Posteroanterior in adults and children and anteroposterior or posteroanterior in infants.
Target-film distance: 200 cm, 150 cm, or 100 cm.

Measurements (Figures 1 through 3; Tables 1 through 3) ▪

L = Long diameter. This line extends from the junction of the superior vena cava and right atrium to the cardiac apex.
B = Broad diameter. This line extends from the junction of the right atrium and the diaphragm to a point on the left heart border at the junction of the pulmonary artery and left atrial appendage.

D = Depth. Represents the greatest horizontal depth of the cardiac shadow.

Calculation of cardiac volume is based on the formula:

$$V = L \times B \times D \times K$$

The constant (K) will vary with the focal-film distances used: 200 cm, K = 0.42; 150 cm, K = 0.39; 100 cm, K = 0.38.

The calculated cardiac volume is correlated with body surface area. (The techniques for calculating body surface area are detailed in the first section of chapter 8, p 309.)

The normal heart volumes for infants correlated with body surface area are shown in Figure 3.

For older children and adults, the variation of normal is sufficiently limited that, for practical purposes, it is adequate to divide the calculated volume by the body surface area and compare with normal standards in Table 3.

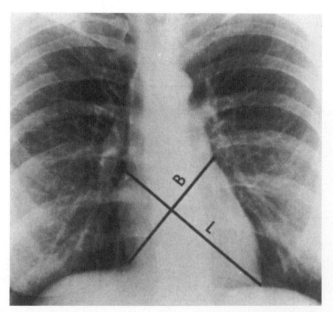

Figure 1 ▪ Measurements for cardiac volume determination from frontal radiograph. (From Keats TE, Enge IP: Radiology 1965; 85:850. Used by permission.)

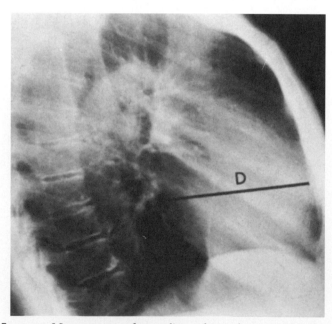

Figure 2 ▪ Measurements for cardiac volume determination from lateral radiograph. (From Keats TE, Enge IP: Radiology 1965; 85:850. Used by permission.)

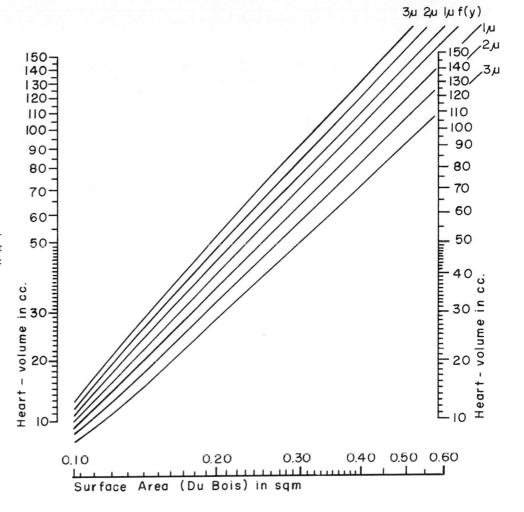

Figure 3 ▪ Predicted normal heart volume compared with calculated heart volumes in infants. (From Lind J: Acta Radiol 1950; suppl 82.

BODY WEIGHT (X) IN POUNDS	CARDIAC VOLUME (Y) OF MALES (cc)			CARDIAC VOLUME (Y) OF FEMALES (cc)		
	Mean	95% Confidence Limits		Mean	95% Confidence Limits	
		Upper Limit	Lower Limit		Upper Limit	Lower Limit
5	27	37	20	29	39	21
10	53	72	40	54	73	39
15	79	107	59	77	105	57
20	104	141	77	101	137	74
25	129	175	95	123	167	91
30	154	209	114	145	197	107
40	204	277	151	189	256	139
50	254	344	187	231	314	170
60	303	411	224	273	370	201
70	352	477	260	314	426	231
80	401	543	296	354	481	261
90	450	610	332	394	535	290
100	498	676	368	434	589	319
110	547	741	404	473	642	348
120	595	807	439	512	695	377
130	644	873	475	550	748	405
140	692	938	510	588	800	433
150	740	1004	545	626	852	461
160	788	1069	580	664	903	489
170	836	1134	616	702	954	516

Table 1 ▪ **Cardiac Volume in Children and Adolescents as Predicted by Body Weight***

*For males $Y = 5.620 \ X^{0.973}$ (linear correlation r = 0.982); for females $Y = 6.628 \ X^{0.907}$ (linear correlation r = 0.980).
From Nghiem QX, Schreiber MH, Harris LC: Circulation 1967; 35:509. Used by permission.

Table 2 ▪ Comparison of Body Surface Area and Body Weight as Predictors of Cardiac Volume*

SAMPLE	NO. OF SUBJECTS	CORRELATION COEFFICIENT (r)	REGRESSION EQUATION	95% CONFIDENCE LIMITS		
				Upper Limit	Lower Limit	% of Mean
Body surface area *(Z)*						
Limited data	261	0.981	$Y = 284Z$	413Z	155Z	±45
Males	132	0.980	$Y = 295Z$	434Z	156Z	±47
Females	129	0.987	$Y = 273Z$	388Z	159Z	±42
Body weight *(X)*						
Limited data	261	0.987	$Y = 5.0X$	6.6X	3.4X	±32
Males	132	0.990	$Y = 5.2X$	6.7X	3.7X	±29
Females	129	0.990	$Y = 4.8X$	6.4X	3.2X	±34
Total data	305	0.985	$Y = 4.9X$	6.6X	3.2X	±34
Males	158	0.985	$Y = 5.1X$	6.8X	3.5X	±32
Females	147	0.989	$Y = 4.7X$	6.3X	3.1X	±34

*The limited data included 261 subjects whose height and weight were known. Y = cardiac volume in cubic cm; X = body weight in pounds; Z = body surface area in square meters.

From Nghiem QX, Schreiber MH, Harris LC: Circulation 1967; 35:509. Used by permission.

Table 3 ▪ Adults: Upper Limits of Normal

$$\frac{\text{HEART VOLUMES}}{\text{BODY SURFACE AREA}} =$$

Females	450–490 cc/m²
Males	500–540 cc/m²

Data from Amundsen P: Acta Radiol 1959, suppl 181.

Cardiac mensuration by volume determination is probably the most accurate method now available.

Source ▪

Nghiem and colleagues studied 305 subjects; 158 were males and 147 were females. Ages ranged from birth to 18 years, 9 months. Body surface area ranged from 0.18 to 1.87 m² and body weight from 6.2 to 167 pounds.[4]

Lind's data on normal heart volumes in infants are based on a study of 293 children under 2 years of age, male and female. All were healthy.[2]

The data on children from 4 to 7, 9 to 12, and 14 to 16 years of age are taken from Carlgren,[5] based on a study of 61 healthy children.

Amundsen's data are based on a study of 87 normal patients (29 males and 58 females).[3]

REFERENCES

1. Keats TE, Enge IP: Cardiac mensuration by the cardiac volume method. Radiology 1965; 85:850–855.
2. Lind J: Acta Radiol 1950; suppl 82.
3. Amundsen P: Acta Radiol 1959, suppl 181.
4. Nghiem QX, Schreiber MH, Harris LC: Cardiac volume in normal children and adolescents. Circulation 1967; 35:509–522.
5. Carlgren LE: Acta Paediatr Scand 1946; 33 (suppl 6).

▪: MEASUREMENT OF CARDIAC STRUCTURES BY CT

▪ ACR Code: 51 (Heart), 56 (Great Vessels)

Technique ▪

1. Varian CT scanner with 3-second scan time. Slice thickness: 10 mm.
2. Scanning was performed in the supine position during suspended moderate inspiration.

3. Studies were performed before and after bolus injection of 20 to 30 ml of Renografin-60 (Squibb).

Measurements (Figure 1 and Table 1) ▪

Structures were measured as the diameter perpendicular to the long axis of a tubular organ (such as aorta or pulmonary

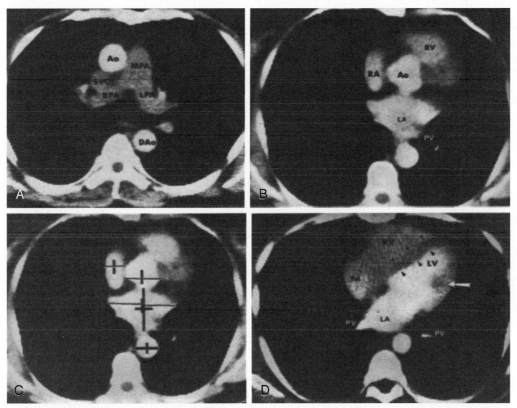

Figure 1 ▪ After contrast administration in different patients 2 to 3 years after bypass graft surgery, with normal hemodynamics and left ventriculogram within 24 hours after study. *A,* Through pulmonary artery bifurcation *(MPA), B,* Plane of section passes through aortic root *(Ao)* and left atrium *(LA)* posteriorly. Low-density fat in pericardial space separates right atrium *(RA)* from aorta. On scans through aortic sinuses *(B),* aorta has cloverleaf configuration. *C* (same as *B*). Location of measurements of right atrium, aortic root, left atrium, and descending aorta. *D,* Through mitral valve. Artifact emanates from sternal wires. Opacified left atrium *(LA)* and left ventricular chamber *(LV)* with protruding papillary muscles *(arrow)* are well seen. Interventricular septum *(arrowheads)* separates right *(RV)* and left *(LV)* ventricles. *RPA* = right pulmonary artery; *LPA* = left pulmonary artery; *SVC* = superior vena cava; *PV* = pulmonary veins; *RA* = right atrium; *RV* = right ventricle; *Ao* = ascending aorta; *DAo* = descending aorta. (From Guthaner DF, et al: AJR Am J Roentgenol 1979; 133:75. Used by permission.)

Table 1 ▪ Cardiac CT Measurements in 15 Normal Patients*

| | SCAN LEVEL | | | | |
STRUCTURE	Arch	Pulmonary Artery Bifurcation	Aortic Root	Mitral Valve	Midventricle
Ascending aorta	3.3 ± 0.6 (N = 4)	3.2 ± 0.5 (N = 12)	3.7 ± 0.3 (N = 12)	—	—
Descending aorta	2.4 ± 0.3 (N = 8)	2.5 ± 0.4 (N = 12)	2.5 ± 0.3 (N = 12)	2.5 ± 0.4 (N = 12)	2.4 ± 0.3 (N = 10)
Arch	1.5 ± 1.2 (N = 6)	—	—	—	—
Right atrium	—	—	1.9 ± 0.8 (N = 12)	3.2 ± 1.2 (N = 12)	2.8 ± 0.4 (N = 6)
Left atrium	—	—	Transverse, 6.6 ± 1.0 (N = 12); AP, 3.8 ± 0.6 (N = 12)	Transverse, 6.9 ± 1.5 (N = 10); AP, 4.0 ± 0.9 (N = 10)	—
Superior vena cava	1.4 ± 0.4 (N = 8)	2.0 ± 0.4 (N = 10)	—	—	—
Main pulmonary artery	—	2.8 ± 0.3 (N = 10)	—	—	—
Left pulmonary artery	—	2.0 ± 0.2 (N = 6)	—	—	—
Right pulmonary artery	—	2.0 ± 0.4 (N = 8)	—	—	—
Right ventricular outflow tract	—	—	2.8 ± 1.1 (N = 10)	—	—
Right ventricle	—	—	—	5.8 ± 1.1 (N = 10)	5.8 ± 1.4 (N = 8)
Interventricular septum	—	—	—	—	0.8 ± 0.6 (N = 6)
Coronary sinus	—	—	—	—	0.9 ± 0.1 (N = 6)
Inferior vena cava	—	—	—	—	2.7 ± 0.6 (N = 5)

*Mean = ± 1 SD; N = number of patients from whom measurements (cm) were taken at the indicated level.
From Guthaner DF, et al: AJR Am J Roentgenol 1979; 133:75. Used by permission.

artery) or the transverse diameter when seen in cross-section.

The widest horizontal diameters of the atria were measured. The longest AP diameter of the left atrium was measured on a line perpendicular to the posterior wall of the aortic root at the level of the pulmonary veins. The right ventricle was measured from the atrioventricular groove at its most anterior extent to the indentation of the right ventricular septum.

Measurements were either by electronic calipers or from hard copies, using appropriate minification correction.

Source ▪

Ten patients without heart disease and with a normal cardiac examination and five patients with normal cardiac catheterization within 24 hours of CT scan, but with a history of aortocoronary bypass surgery 2 or more years earlier.

REFERENCE

1. Guthaner DF, Wexler L, Harell G: CT demonstration of cardiac structures. AJR Am J Roentgenol 1979; 133:75–81.

▪: MEASUREMENT OF THE LEFT ATRIUM ON THE FRONTAL FILM[1]
▪ ACR Code: 522 (Left Atrium)

Technique ▪

Central ray: Centered over midchest, perpendicular to film.
Position: Posteroanterior.
Target-film distance: 182.9 cm.

Measurements (Figure 1 and Table 1) ▪

The left atrium is measured from the midpoint of the curvilinear margin of the double density to the midpoint of the inferior wall of the left bronchus.

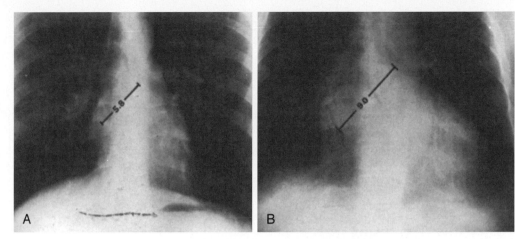

Figure 1 ▪ Measurement of the left atrium. (From Higgins CB, et al: AJR Am J Roentgenol 1978; 130:251. Used by permission.)

Table 1 ▪ Left Atrial Dimension for Normal and Abnormal Groups

GROUP	MALES			FEMALES		
	Mean	SD	Range	Mean	SD	Range
Normal						
Decade 3	6.3	±0.6	5.1–7.4	5.9	±0.6	4.3–7.4
Decade 4	6.1	±0.6	5.0–7.4	6.1	±0.7	5.3–7.1
Decade 5	6.5	±0.9	5.6–7.6	5.8	±0.7	5.2–7.6
Decade 6	5.9	±0.9	5.5–6.6	6.1	±0.8	5.5–6.8
Abnormal	9.1	±1.5	6.6–12.4	8.2	±1.0	6.0–10.4

From Higgins CB, et al: AJR Am J Roentgenol 1978; 130:251. Used by permission.

The measurement is less than 7.0 cm in 98% of normal patients and greater than 7.0 cm in 90% of patients with left atrial enlargement. The measurement is less reliable in children.

Source ▪

One hundred forty-eight normal volunteers and 48 patients in whom there was echocardiographic left atrial enlarge-ment. The study also included 30 pediatric patients with left atrial enlargement secondary to ventricular septal defect.

REFERENCE

1. Higgins CB, Reinke RT, Jones NE, Broderick T: Left atrial dimension on the frontal thoracic radiograph: A method for assessing left atrial enlargement. AJR Am J Roentgenol 1978; 130:251–255.

▪▪ MEASUREMENT OF THE LEFT ATRIUM IN THE LATERAL PROJECTION[1]
▪ ACR Code: 522 (Left Atrium)

Technique ▪

Central ray: Perpendicular to plane of film centered over midpoint of chest.
Position: Upright lateral.
Target-film distance: 6 feet.

Measurements (Figure 1) ▪

To approximate the position of the anterior left atrial wall, a line is drawn downward from the anterior wall of the right pulmonary artery parallel to the long axis of the barium-filled esophagus. The maximum perpendicular dis-

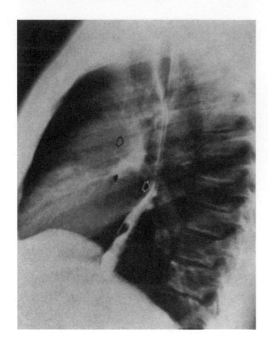

Figure 1 ▪ Measurement of the left atrium in a normal patient. The right pulmonary artery *(open black arrow)* is seen as an oval density anterior to the major bronchi and slightly caudal to the left pulmonary artery *(curved arrow)*. (From Westcott JL, Ferguson P: Radiology 1976; 118:265. Used by permission.)

Table 1 ▪ Left Atrial Diameter (mm)		
	FEMALE	MALE
Normal	<36	<40
Borderline	36–38	40–42
Enlarged	>38	>42

From Westcott JL, Ferguson P: Radiology 1976; 118:265. Used by permission.

tance from the line to the esophagus represents the left atrial diameter. Normal values are given in Table 1.

Source ▪

Data based on study of 82 adult patients.

REFERENCE

1. Westcott JL, Ferguson D: The right pulmonary artery–left atrial axis line. A method for measuring left atrial size on lateral chest radiographs. Radiology 1976; 118:265–274.

▪: MEASUREMENT OF THE INFUNDIBULUM OF THE RIGHT VENTRICLE
▪ ACR Code: 523 (Right Ventricle)

Technique ▪

Central ray: Perpendicular to plane of film centered over midchest.
Projection: True lateral angiocardiograms.
Target-film distance: Immaterial.

Measurements (Figure 1) ▪

1. *The infundibular/bulb ratio.* Several bulb measurements are averaged, and the ratio of the minimum systolic diameter to the average pulmonary diameter is obtained. The critical ratio is 0.4. Figures below this level indicate significant systolic narrowing.

Normal range: 0.45 to 0.83. *Average*: 0.63 ± 0.08.[1]
2. *The infundibular systolic/diastolic ratio.* Measurements are made of the infundibulum at its narrowest point in the systole and at the same point in the diastole. In all cases of tetralogy of Fallot, the ratio is greater than 0.33; in all cases of valvular stenosis, the ratio is less than 0.30. An infundibulum with significant obstruction, as measured by the infundibular/bulb ratio, and an infundibular systolic/diastolic ratio greater than 0.30 may not regress following valvulotomy.

The infundibular systolic/diastolic ratio:
In *tetralogy of Fallot*: 0.33 to 1.00. Average, 0.56.
In *pulmonic valvular stenosis*: 0.11 to 0.30. Average, 0.25.

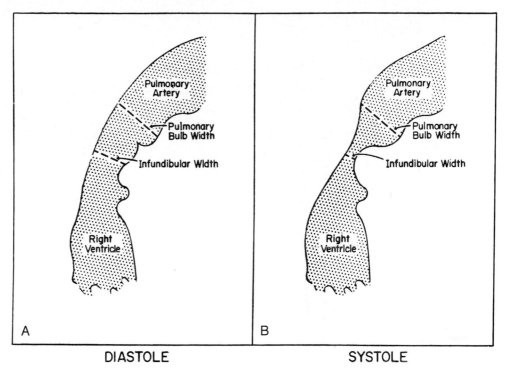

Figure 1 ▪ Measurement of the right ventricular outflow tract from lateral angiocardiograms. (From Little TB, et al: Circulation 1963; 28:182. Used by permission.)

DIASTOLE   SYSTOLE

Source ▪

The data on the infundibular/bulb ratio are based on a study of 13 patients with pulmonary valvular stenosis and 30 control subjects.

The infundibular systolic diameter/infundibular diastolic ratio is based on a study of 42 patients with tetralogy of Fallot and 19 patients with pulmonic valvular stenosis.

References

1. Little TB, et al: Circulation 1963; 28:182.
2. Lester RG, et al: AJR Am J Roentgenol 1965; 94:78.

▪: THICKNESS OF THE NORMAL PERICARDIUM
▪ ACR Code: 55 (Pericardium)

Technique ▪

Moncada and colleagues used an Omni 6000 CT scanner (manufacturer not given), 1.0-cm slice thickness, and 5-sec scan time to make axial scans of the heart.[1] Silverman and Harell performed chest CT with an 8800 machine (General Electric Medical Systems, Milwaukee, WI) and 1.0-cm slice thickness.[2] Ling and colleagues used 5.0- to 7.0-MHz transesophageal transducers and unspecified ultrasound units to perform transesophageal echocardiography (TEE) in standard planes.[3] Bogaert and Duerinckx performed cardiac MRI in the prone position using a 1.5-T Magnetom SP machine (Siemens, Erlangen, Germany) and an elliptic spine coil. Fast-gradient-recalled, ECG-gated, breath-hold sequences were used to produce images in four planes. This technique is typically used for MR coronary angiography.[4] Sechtem and colleagues used a 0.35-T unit (manufacturer not specified) to perform axial scanning of the heart with ECG gating (TR = 750-1250) and dual spin-echo (30, 60) technique.[5]

Measurements ▪

Silverman and Harell measured the thinnest visible portion of the pericardium, using a calibrated grid.[2] Videotaped TEE examinations were selectively digitized and measurements done on a Dextra D-200 analyzer at multiple locations.[3] Bogaert and Duerinckx divided the pericardium at multiple anatomically defined segments, and if any segment had variable thickness they averaged several measurements.[4] Sechtem and colleagues made measurements using a standard grid over the right ventricle at different phases of the cardiac cycle and on first and second echo images.[5] Figure 1 shows the anatomy and a typical measurement location. Table 1 gives the reported normal values and ranges for pericardial thickness.[1-5]

Source ▪

Moncada's subjects consisted of 100 adults (61 men, 39 women, age range 24 to 79 years, mean age 54 years) without cardiac or pericardial disease.[1] Silverman and Harell studied 100 patients without pericardial disease or any condition or surgery that might affect the pericardium. Of these, the pericardium was visible in 95 (46 males, 49 females, age range 1 to 81 years). Only 2 were less than 21 years old.[2] Ling's subjects were 21 normal adults (8 men, 13 women, age range 47 to 75 years, mean age 58 years) without cardiac problems.[3] Bogaert and Duerinckx studied

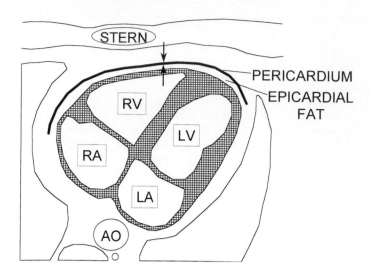

Figure 1 ▪ Measurement of pericardial thickness. Drawing depicts the heart in the axial plane through the atrioventricular valves. STERN = sternum, AO = aorta, chambers labeled with standard nomenclature. The fibrous or parietal pericardium *(heavy solid line)* is usually separated from the myocardium by epicardial fat, rendering it visible in most patients for at least a portion of its length. Measurements *(arrows)* were made at several positions and averaged or at the thinnest visible part.

Table 1 ▪ Thickness of the Normal Pericardium

RESEARCHER	MODALITY	POPULATION	COMMENTS	NO.	PERICARDIAL THICKNESS (mm)	
					Mean ± SD	Range
Moncada	CT	Normal adult		100	—	1–2 (70% of cases) 3–4 (caudally, sometimes)
Silverman	CT	Normal male	Thinnest part	46	2.0 ± 0.6	≤4
	CT	Normal female	Thinnest part	49	2.3 ± 0.5	≤4
	CT	Combined sexes	Thinnest part	95	2.2 ± 0.6	≤4
Ling	TEE	Normal adult	Average of several places	21	1.2 ± 0.4	≤2.5
Bogaert	MRI	Normal adult	Transverse	23	1.5 ± 0.9	—
	MRI	Normal adult	Sagittal	23	2.0 ± 0.9	—
	MRI	Normal adult	Combined	23	1.7	1.5–2.0
Sechtem	MRI	Normal adult	Diastole	18	1.2 ± 0.5	0.8–2.1
	MRI	Normal adult	Systole	18	1.7 ± 0.5	0.8–2.8
	MRI	Normal adult	1st echo	18	2.1 ± 0.5	—
	MRI	Normal adult	2nd echo	18	2.5 ± 0.6	—

TEE = transesophageal echocardiography, SD = standard deviation.[1-5]

23 individuals (21 men, 2 women, age range 18 to 70 years). These were 17 healthy volunteers and 6 patients without pericardial disease.[4] Normal adult volunteers (n = 9) and nine patients without pericardial disease (n = 18, age range 26 to 86 years, mean age 38 years) were included in Sechtem's subjects.[5]

Comments ▪

Most workers stated that there was considerable variability between patients in how much of the pericardium was visible. For the most part, the pericardium was best seen along the anterior border of the heart over the right ventricle, the right atrium, and the left ventricular apex.[1, 2, 4, 5] Bogaert and Duerinckx did not give measurements for different cardiac phases but state that the pericardial thickness never changed more than 2.0 mm during the cycle.[4] Ling's study included a population of 11 patients with surgically proved constrictive pericarditis and reported sen-

sitivity of 95% and specificity of 86%, using 3.0 mm as a cut-off in detecting true thickening with TEE.[3] Sechtem and colleagues suggest a cut-off of 4.0 mm in a companion paper analyzing various pericardial abnormalities.[6]

REFERENCES

1. Moncada R, Baker M, Salinas M, et al: Diagnostic role of computed tomography in pericardial heart disease: Congenital defects, thickening, neoplasms, and effusion. Am Heart J 1982; 103:263–282.
2. Silverman PM, Harell GS: Computed tomography of the normal pericardium. Invest Radiol 1983; 18:141–144.
3. Ling LH, Oh JK, Tei C, et al: Pericardial thickness measured with transesophageal echocardiography: Feasibility and potential clinical usefulness. J Am Coll Cardiol 1997; 29(6):1317–1323.
4. Bogaert J, Duerinckx AJ: Appearance of the normal pericardium on coronary MR angiograms. J Magn Reson Imaging 1995; 5(5):579–587.
5. Sechtem U, Tscholakoff D, Higgins CB: MRI of the normal pericardium. AJR Am J Roentgenol 1986; 147:239–244.
6. Sechtem U, Tscholakoff D, Higgins CB: MRI of the abnormal pericardium. AJR Am J Roentgenol 1986; 147:245–252.

•: MEASUREMENT OF THE PEDIATRIC AORTA BY CT[1]
■ ACR Code: 56 (Aorta)

Technique ■

1. Dynamic scanning was performed on a 9800 GE CT scanner.
2. Sixty percent iodinated contrast material was injected as a bolus with a dose of 3 ml/kg.
3. Scans were performed at 5- or 10-mm levels with the patient breathing quietly. Two-second scans were obtained.

Measurement (Figure 1) ■

Measurement of the aorta was obtained perpendicular to the long axis of the aorta at three levels with direct reading calipers. Level *A* was placed 1 cm caudal to the top of the aortic arch. Level *B* was 1 cm cranial to the aortic root. Level *C* was approximately 1 cm cranial to the dome of the right hemidiaphragm (Figure 2).

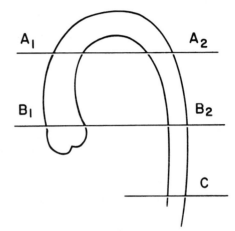

Figure 1 ■ Illustration of the thoracic aorta depicts the approximate levels of aortic measurement. (From Fitzgerald SW, et al: Radiology 1987; 165:667–669. Used by permission.)

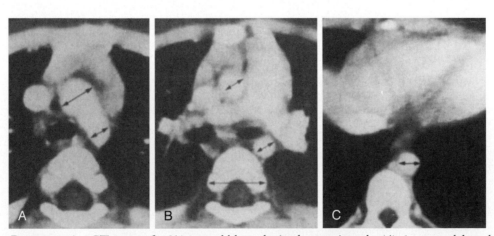

Figure 2 ■ Representative CT scans of a 2½-year-old boy obtained approximately *(A)*, 1 cm caudal to the top of the aortic arch. *B*, 1 cm cranial to the aortic root. *C*, At the level of the dome of the right hemidiaphragm. The thoracic vertebral body width was measured coronally at level B. *Arrows* indicate sites of measurement. (From Fitzgerald SW, et al: Radiology 1987; 165:667–669. Used by permission.)

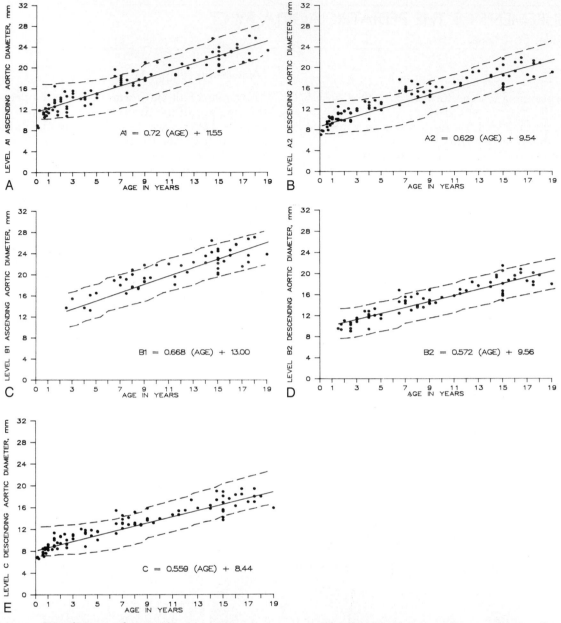

Figure 3 ▪ Distributions of aortic diameters plotted versus age. The *solid lines* represent linear regression lines, and the *dashed lines* represent 95% confidence bands. (*A*) A₁ (ascending aortic diameter). (*B*) A₂ (descending). (*C*) B₁ (ascending). (*D*) B₂ (descending). (*E*) C (descending). (From Fitzgerald SW, et al: Radiology 1987; 165:667–669. Used by permission.)

The distribution of aortic diameters as a function of age is shown in Figure 3.

Source ▪

Data are based on a CT study of 97 patients ranging in age from 2 weeks to 19 years.

Reference

1. Fitzgerald SW, Donaldson JS, Poznanski AK: Pediatric thoracic aorta; normal measurements determined with CT. Radiology 1987; 165:667–669.

∴ THORACIC AORTA DIAMETERS IN ADULTS
- ACR Code: 56 (Aorta)

Technique ▪

Chest CT scans were done with EMI 7070 and DR3 scanners (Siemens Medical Systems, Iselin, NJ), using 8- to 10-mm slice thickness and 10-mm intervals.[1]

Measurements ▪

The coronal diameter of the thoracic aorta was measured in five locations from hard copy images with a caliper corrected for image magnification. The ascending and de- scending aorta was measured on the scans 1 cm caudal to the arch and 1 cm cephalic to the aortic valve. The de- scending aorta was also measured above the diaphragm.[1] Figure 1 shows the measurement locations. Table 1 lists the results by age and gender as well as for the entire group.

Source ▪

The study included 102 patients and all were free of cardio- vascular disease, hypertension, diabetes, or renal problems.

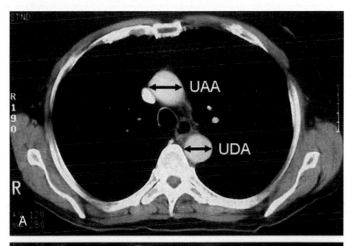

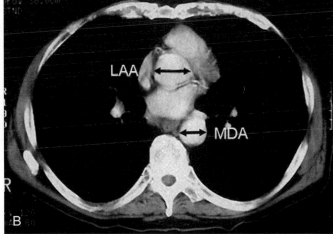

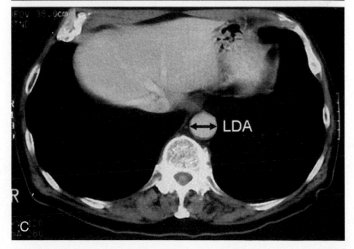

Figure 1 ▪ Measurement of the thoracic aorta from CT scans. Three scan levels were used: 1 cm below the arch (*A*), 1 cm above the aortic valve (*B*), and above the diaphragm (*C*). The transverse (coronal) diameter was measured at five locations:

UAA = upper ascending aorta
UDA = upper descending aorta
LAA = lower ascending aorta
MDA = mid-descending aorta
LDA = lower descending aorta

Table 1 ▪ Diameters of the Thoracic Aorta in Adults

GENDER/AGE RANGE	ASCENDING AORTA DIAMETER (cm)		DESCENDING AORTA DIAMETER (cm)		
	Lower	Upper	Upper	Mid	Lower
Men 21–40 yr	3.47	3.28	2.21	2.25	2.12
Men 41–60 yr	3.63	3.64	2.64	2.39	2.43
Men >60 yr	3.91	3.80	3.14	2.98	2.98
Women 21–40 yr	3.36	2.80	2.06	1.91	1.89
Women 41–60 yr	3.72	3.47	2.63	2.45	2.43
Women >40 yr	3.50	3.68	2.88	2.64	2.40
All subjects (mean)	3.6	3.51	2.63	2.48	2.42
All subjects (±2 SD)	0.76	0.87	0.72	0.61	0.55
All subjects (range)	2.4–4.7	2.2–4.6	1.8–4.0	1.6–3.7	1.4–3.3

The ± 2 SD values for all subjects may be applied to the individual gender/age group means.
From Aronberg DJ, Glazer HS, Madson K, et al: J Comput Assist Tomogr 1984; 8:247–250. Used by permission.

The subjects were divided into three age ranges: 21 to 40 years (n = 36), 41 to 60 years (n = 33), and over 60 years (n = 33). The oldest was 89 years old.[1]

Comments ▪

The diameter of the aorta was significantly smaller in women than in men. In men, the descending aorta diameter increased by about 0.1 cm per decade. The investigators suggest three guidelines for evaluating the thoracic aorta size. First, on any given scan level, the descending aorta should not be larger than the ascending aorta. Second, the ratio of ascending to descending coronal aortic diameter may be as high as 2.2 in young women and is usually 1 to 1.5 for other groups. Third, the size of the aorta varies widely, and an individual measurement should not be considered abnormal unless it exceeds the mean for gender and age group by at least 2 standard deviations.[1]

REFERENCE

1. Aronberg DJ, Glazer HS, Madson K, et al: Normal thoracic aortic diameters by computed tomography. J Comput Assist Tomogr 1984; 8:247–250.

▪: MEASUREMENT OF THE AORTIC NIPPLE[1]
▪ ACR Code: 562 (Aortic Arch)

Technique ▪

Central ray: Perpendicular to plane of film centered to midchest.
Position: Posteroanterior erect.
Target-film distance: 72 inches.

Measurement (Figure 1) ▪

The diameter of the aortic nipple is taken as the horizontal distance from the lateral wall of the aortic knob to the lateral wall of the nipple, through the midplane of the nipple.
The normal nipple ranges in size from 1 to 4 mm, taking the mean plus 2 SD as the upper limit of normal; dilatation of the vein beyond 4.5 mm is a useful sign of a circulatory abnormality. Dilatation may be due to absence of the inferior vena cava, hypoplasia of the left innominate vein, congestive failure, portal hypertension, Budd-Chiari syndrome, or superior or inferior vena caval obstruction.

Source ▪

Five hundred consecutive chest films of patients without known cardiovascular or pulmonary disease were reviewed. Children under the age of 10 years were excluded. Seven of these demonstrated an aortic nipple. In addition, nine aortic nipples previously encountered in normal patients were used in calculating the normal diameter.

REFERENCE

1. Friedman AC, Chambers E, Sprayregen S: The normal and abnormal left superior intercostal vein. AJR Am J Roentgenol 1978; 131:599–602.

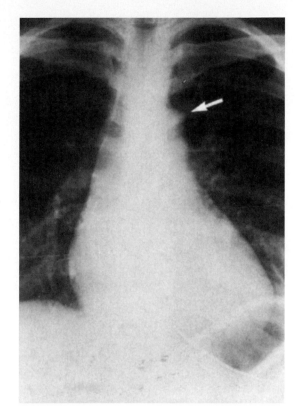

Figure 1 ▪ Normal aortic nipple *(arrow)*. (From Friedman AC, et al: AJR Am J Roentgenol 1978; 131:599. Used by permission.)

▪: DIAMETERS OF THE AORTA AND PULMONARY ARTERIES IN CHILDREN
- ACR Code: 56 (Arteries, Veins of Thorax)

Technique ▪

Calibrated probes (in 1-mm gradations) were used to size the vessels in postmortem specimens within 24 hours of death.[1]

Measurements ▪

The internal diameters of the aorta (four positions), the pulmonary artery (two positions), the right pulmonary artery, and the left pulmonary artery were determined by noting the diameter of the largest probe that could fit within the lumen. The length (in centimeters) of each subject was also noted.[1] Figure 1 shows the sites of measurement. Figures 2 and 3 give the diameter of the aorta and pulmonary arteries related to body length based on linear regression analysis. Table 1 lists the diameters for each vessel in smaller/younger (average length 52 cm) and larger/older (average length 100 cm) subjects. The annotations on Figure 1 correspond to the numbers on the other figures.

Source ▪

Hearts and great arteries of 126 fetuses, infants, and children whose ages ranged from 21 weeks of gestation through 10 years at time of death were examined. All subjects died from noncardiovascular causes.

Comments ▪

Van Meurs–van Woezik and colleagues felt that body length was superior to age, weight, or body surface area (BSA) in establishing normative criteria, partly because weight and

BODY LENGTH (cm)	ASC. AO (1)	AO. OSTIUM (2)	AO. ISTHMUS (3)	DESC. AO. (4)	MPA (5)	PULM. OSTIUM (6)	RPA (7)	LPA (8)
52	8.0 ± 1.22	7.5 ± 1.22	5.5 ± 1.52	6.0 ± 1.22	8.5 ± 1.83	8.0 ± 1.83	5.0 ± 1.83	4.5 ± 1.22
100	14.5 ± 1.22	14.0 ± 1.22	10.5 ± 1.52	10.0 ± 1.22	18.0 ± 1.83	17.0 ± 1.83	12.0 ± 1.83	11.5 ± 1.22

Table 1 ▪ Internal Diameters of the Aorta and Pulmonary Arteries

All measurements are in millimeters (mean ± standard deviation). Vessel abbreviations and numbers correspond to those given in Figure 1.
From van Meurs–van Woezik H, Debets T, Klein HW: Int J Cardiol 1989; 23(3):303–308. Used by permission.

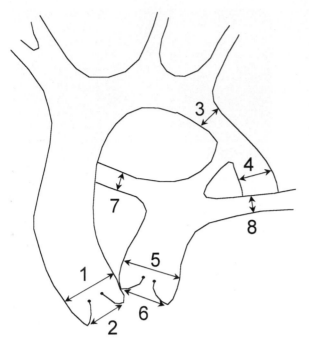

Figure 1 ▪ Sites of measurements of the aorta and pulmonary arteries.

1 = ascending aorta (1 cm above valve)
2 = aortic ostium
3 = aortic isthmus
4 = descending aorta
5 = pulmonary artery (1 cm above valve)
6 = pulmonary ostium
7 = right pulmonary artery (1 cm from bifurcation)
8 = left pulmonary artery (1 cm from bifurcation)

(From van Meurs–van Woezik H, Debets T, Klein HW: Int J Cardiol 1989; 23(3):303–308. Used by permission.)

Figure 2 ▪ Diameters of the aorta at four sites. The numbers correspond to locations in Figure 1. (From van Meurs–van Woezik H, Debets T, Klein HW: Int J Cardiol 1989; 23(3):303–308. Used by permission.)

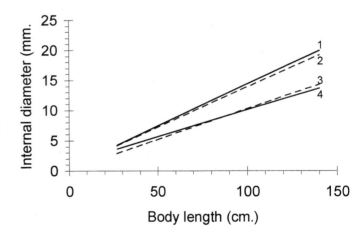

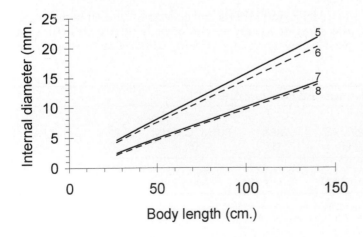

Figure 3 ▪ Diameters of the pulmonary arteries at four sites. The numbers correspond to locations in Figure 1. (From van Meurs–van Woezik H, Debets T, Klein HW: Int J Cardiol 1989; 23(3):303–308. Used by permission.)

BSA (calculated with weight) can change rapidly in sick children. Likewise, heart disease often causes growth delay or arrest, making age unsuitable.[1] They found generally good correlation between their findings and studies using M-mode echocardiography and state that these normative data are potentially useful in imaging studies of congenital heart disease and in surgical planning.[1]

REFERENCE

1. van Meurs–van Woezik H, Debets T, Klein HW: Internal diameters of the ventriculo-arterial junctions and great arteries of normal infants and children: A data base for evaluation of congenital cardiac malformations. Int J Cardiol 1989; 23(3):303–308.

▪▪ MEASUREMENT OF THE NORMAL PULMONARY ARTERIES
▪ ACR Code: 564 (Pulmonary Artery)

In Children ▪

Technique

Central ray: Perpendicular to plane of film centered over midchest.
Position: Posteroanterior.
Target-film distance: 6 feet.

Measurements (Figure 1)

The right lower lung field is utilized. A horizontal line is drawn from the descending branch of the right pulmonary artery just below the right hilar shadow to the lateral chest wall. A perpendicular line is then drawn inferiorly from the midpoint of this line to meet a horizontal line drawn bisecting the distance from the upper line and the cardiophrenic reflection. In this way, a central, square-shaped area and a peripheral L-shaped area are obtained. Three measurements are made: (1) the diameter of the right descending pulmonary artery is measured as it appears below the right hilus; (2) the diameter of the widest-caliber secondary arterial branch is measured in the central area; (3) the widest tertiary branch is then measured in the peripheral area. Normal measurements on function of age

Figure 1 ▪ Location for measurements of right pulmonary arteries in children. Locations (from top to bottom) for measuring main, secondary, and tertiary branch vessels are shown. (From Leinbach LB: AJR Am J Roentgenol 1963; 89:995. Used by permission.)

and surface area are shown in Figure 2. Methods for determining body surface area are found in the first section of Chapter 8, p 309.

Source

The data are based on a study of 243 children ranging in age from infancy to 14 years. Each chest film used was interpreted as normal if the diaphragmatic level was the ninth posterior rib.

In Adults ▪

Technique

Central ray: Perpendicular to plane of film centered over midchest.
Position: Posteroanterior.
Target-film distance: 6 feet.

Measurements (Figure 3)

All films are obtained in deep inspiration and forceful expiration. The right descending pulmonary artery is measured on both inspiratory and expiratory films at its widest point near the bifurcation of the artery from the lateral segment of the right middle lobe and above the branching of the middle basilar artery. This measurement point usually lies between the right eighth and ninth ribs posteriorly in deep inspiration. On expiration, it usually lies just below or over the right eighth rib posteriorly.

Normal values are shown in Table 1. Values greater than those shown are abnormal, and pulmonary hypertension is most likely present.[1] The expiratory measurement is always smaller than the inspiratory, and it is helpful in borderline cases.

These measurements are also useful in the diagnosis of pulmonary infarction.[2] With infarction, values ranging from 17 to 22 mm are noted on the right, and from 17 to

Table 1 ▪ Normal Right Lower Lobe Pulmonary Diameters		
		RANGE OF DIFFERENCE BETWEEN INSPIRATION
INSPIRATION (mm)	**EXPIRATION** (mm)	**AND EXPIRATION** (mm)
Men 16	15	1–3
Women 15	14	1–3

From Chang CH: AJR Am J Roentgenol 1962; 87:929. Used by permission.

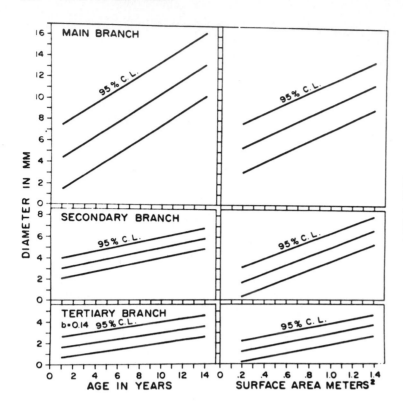

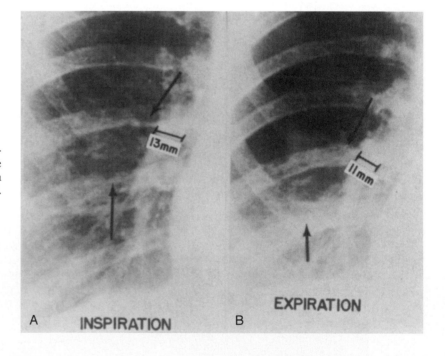

Figure 2 ▪ Normal values for right pulmonary artery diameters in children by age and body surface area. Mean and 95% confidence intervals are shown for the main, secondary, and tertiary branch vessels. (From Leinbach LB: AJR Am J Roentgenol 1963; 89:995. Used by permission.)

Figure 3 ▪ Locations for measuring the right pulmonary artery in adults are shown on radiographs made during inspiration *(A)* and expiration *(B)*. (From Chang CH: AJR Am J Roentgenol 1962; 87:929. Used by permission.)

26 mm on the left, on inspiration. This dilatation usually appears within 24 hours of the onset of chest pain, and maximum dilatation occurs in 2 to 3 days.

Source

The data on normal size are based on a study of 1085 normal adults, including 432 men ranging in age from 18 to 70 years and 652 women ranging in age from 18 to 72 years.

Figures for pulmonary infarction are based on a study of 23 patients with pulmonary infarction.

REFERENCES

1. Chang CH: AJR Am J Roentgenol 1962; 87:929.
2. Chang CH, Davis WC: Clin Radiol 1965; 16:141.

▪: RATIO OF PULMONARY ARTERY DIAMETER TO TRACHEA FOR ASSESSMENT OF PULMONARY VASCULARITY IN CHILDREN[1]

▪ ACR Code: 564 (Pulmonary Artery)

Technique ▪

Central ray: Perpendicular to plane of film.
Position: Posteroanterior or anteroposterior.
Target-film distance: Immaterial.

Measurements (Figure 1) ▪

The diameter of the right descending pulmonary artery was measured at the level where it parallels the right main bronchus and crosses the pulmonary vein, draining the right upper lobe. The diameter of the trachea was measured just above the impression of the aorta.

It was found that when a left-to-right shunt was present, the right descending pulmonary artery never had a diameter less than that of the trachea.

Source ▪

Data were derived from chest films of 112 normal children and 102 children with left-to-right shunts. Ages ranged from 6 months to 14 years.

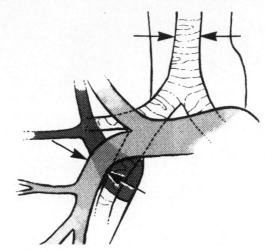

Figure 1 ▪ Sites of measurement of right descending pulmonary artery and tracheal diameters. (From Coussement AM, Gooding CA: Radiology 1973; 109:649. Used by permission.)

REFERENCE

1. Coussement AM, Gooding CA: Objective radiographic assessment of pulmonary vascularity in children. Radiology 1973; 109:649–654.

▪: DIAMETER OF THE PULMONARY ARTERY ON CT

▪ ACR Code: 564 (Pulmonary Artery)

Technique ▪

Unenhanced axial CT of the chest was performed with a Somatom Plus 4A machine (Siemens, Erlangen, Germany), 10-mm slice thickness, 15-second breath-hold spiral technique, pitch of 1.5, rotation time of 0.75 sec, and 10-mm reconstruction.[1]

Measurements ▪

The CT section through the pulmonary artery bifurcation was magnified to full screen on the operator's console, and the diameter of the main pulmonary artery was measured with electronic calipers perpendicular to its long axis. Measurements were done with images displayed at mediastinal window (W = 400/L = 20) settings.[1] Figure 1 shows the measurement location. The main pulmonary artery diameter in the normal subjects was 2.27 ± 0.3 cm (mean ± SD). There was no significant change in the measurement with advancing age.[1]

Source ▪

There were 100 adult subjects (61 men, 39 women, age range 11 to 90 years) who had no history of cardiothoracic disease, mediastinal disease, or radiation therapy. A second group of 12 patients (5 men, 7 women, age range 29 to 70 years) had established pulmonary hypertension by right heart catheterization. The mean pulmonary artery pressure in these 12 patients ranged from 33 to 63 mm Hg, with a mean of 49 mm Hg.[1]

Comments ▪

The main pulmonary artery diameter in the pulmonary hypertension patients was 3.47 ± 0.33 (mean ± SD). The

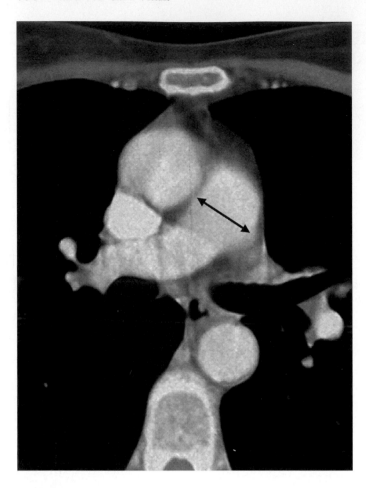

Figure 1 ▪ Measurement of the pulmonary artery from axial CT. The diameter of the main pulmonary *(arrows)* was measured at the level of the bifurcation and perpendicular to its long axis. The authors used unenhanced scans.

difference in the means was significant (p < .001). Using a cut-off of 3.32 cm (normal mean + 2 SD), the sensitivity was 95% and the specificity was 58% for detecting pulmonary artery hypertension.[1]

REFERENCE

1. Edwards PD, Bull RK, Coulden R: CT measurement of main pulmonary artery diameter. Br J Radiol 1998; 71:1018–1020.

▪: PULMONARY ARTERY-TO-BRONCHUS RATIO
▪ ACR Code: 564 (Pulmonary Artery)

Technique ▪

Posteroanterior (PA) upright chest radiographs were performed with a target-to-film distance of 6 feet (183 cm), and supine anteroposterior (AP) radiographs were done with target-to-film distances of from 46 to 56 inches (116–142 cm).[1]

Measurements ▪

The chest radiographs were divided into upper and lower zones at the right hilar angle. Where possible, a segmental pulmonary artery and bronchus pair seen end-on was chosen from the upper and lower zone perihilar areas for measurement. If segmental artery–bronchus pairs were not visible, a subsegmental bundle was chosen. Using a hand-held magnifying lens (X2–X4), calipers, and a millimeter rule, the external diameters of each artery and bronchus were measured. The artery-bronchus ratio (ABR) was formed by dividing the arterial diameter by the bronchial diameter. Figure 1 shows typical examples of measurements of segmental and subsegmental ABR. Table 1 lists the numeric results (mean, standard deviation, and range in each group), as well as the typical visual patterns.[1]

Source ▪

Two groups of adult patients (30 each) had PA and AP radiographs. Those with PA radiographs usually were having routine physical examinations; those with AP radiographs were examined mostly for skeletal trauma. There was no history of cardiopulmonary disease, and the radiographs were interpreted as normal. Another 30 adult patients with clinical findings and history of pulmonary plethora without edema had PA radiographs. The causes included renal failure, iatrogenic volume overload, volume overload related to pregnancy, high-output failure from sickle cell disease, and overcirculation from congenital heart disease. Adult patients with clinical evidence of decompensated congestive heart failure (CHF) had PA and AP radiographs (30 each). The cause of CHF was chronic ischemic heart disease or mitral valve disease in the patients

Table 1 ▪ Pulmonary Artery and Bronchial Diameter Relationships

GROUPS (n = 30 each)	POSITION	UPPER ZONE A/B		LOWER ZONE A/B		VISUAL PATTERN	
		Mean ± SD	Range	Mean ± SD	Range	Upper Zone	Lower Zone
Normal	Upright PA	0.85 ± 0.15	0.63–1.14	1.34 ± 0.25	1.00–2.00	A≤B	A>B
Plethora	Upright PA	1.62 ± 0.31	1.24–2.43	1.56 ± 0.28	1.16–2.33	A>B	A>B
CHF	Upright PA	1.50 ± 0.25	1.10–2.03	0.87 ± 0.20	0.63–1.56	A>B	A<B
Normal	Supine AP	1.01 ± 0.13	0.79–1.31	1.05 ± 0.13	0.85–1.45	A = B	A = B
CHF	Supine AP	1.49 ± 0.31	0.86–2.50	0.96 ± 0.31	0.53–1.91	A>B (22) A>B (7) A = B (1)	A<B (22) A>B (7) A = B (1)

Visual patterns refer to relative sizes of A and B. There were three distinct patterns on AP radiographs of patients with CHF (numbers in parentheses). A = artery, B = bronchus, CHF = congestive heart failure, SD = standard deviation.[1]

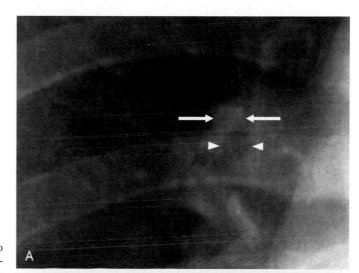

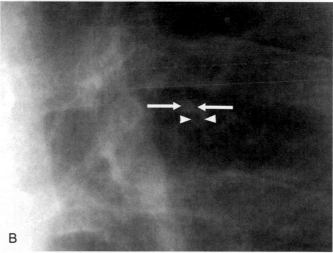

Figure 1 ▪ Measurement of pulmonary artery to bronchus ratio (ABR). Segmental *(A)* and subsegmental *(B)* bronchovascular bundles are depicted, with the arterial *(arrows)* and bronchial *(arrowheads)* diameters shown. The ABR is formed by dividing the arterial by the bronchial diameter in each pair.[1]

having PA radiographs and mostly acute myocardial infarction in those having AP radiographs.[1]

Comments ▪

The positive predictive value for abnormal vascular patterns on the PA radiographs was 100%, and the negative predictive value was 97%. The vascular pattern allowed distinction between pulmonary plethora and CHF with 93% accuracy. On the AP supine radiographs, the positive and negative predictive values of abnormal vascular patterns were the same as for PA radiographs, but because of a mixture of types of patterns for the CHF patients, Woodring speculates that distinction between plethora and frank CHF would not be possible.[1]

REFERENCE

1. Woodring JH: Pulmonary artery–bronchus ratios in patients with normal lungs, pulmonary vascular plethora, and congestive heart failure. Radiology 1991; 179:115–122.

▪: MEASUREMENT OF THE SIZE OF THE ARCH OF THE AZYGOS VEIN[1]

- ACR Code: 567 (Azygos Vein)

In Children ▪

Technique

Central ray: Perpendicular to plane of film centered over midchest.
Position: Supine and upright: AP and PA in infants aged birth to 6 months; others PA upright.
Target-film distance: 72 inches.

Measurements (Table 1; Figure 1)

Measurements were made from the outer margin of the vein and the inner margin of the tracheal wall at its greatest width.

Source

Data were based on routine chest wall radiographs in 429 children ranging in age from birth to 14 years.

Wishart states that respiratory activity, posture, and anatomic arrangement may cause changes in azygos vein width, making clinicoradiologic correlation uncertain.[1]

In Adults ▪

Technique

Central ray: Perpendicular to plane of film centered over midchest.
Position: Posteroanterior, upright; inspiratory phase of respiration.
Target-film distance: 72 inches.

Measurements (Table 2; see Figure 1)

The width of the azygos arches is measured perpendicularly to the trachea in the greatest transverse dimension of the arch. Measurement includes the wall of the trachea.

The normal ranges are exceeded in pregnancy, conges-

Table 1 ▪ Azygos Vein Width in Children				
AGE	**BIRTH TO 6 MON**	**6 TO 24 MON**	**2 TO 7 YR**	**8 TO 14 YR**
Position	AP and PA supine and upright	PA upright	PA upright	PA upright
Mean ± 1 standard deviation	3.5 ± 1.3 mm	4.1 ± 1.0 mm	4.6 ± 1.2 mm	5.1 ± 1.6 mm

From Wishart DL: Radiology 1972; 104:115. Used by permission.

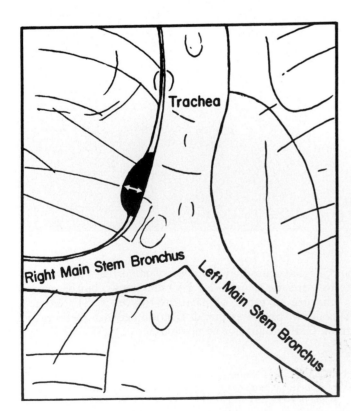

Figure 1 ▪ Measurement of the azygos vein width. See text for details. (From Keats TE, Lipscomb G: Radiology 1968; 90:990. Used by permission.)

tive heart failure, portal hypertension, and obstructions of the superior or inferior vena cava.

Source

The data are based on a study of 200 normal adults, equally divided between men and women aged 20 to 60 years.

REFERENCES

1. Wishart DL: Normal azygos vein width in children. Radiology 1972; 104:115–118.
2. Keats TE, Lipscomb GE, Betts CS 3d: Mensuration of the arch of the azygos vein and its application to the study of cardiopulmonary disease. Radiology 1968; 90: 990–994.

▪: WIDTH OF THE AZYGOS VEIN RELATED TO CENTRAL VENOUS PRESSURE[1]
- ACR Code: 567 (Azygos Vein)

Technique ▪

Central ray: Perpendicular to plane of film centered over midchest.
Position: Anteroposterior. Patient supine on bed rolled flat. Maximum inspiration phase of respiration.
Target-film distance: 40 inches.

Measurements (Table 1; see Figure 1 in preceding section) ▪

The azygos vein width is measured at its greatest diameter, perpendicular to the wall of the trachea. This measurement includes the mediastinal pleural reflection laterally and the tracheal wall medially.

Source ▪

Fifty-four adult patients ranging in age from 23 to 77 years of age. In this group were patients with congestive heart failure, patients recovering from thoracic surgery, and recipients of renal transplants.

REFERENCE

1. Preger L, Hooper TI, Steinbach HL, Hoffman JI: Width of azygos vein related to central venous pressure. Radiology 1969; 93:521–523.

Table 1 ▪ Azygos Vein Width as Related to Central Venous Pressure		
WIDTH OF AZYGOS VEIN (mm)	ESTIMATED CVP (to nearest cm)	95% CONFIDENCE LIMITS (to nearest cm)
4	3	0–10
6	5	0–12
8	8	1–15
10	11	4–18
12	14	7–21
14	17	10–24
16	19	12–26
18	22	15–29
20	25	18–32
22	28	21–35
24	31	24–38
26	33	26–40
28	36	29–43

CVP = central venous pressure.
From Preger L, et al: Radiology 1969; 93:521. Used by permission.

CHAPTER 10

Thorax: Lungs, Mediastinum, and Pleura

▪ ▪
▪

▪ SCORING SYSTEM FOR CYSTIC FIBROSIS
▪ ACR Code: 60 (Lung)

Technique ▪

Posteroanterior (PA) and lateral (LAT) radiographs were performed and analyzed in all studies.

Measurements ▪

The Brasfield scoring system is a forced-choice system requiring graded responses in five aspects of radiographic manifestations of cystic fibrosis. The numbers obtained in each category are summed and subtracted from 25. Possible scores range from 25 (no disease manifestations) to 3 (most severe manifestations in all five categories).[1] Table 1 shows the scoring system.

For the validation study by Brasfield and colleagues, copies of the films were sent to five large and ten small medical centers to be scored by radiologists (large centers) and pediatricians (large and small centers). Films were also scored at the University of Alabama at Birmingham. Each reader read each film twice (first and second review) in random order and separated by several weeks. Table 2 shows the inter- and intraobserver correlations for the total score and the correlations between all observers for each of the five categories.[2]

In Rosenberg's study, two readers scored the films with the Brasfield method.[2] The two scores were averaged and compared with spirometry data using standard regression methodology. Correlations were as follows: $FEV_1 = 0.63$, percent predicted $FEV_1 = 0.68$, $FVC = 0.55$, percent

Table 1 ▪ Scoring System for Cystic Fibrosis from Chest Radiographs

CATEGORY	DEFINITION	SCORE	MEANING
I. Air trapping	Generalized pulmonary overdistention (sternal bowing, depression of diaphragm, or thoracic kyphosis)	0 1–3 4	Absent Increasing severity Most severe
II. Linear markings	Linear opacifications due to prominence of bronchi; may be seen as parallel line densities, sometimes branching, or as end-on circular densities (bronchial wall thickening)	0 1–3 4	Absent Increasing severity Most severe
III. Nodular cystic lesions	Multiple discrete, rounded densities, ≥0.5 cm in diameter, with either radiopaque or radiolucent centers (bronchiectasis); does not refer to irregular linear markings; confluent nodules not classified as large lesions	0 1 2 3 4	Absent 1 quadrant involved 2 quadrants involved 3 quadrants involved 4 quadrants involved
IV. Large lesions	Segmental or lobar atelectasis or consolidation, including acute pneumonia	0 3 5	Absent Segmental or lobar atelectasis and pneumonia Multiple atelectasis and pneumonia
V. General severity	Impression of overall severity of changes on radiograph	0 1–4 5	Absent Increasing severity Complications (e.g., cardiac enlargement, pneumothorax)

The scores from each category are summed and subtracted from 25.[1]

Table 2 ▪ Inter- and Intra-observer Reliability of Brasfield Scores

CORRELATION TYPE	REVIEW	CENTER SIZE	OBSERVER TYPE	AVERAGE COEFFICIENT
Between Birmingham and other centers	First	Small	Pediatrician	0.79 ± 0.07
	First	Large	Pediatrician	0.85 ± 0.05
	First	Large	Radiologist	0.88 ± 0.02
	Second	Small	Pediatrician	0.85 ± 0.05
	Second	Large	Pediatrician	0.85 ± 0.02
	Second	Large	Radiologist	0.86 ± 0.04
Between first and second review	—	Small	Pediatrician	0.78 ± 0.10
	—	Large	Pediatrician	0.84 ± 0.07
	—	Large	Radiologist	0.86 ± 0.03
By category	First	All	Both	I = 0.69, II = 0.74, III = 0.70, IV = 0.49, V = 0.78
By category	Second	All	Both	I = 0.66, II = 0.78, III = 0.73, IV = 0.52, V = 0.82

Birmingham = reference center, 10 small centers, 5 large centers.[2]

predicted FVC = 0.65, FEV$_1$/FVC = 0.47. All correlations were significant to p < .001.[3] Figure 1 is a scatterplot of Brasfield score and percent predicted FEV$_1$.

Cleveland and colleagues also found a strong relationship between Brasfield scores and spirometry results, with age-related rates of decline of normalized values nearly paralleling each other. They produced graphs of Brasfield score by age, which are shown in Figures 2 and 3. These data are useful in assessing the severity of lung disease at presentation, predicting rate of disease progression, and assessing response to new treatments.[4] Cleveland and colleagues found an average annual rate of decline with age in Brasfield score of 0.18 point/year for males and 0.17 point per year for females. Equations for predicting Brasfield score from age are as follows:

Brasfield score (males) =
$$22.6 - (0.18 \times age) - (0.00024 \times age^2)$$

Brasfield score (females) =
$$22.8 - (0.17 \times age) - (0.00024 \times age^2)$$

In addition to male sex, a score of 1 or greater for air trapping or cystic nodular lesions (categories I or III) during the first 5 years of life predicted more severe disease later, with the overall Brasfield score being 1.62 and 2.21 points lower than the mean for all ages.[5]

Source ▪

Brasfield used 40 pairs (PA and LAT) of chest radiographs of patients of varying ages with different severity of cystic fibrosis to validate a scoring system developed by himself and colleagues at the University of Alabama at Birmingham.[1, 2] Rosenberg and colleagues evaluated 66 radiographs from 27 patients with cystic fibrosis (20 men, 7 women, age range 18 to 40 years, mean age 25.8). Results of spirometry done within 3 months of the radiographs were available in all cases.[3] Cleveland and colleagues studied 3038 radiographs from 230 patients (106 males, 124 females, age range 3 days to more than 50 years). There was an average of 13 radiographs per patient. The average time interval between examinations was 1.5 years, and the

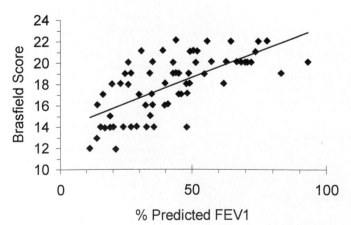

Figure 1 ▪ Scatterplot of Brasfield score versus percent predicted forced expiratory volume at 1 second (FEV$_1$) at spirometry. A linear regression line is shown. (From Rosenberg SM, Howatt WF, Grum CM: Chest 1992; 101:961–964. Used by permission.)

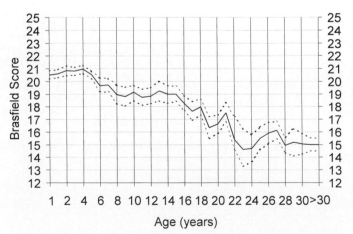

Figure 2 ▪ Brasfield score versus age. Mean values (solid line) and ± 2 standard deviations (dotted lines) are shown. (From Cleveland RH, Neish AS, Zurakowski D, et al: AJR Am J Roentgenol 1998; 170:1067–1072. Used by permission.)

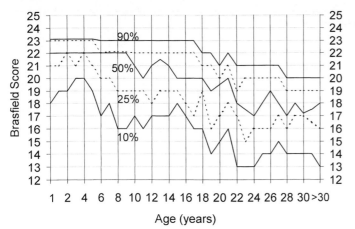

Figure 3 ▪ Brasfield score versus age. Quartile cut-offs as well as 10th and 90th percentiles are shown. (From Cleveland RH, Neish AS, Zurakowski D, et al: AJR Am J Roentgenol 1998; 170:1067–1072. Used by permission.)

average time span during which radiographs were available was 9 years and 8 months.[4, 5] Spirometry results (n = 1433) were obtained for 27 patients that were correlated with 458 radiographs.[4]

Comments ▪

Several scoring systems for the severity of cystic fibrosis on chest radiographs have been proposed. In a comparison with three such systems, Sawyer and colleagues[6] found the Brasfield system to perform equally with the chest radiograph portion of the National Institutes of Health clinical score[7] in terms of precision, reproducibility, and correlation with spirometry. The system developed at the Royal Children's Hospital[8] proved to be less reliable. The Brasfield score has been recommended as the standard for use in the USA.[9]

REFERENCES

1. Brasfield D, Hicks G, Soong S, Tiller RE: The chest roentgenogram in cystic fibrosis: A new scoring system. Pediatrics 1979; 63:24–29.
2. Brasfield D, Hicks G, Soong SJ, et al: Evaluation of scoring system of the chest radiograph in cystic fibrosis: A collaborative study. AJR Am J Roentgenol 1980; 134:1195–1198.
3. Rosenberg SM, Howatt WF, Grum CM: Spirometry and chest roentgenographic appearance in adults with cystic fibrosis. Chest 1992; 101:961–964.
4. Cleveland RH, Neish AS, Zurakowski D, et al: Cystic fibrosis: A system for assessing and predicting progression. AJR Am J Roentgenol 1998; 170:1067–1072.
5. Cleveland RH, Neish AS, Zurakowski D, et al: Cystic fibrosis: Predictors of accelerated decline and distribution of disease in 230 patients. AJR Am J Roentgenol 1998; 171:1311–1315.
6. Sawyer SM, Carlin JB, DeCampo M, Bowes G: Critical evaluation of three chest radiograph scores in cystic fibrosis. Thorax 1994; 49:863–866.
7. Taussig LM, Kattwinkel J, Friedewald WT, di Sant'Agnese PA: A new prognostic score and clinical evaluation system for cystic fibrosis. J Pediatr 1973; 82:380–390.
8. Holzer FJ, Olinsky A, Phelan PD: Variability of airways hyper-reactivity and allergy in cystic fibrosis. Arch Dis Child 1981; 56:455–459.
9. Wood RE, Farrell PM: Cystic fibrosis patient evaluations and scoring systems. In Wood RE, Farrell PM (eds): Cystic Fibrosis Foundation Conference Report, 1978, vol 2.

▪▪ CONTRAST ENHANCEMENT OF PULMONARY NODULES
▪ ACR Code: 60 (Lung Nodule)

Technique ▪

Dynamic enhanced CT of the chest, targeted to the solitary pulmonary nodule (SPN) in question, was performed as outlined in Tables 1 and 2 by Swensen and Yamashita and colleagues[2–4] Data from Swensen's original preliminary report[1] are included in the second work,[2] and a new set of patients (many evaluated with spiral scans) is outlined in Swensen's most recent paper.[3] Careful breathing instructions were given so as to scan the nodule in the same plane each time (usually at end-tidal phase). Swensen and colleagues described the instruction as follows: "Take a small breath in and hold it." This was especially important for single-level studies.

Measurements ▪

For all types of studies (single-level, incremental dynamic, and spiral), preliminary thin-section scanning through the nodule was done to allow determination of unenhanced

Table 1 ▪ CT Scanning Protocols

REFERENCE	SCANNER TYPE	SCAN TYPE	Thickness (mm)	Time (sec)	kVp	mA	RECONSTRUCTION
Swensen et al[2]	9800 Quick (n = 74)	Single level	1.5	—	120	—	—
	1200SX (n = 132)	Single level	2.0	—	130	—	—
	C-100 (n = 12)	Single level	3.0	—	130	—	—
Swensen et al[3]	HiSpeed Advantage (n = 97)	Spiral	3.0	5	120	280	1.0 mm, 13 slices
	1200SX (n = 44)	Single level	2.0	1	130	200	—
Yamashita et al[4]	Quantex (n = 47)	Incremental	2.0	25	—	—	2.0 mm, 6 slices

9800 Quick and HiSpeed Advantage (GE Medical Systems), 1200SX (Picker International), C-100 (Imatron), Quantex (GE–Yokokawa Medical Systems). Number of patients studied on each type of scanner in parentheses. kVp = kilovoltage, mA = milliamps.

Table 2 ▪ Contrast Enhancement Protocols

REFERENCE	CONTRAST TYPE	CONTRAST DOSE (ml)	INJECTION RATE (ml/sec)	POSTCONTRAST SCAN TIMING (sec)
Swensen et al[2]	Omnipaque 300	100	2.0	60, 120, 180, 240, 300 (n = 52)
				30, 60, 90, 120, 180, 210 (n = 166)
Swensen et al[3]	Isovue 300	100 (n = 44)	2.0	60, 120, 180, 240 (n = 141)
		50–175 (n = 97)		
Yamashita et al[4]	Omnipaque 300	100–150	2.0	30, 120, 300 (n = 47)

density and to find the optimal section through the center of the nodule for subsequent single-level postcontrast scans. For spiral and incremental dynamic scan techniques, the same range was scanned for each postcontrast interval. Swensen and colleagues used the image closest to the equator of the nodule on the unenhanced series and on spiral postcontrast scans for density measurement. For single-level postcontrast scans, only one slice was available, and this was used for density determination. On the chosen slice, a single region of interest occupying about 60% of the central portion nodule area was constructed and the reported mean Hounsfield unit (HU) recorded.[2, 3] Yamashita and colleagues used 1 to 3 sections (depending on nodule size) showing the maximum nodule diameter from pre- and postcontrast series for density determination. A circular region of interest enclosing about 60% of the central nodule was constructed and the mean HU recorded. If the individual values were within 10 HU of each other the average was taken, and if not, the median was used.[4] The nodule diameter (in centimeters) was measured and recorded in all cases.[2-4]

Nodule enhancement was defined as the maximum difference in HU values between precontrast and postcontrast scans. This usually occurred at about 2 minutes, but Swensen and colleagues decided to extend postcontrast scanning time to 4 minutes because of Yamashita's observation of 11 of 18 cases of lung cancer with later peak enhancement.[3, 4] Table 3 gives enhancement and nodule diameter data for malignant nodules, granulomata, and benign neoplastic nodules from each study. Table 4 lists

the test performance from each study (and the calculated combined performance) using a cut-off of over 19 HU enhancement for test positive.[2-4]

Source ▪

Swensen and colleagues initially scanned a total of 218 adult patients with SPN, of whom 163 had satisfactory scans and definitive diagnosis and/or follow-up was available for analysis.[1, 2] They subsequently studied 141 similar patients,[107] of whom 107 were included in the analysis.[3] Specific inclusion criteria included size up to 4.0 cm, homogeneous appearance, roughly spherical shape, and lack of significant calcification or fat density.[1-3] Yamashita and colleagues studied 47 adult patients with SPN, excluded 15, and analyzed 32.[4] Inclusion criteria were size less than 3.0 cm and lack of benign calcification by standard criteria.[5]

Comments ▪

Swensen and colleagues made specific note of the one false-negative result from their two series. This was a 1.5-cm diameter, spiculated nodule in a 59 year old man who was a heavy smoker, which enhanced only by 11 HU.[2] No other false-negatives have been reported. Because of some overlap in the ranges of enhancement between benign and malignant nodules, Swensen and group suggest that nodules that enhance 16 to 24 HU be considered indeterminate.[2] From the three papers cited here, 26 of 302 (8.6%) of patients would fall into this category, but this tactic still would not eliminate the one false-negative case.

Table 3 ▪ Nodule Enhancement and Diameter Results

REFERENCE	LESION TYPE	NO.	LESION ENHANCEMENT (HUmax—HUpre) Mean ± SE	Range	LESION DIAMETER (mm) Mean ± SE	Range
Swensen et al[2]	Malignant	111	42.2 ± 1.30	20–108	19.6 ± 0.70	8–40
	Granuloma	43	10.9 ± 1.84	−4–48	14.0 ± 0.85	6–30
	Benign neoplasm	9	31.7 ± 6.00	5–58	13.3 ± 1.66	6–20
Swensen et al[3]	Malignant	52	49.5 ± 3.2	11–110	17.3 ± 0.90	7–30
	Granuloma	51	16.1 ± 3.2	−10–94	14.2 ± 0.70	7–29
	Benign neoplasm	4	11.8 ± 7.50	−5–25	13.5 ± 7.50	11–20
			Mean ± SD	Range	Mean ± SD	Range
Yamashita et al[4]	Malignant	18	40 ± 10	28–56	19.0 ± 8.02	6–30
	Granuloma	10	3 ± 6	−7–12	14.5 ± 4.65	10–23
	Hamartoma	3	2 ± 4	−2–5	12.7 ± 4.04	8–15
	Hamartoma	1	71	—	—	10

HU = Hounsfield units, max = maximum postcontrast, pre = precontrast, Humax—Hupre = maximum enhancement attenuation—precontrast attenuation, SE = standard error, SD = standard deviation.

Table 4 ▪ **Test Performance Statistics**

REFERENCE	PREVALENCE OF MALIGNANCY (%)	SENSITIVITY (%) (95% CI)	SPECIFICITY (%) (95% CI)	PPV (%) (95% CI)	NPV (%) (95% CI)
Swensen[2]	68.1	100 (96.7–100)	76.9 (63.2–87.5)	90.2 (83.6–94.9)	100 (91.2–100)
Swensen[3]	49	98 (90–100)	73 (59–84)	77 (65–87)	98 (87–100)
Swensen[2, 3]	60	99 (97–100)	75 (66–82)	86 (80–90)	99 (93–100)
Yamashita[4]	58	100	93	95	100
Combined[2–4]	53.6	99.4	76.9	86.5	98.9

In all series and combined, test positive defined as greater than 19 Hounsfield unit nodule enhancement. PPV = positive predictive value, NPV = negative predictive value, CI = confidence intervals.

When considering postcontrast scan timing, it is probably adequate to scan at 1-minute intervals if incremental dynamic or spiral technique is used. However, if single-level scans are done, 30-second intervals are still useful to compensate for misregistration due to breathing, which often leads to one or more scans not including the nodule.

REFERENCES

1. Swensen SJ, Morin RL, Schueler BA, et al: Solitary pulmonary nodule: CT evaluation of enhancement with iodinated contrast material—a preliminary report. Radiology 1992; 182:343–347.
2. Swensen SJ, Brown LR, Colby TV, Weaver AL: Pulmonary nodules: CT evaluation of enhancement with iodinated contrast material. Radiology 1995; 194:393–398.
3. Swensen SJ, Brown LR, Colby TV, et al: Lung nodule enhancement at CT: Prospective findings. Radiology 1996; 201:447–455.
4. Yamashita K, Matsunobe S, Tsuda T, et al: Solitary pulmonary nodule: Preliminary study of evaluation with incremental dynamic CT. Radiology 1995; 194:399–405.
5. Siegelman SS, Khouri NF, Leo FP, et al: Solitary pulmonary nodules: CT assessment. Radiology 1986; 160:307–312.

▪▪ BAYESIAN ANALYSIS OF THE SOLITARY PULMONARY NODULE
▪ ACR Code: 60 (Lung Nodule)

Technique ▪

Chest radiographs, x-ray tomography, CT for morphologic analysis, CT for nodule size determination, and CT nodule densitometry with a standard reference phantom were evaluated. For each case, all available studies of these types were utilized.

Measurements ▪

Gurney analyzed the current literature concerning radiologic evaluation of solitary pulmonary nodules (SPNs) and used bayesian analysis techniques to quantify different nodule characteristics and patient demographic information.[1] This was done using the concept of the likelihood ratio (LR) as described in reference 2. He then with his colleagues compared the qualitative (rating scale) judgment concerning the likelihood of malignancy by four expert readers with quantitative determination of probability of malignancy by applying pertinent LRs to a standard prior probability.[3]

Figure 1 shows how calculations of LR and the odds of cancer for an individual case are done. The prevalence of malignancy in SPNs varies from 10% to 70%, but a reasonable estimate of 22% (70/323) may be obtained from a large series done in a midwestern clinic, and this was used by Gurney.[1, 4] This yields prior odds of malignancy of 0.28:1 (0.22/0.78). Figure 2 depicts nodule edge characteristics that were applied to radiographs or CT studies for LR determination.[5–7] Figure 3 shows x-ray tomographic appearances used to generate LR numbers.[4] Figure 4 de-

Figure 1 ▪ Calculation of adjusted prevalence of cancer in an SPN using Bayesian analysis in the form of likelihood ratios (LR). Subscript N refers to the LR and test sensitivity/specificity for each characteristic to be used (equation 2). Numbers in subscript (equation 3) refer to each pertinent LR to be applied to the prior odds of cancer. A reasonable prior odds of cancer may be 0.28, as outlined in the text. (From Gurney JW: Radiology 1993; 186:405–413. Used by permission.)

$$(1) \quad \text{PRIOR ODDS OF CANCER} = \frac{\text{PREVALENCE OF CANCER}}{1 - \text{PREVALENCE OF CANCER}}$$

$$(2) \quad \text{LIKELIHOOD RATIO}_N = \frac{\text{TEST}_N \text{ SENSITIVITY}}{1 - \text{TEST}_N \text{ SPECIFICITY}}$$

$$(3) \quad \text{ODDS OF CANCER} = \text{PRIOR ODDS OF CANCER} \times \text{LIKELIHOOD RATIO}_1 \times \text{LIKELIHOOD RATIO}_2 \cdots$$

$$(4) \quad \text{PROBABILITY OF CANCER} = \frac{\text{ODDS OF CANCER}}{\text{ODDS OF CANCER} + 1}$$

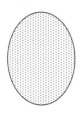
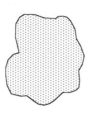
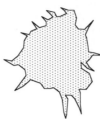

WELL DEFINED SMOOTH   **WELL DEFINED LOBULAR**   **ILL DEFINED SPICULATED**

Figure 2 ▪ Edge characteristics of SPN as defined for CT and radiography.

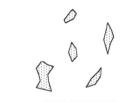

LINEAR   **ANGULAR**   **MULTIPLE**

Figure 3 ▪ Nodule appearances on x-ray tomography. Linear, angular, and multiple tiny opacities were defined as benign. Round, irregular, or cavitated lesions were defined as indeterminate. Spiculated masses were defined as malignant.

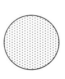

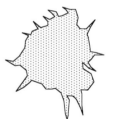

ROUND   IRREGULAR   CAVITATED   MALIGNANT

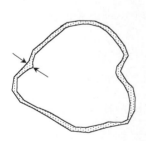
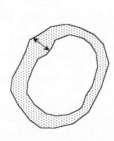
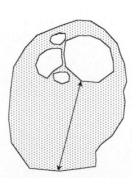

WALL ≤ 4 MM.   **WALL 5-15 MM.**   **WALL ≥ 16 MM.**

Figure 4 ▪ Maximal thickness of the border of cavitary lesions on chest radiographs. Three ranges of measurement are shown *(arrows)*.

Table 1 ▪ Likelihood Ratios for Malignancy in Solitary Pulmonary Nodules

CRITERION	CHARACTERISTIC	LR FOR MALIGNANCY	CONFIDENCE INTERVAL OF LR	COMMENTS
Size (data from CT)	0–1 cm	0.52	0.43–0.62	
	1.1–2.0 cm	0.74	0.66–0.82	
	2.1–3.0 cm	3.67	3.46–3.87	
	>3.0 cm	5.23	5.11–5.34	
Edge on chest radiograph*	Ill-defined	2.51	1.77–3.56	(See Figure 2)
	Well-defined, lobular	1.27	0.75–2.15	
	Well-defined, smooth	0.36	0.20–0.65	
Edge on CT*	Smooth	0.30	0.20–0.41	(See Figure 2)
	Lobulated	0.74	0.64–0.84	
	Irregular/spiculated	5.54	5.46–5.63	
Tomographic appearance*	Malignant	37.20	17.20–80.83	(See Figure 3)
	Indeterminate	0.73	0.56–0.94	
	Benign	0	0–0.02	
Calcification at CT	Calcified (264 HU)	0.01	0–0.03	Done with dedicated
	Calcified (185 HU)	0.07	—	reference phantom
	Not calcified	2.20	2.14–2.26	
Growth rate	<7 days	0	0–0.02	Volume doubling time
	7–465 days	3.40	2.48–4.66	
	>465 days	0.01	0–0.04	
Location	Upper/middle lobe	1.22	0.91–1.64	
	Lower lobe	0.66	0.49–0.89	
Cavity wall thickness	≤4 mm	0.07	0.03–0.14	(See Figure 4)
	5–15 mm	0.72	0.50–4.03	
	≥16 mm	37.97	13.07–110.30	
Enhancement at CT	≤19 HU	0.03	0–0.19	Gurney JW (personal
	>19 HU	3.60	2.33–5.55	communication)

*Only one of these should be used (preferably CT). HU = Hounsfield units, LR = likelihood ratio.
From Gurney JW: Radiology 1993; 186:405–413. Used by permission.

picts measurement of cavity wall thickness.[8, 9] CT nodule densitometry with and without the use of a reference phantom has been extensively described.[10–14] Nodule size on CT was defined as the average of the largest and smallest diameters measured from the slice on which the nodule appeared—the largest using lung window settings.[6, 7, 15]

Table 1 lists the LR numbers for each radiographic characteristic of SPN, and Table 2 lists LRs for patient demo-graphic criteria.[1] The four expert readers using qualitative judgment of probability of malignancy in SPNs had an accuracy rate of 63% and error rate of 37%. Quantitative determination of probability of malignancy using LRs and bayesian analysis was accurate to 78% and had an error rate of 16%.[2] Contrast enhancement at CT was not evaluated; it is covered in a separate section in this chapter, and the LR numbers are included in Table 1 for completeness.

Table 2 ▪ Likelihood Ratios (LR) for Malignancy in Solitary Pulmonary Nodules

CRITERION	CHARACTERISTIC	LR FOR MALIGNANCY	CONFIDENCE INTERVAL OF LR
Age	20–29 yr	0.05	0.01–0.09
	30–39 yr	0.24	0.14–0.35
	40–49 yr	0.94	0.87–1.01
	50–59 yr	1.90	1.73–2.07
	60–69 yr	2.64	2.44–2.83
	≥70 yr	4.16	3.97–4.35
Smoking history*	Never smoked	0.19	0.18–0.20
	Current cigarette	2.27	2.17–2.37
	Current pipe/cigar	1.00	0.96–1.04
	Ex-cigarette	0.92	0.88–0.96
	Ex-pipe/cigar	0.55	0.53–0.57
Amount smoked*	1–10 cigs./day	0.39	—
	11–20 cigs./day	0.88	—
	21–30 cigs./day	1.25	—
	31–40 cigs./day	1.53	—
	>40 cigs./day	1.57	—
Hemoptysis	Positive	5.08	3.55–7.27
Previous malignancy	Positive	4.95	4.13–5.93

*Only one of these should be used (preferably amount smoked if current cigarette smoker).
From Gurney JW: Radiology 1993; 186:405–413. Used by permission.

Source ▪

Patients (n = 66) with SPNs, who had suitable radiographic studies, pathologic proof of benign or malignant etiology, and/or long-term follow-up for presumed benign disease.

Comments ▪

The problem of analyzing a SPN can be daunting and confusing at times. The methods articulated by Gurney outline a useful framework for organizing one's thinking about such cases. Black's article on LR provides a clear description, with examples of how to perform the calculations, and is recommended.[2]

REFERENCES

1. Gurney JW: Determining the likelihood of malignancy in solitary pulmonary nodules with bayesian analysis. Part I. Theory. Radiology 1993; 186:405–413.
2. Black WC, Armstrong P: Communicating the significance of radiologic test results: The likelihood ratio. AJR Am J Roentgenol 1986; 147:1313–1318.
3. Gurney JW, Lyddon DM, McKay JA: Determining the likelihood of malignancy in solitary pulmonary nodules with bayesian analysis. Part II. Application. Radiology 1993; 186:415–422.
4. Huston J, Muhm JR: Solitary pulmonary opacities: Plain tomography. Radiology 1987; 163:481–485.
5. Bateson EM: An analysis of 155 solitary lung lesions illustrating the differential diagnosis of mixed tumors of the lung. Clin Radiol 1965; 16:51–65.
6. Siegelman SS, Khouri NF, Leo FP, et al: Solitary pulmonary nodules: CT assessment. Radiology 1986; 160:307–312.
7. Zerhouni EA, Stitik FP, Siegelman SS, et al: CT of the pulmonary nodule: A cooperative study. Radiology 1986; 160:319–327.
8. Woodring JH, Fried AM, Chuang VP: Solitary cavities of the lung: Diagnostic implications of cavity wall thickness. AJR Am J Roentgenol 1980; 135:1269–1271.
9. Woodring JH, Fried AM: Significance of wall thickness in solitary cavities of the lung: A follow-up study. AJR Am J Roentgenol 1983; 140:473–474.
10. Siegelman SS, Zerhouni EA, Leo FP, et al: CT of the solitary pulmonary nodule. AJR Am J Roentgenol 1980; 135(1):1–13.
11. Zerhouni EA, Boukadoum M, Siddiky MA, et al: A standard phantom for quantitative CT analysis of pulmonary nodules. Radiology 1983; 149(3):767–773.
12. deGeer G, Gamsu G, Cann C, Webb WR: Evaluation of a chest phantom for CT nodule densitometry. AJR Am J Roentgenol 1986; 147:21–25.
13. Khan A, Herman PG, Vorwerk P, et al: Solitary pulmonary nodules: Comparison of classification with standard, thin section, and reference phantom CT. Radiology 1991; 179:477–481.
14. Swensen SJ, Harms GF, Morin RL, Myers JL: CT evaluation of solitary pulmonary nodules: Value of 185-H reference phantom. AJR Am J Roentgenol 1991; 156(5):925–929.
15. Proto AV, Thomas SR: Pulmonary nodules studied by computed tomography. Radiology 1985; 156:149–153.

▪: VOLUME OF PLEURAL EFFUSION
▪ ACR Code: 66 (Pleura)

Technique ▪

Ultrasound (U/S) of the chest with the patient supine was performed with 3.5-MHz curved array or 6.3-MHz annular array using an Ultramark 9 machine (ATL, Bothell, WA). Transverse scans were done in maximal inspiration just above the lung base before and during aspiration of pleural effusions with a vanSonnenberg drainage catheter (Meditech/Boston Scientific, Watertown, MA) placed under U/S guidance. Lateral decubitus chest radiographs (LDX-ray) were obtained prior to drainage, with the effusion side down, a film-focus distance of 150 cm, and 120-kV technique.[1]

Measurements ▪

The maximum thickness of layering pleural fluid was measured from radiographs to the nearest millimeter. The maximum distance between the pleural surface and the lung edge (with pleural fluid intervening) was measured in millimeters from frozen U/S images, as shown in Figure 1. Although the radiographic measurement was made only prior to drainage, U/S measurements of fluid thickness were made prior to and during the drainage (after every 200 ml was removed). By knowing the final volume of fluid removed and subsequent subtraction, the volume of pleural fluid during each of 331 U/S measurements could be inferred. Table 1 gives results of U/S fluid thickness measurements versus known fluid volumes.[1]

Figure 1 ▪ Measurement of pleural fluid thickness from transverse lateral chest ultrasound with the patient supine and at maximal inspiration. The maximal distance between parietal pleura and the lung edge is measured (arrows) in mm.

Source ▪

Subjects included 51 patients (21 men, 41 women, age range 26 to 82 years, mean age 61 years) who had drainage of nonloculated, simple pleural effusions. Complete drainage was documented by postprocedure sonography and chest radiograph. Of the 64 patients initially enrolled in the study, 16 were excluded because of incomplete drainage.[1]

Table 1 ▪ Pleural Effusion Volume Predicted by Ultrasound Fluid Thickness

MAXIMUM THICKNESS (mm)	NO.	VOLUME (ml) Mean ± SD	PERCENT ERROR SD/Mean × 100	RANGE (ml)
0	53	5 ± 15	—	0–90
5	20	80 ± 35	44	20–170
10	24	170 ± 55	32	50–300
15	29	260 ± 100	38	90–420
20	41	380 ± 130	34	150–660
25	41	580 ± 230	40	250–1,080
30	40	550 ± 200	36	210–1,060
35	33	780 ± 260	33	410–1,400
40	18	1,000 ± 330	33	490–1,670
45	13	1,020 ± 250	25	730–1,500
50	9	1,420 ± 380	27	650–1,840
55	5	1,430 ± 430	30	850–1,900
≥60	5	1,640 ± 590	36	950–2,150

Number refers to individual measurements (total n = 331) correlated with known fluid volume in 51 patients.
From Eibenberger KL, Dock WI, Ammann ME, et al: Radiology 1994; 191:681–684. Used by permission.

Comments ▪

Linear correlation of aspirated fluid volume with preprocedure U/S and LDX-ray pleural fluid thickness measurements yielded the following formulas:

Volume (ml) =
45.5 × (fluid thickness on LDX-ray in mm) − 403
(r = 0.58, mean prediction error = 465 ml).

Volume (ml) = 47.6 × (fluid thickness at U/S) − 837
(r = 0.80, mean prediction error = 263 ml).

Eibenberger and colleagues found that the mean values for fluid volume versus U/S thickness based on the 331 experimental measurements (Figure 1) were the most accurate at predicting total aspirated fluid volume from each patient based on preprocedure U/S thickness (mean prediction error was 224 ml). They stress the importance of having the transducer in true transverse orientation so as to avoid overestimating fluid thickness with oblique scanning.[1]

REFERENCE

1. Eibenberger KL, Dock WI, Ammann ME, et al: Quantification of pleural effusions: Sonography versus radiography. Radiology 1994; 191:681–684.

▪: MEASUREMENT OF TRACHEA DIAMETER IN THE NEWBORN INFANT[1]
▪ ACR Code: 671 (Trachea)

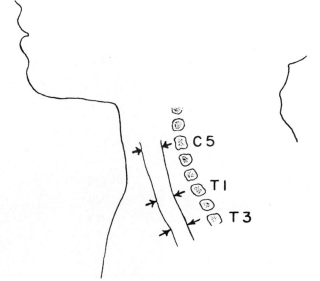

Figure 1 ▪ Measurement of anteroposterior tracheal diameter from lateral radiographs. The same levels are used for transverse (lateral) diameter from frontal radiographs.

Table 1 ▪ Normal Tracheal Diameters in the Newborn			
	C5	T1	T3
Anteroposterior diameter of trachea			
Average diameter (mm)	4.5	3.9	3.5
Lateral diameter of trachea*			
Minimum diameter (mm)	2	1	1
Maximum diameter (mm)	7	6	5

*Donaldson and Tompsett found that this diameter was quite variable. Also, they considered a 3-mm anteroposterior diameter in the upper thorax to be the lower limit of normal.

Technique ▪

Central ray: Anteroposterior to fourth thoracic vertebra.
    Left lateral: To fourth thoracic vertebra on midcoronal plane.
Position: Anteroposterior, left lateral.
Target-film distance: 36 inches.
Films taken in maximum inspiration.

Measurements (Figure 1 and Table 1) ▪

Source ▪

Studies of 350 normal infants were made within 24 hours after birth.

REFERENCE

1. Donaldson SW, Tompsett AC: AJR Am J Roentgenol 1952; 67:785.

▪: DIMENSIONS OF THE NORMAL TRACHEA[1]
▪ ACR Code: 671 (Trachea)

Technique ▪

Central ray: Perpendicular to plane of film.
Position: Posteroanterior and lateral with maximum inspiration.
Target-film distance: 10 feet (3.05 m). Magnification factor 1.08.

Measurements (Figure 1) ▪

The internal diameter of the tracheal air column was measured at a level 2 cm above the projected top of the aortic arch on both PA and lateral films. Measurements were made of the air column alone, excluding the tracheal wall.

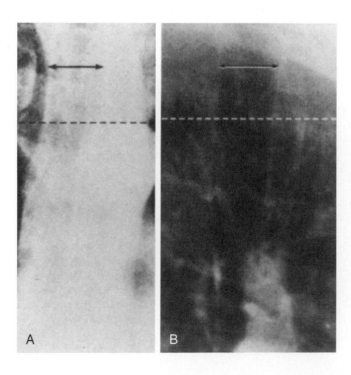

Figure 1 ▪ Level of measurement *(solid line)* of coronal *(A)* and sagittal *(B)* tracheal diameters, 2 cm above projected top of aortic arch *(broken line)*. (From Breatnach E, et al: AJR Am J Roentgenol 1984; 142:903–906. Used by permission.)

Table 1 • Mean Coronal and Sagittal Tracheal Diameters in Normal Subjects by Gender and Age*

| AGE GROUP (YR) | MALE | | | FEMALE | | |
| | No. of Subjects | Tracheal Diameter (mm): Mean ± SD | | No. of Subjects | Tracheal Diameter (mm): Mean ± SD | |
		Coronal	Sagittal		Coronal	Sagittal
10–19	26	15.5±2.8	15.4±3.1	22	14.4±1.6	14.5±1.3
20–29	81	18.7±2.0	19.3±2.0	98	15.7±1.6	15.6±1.7
30–39	72	19.2±2.1	19.7±2.4	64	16.0±1.8	16.3±2.3
40–49	69	19.5±2.3	20.3±2.2	45	16.6±2.0	16.8±2.2
50–59	80	19.2±2.3	20.4±2.6	65	16.5±1.6	17.0±2.0
60–69	71	19.5±2.2	20.7±2.5	48	16.8±2.0	17.2±2.3
70–79	31	19.7±2.2	20.8±1.8	36	16.4±2.4	16.5±2.3

*Coronal and sagittal tracheal diameters were defined as the internal diameters of the tracheal air column as measured at a level 2 cm above the projected top of the aortic arch on posteroanterior and lateral radiographs, respectively.
From Breatnach E, et al: AJR Am J Roentgenol 1984; 142:903–906. Used by permission.

The dimensions of the trachea related to age are given in Table 1.

Source •

Data are based on studies of chest films of 808 patients with no clinical or radiologic evidence of respiratory disease. There were 430 men and 378 women, ranging in age from 10 to 79 years.

REFERENCE

1. Breatnach E, Abbott GC, Fraser RG: Dimensions of the normal human trachea. AJR Am J Roentgenol 1984; 142:903–906.

•: MEASUREMENT OF TRACHEAL DIMENSIONS
• ACR Code: 671 (Trachea, Bronchi)

Technique •

Griscom and Wohl used GE 8800 or 9800 CT scanners (GE Medical Systems, Milwaukee, WI) to examine the trachea. Anteroposterior (AP) and lateral (LAT) scout views were taken first, followed by contiguous 10-mm axial slices through the chest. The youngest patients were asleep; slightly older patients were sedated and breathing quietly or awake and scanned near functional residual capacity. Those over 6 years of age were scanned at full inspiration.[1, 2]

Measurements •

Griscom has standardized a method of measuring tracheal dimensions during previous work.[3, 4] The length between the vocal cords and carina is measured directly from the AP scout with electronic calipers at the operator's console. This is shown in Figure 1. The AP diameters, transverse (TRV) diameters, and areas were measured on all sections containing the trachea (mean 6, range 3 to 10). The method used is meant to correct for the variability in apparent tracheal size depending on window/level selection.[5] All subsequent steps are done at the operator's console with magnified images through the trachea. Using region of interest (ROI) cursors, the average CT number in Hounsfield units (HU) is determined within the tracheal air column and in the paratracheal tissues. The midpoint between these two HU values was set as the level, and the pixels within 75 HU of that value were highlighted using the "blink" mode of the machine. These pixels outlined the tracheal lumen, allowing measurement of AP dimension, TRV dimension, and area using the measure distance and trace functions. Figure 2 shows these measurement techniques.

Two corrections were made to the area measurements. First, one half of the area of the highlighted pixels was added since the traced area did not include them. Table 1 gives approximate values for these corrections.[4] Second, correction for the anterior angulation of the trachea in the cephalad direction was done by multiplying the area by the cosine of the angle (determined from the LAT scout). This angle averages 11.5 degrees, and the cosine is 0.98.[3] The linear dimensions and areas from each examination were

Table 1 • Correction of Tracheal Area for Air–Soft Tissue Interface

AREA RANGE (sq cm)	CORRECTION (sq cm)
<0.20	0.04
0.20–0.40	0.05
0.40–0.60	0.06
0.60–0.80	0.07
0.80–1.05	0.08
1.05–1.35	0.09
1.35–1.65	0.10
1.65–1.20	0.11
1.20–1.35	0.12
2.35–2.70	0.13
2.70–3.05	0.14

The correction is added to measured areas.[3]

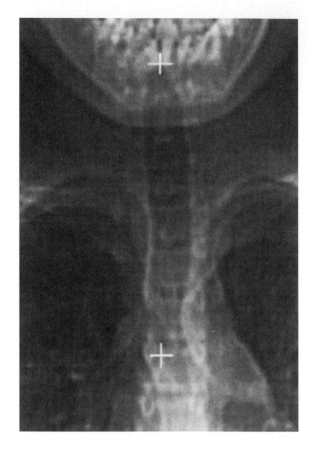

Figure 1 ▪ Measurement of tracheal length from AP scout film obtained during CT examination. Cursors were placed over the vocal cords and the carina to obtain the distance. (From Griscom NT: Radiology 1982; 145(2):361–364. Used by permission.)

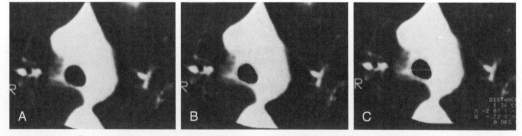

Figure 2 ▪ *A*, Magnified 10 mm section through the trachea. The window is 1000 HU and the level is −500 HU. *B*, Same section, with pixels within 75 HU of the value between the air column and peritracheal soft tissue highlighted. *C*, Transverse diameter measured using the highlighted pixels as the border. AP diameter and area are traced in similar fashion. (From Griscom NT: Radiology 1982; 145(2):361–364. Used by permission.)

Table 2 ▪ Tracheal Dimensions in Children and Adolescents

AGE RANGE (yr)	NO. FEMALES	NO. MALES	AVERAGE AGE (yr)	LENGTH (cm)	AP (cm)	TRV (cm)	AREA (sq cm)	VOLUME (cc)
0–2	5	8	1.0	5.4±0.7	0.53±0.10	0.64±0.12	0.28±0.09	1.57±0.67
2–4	6	9	3.2	6.4±0.5	0.74±0.08	0.81±0.07	0.48±0.08	3.11±0.61
4–6	4	4	4.9	7.2±0.8	0.80±0.06	0.90±0.09	0.58±0.10	4.16±0.86
6–8	6	5	6.5	8.2±0.7	0.92±0.11	0.93±0.08	0.69±0.11	5.67±1.20
8–10	4	7	9.2	8.8±0.9	1.05±0.05	1.07±0.06	0.89±0.09	7.87±1.45
10–12	4	4	11.2	10.0±1.0	1.16±0.10	1.18±0.09	1.10±0.18	11.1±2.3
12–14	7	8	13.2	10.8±1.5	1.30±0.18	1.33±0.16	1.39±0.36	15.4±6.0
14–16	6	—	15.1	11.2±1.2	1.39±0.07	1.46±0.07	1.62±0.14	18.2±2.2
16–18	13	—	16.7	12.2±1.1	1.37±0.17	1.40±0.12	1.54±0.29	18.8±4.3
18–20	4	—	18.6	11.8±1.0	1.42±0.18	1.39±0.11	1.59±0.29	18.9±4.2
14–16	—	6	15.0	12.4±0.6	1.45±0.08	1.43±0.06	1.62±0.13	20.2±2.4
16–18	—	13	16.8	12.4±1.3	1.57±0.14	1.59±0.16	2.01±0.30	25.1±5.2
18–20	—	7	19.2	13.1±0.9	1.75±0.17	1.66±0.16	2.30±0.39	30.3±5.9

Males and females shown separately at age 14 years and older.
All measurements are mean ± standard deviation. cm = centimeters, sq cm = square centimeters, cc = cubic centimeters.
From Griscom NT, Wohl ME: AJR Am J Roentgenol 1986; 146:233–237. Used by permission.

averaged and the average area multiplied by length to obtain volume.[1, 2]

Table 2 lists the measurements obtained by age and gender (from 0 to 20 years). There was no significant difference between genders before age 14 years. Table 3 lists the results of multiple regression of logarithms of the various dimensions and logarithm of height. Figures 3, 4, and 5 show tracheal dimensions based on height calculated from the "All subjects" rows from Table 3.

Source ▪

In a study of tracheal dimensions related to age and gender, 130 children and adolescents (age and gender distribution shown in Table 2) with no disease or condition affecting the airway were included.[1] In a separate study of tracheal dimensions related to body height, 100 children and adolescents (45 males, 55 females, age range 9 days to 20 years) had chest CT scans. These patients had no intrathoracic

Table 3 ▪ Relationship Between Tracheal Dimensions and Body Height

DIMENSION/ GROUP	a	b	95% CI FOR b	CORRELATION WITH HEIGHT (r)
Length (cm)				
All subjects	−3.80	1.22	1.08–1.36	0.88
Males	−3.58	1.18	1.04–1.32	0.92
Females	−4.52	1.37	1.05–1.69	0.80
AP diameter (cm)				
All subjects	−6.65	1.37	1.22–1.52	0.89
Males	−6.74	1.39	1.23–1.55	0.93
Females	−6.26	1.29	0.96–1.62	0.78
TRV diameter (cm)				
All subjects	−5.88	1.22	1.09–1.35	0.89
Males	−5.70	1.19	1.03–1.35	0.91
Females	−6.40	1.32	1.06–1.56	0.87
Area (sq cm)				
All subjects	−12.7	2.58	2.33–2.83	0.90
Males	−12.7	2.57	2.29–2.85	0.93
Females	−12.7	2.57	2.04–3.10	0.83
Volume (cc)				
All subjects	−16.5	3.80	3.48–4.12	0.92
Males	−16.3	3.76	3.41–4.11	0.95
Females	−17.2	3.92	3.23–4.61	0.88

The equation used is $\ln(\text{dimension}) = a + b \times \ln(\text{body height in cm})$. This simplifies to $\text{dimension} = e^a \times \text{height}^b$.
cm = centimeters, sq cm = square centimeters, cc = cubic centimeters.
From Griscom NT, Wohl MEB: Am Rev Respir Dis 1985; 131:840–844. Used by permission.

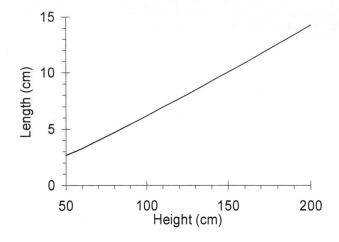

Figure 3 ▪ Length of the trachea versus body height. Calculated from regression equation and reported coefficients.[2]

Figure 4 ▪ Tracheal diameters (anteroposterior = AP and transverse = TRV) versus body height. Calculated from regression equation and reported coefficients.[2]

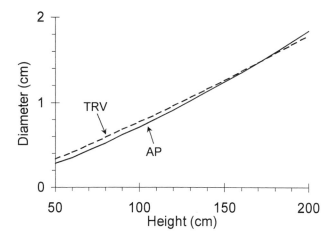

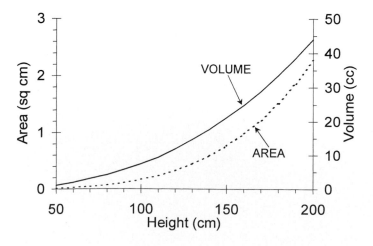

Figure 5 ▪ Tracheal area and volume versus body height. Calculated from regression equation and reported coefficients.[2]

abnormalities likely to distort the trachea, and most were well grown with only six falling just below the 5th percentile for height.[2]

REFERENCES

1. Griscom NT, Wohl ME: Dimensions of the growing trachea related to age and gender. AJR Am J Roentgenol 1986; 146:233–237.

2. Griscom NT, Wohl MEB: Dimensions of the growing trachea related to body height. Am Rev Respir Dis 1985; 131:840–844.
3. Griscom NT: Computed tomographic determination of tracheal dimensions in children and adolescents. Radiology 1982; 145(2):361–364.
4. Griscom NT: CT measurement of the tracheal lumen in children and adolescents. AJR Am J Roentgenol 1991; 156:371–372.
5. Baxter BS, Sorenson JA: Factors affecting the measurement of size and CT number in computed tomography. Invest Radiol 1981; 16:337–341.

▪: THE LEVEL OF BIFURCATION OF THE TRACHEA IN ADULT AND CHILD[1]
▪ ACR Code: 671 (Trachea, Bronchi)

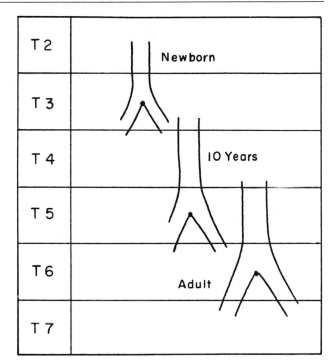

Figure 1 ▪ Vertebral levels of tracheal bifurcation.

Technique ▪

Central ray: To fourth thoracic vertebra.
Position: Posteroanterior.
Target-film distance: 72 inches.

Measurements (Figure 1) ▪

Newborn, third thoracic vertebra; 10-year-old, fifth thoracic vertebra; adult, sixth thoracic vertebra.

Source ▪

Caffey quotes the work of Mehnert.[2] The number of cases studied by Mehnert is not known.

REFERENCES

1. Caffey J: Pediatric X-ray Diagnosis, ed 3. Year Book Medical Publishers, Chicago, 1956.
2. Mehnert E: Über topographische Alterveränderungen des Atmungsapparates. Jena, 1901.

▪: ANGLE OF TRACHEAL BIFURCATION[1]
▪ ACR Code: 671 (Trachea, Bronchi)

Technique ▪

Central ray: To the fourth thoracic vertebra.
Position: Posteroanterior.
Taget-film distance: 40 inches for patients under age 1 year; 72 inches for all other patients.

Measurements (Figure 1) ▪

Draw a straight line in the middle of each bronchus parallel to the walls of the bronchus.

Bifurcation angle θ is given in Figures 2 and 3. Mean and 95% confidence limits are shown.

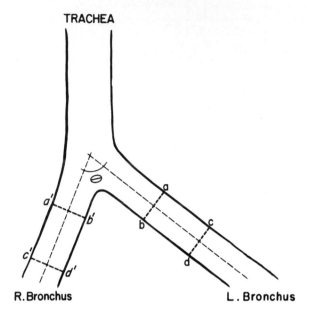

Figure 1 ▪ Measurement of the tracheal bifurcation angle from a frontal radiograph. Straight lines are drawn through the middle of each bronchus and that angle is measured at their intersection.

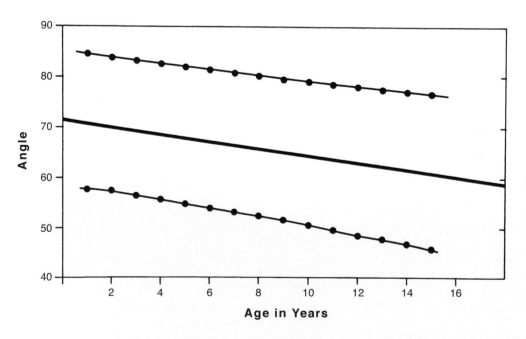

Figure 2 ▪ Ninety-five percent confidence band for people under 16 years of age. Regression equation based on male and female data.

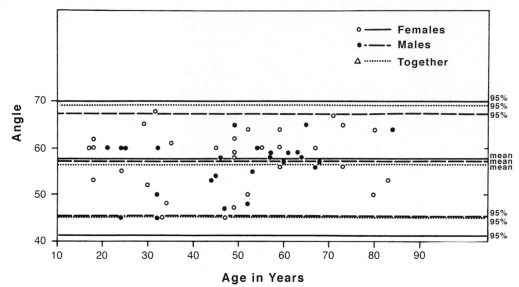

Figure 3 ▪ Ninety-five percent confidence band for people over 16 years of age.

Source ▪

Eighty-seven patients whose chest roentgenograms were interpreted as normal. Forty-one males and 46 females were in the study. Twenty-nine of the patients were under 16 years of age.

REFERENCE

1. Alavi SM, Keats TE, O'Brien WM: The angle of tracheal bifurcation: Its normal mensuration. AJR Am J Roentgenol 1970; 108:546–549.

▪▪ INTERBRONCHIAL AND SUBCARINAL ANGLES
▪ ACR Code: 671 (Trachea, Bronchi)

Technique ▪

Posteroanterior (PA) inspiratory chest radiographs with a target-to-film distance of 72 inches (182 cm) and standard high-voltage technique were performed.[1–3] Echocardiography with a Sonus 700 machine (Hewlett-Packard, Andover, MA), using a 2.5-MHz probe and standard views, was done to assess left atrial dimension.[2] Taskin's study included both standard PA (as above) and portable films.[4]

Measurements ▪

The interbronchial angle (IA) was defined by drawing lines through the middle of each main stem bronchus and was measured in degrees with a goniometer from the film.[1, 2, 4] The subcarinal angle (SA) was defined by drawing lines through the inferior walls of each bronchus and was measured as well.[1, 2, 3] Figure 1 shows these angles and Table 1 lists reported values.

Table 1 ▪ Interbronchial and Subcarinal Angles

REFERENCE	SUBJECT TYPE	AGE RANGE (yr)	NO.	INTERBRONCHIAL ANGLE (degrees)	SUBCARINAL ANGLE (degrees)
Haskin (normative)	Normal	21–30	22	62.6 ± 7.49	64.2 ± 10.03
	Normal	31–40	17	57.2 ± 11.35	58.9 ± 13.36
	Normal	41–50	17	61.2 ± 9.46	61.9 ± 11.61
	Normal	51–60	21	62.5 ± 9.72	63.1 ± 11.96
	Normal	>60	23	54.8 ± 9.01	55.9 ± 11.30
	Normal	all patients	100	59.6 ± 9.74	60.8 ± 11.80
Murray (left atrium)	Normal	27–85	65	70.4 ± 14.3	62.6 ± 14.8
	Enlarged	27–79	43	80.5 ± 17.0	73.0 ± 18.9
Chen (pericardial effusion)	Before	8–75	14	—	62.3 ± 8.6
	Maximum	8–75	54	—	81.0 ± 10.3
	Resolving	8–75	27	—	64.4 ± 9.5
	After	8–75	21	—	56.7 ± 7.7

Measurements are given as mean ± standard deviation.

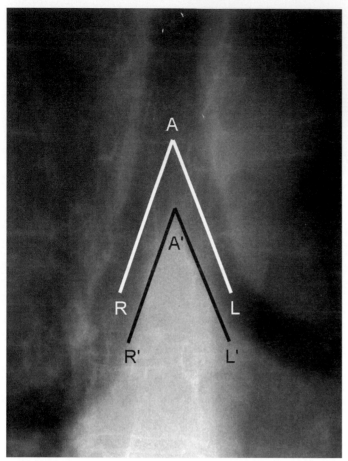

Figure 1 ▪ Measurement of interbronchial (IA) and subcarinal (SA) angles from a chest radiograph. The IA *(RAL)* is measured between lines *(white)* drawn through the middle of the right and left main bronchi. The SA *(R′A′L′)* is measured between lines *(black)* drawn through the lower borders of the right and left main bronchi. The airway has been enhanced in this radiograph for clarity.

Source ▪

Haskin and Goodman studied 100 healthy subjects (47 men, 53 women, age range 21 to 80 years) to determine normal tracheal bifurcation angles.[1] Murray and colleagues evaluated 108 patients (53 men, 55 women, age range 27 to 85 years, mean age 64 years), of whom 65 had normal left atrial dimensions and 43 had left atrial enlargement (LAE) by echocardiography. This was determined by the distance between the posterior aortic root and the posterior left atrial wall at end-systole, and 4.0 cm was used as the cut-off value.[2] Chen and colleagues studied 48 adults (22 men, 26 women, age range 20 to 75 years) and 6 children (5 boys, 1 girl, age range 8 to 15 years) with pericardial effusion for various reasons. The presence of effusion was confirmed by surgery, autopsy, pericardiocentesis, or echocardiography. Radiographs were divided into four groups (before, maximum, resolving, after), depending on timing with respect to the episode of effusion.[3] Taskin and colleagues reviewed echocardiogram reports and evaluated chest radiographs of 70 patients (33 men, 37 women, age range 18 to 87 years, mean age 56 years) with LAE (diameter >4.5 cm). A group of 35 age-paired controls were also studied.[4]

Comments ▪

The reported limits of normal (95% confidence intervals) for the adult IA are 45 to 69, 40 to 80, and 40 to 99 degrees.[1, 2, 5] The 95% confidence limits of the SA from the two sizable studies cited here are 37 to 84 and 33 to 92 degrees.[1, 2] Murray and colleagues found that an IA of 76.4 degrees was the best cut-off for predicting LAE (sensitivity 61%, specificity 63%), and the best cut-off for SA was 65.4 degrees (sensitivity 51%, specificity 66%). They felt that neither angle was particularly useful in predicting LAE.[2] Taskin and colleagues did not report values but stated that an IA of greater than 100 degrees confidently predicts the presence of LAE (>5.0 cm) on echocardiography.[4] Chen and colleagues state that widening of the SA is a late and insensitive sign for LAE, whereas it may be an important clue to pericardial effusion.

REFERENCES

1. Haskin PH, Goodman LR: Normal tracheal bifurcation angle: A reassessment. AJR Am J Roentgenol 1982; 139:879–882.
2. Murray JG, Brown AL, Anagnostou EA, Senior R: Widening of the tracheal bifurcation on chest radiographs: Value as a sign of left atrial enlargement. AJR Am J Roentgenol 1995; 164:1089–1092.
3. Chen JTT, Putman CE, Hedlund LW, et al: Widening of the subcarinal angle by pericardial effusion. AJR Am J Roentgenol 1982; 139:883–887.
4. Taskin V, Bates MC, Chillag SA: Tracheal carinal angle and left atrial size [see comments]. Arch Intern Med 1991; 151(2):307–308.
5. Alavi SM, Keats TE, O'Brien WM: The angle of tracheal bifurcation: Its normal mensuration. AJR Am J Roentgenol 1970; 108:546–549.

▪: MEASUREMENT OF THE RIGHT PARATRACHEAL STRIPE IN CHILDREN AND ADULTS[1, 2]

▪ ACR Code: 671 (Trachea)

Technique ▪

Central ray: Projected through the midchest.
Position: Posteroanterior.
Target-film distance: 72 inches.

Measurements (Figure 1) ▪

The right paratracheal stripe in normal children measures 0.5 to 3 mm, and any stripe 4 mm or wider is reliable evidence of disease affecting the trachea, mediastinum, or pleura.

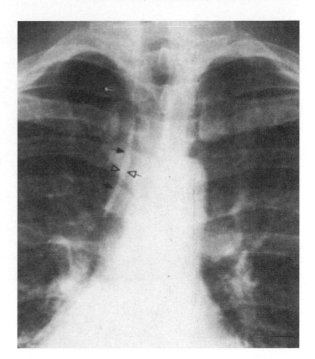

Figure 1 ▪ The right paratracheal stripe. The *open arrows* outline the stripe at a level 2 cm above the superior extent of the azygos arch. *Arrows* 1 cm above and 1 cm below indicate the range within which the width of the stripe was measured. (From Savoca CJ, et al: Radiology 1977; 122:295. Used by permission.)

The right paratracheal stripe in a normal adult measures 1 to 4 mm. A measurement of 5 mm or more is reliable evidence of disease.

Source ▪

Data for children were derived from 50 children aged 5 months to 15 years. Adult data were derived from end-inspiration chest films of 1259 normal subjects.

References

1. Savoca CJ, Brasch RC, Gooding CA, Gamsu G: The right paratracheal stripe in children. Pediatr Radiol 1978; 6:203–207.
2. Savoca CJ, Austin JH, Goldberg HI: The right paratracheal stripe. Radiology 1977; 122:295–301.

▪: MEASUREMENT OF THE POSTERIOR TRACHEAL BAND[1]
▪ ACR Code: 671 (Trachea)

Technique ▪

Central ray: Perpendicular to plane of film centered over midchest.
Position: Lateral upright.
Target-film distance: 72 inches.

Measurements (Figure 1) ▪

The posterior tracheal band is uniform in width, measuring up to 3 mm (rarely to 4 mm) in thickness. Width greater than 4.5 mm is considered pathologic in a follow-up study by Putman et al.[2]

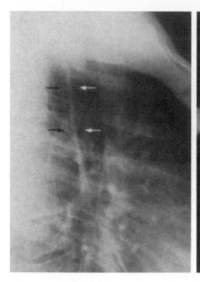 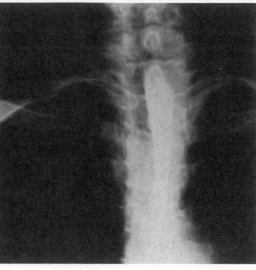

Figure 1 ▪ The normal posterior tracheal band. (From Bachman AL, Teixidor HS: Br J Radiol 1975; 48:352. Used by permission.)

Source ▪

Based on a study of 200 normal individuals in whom 182 posterior tracheal bands could be visualized.

REFERENCES

1. Bachman AL, Teixidor HS: The posterior tracheal band: A reflector of local superior mediastinal abnormality. Br J Radiol 1975; 48:352–359.
2. Putman CE, Curtis AM, Westfried M, McLoud TC: Thickening of the posterior tracheal stripe: A sign of squamous cell carcinoma of the esophagus. Radiology 1976; 121(3 Pt.1):533–536.

▪: MEASUREMENT OF RETROSTERNAL SOFT TISSUE[1]
▪ ACR Code: 673 (Anterior Mediastinum)

Technique ▪

Central ray: Perpendicular to plane of film centered over midchest.
Position: True lateral upright.
Target-film distance: 180 cm.

Measurements (Table 1) ▪

Measurements made 2, 4, and 6 cm below the sternal margin of the manubriosternal sternal joint. These measurements are useful in detecting abnormalities of the retrosternal soft tissues.

Table 1 ■ Width of the Retrosternal Soft Tissue

GENDER	AGE RANGE (Yr)	MEAN AGE (Yr)	DISTANCE FROM MANUBRIOSTERNAL JOINT (cm)*	NO. OF CASES	MEAN (mm)	SD (mm)	SE (mm)
Normal subjects	20–39	28.4	2	43	2.35	1.00	0.15
Men			4	43	2.35	1.34	0.20
			6	41	2.68	1.52	0.24
	42–59	49.2	2	33	2.64	1.11	0.19
			4	33	2.64	0.99	0.17
			6	31	3.03	1.30	0.23
	61–72	64.3	2	12	3.42	1.38	0.40
			4	13	3.46	1.61	0.45
			6	13	4.46	1.61	0.45
Women	20–40	29.7	2	33	2.12	1.16	0.20
			4	33	2.33	1.36	0.23
			6	33	2.88	1.34	0.23
	41–59	49.9	2	23	2.26	1.48	0.31
			4	22	2.59	1.56	0.33
			6	23	3.17	1.77	0.37
	63–78	69.2	2	8	2.38	1.19	0.42
			4	8	2.25	0.71	0.25
			6	8	3.25	1.49	0.53
All measurements analyzed together		41.5		453	2.67	1.38	0.065
Subjects with obstructive emphysema							
Men	22–78	57.7	2	8	1.75	0.89	0.31
			4	8	1.63	0.92	0.32
			6	8	1.63	1.30	0.46

*Indicates the point at which the measurement was taken.
From Jemelin C, Candardjis G: Radiology 1973; 109:7–11. Used by permission.

Source ■

Data based on a study of 380 chest films of normal patients, men and women, ranging in age from 20 to 78 years.

REFERENCE

1. Jemelin C, Candardjis G: Retrosternal soft tissue; Quantitative evaluation and clinical interest. Landmarks between normal and pathological aspects. Radiology 1973; 109:7–11.

■: THYMIC SIZE FROM BIRTH THROUGH 2 YEARS
■ ACR Code: 675 (Thymus)

Technique ■

Parasternal and suprasternal ultrasound of the anterior chest was done with real-time equipment (machine and transducer details not listed).[1]

Measurements ■

The thymus gland was identified on transverse and longitudinal images. The transverse diameter of the thymus was measured from frozen images with electronic calipers (Figure 1A). The perimeter of the thymus was drawn on a frozen longitudinal image, and the area subtended was calculated (Figure 1B). The thymic index was defined as the product of the longitudinal area (in square centimeters) and the transverse diameter (in centimeters). Table 1 lists the thymic index by age and feeding status (exclusive breast feeding, breast and bottle feeding, and exclusive bottle feeding).[1]

Source ■

The study included 37 healthy infants scanned at birth and then at 4, 8, 10, and 12 months of age. Of these, 34 were able to return at 2 years for a last examination. Feeding status, gender, length, and weight were recorded. Exclusive breast feeding was defined as reported intake of less than 1 bottle of formula per week at the date of the 4-month examination.[1]

Comments ■

The thymic index has been shown to correlate well with thymic weight and volume in a postmortem study.[2] Inter- and intraobserver variability have been evaluated (1.47 and 1.13, respectively) and the measurement determined to be reproducible.[3] Exclusively breast-fed infants had a significantly larger thymic index (p = .0002) at 4 months and again (p = .014) at 10 months.[1] A positive history for one or more febrile illnesses between 10 and 12 months was

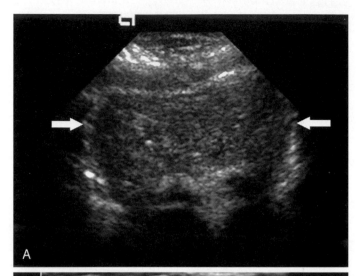

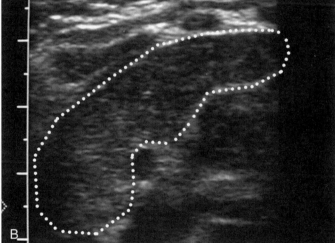

Figure 1 • Thymic index determination from ultrasound done from birth to 2 years. *A*, Transverse image showing transverse diameter *(arrows)* measurement. *B*, Longitudinal image with perimeter *(dotted line)* traced for area determination. The thymic index was defined as the product of these two measurements.

Table 1 • Thymic Index from Birth to 2 Years by Age and Feeding Status

	BIRTH	4 MON	8 MON	10 MON	12 MON	24 MON
Median	11.8 (8.3–13.6)	25.7	29.0	18.9	17.3	21.2
Overall mean	11.9	26.3	26.6	18.9	18.3	21.1
Exclusively breast-fed infants		36.34 (27.6–56.1)	27.41 (23.7–36.9)	23.52 (18.4–35.9)	17.7 (14.5–37.4)	22.2 (20.1–29.6)
Partially breast-fed infants		26.50 (20.3–27.6)	23.76 (14.4–29.6)	16.53 (12.4–17.8)	21.0 (12.4–25.8)	19.7 (11.0–24.1)
Exclusively formula-fed infants		18.89 (14.4–28.3)	28.99 (23.5–40.0)	17.33 (13.7–23.6)	16.5 (8.7–25.3)	21.6 (16.8–21.0)
Feeding status p values		0.0002	0.5387	0.0140	0.4662	0.4218

5th and 95th percentiles are given in parentheses.
From Hasselbalch H, Ersboll AK, Jeppesen DL, Nielsen MB: Acta Radiol 1999; 40:41–44. Used by permission.

correlated with a smaller thymic index measured at 12 months. The median and range were 17.0 and 7.4 to 26.0 compared with 24.2 and 8.8 to 53.0 for those without a history of fever.[4] Hasselbalch and colleagues[5] have also derived a formula for predicting thymic index in healthy neonates based on weight as follows:

$$\ln \text{(thymic index)} = 1.216 + 0.00034 \text{ (weight in grams)}, \text{ r squared} = 0.18, p = .0003.$$

REFERENCES

1. Hasselbalch H, Ersboll AK, Jeppesen DL, Nielsen MB: Thymus size in infants from birth until 24 months of age evaluated by ultrasound. A longitudinal prediction model for the thymic index. Acta Radiol 1999; 40:41–44.
2. Hasselbalch H, Jeppesen DL, Ersboll AK, Nielsen MB: Thymus size in preterm infants evaluated by ultrasound: A preliminary report. Acta Radiol 1999; 40:37–40.
3. Hasselbalch H, Nielsen MB, Jeppesen DL, et al: Sonographic measurements of the thymus in infants. Eur Radiol 1996; 6:700–703.
4. Hasselbalch H, Jeppesen DL, Ersboll AK, et al: The size of the thymus evaluated by sonography: A longitudinal study in infants during the first year of life. Acta Radiol 1997; 38:222–227.
5. Hasselbalch H, Jeppesen DL, Ersboll AK, et al: Sonographic measurements of the thymic size in healthy neonates: Relation to clinical variables. Acta Radiol 1997; 38:95–98.

▪: MEASUREMENT OF THE NORMAL THYMUS BY CT[1]
▪ ACR Code: 675 (Thymus)

Technique ▪

1. CT scans were performed on a GE 8800 scanner using a scan time of 5.6 sec and a 2.5-sec interscan delay.
2. Contiguous 1-cm-thick slices were obtained at full inspiration. Contrast infusion was administered by bolus.

Measurements ▪

The craniocaudal extent, maximum AP and transverse dimensions, and thickness were measured as shown in Figure 1.

The normal measurements are given in Table 1.

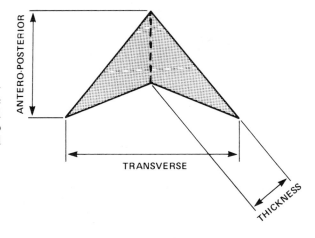

Figure 1 ▪ Measurement of thymic dimensions from the CT slice best depicting the gland. Anteroposterior and transverse dimensions of the whole gland as well as thickness of each lobe may be measured. The cephalocaudal extent is determined by subtracting table positions of scans showing the top and bottom of the gland. (From Francis IR, et al: AJR Am J Roentgenol 1985; 145:249–254.)

Table 1 ▪ Thymic Measurements in Patients with Normal Glands

AGE GROUP (Yr)	NO. OF PATIENTS	MEAN DIMENSION IN CM (SD)			
		Thickness	Anteroposterior	Craniocaudal	Transverse
0–10	23	1.50 (0.46)	2.52 (0.82)	3.53 (0.99)	3.13 (0.85)
10–20	31	1.05 (0.36)	2.56 (0.88)	4.99 (1.25)	3.05 (1.17)
20–30	13	0.89 (0.16)	2.38 (0.72)	5.38 (1.80)	2.87 (0.86)
30–40	8	0.99 (0.34)	2.48 (0.86)	5.00 (1.12)	3.38 (1.37)
40–50	3	0.93 (0.58)	2.23 (0.93)	6.67 (2.08)	3.17 (0.76)
50–60	4	0.58 (0.33)	0.58 (0.33)	2.00 (1.15)	1.43 (0.48)

From Francis IR, et al: AJR Am J Roentgenol 1985; 145:249–254. Used by permission.

Source ▪

Data based on CT examination of 309 normal patients ranging in age from 6 weeks to 81 years.

REFERENCE

1. Francis IR, Glazer GM, Bookstein FL, Gross BH: The thymus: Reexamination of age-related changes in size and shape. AJR Am J Roentgenol 1985; 145:249–254.

⠆ DIMENSIONS OF THE NORMAL THYMUS
- ▪ ACR Code: 675 (Thymus)

Technique ▪

Baron and colleagues performed CT of the chest with a 7070 (EMI) machine using 1-cm slice thickness with 3-sec scan time. St. Amour and colleagues used EMI 7070 or DR3 machines (Siemens, Erlangen, Germany) with 3- to 4-sec scan times and 1-cm intervals.[2] Most scans were done without contrast in both CT studies. Siegel and colleagues used 0.35- or 0.5-T Magnetom MR scanners (Siemens) to make axial T1 (300-700/17-35) and T2 (1500-3200/70-90) images through the chest.[3] Adam and Ignotus performed ultrasound of the thymic bed using a DRF unit (Diasonics,

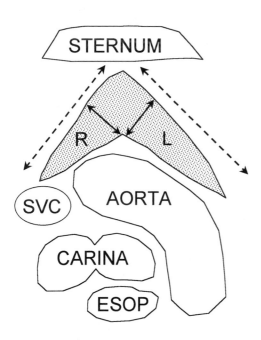

Figure 1 ▪ Measurement of individual lobes (*R = right, L = left*) of the thymus gland (*shaded*). The width (*dotted lines and arrowheads*) and thickness (*solid lines with arrowheads*) of each lobe were measured. SVC = superior vena cava, ESOP = esophagus.

Table 1 ▪ Dimensions of the Right and Left Lobes of the Normal Thymus

REFERENCE (Modality)	AGE RANGE (Yr)	NO.	RIGHT LOBE (cm) Width	RIGHT LOBE (cm) Thickness	LEFT LOBE (cm) Width	LEFT LOBE (cm) Thickness
Baron (CT)	6–19	11	2.0±0.55	1.0±0.39	3.3±1.10	1.1±0.40
	20–29	11	1.9±0.83	0.7±0.24	2.3±1.00	0.8±0.14
	30–39	13	1.3±0.51	0.5±0.14	2.0±0.95	0.7±0.21
	40–49	14	1.4±0.66	0.6±0.23	1.9±0.76	0.6±0.20
	>49	16	1.4±0.90	0.5±0.15	1.4±0.59	0.5±0.27
St. Amour (CT)	0–5	14	2.7±0.7	0.9±0.3	3.6±0.9	1.4±0.5
	6–10	12	2.5±0.7	1.0±0.5	3.9±1.2	1.0±0.4
	11–15	22	2.7±0.7	0.8±0.3	4.5±0.7	1.0±0.5
	16–19	23	2.5±0.7	0.7±0.2	4.2±0.9	0.8±0.4
	0–19	71	2.6±0.7	0.9±0.3	4.2±0.9	1.1±0.4
Siegel (MRI)	0–1	11	2.68±0.7	1.51±0.4	2.97±0.7	1.62±0.3
	1.1–5	16	2.71±0.6	1.51±0.6	3.01±0.7	1.47±0.4
	5.1–10	7	2.60±0.9	0.98±0.3	3.42±0.7	1.58±0.4
	10.1–15	10	3.13±0.6	1.14±0.3	3.60±0.6	1.51±0.2
	15.1–18	3	2.50	1.45	2.80	1.37
Adam (U/S)	2–8	50	2.5 (1.54–4.02)	1.4 (0.81–2.35)	2.9 (1.79–4.1)	1.4 (0.78–2.47)

Measurements given as mean ± standard deviation except for Adam, where the mean and range (in parentheses) are listed.[1-4]

Milpitas, CA) and a 7.5-MHz sector transducer. The patients were supine, and intercostal bilateral parasternal windows were used to visualize the thymus.[4]

Measurements ▪

Each lobe of the thymus was evaluated on axial CT and MRI images showing it to best advantage. The thickness and width on each side were measured using electronic calipers on the operator's console or with calipers from filmed images.[1-3] Thickness and width of each lobe were measured from frozen ultrasound images made through the ipsilateral parasternal window that best showed it.[4] Figure 1 depicts the thymus and surrounding structures and shows the measurements. Table 1 lists measurements of width and thickness of each lobe from each study by age group.[1-4]

Source ▪

Subject age ranges and sample sizes are given in Table 1. All subjects were free of disease or condition that might cause thymic enlargement or premature involution, including lymphoproliferative disorder, myasthenia gravis, thyroid disease, acute infections, and steroid therapy.[1-4]

Comments ▪

Baron and group found that the gland was seen on CT in all patients under the age of 30 years, 73% of patients between 30 and 49 years, and 17% of those over 49 years old. They noted three gland configurations: triangular or arrowhead shaped in 62%, distinctly separate lobes in 32%, and only one lobe seen in 6%.[1] St. Amour described a change in shape with age, from a lobular quadrilateral structure with biconvex outlines to a smoother triangular shape with biconvex outlines.[2]

The CT density of the gland changes with age from near-muscle density (>30 HU) in patients under 20 years of age to near-fat density (<10 HU) in patients over 49 years of age.[1] Similar changes were noted by St. Amour.[2] On MRI, the signal intensity of the normal thymus was homogeneous, slightly greater than muscle, and less than fat on T1 weighting, and moderately greater than muscle and slightly less than fat on T2-weighted sequences.[3] At ultrasound, the echoarchitecture of the gland closely resembled that of hepatic parenchyma.[4]

REFERENCES

1. Baron RL, Lee JKT, Sagel SS, Peterson RR: Computed tomography of the normal thymus. Radiology 1982; 142:121–125.
2. St. Amour TE, Siegel MJ, Glazer HS, Nadel SN: CT appearances of the normal and abnormal thymus in childhood. J Comput Assist Tomogr 1987; 11:645–650.
3. Siegel MJ, Glazer HS, Wiener JI, Monlina PL: Normal and abnormal thymus in childhood: MR imaging. Radiology 1989; 172:367–371.
4. Adam EJ, Ignotus PI: Sonography of the thymus in healthy children: Frequency of visualization, size, and appearance. AJR Am J Roentgenol 1993; 161(1):153–155.

▪: SIZE AND NUMBER OF HILAR NODES AT AUTOPSY
▪ ACR Code: 677 (Hilar Lymph Node)

Technique ▪

Lungs were resected en bloc, distended with 10% formalin, and immersed in the same solution. For each defined hilar region (Figure 1), the nodes were counted and the sizes measured.

Measurements ▪

The nodes were measured in the transverse plane to correlate with sizes obtained at CT or MR imaging. The short and long transverse diameters were measured to the nearest 0.1 mm. From prior work by the same investigators, the

Table 1 ▪ Number and Size of Hilar Nodes in 30 Cadavers

STATION	NUMBER WITH NODES (%)	NUMBER PER CADAVER		TOTAL NODES	SHORT TRANSVERSE DIAMETER (mm)		LONG TRANSVERSE DIAMETER (mm)	
		Mean	Maximum		Mean ± SD	Range	Mean ± SD	Range
Right								
AUL	30 (100)	1.8	4	53	6.4±2.9	1.6–14.6	10.0±4.6	2.8–21.5
LUL/PUL	13 (43)	0.5	1	13	3.2±1.5	1.9–7.8	4.9±2.5	2.2–12.3
SIL	30 (100)	1.7	3	51	5.7±2.5	2.1–14.7	9.4±4.2	3.5–18.8
IIL	30 (100)	1.6	3	49	6.4±2.7	1.4–13.2	9.5±3.5	2.7–16.9
ML	9 (30)	0.3	2	10	3.5±1.6	1.8–6.0	6.4±3.8	1.8–14.6
LLL	26 (87)	1.3	3	38	4.0±1.5	1.6–7.0	6.1±2.3	1.7–11.9
MLL	27 (90)	1.5	5	44	4.7±2.0	1.8–9.0	6.6±2.6	1.8–12.8
Left								
AUL	30 (100)	1.6	4	49	5.7±2.7	1.4–12.6	9.1±4.0	2.8–19.4
LUL	9 (30)	0.3	1	9	4.5±1.7	2.4–7.7	6.9±3.2	4.0–14.8
SIL	30 (100)	2.0	4	59	4.7±1.6	2.1–10.2	7.6±2.8	3.3–13.3
IIL	30 (100)	1.5	4	46	6.3±2.3	1.8–11.0	8.9±2.9	2.6–16.5
LLL	26 (87)	1.0	3	30	3.8±1.9	1.6–9.5	5.5±1.8	3.0–9.5
MLL	21 (70)	1.1	3	32	3.8±1.3	1.7–6.6	5.4±2.6	2.3–10.0

Nodal location abbreviations as in Figure 1.
From Kiyono K, Sone S, Izuno I, et al: Acta Radiol 1989; 30(5):471–474. Used by permission.

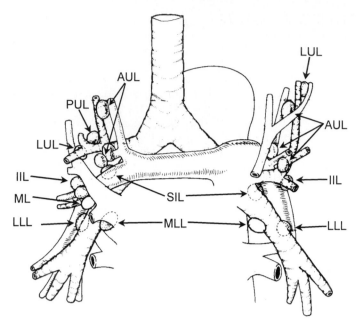

Figure 1 ■ Nodal location nomenclature:

AUL = anterior upper lobe
PUL = posterior upper lobe
LUL = lateral upper lobe
IIL = inferior interlobar
SIL = superior interlobar
ML = middle lobe
LLL = lateral lower lobe
MLL = medial lower lobe

(From Sone S, Higashihara T, Morimoto S, et al: AJR Am J Roentgenol 1983; 140:887–892. Used by permission.)

estimated shrinkage after fixation was 2% so correction was not applied.[2] Figure 1 depicts the nomenclature used for nodal locations.[3] Table 1 lists the numbers and sizes of nodes, and Table 2 lists suggested normal maximal sizes.[1]

Table 2 ■ Standard Maximal Normal Sizes of Hilar Lymph Nodes

SHORT TRANSVERSE DIAMETER		LONG TRANSVERSE DIAMETER	
Maximum Normal Size (mm)	Regions	Maximum Normal Size (mm)	Regions
8	All except below	12	All except below
		14	ML, L-SIL, L-IIL
10	R-SIL, L-AUL, L-IIL	16	R-IIL
12	R-AUL, R-IIL	18	R-AUL, L-AUL, R-SIL

Abbreviations of nodal locations as in Figure 1, with prefixes R = right and L = left.[1]

Source ■

Cadavers of 18 men (age range 34 to 82 years, mean age 64 years) and 12 women (age range 39 to 76 years, mean age 64 years) who had no history or pathologic findings of intrathoracic malignancy or infection were studied.[1]

Comments ■

There were no significant differences in size of nodes between male and female subjects. Using the maximal size criteria (Table 2) proposed by Kiyono and colleagues yielded 5 of 483 (1%) nodes larger than the standards that were found in 5 of 30 (17%) of the cadavers. These were usually anthracotic nodes.[1]

REFERENCES

1. Kiyono K, Sone S, Izuno I, et al: Size of normal hilar lymph nodes measured in autopsy specimens. Acta Radiol 1989; 30(5):471–474.
2. Kiyono K, Sone S, Sakai F, et al: The number and size of normal mediastinal lymph nodes: A postmortem study. Radiology 1988; 150:771–776.
3. Sone S, Higashihara T, Morimoto S, et al: CT anatomy of hilar lymphadenopathy. AJR Am J Roentgenol 1983; 140:887–892.

■: SIZE AND DISTRIBUTION OF NORMAL HILAR NODES
■ ACR Code: 677 (Hilar Lymph Node)

Technique ■

Spiral CT of the hilar region was done with a Somatom Plus S machine (Siemens, Erlangen, Germany), with 5-mm columnation, 1:1 pitch, and reconstruction at 3-mm intervals. Scanning was begun 5 to 14 seconds after the start of an intravenous bolus of 90 to 120 ml of contrast at 4- to 5-ml/sec injection rate. Various types of contrast were used.[1]

Measurements ■

A nomenclature for hilar node stations was developed consisting of four levels on each side, which complements standard numeric nomenclature of bronchopulmonary segmental anatomy.[2, 3] Table 1 lists the standard numbering of segmental anatomy, and Figures 1 and 2 depict the proposed hilar node location nomenclature. Scans at each

defined level on the right (n = 42) and left (n = 45) were evaluated to determine the number of patients with visible nodes at each station. The length of the maximal short axis of each visible node was also measured and recorded. Table 2 lists the numbers (and percentages) of nodes falling within three size ranges at each level on both sides.[1]

Source ■

The study group consisted of 50 patients (37 men, 13 women, age range 25 to 81 years, mean age 45 years) scanned to exclude pulmonary embolism (n = 32) or other reasons (n = 18). There were 27 current and 5 former smokers, and the number of packs smoked per year ranged from 3 to 108. Care was taken to exclude any patients with a history of disease or condition that would cause nodal enlargement, and the scans were all read as having normal hila.

Table 1 ▪ Standard Numeric Nomenclature of Bronchopulmonary Segments

RIGHT LOBE/SEGMENT	NO.	LEFT LOBE/SEGMENT	NO.
Upper		Upper	
Apical	1	Apical-posterior	1, 3
Anterior	2	Anterior	2
Posterior	3		
Middle		Lingula	
Lateral	4	Superior	4
Medial	5	Inferior	5
Lower		Lower	
Superior	6	Superior	6
Medial	7	Medial	7
Anterior	8	Anterior	8
Lateral	9	Lateral	9
Posterior	10	Posterior	10

Letters are placed in front of the number of identify nodes *(N)*, pulmonary arteries *(A)*, veins *(V)*, and bronchi *(B)* in Figures 1 and 2.[2, 3]

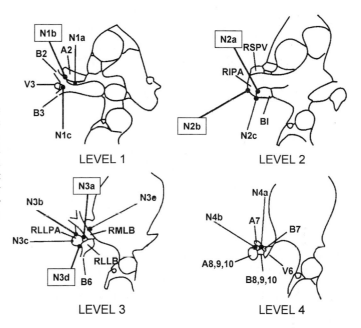

Figure 1 ▪ Right hilar nodal stations are identified with N#x, where # is the level number and x is the location (a, b, . . .). The labels with a box around them identify locations where more than 25% of normal patients had visible nodes. Bronchopulmonary segmental structures are labeled with standard nomenclature as described in Table 1. RSPV = right superior pulmonary vein, RIPA = right inferior pulmonary artery, RLLPA = right lower lobe pulmonary artery, RMLB = right middle lobe bronchus, RLLB = right lower lobe bronchus. (From Remy-Jardin M, Duyuck P, Remy J, et al: Radiology 1995; 196:387–394. Used by permission.)

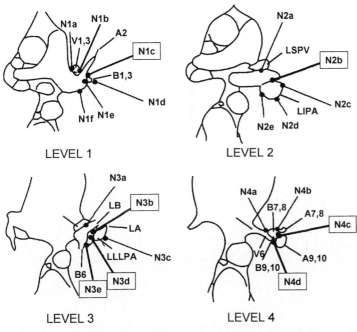

Figure 2 ▪ Left hilar nodal stations are identified with N#x, where # is the level number and x is the location (a, b, . . .). The labels with a box around them identify locations where more than 25% of normal patients had visible nodes. Bronchopulmonary segmental structures are labeled with standard nomenclature as described in Table 1. LSPV = left superior pulmonary vein, LIPA = left inferior pulmonary artery, LLLPA = left lower lobe pulmonary artery, LB = lingular bronchus, LA = lingular artery. (From Remy-Jardin M, Duyuck P, Remy J, et al: Radiology 1995; 196:387–394. Used by permission.)

Table 2 ▪ Size of Normal Hilar Nodes

SIDE/LEVEL	NO. OF NODES	NUMBER (%) HAVING MAXIMUM SHORT AXIS OF:		
		<3 mm	3–5 mm	5–7 mm
Right				
1	46	32 (70)	7 (15)	7 (15)
2	43	27 (62)	8 (19)	8 (19)
3	66	39 (59)	21 (32)	6 (9)
4	19	16 (84)	1 (5)	2 (11)
Left				
1	39	24 (62)	8 (20)	7 (18)
2	53	39 (73)	10 (18)	5 (9)
3	61	22 (36)	25 (41)	14 (23)
4	45	36 (80)	7 (16)	2 (4)

Levels same as in Figures 1 and 2. Maximum short axis diameter given as numbers and percentages falling within three ranges.
From Remy-Jardin M, Duyuck P, Remy J, et al: Radiology 1995; 196:387–394. Used by permission.

Comments ▪

The authors found that their findings matched previously described anatomic descriptions that have emphasized the lack of nodes along the lateral walls of pulmonary arteries in the lower lobes.[1]

REFERENCES

1. Remy-Jardin M, Duyuck P, Remy J, et al: Hilar lymph nodes: Identification with spiral CT and histologic correlation. Radiology 1995; 196:387–394.
2. Boyden EA: Segmental Anatomy of the Lungs. McGraw-Hill, New York, 1955.
3. Jackson CL, Huber JF: Correlated applied anatomy of bronchial tree and lungs with system of nomenclature. Dis Chest 1943; 9:319–326.

▪▪ MEASUREMENT OF THE HILA[1]
▪ ACR Code: 679 (Hila)

Technique ▪

Central ray: To fourth thoracic vertebral body.
Position: Posteroanterior chest.
Target-film distance: 72 inches.

Measurements (Figure 1) ▪

Mean width for right and left hila: 5.56 ± 0.12 cm. Minimum width, 3.5 cm; maximum width, 7.0 cm.

Sum of transverse diameters of right and left hila = 11.0 ± 0.03 cm.

In at least 84% of the cases, the difference between the right and left hila did not exceed 1.0 cm.

The lateral border of the hilum is the margin farthest from the midline (midline to *b* and to *a* in Figure 1) but not including the first branchings of each pulmonary artery. Rigler and his coworkers found that in 100 patients with proved bronchogenic carcinoma, the mean sum of the hilar diameters was 13 cm.[1] If either hilum is more than 7.0 cm or if the sum of the diameters is 13 cm, the chance of abnormality is about 90%.

However, in a study of 541 cases of proved bronchogenic

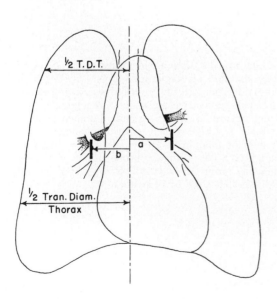

Figure 1 ▪ Measurements of the hila from frontal radiographs. See text for details.

carcinoma, Lodwick and colleagues found that only 31.9% of the cases had a total transverse diameter greater than 13 cm; only 36.8% of the cases had a unilateral measurement greater than 7.0 cm; 13.5% had a total transverse diameter of less than the mean normal diameter of 11 cm.[2]

In the very early bronchogenic cancer cases, hilar measurements were abnormal in only 19.4% of the cases.

Source ▪

Chest roentgenograms of 100 consecutive patients over 40 years of age, made as hospital routine on admission, were studied.

REFERENCES

1. Rigler LG, O'Laughlin BJ: Radiology 1952; 59:683.
2. Lodwick G, Keats TE, Dorst J: Radiology 1958; 71:370.

▪▪ MEASUREMENT OF THE HILAR HEIGHT RATIO FOR DETECTION OF HILAR DISPLACEMENT[1]
- ACR Code: 679 (Hila)

Technique ▪

Central ray: Perpendicular to plane of film centered over midchest.
Position: Posteroanterior, inspiratory phase.
Target-film distance: 72 inches.

Measurements (Figure 1) ▪

A line parallel to the thoracic spine is drawn from the highest point of the pulmonary apex to the diaphragm. An intersecting line is drawn from the midpoint of the hilum, perpendicular to the vertical line. The lateral angle, designated by the midpoint of the right hilum, is joined by the right upper lobe pulmonary vein *(PV)* crossing the right basal pulmonary artery *(PA)*. The left hyparterial bronchus *(H)* must be identified in order to determine the midpoint of the left hilum (*). The right hilar height ratio = *a/b*; left hilar height ratio = *c/d*.

In normal patients, the right hilum is positioned in the lower half of the hemithorax, whereas the left hilum is positioned in the upper half of its hemithorax. The normal right hilar height ratio, therefore, should be greater than 1 and the left hilar height ratio less than 1. When these values are abnormal, pulmonary volume changes or intrapulmonary and subphrenic abnormal processes are present.

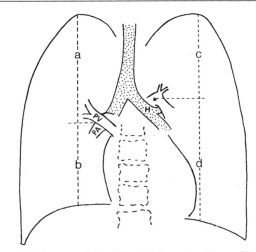

Figure 1 ▪ Calculation of the hilar height ratio. (From Homer MJ: Radiology 1978; 129:11. Used by permission.)

Source ▪

Data were obtained from films of 90 normal patients. There was no significant difference between men and women.

REFERENCE

1. Homer MJ: The hilar height ratio. Radiology 1978; 129:11–16.

▪▪ MEASUREMENT OF NORMAL MEDIASTINAL LYMPH NODES BY CT[1]
- ACR Code: 679 (Mediastinal Lymph Nodes)

Technique ▪

1. CT scans performed using a GE 8800 scanner with a scan time of 5.6 seconds.
2. Contiguous 1.0-cm-thick sections from the pulmonary apices to the lung bases are obtained in the supine position at full inspiration. Scans are obtained after bolus injection of 50 to 75 ml of iothalamate (Conray 60%).

Measurement ▪

The number and size of lymph nodes were recorded at defined sites using the node-mapping scheme of the American Thoracic Society (Figure 1 and Table 1).

Nodes in locations X, 9, and 11 were not analyzed. The longest and shortest node diameters in the transverse plane were recorded. The number and size of normal mediastinal lymph nodes are shown in Table 2.

Table 1 ▪ American Thoracic Society Definitions of Regional Nodal Stations

X   Supraclavicular nodes.

2R   Right upper paratracheal nodes; nodes to the right of the midline of the trachea, between the intersection of the caudal margin of the innominate artery with the trachea and the apex of the lung.

2L   Left upper paratracheal nodes: nodes to the left of the midline of the trachea, between the top of the aortic arch and the apex of the lung.

4R   Right lower paratracheal nodes: nodes to the right of the midline of the trachea, between the cephalic border of the azygos vein and the intersection of the caudal margin of the brachiocephalic artery with the right side of the trachea.

4L   Left lower paratracheal nodes: nodes to the left of the midline of the trachea, between the top of the aortic arch and the level of the carina, medial to the ligamentum arteriosum.

5   Aortopulmonary nodes: subaortic and para-aortic nodes, lateral to the ligamentum arteriosum or the aorta or left pulmonary artery, proximal to the first branch of the left pulmonary artery.

6   Anterior mediastinal nodes: nodes anterior to the ascending aorta or the innominate artery.

7   Subcarinal nodes: nodes arising caudal to the carina of the trachea but not associated with the lower lobe bronchi or arteries within the lung.

8   Paraesophageal nodes: nodes dorsal to the posterior wall of the trachea and to the right or left of the midline of the esophagus.

9   Right or left pulmonary ligament nodes: nodes within the right or left pulmonary ligament.

10R   Right tracheobronchial nodes: nodes to the right of the midline of the trachea, from the level of the cephalic border of the azygos vein to the origin of the right upper lobe bronchus.

10L   Left peribronchial nodes: nodes to the left of the midline of the trachea, between the carina and the left upper lobe bronchus, medial to the ligamentum arteriosum.

11   Intrapulmonary nodes: nodes removed in the right or left lung specimen, plus those distal to the main stem bronchi or secondary carina.

From Tisi GM, et al: Am Rev Resp Dis 1983; 127:659–664. Used by permission.

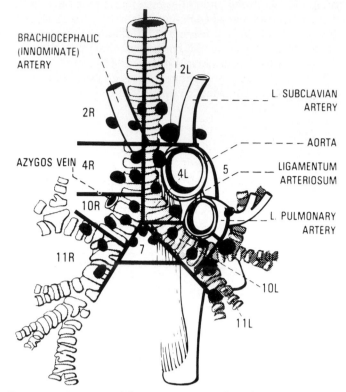

Figure 1 ▪ American Thoracic Society lymph node mapping scheme. Locations of regions 6, 8R, and 8L are not illustrated because they lie in front of or behind other regions in the drawing. Definitions of all regions are listed in Table 1. (From Tisi GM, et al: Am Rev Resp Dis 1983; 127:659–664. Used by permission.)

Table 2 ▪ Numbers and Sizes of Normal Mediastinal Lymph Nodes in 56 Patients

REGION	NO. OF PATIENTS WITH NODES VISIBLE IN REGION	NODES			
		No. (Mean ± SD)	Maximum No.	Shortest Diameter, mm (Mean ± SD)	Sum of Diameters, mm (Mean ± SD)
2R	53	2.1±1.3	6	3.5±1.3	8.0±3.1
2L	42	1.9±1.6	6	3.3±1.6	7.6±4.0
4R	56	3.2±2.0	10	5.0±2.0	11.1±3.9
4L	47	2.1±1.6	7	4.7±1.9	10.8±4.2
5	33	1.2±1.1	3	4.7±2.1	11.8±5.0
6	48	4.8±3.5	12	4.1±1.7	10.3±4.2
7	53	1.7±1.1	6	6.2±2.2	14.3±4.6
8R	32	1.0±1.1	4	4.4±2.6	10.1±6.1
8L	25	0.8±1.2	6	3.8±1.7	8.9±3.9
10R	56	2.8±1.3	7	5.9±2.1	13.6±4.0
10L	39	1.0±0.8	3	4.0±1.2	9.4±2.3

From Glazer GM, et al: AJR Am J Roentgenol 1985; 144:261–265. Used by permission.

Source ▪

Data are based on CT studies of 56 adult patients with no evidence of neoplasia. The group included 31 men, 21 to 75 years of age, and 25 women, 18 to 82 years of age.

REFERENCES

1. Glazer GM, Gross BH, Quint LE, et al: Normal mediastinal lymph nodes: Number and size according to American Thoracic Society mapping. AJR Am J Roentgenol 1985; 144:261–265.
2. Tisi GM, Friedman PJ, Peters RM, et al: Clinical staging of primary lung cancer: Official statement of the American Thoracic Society. Am Rev Resp Dis 1983; 127:659–664.

▪: NUMBER AND SIZE OF MEDIASTINAL NODES AT AUTOPSY
- ACR Code: 679 (Mediastinal Lymph Nodes)

Table 1 ▪ American Thoracic Society Nodal Stations[2]

STATION	DESCRIPTION
X	Supraclavicular
2 (R or L)	Upper paratracheal
4 (R or L)	Lower paratracheal
5	Aortopulmonary
6	Anterior mediastinal
7	Subcarinal
8 (R or L)	Paraesophageal
9 (R or L)	Pulmonary ligament
10 (R or L)	Tracheobronchial (R) Parabronchial (L)
11	Intrapulmonary

Table 3 ▪ Standard Maximum Normal Sizes of Mediastinal Lymph Nodes

SHORT TRANSVERSE DIAMETER		LONG TRANSVERSE DIAMETER	
Maximum Normal Size (mm)	Regions	Maximum Normal Size (mm)	Regions
8	2, 5, 6, 8, 9, 10L	10	2, 8, 9
10	4, 10R	15	4, 6, 10L
		20	5, 10R
12	7	25	7

Nodal station abbreviations are detailed in Table 1.
From Kiyono K, Sone S, Sakai F, et al: Radiology 1988; 150:771–776. Used by permission.

Technique ▪

The mediastinum was resected en bloc and fixed in 10% formalin. The number and size of nodes in each region (American Thoracic Society) were determined.[1]

Measurements ▪

The nodes were measured in the transverse plane to correlate with sizes obtained at CT or MR imaging. The short and long transverse diameters were measured to the nearest 0.1 mm. A subset of 20 nodes from two cadavers showed only 2% shrinkage after fixation so correction was not applied.[1] Table 1 is a brief listing of the American Thoracic Society nodal location nomenclature.[2] Table 2 lists the numbers and sizes of nodes, and Table 3 gives standard maximum sizes for both long and short transverse diameters.[1]

Source ▪

Subjects were 40 adults (25 men with an average age of 58 years, 15 women with an average age of 64 years) who had no history or postmortem evidence of chest malignancy or infection.[1]

Table 2 ▪ Number and Size of Mediastinal Lymph Nodes in 40 Cadavers

STATION	NUMBER WITH NODES (%)	NUMBER PER CADAVER		TOTAL NODES	SHORT TRANSVERSE DIAMETER (mm)		LONG TRANSVERSE DIAMETER (mm)	
		Mean	Maximum		Mean ± SD	Range	Mean ± SD	Range
2R	32 (80)	2.5	11	99	3.7 ± 2.1	1.3–8.6	4.8 ± 3.2	1.3–16.0
2L	27 (68)	2.1	7	82	2.9 ± 1.4	1.2–6.0	3.9 ± 2.2	1.2–10.8
4R	39 (98)	4.8	11	191	4.0 ± 2.6	1.0–13.4	6.0 ± 5.0	1.3–16.2
4L	39 (98)	4.5	16	178	4.1 ± 2.6	1.0–14.0	6.2 ± 4.6	1.0–18.5
5	23 (58)	1.1	6	43	3.6 ± 2.5	0.8–8.7	6.1 ± 6.3	1.5–21.6
6	34 (85)	4.7	15	186	3.3 ± 2.0	1.0–9.5	5.3 ± 4.2	1.0–16.6
7	40 (100)	2.9	6	115	5.6 ± 3.4	1.3–14.0	10.0 ± 8.4	1.3–33.0
8R	23 (58)	1.2	6	46	3.7 ± 2.3	1.0–7.7	5.6 ± 2.9	2.4–11.2
8L	20 (50)	1.1	5	43	2.9 ± 1.6	1.0–7.1	4.3 ± 3.4	1.2–10.0
9R	4 (10)	0.1	2	5	2.4 ± 0.8	1.8–3.0	4.8 ± 1.3	3.6–6.0
9L	14 (35)	0.5	3	20	3.2 ± 1.7	1.6–7.0	4.8 ± 2.5	2.3–9.2
10R	38 (95)	3.5	10	140	4.5 ± 3.2	1.2–14.8	7.9 ± 6.5	1.5–25.6
10L	36 (90)	2.4	7	95	3.5 ± 1.7	1.0–8.7	6.1 ± 3.5	2.0–17.4

Nodal station abbreviations are given in Table 1.
From Kiyono K, Sone S, Sakai F, et al: Radiology 1988; 150:771–776. Used by permission.

Comments ▪

Only 5 of 40 cadavers (12.5%) had any nodes that exceeded the standard maximum values (Table 3) by 20% (2 mm for the short diameter and 3 mm for the long diameter).[1]

REFERENCES

1. Kiyono K, Sone S, Sakai F, et al: The number and size of normal mediastinal lymph nodes: A postmortem study. Radiology 1988; 150:771–776.
2. Tisi GM, Friedman PJ, Peters RM, et al: Clinical staging of primary lung cancer: Official statement of the American Thoracic Society. Am Rev Resp Dis 1983; 127:659–664.

▪: MEASUREMENT OF THE STRAIGHT-BACK SYNDROME[1]
- ▪ ACR Code: 32/69 (Thoracic Spine, Bony Thorax)

Absence of the normal thoracic kyphosis is a recently accepted cause of "pseudo heart disease." Roentgenographically, the heart is usually normal in size and configuration, but in some patients it is "pancake" in appearance, and in other patients it is displaced to the left with prominence of the pulmonary arteries.

Technique ▪

Central ray: PA chest: to fourth thoracic vertebral body. Lateral chest: centered over midchest.
Position: Posteroanterior and true lateral.
Target-film distance: Posteroanterior: 72 inches. Lateral: 72 inches.

Measurements (Table 1) ▪

Source ▪

Twenty-four men and women in whom loss of thoracic kyphosis was the only somatic fault.

Table 1 ▪ Chest Dimensions in Normals and Those with Straight Back Syndrome

	NO.	AP CHEST DIAM (cm)	AP/TRANSTHORACIC RATIO (%)
Straight-back syndrome patients			
Males	12	10.6	35.8
Females	12	9.8	37.3
Normal patients			
Males	50	14.2	47.0
Females	50	12.0	45.7

REFERENCE

1. Twigg HL, De Leon A, Perloff JK, Maid M: The straight-back syndrome: Radiographic manifestations. Radiology 1967; 88:274–277.

▪: MEASUREMENTS FOR RADIOLOGIC EVALUATION OF FUNNEL CHEST
- ▪ ACR Code: 472/69 (Sternum, Bony Thorax)

Technique ▪

Central ray: Perpendicular to plane of film centered over midchest.
Position: True lateral.

Target-film distance: Immaterial.

Measurements (Figures 1 and 2) ▪

The vertebral index indicates the percentage ratio between the minimum sagittal diameter of the chest, measured from

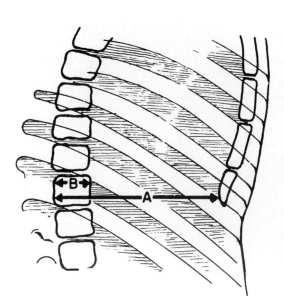

Figure 1 ▪ Measurements used to calculate the vertebral index (A/B). See text for details. (Adapted from Backer O, et al: Acta Radiol 1961; 55:249.)

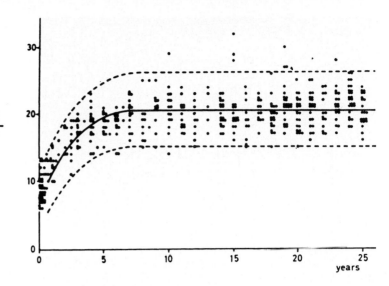

Figure 2 ▪ Normal vertebral index plotted against age. Dots represent individual subject measurements, the mean *(solid)* and 95% confidence intervals *(dotted lines)* from regression analysis are shown. (From Backer O, et al: Acta Radiol 1961; 55:249. Used by permission.)

the posterior surface of the vertebral body to the nearest point on the body of the sternum *(A)*, and the sagittal diameter of the vertebral body at the same level *(B)*. Figure 2 shows the vertebral index in normal persons. The *solid line* represents the mean curve. The 95% range lies between the *broken lines.* This method is applicable in assessment of the late results of operation, which heretofore has been based on subjective estimation.

Source ▪

The data are based on a normal series of 445 subjects, 197 males and 248 females, about equally distributed in 5-year age groups from 0 to 25 years.

REFERENCE

1. Backer O, et al: Acta Radiol 1961; 55:249.

▪▪ DIAPHRAGMATIC MOTION
▪ ACR Code: 69 (Diaphragm)

Technique ▪

Five studies are abstracted here, representing fluoroscopic, ultrasound (U/S), and MRI techniques to quantify diaphragmatic motion.[1-5] Table 1 details the subject position, modality, and type of breathing assessed.

Measurements ▪

Measurements were made to the nearest millimeter at or near the dome of the diaphragms, with methods appropriate to the modality being used. Figure 1 shows real-time ultrasound for measuring excursions since this is the most available and accurate means of making such measurements. Table 2 lists the respiratory excursions of the right and left diaphragms as reported in each study.[1-5]

Source ▪

Figure 1 lists patient demographics for each study.[1-5] All subjects were either normal volunteers or patients without any history or finding of disease or condition that might affect diaphragmatic function. Harris and colleagues recorded weight, height, and calculated body surface area in addition to gender and age for subsequent correlation with respiratory excursion of the diaphragm.[3]

Comments ▪

Harris and group found that males had significantly greater excursions than females (p = .006). There was also a strong positive correlation between body weight and diaphragm

Table 1 ▪ Details of Studies of Diaphragmatic Motion

REFERENCE	MALES/FEMALES (Total)	AGE RANGE (Yr)	PATIENT POSITION	TYPE OF BREATHING	MODALITY	COMMENTS
Wade[1]	10/0 (10)	24–36	Supine/upright	Quiet & deep	Fluoro	Fluoroscopic tracking mechanism
Alexander[2]	80/47 (127)	Not given	Upright	Deep	Fluoro	Direct measurement from fluoro screen
Harris et al[3]	29/21 (50)	19–57	Supine	Deep	U/S	B-mode
Houston et al[4]	30/25 (55)	27–97	Supine	Quiet & deep	U/S	Real-time sector
Gierada et al[5]	6/4 (10)	25–35	Supine	Deep	MRI	GRE (9.2/4.2/20°) coronal/sagittal

GRE = gradient echo, B-mode = brightness mode ultrasound.

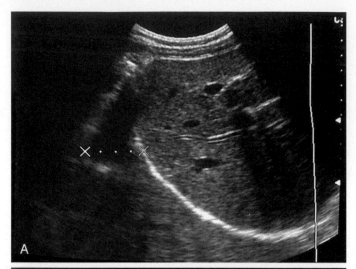

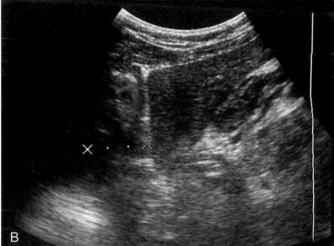

Figure 1 • Measurement of diaphragm excursion from real-time sector ultrasound. *A*, Right diaphragm, *B*, Left diaphragm. Both are subcostal longitudinal sector scans at deep inspiration. Measurements are made on each side between the dome of the diaphragm and a cursor previously deposited over the dome at end-tidal volume, with the transducer in the same position. Using forced expiration is often problematic because the dome may not be visible.

Table 2 • Diaphragmatic Excursions

AUTHOR/ MODALITY-GROUP	NO.	RIGHT (cm)		LEFT (cm)		R/L RATIO	
		Mean ± SD	Range	Mean ± SD	Range	Mean ± SD	Range
Wade—fluoro							
males (deep/upright)	10	9.2 ± 2.2	6.8–13.3	10.5 ± 1.9	8.8–13.5	0.97 ± 0.08	0.76–0.98
males (deep/supine)	10	9.3 ± 1.6	7.5–11.8	9.9 ± 1.6	7.5–11.8	0.95 ± 0.11	0.68–1.09
males (quiet/upright)	10	1.6 ± 0.2	1.5–2.0	1.7 ± 0.3	1.3–2.3	1.0 ± 0.14	0.78–1.20
males (quiet/supine)	10	1.7 ± 0.3	1.3–2.0	1.8 ± 0.2	1.5–2.3	0.97 ± 0.18	0.71–1.33
Alexander—fluoro							
adults (quiet)	127	2.75		3.15		0.89*	0.53–1.4
Harris—U/S							
males (deep)	29	5.4 ± 1.7	3.0–9.0				
females (deep)	21	4.0 ± 1.2	2.0–6.2				
adults (deep)	50	4.8 ± 1.6	1.9–9.0				
Houston—U/S							
adults (quiet)	55	2.2 ± 0.61	0.9–3.9	2.0 ± 0.75	0.7–4.5	1.2 ± 0.44	0.5–2.5
adults (deep)	55	5.3 ± 1.64	2.6–9.7	4.6 ± 1.24	2.3–8.7	1.1 ± 0.28	0.5–1.6
Gierada—MRI							
males (deep)	10	4.4 ± 1.26	2.1–5.6	4.2 ± 0.95	3.1–5.3		

*Done on a subset of 81 subjects.
R/L ratio = right excursion divided by left excursion.

excursion.[3] Linear regression of the right mid-diaphragm deep breathing excursion yielded the following equation:

Right diaphragm excursion (cm) =
$$0.077 \text{ (weight kg)} - 0.389 \text{ (r = 0.78)}.$$

He postulated that the weight difference explained the gender difference. Height and body surface area were not significantly correlated with diaphragmatic excursions.

Both Houston and colleagues and Alexander reported ratios between the right and left motion, and the ratios were calculated from Wade's tables.[1, 2, 4] These data are included in Table 2. Houston and group found that the right side moved more (mean R/L > 1), whereas Alexander found that the left side moved more (mean R/L < 1). Probably more important was the range of ratios reported, which yields a useful "rule of thumb" that if the difference in sides is greater than 2:1 (R/L < 0.5 or > 2.0), then the side with decreased motion is abnormal. Qualitative observations of the motion during quiet breathing, deep breathing, and rapid breathing (sniff test) are also important to reveal paradoxic and/or delayed motions.[2] M-mode ultrasound and dynamic MRI can produce tracings

of position versus time during the respiratory cycle, which may be useful in characterizing the motion better.[4, 6-8]

REFERENCES

1. Wade OL: Movements of the thoracic cage and diaphragm in respiration. J Physiol 1954; 124–193.
2. Alexander C: Diaphragm movements and the diagnosis of diaphragmatic paralysis. Clin Radiol 1966; 17:79–83.
3. Harris RS, Giovannetti M, Kim BK: Normal ventilatory movement of the right hemidiaphragm studied by ultrasonography and pneumotachography. Radiology 1983; 146:141–144.
4. Houston JG, Morris AD, Howie CA, et al: Technical report: Quantitative assessment of diaphragmatic movement—a reproducible method using ultrasound. Clin Radiol 1992; 46:405–407.
5. Gierada DS, Curtin JJ, Erickson SJ, et al: Diaphragmatic motion: Fast gradient-recalled-echo MR imaging in healthy subjects. Radiology 1995; 194(3):879–884.
6. Davies SC, Hill AL, Holmes RB, et al: Ultrasound quantitation of respiratory organ motion in the upper abdomen. Br J Radiol 1994; 67:1096–1102.
7. Korin HW, Ehman RL, Riederer SJ, et al: Respiratory kinematics of the upper abdominal organs: A quantitative study. Magn Reson Med 1992; 23(1):172–178.
8. Holland AE, Goldfarb JW, Edelman RR: Diaphragmatic and cardiac motion during suspended breathing: Preliminary experience and implications for breath-hold MR imaging. Radiology 1998; 209:483–489.

CHAPTER 11

Gastrointestinal System

∵ ∴

∵ MEASUREMENT OF CRICOPHARYNGEAL DIAMETER
- ACR Code: 711 (Pharyngoesophageal Sphincter)

Technique ▪

Central ray: Spot roentgenograms are used.
Position: Lateral neck. Erect or recumbent position. Barium-filled esophagus.
Target-film distance: Variable. Roentgenographic measurements must be corrected before comparison is made with Table 1.

Measurements ▪

The cricopharyngeal diameter was found to be the narrowest point. Range of measurements is shown in Table 1.

Source ▪

Fresh esophageal specimens were obtained from 28 cadavers. Direct measurement of mucosa was made. In no case

Table 1 ▪ Measurement Made at the Level of the Cricopharyngeus Muscle	
AGE	**ANATOMIC DIAM. (mm)**
9 days–4 weeks	6
1–9 months	7–8
10 months–7 years	8–11
7–16 years	9–13

From Haase FR, Brenner A: Arch Otolaryngol 1963; 77:119. Used by permission.

was the cause of death due to an abnormality of the esophagus.

REFERENCE

1. Haase FR, Brenner A: Arch Otolaryngol 1963; 77:119.

∵ MEASUREMENT OF THE LOWER ESOPHAGEAL RING
- ACR Code: 714 (Lower Esophagus)

Technique ▪

Central ray: Spot roentgenograms are used.
Position: Erect or recumbent.
Target-film distance: Variable. Target-tabletop distance: 18 inches.

Measurements ▪ (Figures 1 and 2)

Maximum diameter of the ring in a barium-filled esophagus. Measured on spot films without consideration of magnification.

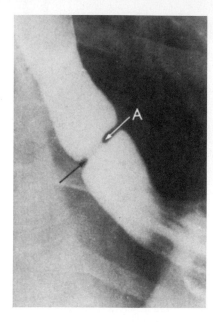

Figure 1 • Measurement of the lower esophageal ring *(arrows, A)*. (From Schatzki R: AJR Am J Roentgenol 1963; 90:805. Used by permission.)

Figure 2 • Relationship between dysphagia and diameter of esophageal rings of various patients. The measurement refers to the maximal diameter of the ring at the time of first demonstration as measured on spot roentgenogram. (From Schatzki R: AJR Am J Roentgenol 1963; 90:805. Used by permission.)

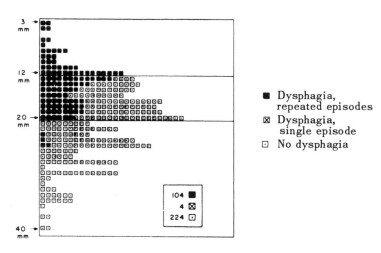

■ Dysphagia, repeated episodes

☒ Dysphagia, single episode

☐ No dysphagia

104 ■
4 ☒
224 ☐

Schatzki and Gary[1] state that the lower esophageal ring:

1. Is not an abnormal contraction.
2. Lies at the junction of esophageal and gastric mucosa and is the junction of esophagus and stomach.
3. Has always been symptomatic in their experience if it has an original diameter of less than 13 mm.

Source •

The data are based on measurements of 104 patients with repeated episodes of dysphagia, 4 patients with one episode of dysphagia, and 224 patients without dysphagia.

Note: This does not include all asymptomatic patients with lower esophageal ring who were seen in this study.

REFERENCE

1. Schatzki R, Gary JW: AJR Am J Roentgenol 1953; 70:911.

•: MEASUREMENT OF THE ADULT STOMACH AND DUODENUM[1]
- ACR Code: 72 (Stomach); 73 (Duodenum)

Technique •

Central ray: Posteroanterior recumbent: to second lumbar vertebra. Right lateral recumbent: 3 inches anterior to midcoronal plane at level of second lumbar vertebra. Left lateral erect: same as right lateral recumbent. Stomach may be lower in position than for recumbent, and fluoroscopic observation is recommended for accurate centering.
Position: Posteroanterior recumbent; right lateral recumbent; left lateral erect.
Target-film distance: 36 inches.

The stomach contained approximately 8 oz of barium sulfate in water. Films were obtained in suspended respiration.

Measurements • (Figure 1 and Table 1)

1 = Distance between top of stomach fundus and diaphragm.
4 = Stomach to anterior spine.
9 = Maximum vertical internal diameter of the duodenal loop.
10 = Minimum measurement of the outer margin of the second portion of the duodenum to the posterior margin of the vertebral bodies.
11 = Maximum horizontal internal diameter of the duodenal loop.
12 = Maximum outer diameter of the second portion of the duodenum.

13 = Distance between pylorus and the outer margin of the spine.
m = Width of base of duodenal bulb.
n = Height of duodenal bulb from apex to pylorus.

Dimension *1* in Figure 1*A* had an average measurement = 0.5 cm; maximum = 1.5 cm.

The diameter of the second portion of the duodenum, Figure 1*A* and *B*, dimension *12*: average = 2.0 cm; minimum = 1.0 cm; maximum = 2.5 cm.

Width of gastric and duodenal rugae: upper stomach, 0.5 cm; lower stomach, 0.3 to 0.5 cm; mid-duodenum, 0.2 to 0.3 cm.

The size of the duodenal bulb in Figure 1*B*, width at base (*m*): average = 3.0 cm, maximum = 3.5 cm; height (*n*): average = 3.0 cm, maximum = 4.0 cm.

Types of Stomachs

1. J-shaped or eutonic stomach: Pylorus and incisura angularis are at the same level.
2. Cascade stomach: Fundus has a posterior pouchlike projection that overlaps the body of the stomach.
3. Fishhook or hypotonic-type stomach: Incisura angularis is considerably lower than pylorus.
4. Steer-horn stomach: Incisura angularis lies above the level of the pylorus.

Weight Groups (Table 1)

Meschan and colleagues divided the patients into three groups according to weight. The Equitable Life Assurance

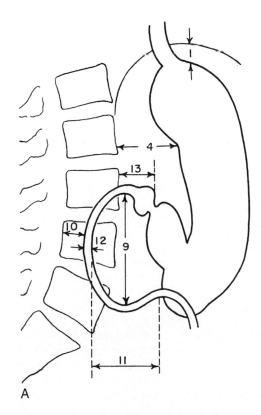

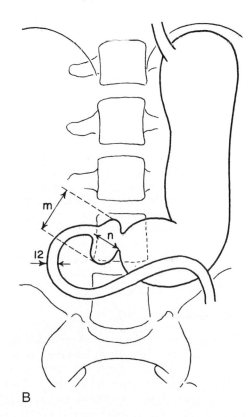

Figure 1 • *A*, Stomach and duodenum in right lateral recumbent or left lateral erect positions. *B*, Stomach and duodenum in posteroanterior recumbent position. (Adapted from Meschan I, et al: South Med J 1953; 46:878.)

A   B

Table 1 ▪ Relationships of Stomach and Duodenum to the Spine in Different Weight and Stomach-Type Groups
(Both Asymptomatic and Symptomatic Summated)

WEIGHT GROUP	STOMACH TYPE	NO. OF CASES (211 Total)	9 R LATERAL		10 R LATERAL		11 R LATERAL		13 R LATERAL	
			Avg. of Medians	Range	Avg. of Medians	Range	Avg. of Medians	Range	Avg. of Medians	Range
Normal	J-shape	58	6.5	4.0–9.5	3.0	1.0–9.0	3.0	0.0–12.5	4.0	0.5–8.0
	Fishhook	10	6.0	4.0–8.0	3.0	2.5–4.0	5.6	3.5–8.0	4.5	2.5–9.0
	Cascade	13	6.0	4.5–6.0	4.3	2.0–9.5	6.6	1.0–11.0	6.0	2.5–9.0
	Steer-horn	9	6.5	5.5–8.0	3.5	0.5–5.0	5.5	1.5–9.0	5.0	2.5–10.0
Underweight	J-shape	56	5.5	2.0–11.0	3.0	0.5–7.0	4.0	0.0–9.0	3.0	0.5–6.5
	Fishhook	21	5.5	3.5–8.0	2.5	0.0–5.0	3.0	1.5–5.0	2.5	1.0–4.0
	Cascade	5	6.0	5.5–6.5	2.5	2.0–3.5	4.5	4.0–5.0	3.0	2.0–5.0
	Steer-horn	3	8.0	8.0	4.5	2.0–6.0	7.0	6.5–8.0	4.0	1.5–5.0
Overweight	J-shape	13	6.5	4.0–9.0	3.3	2.0–7.0	4.5	3.5–9.0	3.5	1.5–9.5
	Fishhook	5	5.0	3.0–7.5	2.5	0.0–4.0	4.5	2.0–9.5	4.6	3.0–6.5
	Cascade	10	7.0	4.0–9.0	4.0	1.0–7.5	5.0	1.5–10.0	5.6	3.0–12.0
	Steer-horn	8	6.0	5.5–8.0	4.0	3.5–5.5	5.0	3.0–7.5	4.5	3.0–7.5

9, 10, 11, and 13 Right lateral are shown in Figure 1.
Data from Meschan I, et al: South Med J 1953;46:878.

Society standards for height and weight were used to establish whether patients were normal weight (plus or minus 10%), overweight, or underweight.

Source of Material ▪

The data are based on a study of 211 adults of all ages between the third and the seventh decade, chosen at random from patients at two Veterans Administration hospitals, the University of Arkansas Hospital, and University of Arkansas medical students.

Of these adults, 107 were asymptomatic, and 104 were symptomatic with no apparent radiographic abnormality in stomach or duodenum.

Gender and age distribution were random.

More than 10,000 measurements were made for this study.

Note: Gastrocolic space (measurement made from inferior aspect of the greater curvature of the stomach to the adjacent transverse colon) has been measured by Moreno and Rivera[2] and by Seymour.[3] Moreno and Rivera proposed a normal limit of 3 cm for the gastrocolic space, but Seymour, who examined 50 patients, found that the 3-cm limit was exceeded in 36% of the patients, in whom the gastrocolic space averaged 8.7 cm.

REFERENCES

1. Meschan I, et al: South Med J 1953; 46:878.
2. Moreno G, Rivera HH: Evaluation of the gastrocolic space in 100 cases of acute pancreatitis. Radiology 1976; 118:535–538.
3. Seymour EQ: Unreliability of an increased gastrocolic measurement in the diagnosis of acute pancreatitis [letter]. Radiology 1977; 123:527.

▪: MEASUREMENTS OF THE PYLORUS FOR HYPERTROPHIC STENOSIS
▪ ACR Code: 724 (Pylorus)

Technique ▪

Though different in some technical details over time, there is general consensus in the literature about how to perform ultrasound to detect pyloric stenosis in infants.[1–12] Real-time sector, curved array, or linear ultrasound is done with 3.5–7.0-MHz transducers over the upper right abdomen. The infant usually is given sweetened electrolyte solution to drink from a bottle during the examination, and right-side-down oblique positioning may be helpful. The pylorus is identified at the end of the stomach, usually near the gallbladder.

Measurements ▪

Measurements of the pylorus are made from frozen images best depicting it (usually in longitudinal orientation). Three measurements may be taken: pyloric muscle thickness *(MT)*, pyloric diameter *(PD)*, and pyloric channel length *(PL)*. Figure 1 shows these measurements. In one paper, the pyloric muscle length was reported separately from the PL.[2] Tables 1, 2, and 3 list reported values of MT, PL, and PD for normal controls, infants without hypertrophic pyloric stenosis (HPS), and those with HPS confirmed. At the bottom of each table the mean, standard deviation (SD), and range of combined measurements from all pertinent series are listed. Various criteria for abnormal MT, PL, and PD have been advocated in these articles, in a review by Haller and Cohen, and in several texts. These range from 3 to 4 mm for MT, 15 to 19 mm for PL, and 10 to 15 mm for PD. A rough consensus based on frequency of citation would seem to be that MT is greater than 3 mm, PL is greater than 16 mm, and PD is greater than 12 mm.

O'Keeffe and colleagues measured the thickness of the antropyloric muscle (APT) in the fluid-distended stomach within 1.5 cm of the pylorus in 145 infants and found it to average less than 2 mm in 99 without HPS, to be greater than 2 mm in 40 with HPS, and to be between 2 and 3

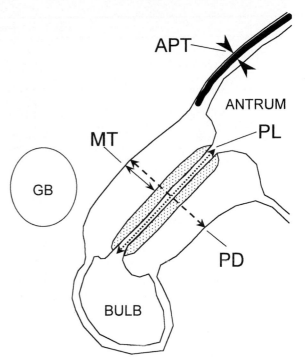

Figure 1 ▪ Measurements using ultrasound of the pylorus in infants. Longitudinal view through the antrum and pylorus is depicted, with measurements shown. MT = muscle thickness *(solid line with arrows)*, PD = pyloric diameter *(dashed line with arrows)*, PL = pyloric length *(dotted line with arrows)*, APT = antropyloric muscle thickness *(arrowheads)*, GB = gallbladder.

mm in 6, of whom 2 had HPS.[10] This is indicated in Figure 1.

Source ▪

The studies abstracted in Tables 1, 2, and 3 are a subset of the numerous published works and were chosen to be representative.[1–9] Infants ranging in age from 1 to 20 weeks were examined for clinical suspicion of HPS because of one or more of the following: prolonged vomiting, dehydration, palpable mass, or signs of base excess in serum chemistry analysis. The diagnosis of HPS was almost always confirmed by surgery; those presumed to have other conditions (pylorospasm, reflux, milk allergy, overfeeding, gastroenter-

Table 1 ▪ Measurements of Pyloric Muscle Thickness

| | | | MUSCLE THICKNESS | |
REFERENCE	CATEGORY	NO.	Mean ± SD	Range
Stunden[1]	No HPS	88	1.6±0.4	1.0–3.0
	HPS	112	3.4±0.7	3.0–5.0
Blumhagen[2]	No HPS	210	1.8±0.4	1.0–3.0
	HPS	108	4.8±0.6	3.5–6.0
Lund Kofoed[3]	Control	34	3.5±1.0	2.0–6.0
	No HPS	5	4.1±1.5	3.0–6.0
	HPS	29	6.4±1.1	5.0–10.0
Westra[4]	Control	28		1.0–3.0
	No HPS	25		1.0–3.0
	HPS	22	4.8±0.1	3.0–7.0
Davies[5]	No HPS	10	2.1±0.6	1.0–3.0
	HPS	15	4.3±0.63	3.0–5.6
van der Schouw[6]	No HPS	45	2.6±0.17	
	HPS	60	5.3±0.31	
Hernandez-Schulman[7]	Spasm	7	2.04±0.45	1.3–2.7
	HPS	66		3.0–7.0
Hallam[8]	Control	92	2.0	1.0–3.0
	No HPS	26	2.4	1.5–3.5
	HPS	21	4.0	2.5–5.5
Cohen[9]	Spasm-minimal	34	0.9±1.0	0.0–2.9
	Spasm-maximal	34	3.8±1.0	1.5–6.0
	HPS	37	5.3±0.9	3.0–7.7
Combined (without refs 8 or 9)	No HPS	355	1.9±0.42	1.0–6.0
Combined	HPS	352	4.8±0.69	2.5–10.0

All measurements are in millimeters. Mean ± standard deviation and ranges are given except for Hallam, which are median values, and van der Schouw (mean ± standard error). HPS = hypertrophic pyloric stenosis; spasm = pylorospasm.

Table 2 ▪ Measurements of Pyloric Channel Length

REFERENCE	CATEGORY	NO.	CHANNEL LENGTH Mean ± SD	CHANNEL LENGTH Range
Stunden[1]	No HPS	88	8.3 ± 2.5	5.0–14.0
	HPS	112	22.3 ± 2.3	18.0–28.0
Blumhagen[2]	No HPS	210	11.3 ± 3.2	5.0–22.0
	HPS	108	17.8 ± 2.6	11.0–25.0
Westra[4]	Control	28	11.6 ± 2.0	8.0–15.0
	No HPS	25	13.0 ± 2.5	9.0–17.0
	HPS	22	19.5 ± 3.1	15.0–26.0
Davies[5]	No HPS	10	10.0 ± 2.4	6.0–12.5
	HPS	15	17.4 ± 2.8	12.0–22.7
van der Schouw[6]	No HPS	45	7.9 ± 0.92	
	HPS	60	18.8 ± 0.53	
Hernandez-Schulman[7]	Spasm	7	12.3 ± 0.15	10.0–14.0
	HPS	66		12.0–30.0
Cohen[9]	Spasm-minimal	34	3.5 ± 3.7	0.0–15.0
	Spasm-maximal	34	14.4 ± 4.7	3.4–27.0
	HPS	37	22.5 ± 3.6	14.0–31.0
Combined (without ref 9)	No HPS	378	10.4 ± 2.7	5.0–22.0
Combined	HPS	420	20.0 ± 2.5	10.0–31.0

All measurements are in millimeters. Mean ± standard deviation and ranges are given except for van der Schouw (mean ± standard error). HPS = hypertrophic pyloric stenosis; spasm = pylorospasm.

itis, or idiopathic) were, for the most part, found to improve on follow-up with nonsurgical treatment. In a few cases, negative results at surgery confirmed the absence of HPS. Additionally, three of the studies included control groups of infants being scanned for other reasons with no gastrointestinal problems.[3, 4, 8]

Comments ▪

There is some controversy about which of the measurements is the most reliable. Haller considered the PD to be least reliable and used critical values of MT-40 mm and PL-18 mm, measured on longitudinal images. Van der Schouw and colleagues performed receiver operating characteristic (ROC) analysis on various clinical, laboratory,

and ultrasound parameters and produced a model that uses age of onset of vomiting, PL, and PD. This yielded an area under the ROC curve of .970. Onset of vomiting under 5 weeks, PL greater than 13 mm, and PD greater than 9 mm were the optimal cut-off points.[6]

Westra and colleagues combined parameters to obtain a volume as follows:

$$\text{Pyloric volume} = 0.25 \times PD^2 \times PL.$$

Infants without HPS had volumes of between 0.4 and 1.3 ml whereas those with HPS ranged between 1.4 and 5.1 ml. The suggested cut-off is 1.4 ml.[4]

Table 3 ▪ Measurements of Pyloric Diameter

REFERENCE	CATEGORY	NO.	PYLORUS DIAMETER Mean ± SD	PYLORUS DIAMETER Range
Stunden[1]	No HPS	88	9.1 ± 1.1	7.7–13.0
	HPS	112	13.3 ± 2.1	9.0–19.0
Lund Kofoed[3]	Control	34	8.5 ± 2.2	4.0–13.0
	No HPS	5	9.8 ± 3.2	6.0–14.0
	HPS	29	14.1 ± 2.4	10.0–21.0
Westra[4]	Control	28	8.2 ± 1.8	5.0–12.0
	No HPS	25	9.0 ± 1.3	7.0–13.0
	HPS	22	14.0 ± 1.7	10.0–18.0
Davies[5]	No HPS	10	7.5 ± 2.5	4.0–12.5
	HPS	15	12.7 ± 2.8	8.0–18.0
van der Schouw[6]	No HPS	45	5.3 ± 0.6	
	HPS	60	13.1 ± 0.4	
Hallam[8]	Control	92	10.0	7.5–14.0
	No HPS	26	11.0	7.0–15.0
	HPS	21	14.0	11.0–17.0
Combined (without ref 8)	No HPS	389	8.0 ± 1.3	4.0–15.0
	HPS	346	13.4 ± 1.8	8.0–21.0

All measurements are in millimeters. Mean ± standard deviation and ranges are given except for Hallam, which are median values, and van der Schouw (mean ± standard error). HPS = hypertrophic pyloric stenosis.

Carver and colleagues modified the pylorus volume calculation and indexed it with patient weight as follows:

Pyloric muscle index =

$$\frac{(\pi \times MT \times PL \times [PD - MT])}{\text{weight in kg}}$$

Infants without HPS had indices of between 0.08 and 0.28 whereas the indices of those with HPS ranged between 0.46 and 1.26. The suggested cut-off is 0.4.[12]

Davies and coworkers combined PL and MT into an index as follows:

$$\text{Pyloric index} = PL + 3.64 \times MT.$$

Infants without HPS had indices of between 10 and 19 whereas the indices of those with HPS ranged between 24 and 99. The suggested cut-off is 25.[5]

Cohen and coworkers cautioned that patients with pylorospasm may have MT and PL values in the same range as those with HPS. The measurements in pylorospasm varied over 5 minutes of continuous real-time observation, whereas they remained fixed in those with HPS.[9]

Most authors stress the importance of ancillary signs, including exaggerated peristalsis in the stomach, lack of gastric emptying of fluid into the duodenum, hypoechoic ring of hypertrophied muscle, and indentation of pyloric muscle into the antrum.

REFERENCES

1. Stunden RJ, LeQuesne GW, Little KE: The improved ultrasound diagnosis of hypertrophic pyloric stenosis. Pediatr Radiol 1986; 16(3):200–205.
2. Blumhagen JD, Maclin L, Krauter D, et al: Sonographic diagnosis of hypertrophic pyloric stenosis. Radiology 1988; 150:1367–1370.
3. Lund Kofoed PE, Host A, Elle B, Larsen C: Hypertrophic pyloric stenosis: Determination of muscle dimensions by ultrasound. Br J Radiol 1988; 61:19–20.
4. Westra SJ, de Groot C, Smits NJ, Staalman CR: Hypertrophic pyloric stenosis: Use of the pyloric volume measurement in early US diagnosis. Radiology 1989; 172:615–619.
5. Davies RP, Linke RJ, Robinson RG, et al: Sonographic diagnosis of infantile hypertrophic pyloric stenosis. J Ultrasound Med 1992; 11(11):603–605.
6. van der Schouw YT, van der Velden MT, Hitge-Boetes C, et al: Diagnosis of hypertrophic pyloric stenosis: Value of sonography when used in conjunction with clinical findings and laboratory data. AJR Am J Roentgenol 1994; 163(4):905–909.
7. Hernandez-Schulman M, Sells LL, Ambrosino MM, et al: Hypertrophic pyloric stenosis in the infant without a palpable olive: Accuracy of sonographic diagnosis. Radiology 1994; 193:771–776.
8. Hallam D, Hansen B, Bodker B, et al: Pyloric size in normal infants and in infants suspected of having hypertrophic pyloric stenosis. Acta Radiol 1995; 36(3):261–264.
9. Cohen HL, Zinn HL, Haller JO, et al: Ultrasonography of pylorospasm: Findings may simulate hypertrophic pyloric stenosis. J Ultrasound Med 1998; 17:705–711.
10. O'Keeffe FN, Stansberry SD, Swischuk LE, Hayden CK Jr: Antropyloric muscle thickness at US in infants: What is normal? Radiology 1991; 178(3):827–830.
11. Haller JO, Cohen HL: Hypertrophic pyloric stenosis: Diagnosis using US. Radiology 1986; 161:335–339.
12. Carver RA, Okorie M, Steiner GM, et al: Infantile hypertrophic pyloric stenosis—Diagnosis from pyloric muscle index. Clin Radiol 1989; 38:625–627.

▪▪ POSITION OF DUODENUM FOR DIAGNOSIS OF MALROTATION
▪ ACR Code: 73 (Duodenum)

Technique ▪

Barium was administered orally or via nasogastric tube with fluoroscopic monitoring with the patient in right decubitus position. When barium reached the second portion of the duodenum, the patient was rolled supine and spot radiographs were made in midinspiration as the bolus reached the level of the ligament of Treitz (LOT). The duodenojejunal flexure (DJF) was then manually pushed to the right with slow deep palpation and a radiograph was made at maximal excursion.[1]

Measurements ▪

On each study the center of the duodenal bulb apex (DBA), the inferior duodenal flexure (IDF), and the duodenojejunal flexure (DJF) were identified and lines drawn between them to form a triangle. The vertical distance between DBA and DJF was measured, as was the base of the triangle (IDF-DJF). Figure 1 shows these measurements. These distances (in centimeters) were corrected by dividing by the arithmetic mean of the T11 interpeduncular distance and the distance between superior end-plates of T11 and T12 (X and Y on Figure 1):

$$\text{Corrected distance} = \text{measured distance}/([X + Y]/2).$$

The lateral mobility of the DJF was measured by noting the rightward displacement (in centimeters) caused by manual manipulation and correcting as noted earlier. Table 1 lists criteria for malrotation. Table 2 gives transverse and cephalocaudal positions of the normal DBA, IDF, DJF, and the pylorus. Table 3 shows cephalocaudal locations of these structures from prior literature as abstracted by the authors. Table 4 gives the normal mobility of the DJF.

Source ▪

A control group of 43 patients (21 male, 22 female, age range 1 day to 17 years, mean age 3.5 years) had upper gastrointestinal (UGI) series performed, including the maneuvers described earlier. None had clinical or radiographic evidence of intestinal malrotation. UGI studies of 35 patients (20 male, 15 female, age range under 6 months

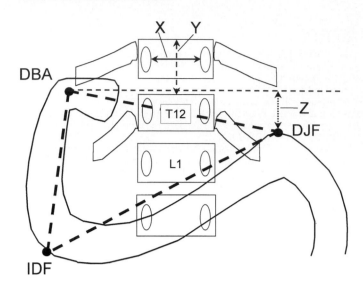

Figure 1 ▪ Measurements of the duodenum from a UGI series for diagnosis of malrotation. Correction of the measurements is done by dividing them by the average of the T11 interpeduncular distance (*X, solid*) and between superior endplates of T11 and T12 (*Y, dashed*). DBA = midlumen at duodenal bulb apex, IDF = inferior duodenal flexure, DJF = duodenojejunal flexure. IDF–DJF should be the longest leg of a triangle drawn between the three points. It is normally 3.5 ± 0.45 cm (corrected), and a length of less than 2.6 cm is abnormal. The vertical distance between DBA and DJF (*Z, dotted*) should be less than 1.3 cm (corrected). (From Katz ME, Siegel MJ, Shackelford GD, McAlister WH: AJR Am J Roentgenol 1987; 148:947–951. Used by permission.)

Table 1 ▪ Criteria for Malrotation on UGF Studies

LANDMARK: ABNORMAL FINDING	NUMBER WITH ABNORMALITY PRESENT	
	Controls (n = 43)	Malrotation (n = 35)
Pylorus:		
1 To left of midline	3 (7%)	16 (37%)
Duodenojejunal flexure:		
2 Below level of L1–L2 disc in child under age 18 yr	1 (2%)	22 (51%)
3 >1.3 corrected distance below apex of bulb	1 (2%)	20 (47%)
4 To right of left pedicle	0	16 (37%)
Segment between inferior flexure and duodenojejunal flexure:		
5 Intervening obstruction	0	21 (49%)
6 Connecting line not longest side of triangle	1 (2%)	24 (56%)
7 Connecting line <2.6 (corrected distance)	1 (2%)	21 (49%)
Jejunum:		
8 Corkscrewing or zigzagging	0	20 (57%)
9 To right of spine	1 (2%)	23 (53%)

Malrotation is diagnosed when three or more criteria are met. From Katz ME, Siegel MJ, Shackelford GD, McAlister WH: AJR Am J Roentgenol 1987; 148:947–951. Used by permission.

Table 2 ▪ Locations of Duodenal Landmarks on UGI Studies

LANDMARK	MEDIOLATERAL (N = 43)				CEPHALOCAUDAL	
	Right of Spine	Right Half of Spine	Left Half of Spine	Left of Spine	Mean Level	Range
Pylorus	24 (56%)	16 (37%)	2 (5%)	1 (2%)	T12–L1	T11–L1/L2
Apex of bulb	33 (77%)	10 (23%)	0	0	T12–L1	T11/T12–L1/L2
Inferior flexure	36 (84%)	7 (16%)	0	0	L3	L2–L3/L4
Duodenojejunal flexure	0	0	6 (14%)	37 (86%)	T12–L1	T11–Superior half L2

From Katz ME, Siegel MJ, Shackelford GD, McAlister WH: AJR Am J Roentgenol 1987; 148:947–951. Used by permission.

Table 3 ▪ Vertebral Levels of Duodenal Landmarks

REFERENCE	AGE RANGE	EXAMINATION POSITION	AVERAGE VERTEBRAL LEVEL OF LANDMARK			
			Pylorus	Duodenal Bulb	Inferior Flexure	Duodenojejunal Flexure
Katz[1]	0–17 yr	Supine	T12–L1	T12–L1	L3	T12–L1
deBacker[2]	0–7 mon	Prone		T12	L3–L3	
Moody[3]	College age	Supine	L2			
		Erect	L3			
		Prone	L3			
Friedman[4]	10–20 yr	Prone		L1	L3	L2
		Erect		L2		L2–L3
	50–80 yr	Prone		L2	L4	L2
Meschan[5]	20–70 yr	Supine		T12–L1		L1–L2

From Katz ME, Siegel MJ, Shackelford GD, McAlister WH: AJR Am J Roentgenol 1987; 148:947–951. Used by permission.

Table 4 ▪ Rightward Mobility of the Normal Duodenojejunal Flexure

AGE	NO.	ACROSS MIDLINE	TO RIGHT OF SPINE	MOBILITY (CORRECTED DISTANCE)	
				Mean ± SD	Range
0–4 mon	13	12 (92%)	9 (69%)	2.03 ± 0.78	0.19–3.37
4–18 mon	12	8 (67%)	2 (17%)	1.43 ± 0.97	0.20–3.35
18 mon–4 yr	6	4 (67%)	0	0.95 ± 0.60	0–1.46
4–18 yr	12	0	0	0.08 ± 0.12	0–0.35

SD – standard deviation.
From Katz ME, Siegel MJ, Shackelford GD, McAlister WH: AJR Am J Roentgenol 1987; 148:947–951. Used by permission.

to 14 years, mean age 3.2 years) with proved intestinal malrotation were retrospectively evaluated.[1]

Comments ▪

The ileocecal position was visible in 22 of 35 patients with malrotation and was in the right lower quadrant in 7 (32%), the right upper quadrant in 7 (32%), the left upper quadrant in 7 (32%) and the left lower quadrant in 1 (4%). Although many cases of malrotation are obvious on UGI series, 10% to 15% are rather more subtle. Katz and colleagues use the criteria in Table 1 and diagnose malrotation when three or more are met.[1]

REFERENCES

1. Katz ME, Siegel MJ, Shackelford GD, McAlister WH: The position and mobility of the duodenum in children. AJR Am J Roentgenol 1987; 148:947–951.
2. deBacker, Van de Putte: Radiological study of the digestive tract in normal infants. Br J Radiol 1926; 31:493–497.
3. Moody RO, Van Nuys RG, Kidder CH: The form and position of the empty stomach in healthy young adults shown in roentgenograms. Anat Rec 1929; 43:359–379.
4. Friedman SM: The position and mobility of the duodenum in the living subject. Am J Anat 1946; 79:147–165.
5. Meschan I, Landsman H, Regnier G, et al: The "normal" radiographic adult stomach and duodenum. South Med J 1953; 46:878–886.

▪: SMALL BOWEL CALIBER IN CHILDREN AND ADULTS[1]
▪ ACR Code: 74 (Small Intestine)

Table 1 ▪ Mean Diameter of Small Bowel*	
AGE	DIAMETER (mm)†
6 mon	12.0
1 yr	13.0
2 yr	15.0
3 yr	16.7
4 yr	18.9
5 yr	19.0
6 yr	19.9
7 yr	20.5
8 yr	21.0
9 yr	21.4
10 yr	21.8
11 yr	22.1
12 yr	22.3
13 yr	22.5
14 yr	22.7
15 yr	23.0

*Adult value is 23.1 mm ± 1.9 (1 SD). Upper limit for adult is 25 mm.
†1 SD = 1.9 mm.
From Haworth EM, et al: Clin Radiol 1967; 18:417. Used by permission.

Technique ▪

Central ray: Perpendicular to plane of film centered over midabdomen.
Position: Anteroposterior, with patient supine.
Target-film distance: Children, 36 inches; adults, 30 inches.

Measurements ▪ (Table 1)

Nonflocculating media that are complex barium sulfate suspensions are used. A 50% dilution in volume of 2 to 8 oz is used according to age in children and according to size of stomach in adults. Three segments of the small bowel that have clearly defined margins and approximately the same caliber as the rest of the small bowel are selected for measurement. The measurements are made at right angles to the parallel margins of the bowel. The average of the three measurements is used.

Source ▪

Small bowel measurements were taken from 61 infants and children aged 9 months to 15.5 years and from 77 adults (37 men and 40 women) aged 19 to 77 years.

REFERENCE

1. Haworth EM, Hodson CJ, Joyce CR, et al: Radiological measurement of small bowel calibre in normal subjects according to age. Clin Radiol 1967; 18:417–421.

■: SIZE OF GAS-FILLED BOWEL LOOPS IN INFANTS[1]
■ ACR Code: 74 (Small Intestine); 75 (Colon)

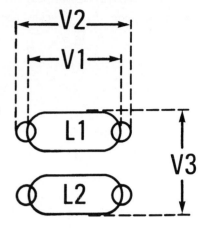

Figure 1 ■ Measurements of the upper lumbar spine elements used in this study. (From Edwards DK: AJR Am J Roentgenol 1980; 135:331. Used by permission.)

Technique ■

Central ray: Perpendicular to plane of film.
Position: Anteroposterior supine.
Target-film distance: Immaterial.

Measurements ■ (Figure 1 and Table 1)

The width of the largest bowel loop was measured. No attempt was made to distinguish large from small bowel. Three dimensions of the upper lumbar spine were made:

V_1 = Width of the first lumbar vertebral body (L_1).
V_2 = Distance between the outer edges of the pedicles of L_1.
V_3 = Total height of L_1 and L_2, including the disc space.

This measurement is the easiest to measure and statistically the most reproducible.

The maximum bowel width is divided by the three vertebral measures to form the three bowel-vertebral ratios.

Source ■

Normal data based on a study of 375 normal patients (Table 1).

REFERENCE

1. Edwards DK: Size of gas-filled bowel loops in infants. AJR Am J Roentgenol 1980; 135:331–334.

Table 1 ■ Ratios of Maximum Bowel Width and Vertebral Body Measures

POPULATION, AGE*/BOWEL-VERTEBRAL RATIO	MEAN VALUE	SD	MEAN ± 2 SD
Normal (n = 375), 0.9			
B:V_1	0.81	0.12	0.56–1.05
B:V_2	0.57	0.11	0.36–0.79
B:V_3	0.61	0.11	0.40–0.83
Suspected NEC† (all) (n = 188), 11.3			
B:V_1	1.27	0.27	
B:V_2	0.90	0.21	
B:V_3	0.96	0.20	
Proved NEC (n = 48), 17.1			
B:V_1	1.40	0.31	
B:V_2	0.97	0.23	
B:V_3	1.05	0.23	
NEC suspected, not proved (n = 140), 9.3			
B:V_1	1.23	0.24	
B:V_2	0.87	0.19	
B:V_3	0.93	0.18	
Congenital obstruction (n = 24), 3.4			
B:V_1	2.16	0.51	
B:V_2	1.59	0.38	
B:V_3	1.63	0.40	

*Mean age at radiograph (days).
†NEC = necrotizing enterocolitis; SD = standard deviation.
From Edwards DK: AJR Am J Roentgenol 1980; 135:331–334. Used by permission.

▪▪ MEASUREMENT OF THE ILEOCECAL VALVE[1]
- ▪ ACR Code: 752 (Cecum, Ileocecal Valve)

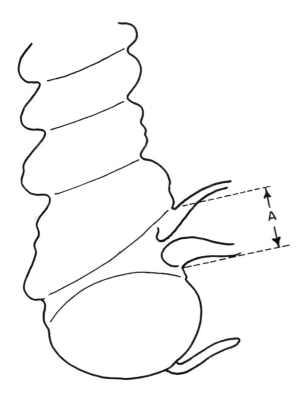

Figure 1 ▪ Measurement of the ileocecal valve (*A*).

Technique ▪

Central ray: Spot roentgenograms made during fluoroscopy.
Position: Posterior and oblique views (found to best demonstrate the valve during fluoroscopy), using graduated pressure over ileocecal valve region.
Target-film distance: Depends on patient thickness.

Measurements ▪ (Figure 1)

Average vertical diameter (*A*) = 2.5 cm.
   Vertical diameter (*A*) of 4.0 cm or more is considered abnormal by Hinkel.[1]

Source ▪

Five hundred consecutive routine barium enema examinations.

Reference

1. Hinkel CL: AJR Am J Roentgenol 1952; 68:171.

▪▪ MEASUREMENT OF CECAL DIAMETER[1]
▪ ACR Code: 752 (Cecum)

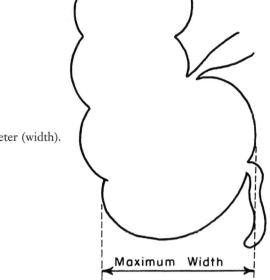

Figure 1 ▪ Measurement of the maximum cecal diameter (width).

Maximum Width

Technique ▪

Central ray: On median plane at level of iliac crests.
Position: Posteroanterior.
Target-film distance: 36 inches.

Measurements ▪ (Figure 1)

The greatest transverse diameter is measured on the prone film of the abdomen.
  Average diameter = 5 to 7 cm.
  A width of 9 cm or greater is a critical diameter beyond which danger of perforation exists.

Source ▪

Artificial distention of the cecum with barium and air was performed on 100 selected patients without intrinsic cecal disease or distal large bowel obstruction. Nineteen cases of cecal distention with distal large bowel obstruction were studied for comparison.

REFERENCE

1. Davis L, Lowman RM: Radiology 1957; 68:542.

▪▪ ULTRASOUND OF THE APPENDIX IN SUSPECTED APPENDICITIS
▪ ACR Code: 751 (Appendix)

Technique ▪

Graded compression ultrasound of the right lower quadrant (RLQ) was done in all studies with various transducers and machines.[1-14] In more recent studies, 5.0-10.0-MHz linear transducers have been favored. Left-side-down oblique or decubitus positioning may be helpful, especially in pregnant patients.[7]

Measurements ▪

The appendix is sought in the RLQ and can be recognized by its relationship to the cecum. It is often draped over the right iliac vessels, anterior to the ileopsoas muscles, and/or posterior to the terminal ileum. Measurements can be made of the maximal diameter (serosa to serosa) or the wall thickness (lumen to serosa). Figure 1 shows the layers of the appendix, which are variably seen, and sites for measurement. Though Figure 1 shows measurements in a plane transverse to the long axis of the appendix, care must be taken not to make them from an oblique section to avoid distortion. Alternatively, a longitudinal image may be used (at least for the diameter). Table 1 gives patient demographics, numbers with and without appendicitis, normal appendices seen, and test performance statistics of ten studies.[1-10] Most studies used measurement of wall thickness or diameter, compressibility of the appendix, and

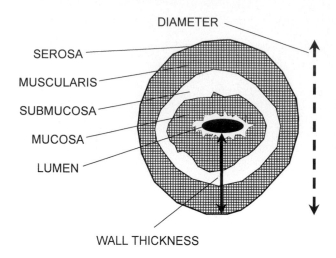

DIAMETER

SEROSA

MUSCULARIS

SUBMUCOSA

MUCOSA

LUMEN

WALL THICKNESS

Figure 1 ▪ Representation of a transverse section through the appendix. Four layers and the lumen are labeled and are variably seen in normal and inflamed appendixes. Wall thickness *(solid line with arrows)* is measured from lumen to serosa, and diameter *(dashed line with arrows)* is measured from serosa to serosa. The maximum thickness or diameter is used.

Table 1 ▪ Results of Studies of Ultrasound to Diagnose Appendicitis

REFERENCE	AGES (yr)	NUMBER − APPY	APPENDIX SEEN	NUMBER + APPY	SENS. (%)	SPEC. (%)	CRITERIA FOR POSITIVE STUDY
Puylaert[1]	11–81	32	0	28	89	100	Noted dilated lumen 3–10 mm
Jeffrey[2]	5–74	60	3 (5%)	30	89	95	Noted wall thickening 3–8 mm
Abu-Yousef[3]	2–64	43	2 (5%)	25	80	95	Noted wall thickening >2 mm
Jeffrey[4]	2–81	156	5 (3%)	89	90	96	Used diameter >6 mm
Vignault[5]	4–18	37	12 (32%)	33	94	89	Used diameter >6 mm (same as in adults)
Rioux[6]	4–73	125	102 (82%)	45	93	94	Used wall thickness >3 mm
Lim[7] all pregnant	21–40	27	1 >6 mm ? <7 mm	15	100	96	Used diameter >7 mm
Sivit[8]	2–19	128	64 (50%)	52	88	96	Used diameter >6 mm
Quillin[9]	1–19	61	8 (13%)	39	87	97	Used diameter >6 mm, also hypervascular wall at color Doppler
Rapp[10]	0–83	144	89 (62%)	59	90	97	Used diameter >6 mm

−Appy = disease negative, +Appy = disease positive; Sens. = sensitivity, Spec. = specificity; Appendix seen = number of disease-negative cases in which the appendix was identified.

a combination of other findings for diagnostic criteria. Table 2 is a composite of the diagnostic criteria for appendicitis.

Source ▪

Numbers of patients with and without appendicitis, as well as age ranges for the studies abstracted here, are given in Table 1.[1–10]

Comments ▪

As equipment and experience improve, the appendix seems to be found more frequently in patients without appendicitis. Criteria based on measurements become more important in light of this fact. These have the same numeric values for both children and adults. Focal or segmental appendicitis (sometimes confined to the distal tip) is a potential pitfall.[10–12] For this reason, attempts should be made to visualize the entire appendix and measurement of the maximum obtainable diameter or wall thickness used for diagnosis. In advanced supportive appendicitis, the lumen may be so distended that the wall is thinned to less than 3 mm, though overall diameter will usually be more than 6 mm. Color Doppler ultrasound can be helpful in

cases in which the appendix is seen and is borderline in terms of size. The normal appendix will have little if any flow associated with the wall, whereas appendicitis often causes hyperemia visible with optimized Doppler settings.[9, 13, 14]

Table 2 ▪ Diagnostic Criteria for Appendicitis at Ultrasound

Appendix—Major Findings
Noncompressible
Maximum diameter >6 mm (6 mm borderline)
Maximum wall thickness >3 mm (3 mm borderline)

Appendix—Secondary Findings
Hypervascular wall at color Doppler
Target pattern, diffuse hypoechogenicity
Fluid in appendiceal lumen
Appendicolith

Ancillary Findings
Complex mass in RLQ
Inflammatory changes in periappendiceal fat
Free fluid or air outside bowel
Point tenderness over appendix
Mesenteric adenopathy (consider adenitis if appendix normal)

REFERENCES

1. Puylaert JBCM: Acute appendicitis: US evaluation using graded compression. Radiology 1986; 158:355–360.
2. Jeffrey RB Jr, Laing FC, Lewis FR: Acute appendicitis: High-resolution real-time US findings. Radiology 1987; 163(1):11–14.
3. Abu-Yousef MM, Bleicher JJ, Maher JW, et al: High-resolution sonography of acute appendicitis. AJR Am J Roentgenol 1987; 149:53–58.
4. Jeffrey RB Jr, Laing FC, Townsend RR: Acute appendicitis: Sonographic criteria based on 250 cases. Radiology 1988; 167(2):327–329.
5. Vignault F, Filiatrault D, Brandt ML, et al: Acute appendicitis in children: Evaluation with US. Radiology 1990; 176(2):501–504.
6. Rioux M: Sonographic detection of the normal and abnormal appendix. AJR Am J Roentgenol 1992; 158(4):773–778.
7. Lim HK, Bae SH, Seo GS: Diagnosis of acute appendicitis in pregnant women: Value of sonography. AJR Am J Roentgenol 1992; 159:539–542.
8. Sivit CJ, Newman KD, Boenning DA, et al: Appendicitis: Usefulness of US in diagnosis in a pediatric population. Radiology 1992; 185:549–552.
9. Quillin SQ, Siegel MJ: Appendicitis: Efficacy of color Doppler sonography. Radiology 1994; 191:557–560.
10. Rapp CL, Stavros AT, Meyers PR: Ultrasound of the normal appendix: The how and why. J Diagn Med Sonogr 1998; 14:195–201.
11. Nghiem HV, Jeffrey RB Jr: Acute appendicitis confined to the appendiceal tip: Evaluation with graded compression sonography. J Ultrasound Med 1992; 11(5):205–207.
12. Lim HK, Lee WJ, Lee SJ, et al: Focal appendicitis confined to the tip: Diagnosis at US. Radiology 1996; 200:799–800.
13. Quillin SP, Siegel MJ: Appendicitis in children: Color Doppler sonography. Radiology 1992; 184:745–747.
14. Lim HK, Lee WJ, Kim TH, et al: Appendecitis: Usefulness of color Doppler US. Radiology 1996; 201:221–225.

▪▪ RECTOSIGMOID INDEX FOR THE EARLY DIAGNOSIS OF HIRSCHSPRUNG DISEASE[1]
▪ ACR Code: 756 (Rectosigmoid Colon)

Technique ▪

Central ray: Perpendicular to plane of film.
Position: Anteroposterior lateral and left posterior oblique.
Target-film distance: Immaterial.

Measurements ▪ (Figure 1)

The widest diameter of the rectum *(RR¹)* was obtained at any level below the third sacral vertebra. The largest measurement of the sigmoid *(SS¹)* was also measured. All measurements were obtained along a transverse axis, vertical to the longitudinal axis of the colon at that point. The rectosigmoid index was obtained by dividing the widest diameter of the rectum by the widest margin of the sigmoid loop when the colon was fully distended.

The data indicate that a rectosigmoid index of less than 1 indicates Hirschsprung disease. An index higher than 1 may indicate a normal colon or a condition mimicking Hirschsprung disease, such as meconium plug syndrome.

Source ▪

Based on a study of 21 infants with biopsy-proved cases of Hirschsprung disease, 10 infants with meconium plug syndrome, 12 term neonates considered normal, and 25 infants with other bowel disorders.

REFERENCE

1. Pochaczevsky R, Leonidas JC: The "rectosigmoid index." A measurement for the early diagnosis of Hirschsprung's disease. AJR Am J Roentgenol 1975; 123:770–777.

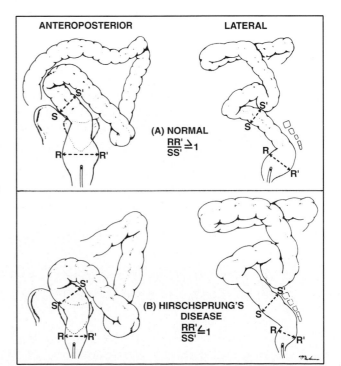

Figure 1 ▪ The rectosigmoid index. (From Pochaczevsky R, Leonidas JC: AJR Am J Roentgenol 1975; 123:770. Used by permission.)

▪: MEASUREMENT OF THE PRESACRAL SPACE IN CHILDREN AND ADULTS
▪ ACR Code: 759 (Presacral Space)

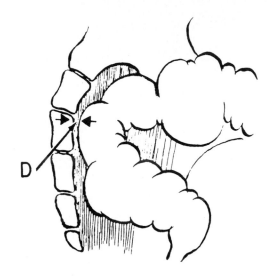

Figure 1 ▪ Measurement of the presacral space in children and adults (*D*). (From Kattan KR, King AY: AJR Am J Roentgenol 1979; 132:437. Used by permission.)

Technique ▪

Central ray: Spot roentgenograms made during fluoroscopy.
Position: Lateral view obtained during barium enema examination.
Target-film distance: Variable; depends on width of patient.

Measurements ▪ (Figure 1)

The shortest distance between the posterior rectum and the sacrum is indicated by *D*.

In children aged 1 to 15 years, the average distance is 3 mm (range = 1 to 5 mm). Measurements over 5 mm should be considered abnormal.

In adults, the average distance is 7 mm (range = 2 to 16 mm). Measurements over 20 mm should be considered abnormal. However, in some normal patients older than 45 years, the presacral space is wider than 15 mm and may even exceed 20 mm.

Source ▪

Eklof and Gierup studied 85 boys and 75 girls in the 1- to 15-year age group who had no evidence of inflammatory bowel disease.[1]

Chrispin and Fry studied 100 patients, selected at random, in whom no bowel abnormality could be demonstrated.[2]

Kattan and King studied 100 men and 87 women, aged 17 to 89 years.[3]

REFERENCES

1. Eklof O, Gierup J: The retrorectal soft tissue space in children; normal variations and appearances in granulomatous colitis. AJR Am J Roentgenol 1970; 108:624–627.
2. Chrispin AR, Fry IK: Br J Radiol 1963; 36:319.
3. Kattan KR, King AY: Presacral space revisited. AJR Am J Roentgenol 1999; 132:437–439.

•: DETERMINATION OF LIVER SIZE IN INFANCY AND CHILDHOOD[1]
- ACR Code: 761 (Liver)

Figure 1 • Measurement of vertical axis of the liver. The lower horizontal line is drawn from the lowest right border of the liver. (From Deligeorgis D, Yannakos D, Doxiadis S: Arch Dis Child 1973; 48:790. Used by permission.)

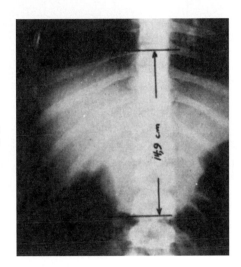

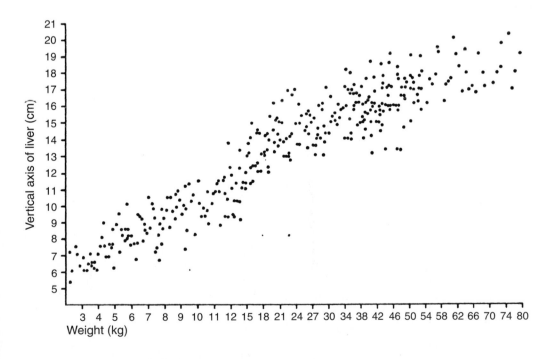

Figure 2 • Vertical axis of the liver related to weight. (From Deligeorgis D, Yannakos D, Doxiadis S: Arch Dis Child 1973; 48:790. Used by permission.)

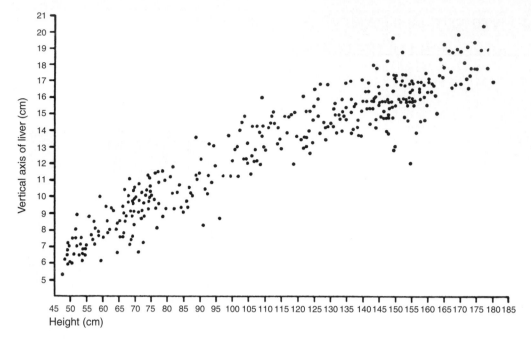

Figure 3 ▪ Vertical axis of the liver related to height. (From Deligeorgis D, Yannakos D, Doxiadis S: Arch Dis Child 1973; 48:790. Used by permission.)

Figure 4 ▪ Vertical axis of the liver related to age. (From Deligeorgis D, Yannakos D, Doxiadis S: Arch Dis Child 1973; 48:790. Used by permission.)

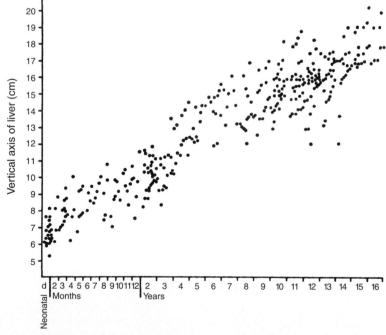

Technique ▪

Central ray: Perpendicular to plane of film.
Position: Anteroposterior supine, filmed at end of expiration.
Target-film distance: 140 cm.

Measurements ▪ (Figure 1)

A horizontal line is drawn across the uppermost region of the liver, just below the dome of the diaphragm, and another is drawn parallel to the first across the lowest right border of the liver. The vertical distance between the two lines is the vertical axis of the liver. Normal values are given in Figures 2 through 4.

Source ▪

Data were derived from studies of 350 healthy Greek infants and children between birth and the age of 16 years.

REFERENCE

1. Deligeorgis D, Yannakos D, Doliadis S: Normal size of liver in infancy and childhood; X-ray study. Arch Dis Child 1973; 48:790.

⁚ LIVER LENGTH IN CHILDREN WITH ULTRASOUND
▪ ACR Code: 761 (Liver)

Table 1 ▪ Length of Right Lobe of Liver in Children Versus Body Height and Age

BODY HEIGHT (cm)	NUMBER	AGE RANGE (Mon)	MEAN ± SD	RANGE	NORMAL LIMITS
47–64	53	1–3	64 ± 10.4	45–90	40–90
54–73	40	4–6	73 ± 10.8	44–92	45–95
65–78	20	7–9	79 ± 8.0	68–100	60–100
71–92	18	12–30	85 ± 10.0	67–104	65–105
85–109	27	36–59	86 ± 11.8	69–109	65–115
100–130	30	60–83	100 ± 13.6	73–125	70–125
110–131	38	84–107	105 ± 10.6	81–128	75–130
124–149	30	108–131	105 ± 12.5	76–135	75–135
137–153	16	132–155	115 ± 14.0	93–137	85–140
143–168	23	156–179	118 ± 14.6	87–137	85–140
152–175	12	180–200	121 ± 11.7	100–141	95–145

All measurements are in centimeters.
From Konus OL, Ozdemir A, Akkaya A, et al: AJR Am J Roentgenol 1998; 171:1693–1698. Used by permission.

Technique ▪

Ultrasound of the abdomen was done with SSA 27A (Toshiba, Tokyo, Japan) and EUB-515 (Hitachi, Tokyo, Japan) machines and 3.5-MHz transducers. Patients were supine without preparation or sedation.

Measurements ▪

From frozen images of longitudinal midclavicular scans over the liver, the cephalocaudal dimension (length) was measured from the uppermost portion of the dome of the diaphragm to the inferior tip. Table 1 lists liver lengths by age and body height of the patients.

Source ▪

Subjects were 307 children (138 boys, 169 girls, age range neonate to 16 years), with no history, clinical findings, or sonographic evidence of liver disease.

Comments ▪

There were no significant differences between genders at any age. The best correlation between liver measurements and patient parameters was for liver length versus body height.

REFERENCE

1. Konus OL, Ozdemir A, Akkaya A, et al: Normal liver, spleen, and kidney dimensions in neonates, infants and children: Evaluation with sonography. AJR Am J Roentgenol 1998; 171:1693–1698.

⁚ MEASUREMENT OF THE NORMAL LIVER, SPLEEN, AND PANCREAS BY ULTRASOUND[1]
▪ ACR Code: 761 (Liver); 775 (Spleen); 770 (Pancreas)

Technique ▪

1. A high-resolution, real-time scanner (Siemens Imager) was used with a 3.5-MHz transducer.
2. Subjects were examined supine, with the right side elevated to demonstrate the porta hepatis, and with the left side elevated to show the longitudinal axis of the spleen.

Length was measured to the nearest millimeter with dividers.

Measurements ▪

Longitudinal scans of the liver were obtained in the midclavicular line and midline, measuring the longitudinal and anteroposterior diameters (Figures 1, 2 and 3).

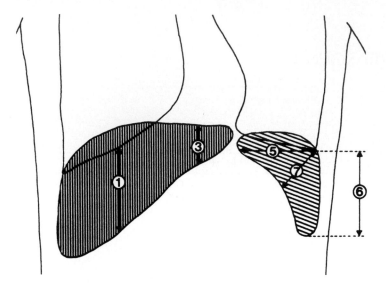

Figure 1 ▪ AP view. *1* = Midclavicular longitudinal diameter of the liver; *3* = midline longitudinal diameter of the liver; *5* = transverse diameter of the spleen; *6* = longitudinal diameter of the spleen; *7* = diagonal diameter of the spleen. The upper regions of the liver and the spleen are located in the dome of the diaphragm and hidden by the air in the lung, so that their longitudinal diameters can be measured only as far as the margin of the lung. (From Niederau C, et al: Radiology 1983; 149:537–540. Used by permission.)

Figure 2 ▪ Lateral view of the liver in the midclavicular plane. *1* = Midclavicular longitudinal diameter; *2* = midclavicular AP diameter, measured at the midpoint of the longitudinal diameter. The upper region of the liver is masked by the air in the lung. (From Niederau C, et al: Radiology 1983; 149:537–540. Used by permission.)

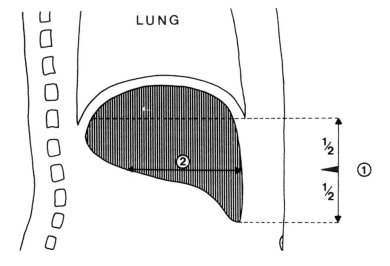

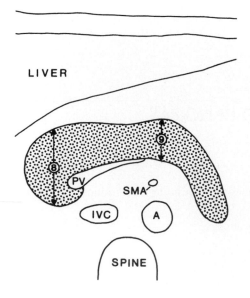

Figure 3 ▪ Transverse scan. *8* = Maximum AP diameter of the head of the pancreas; *9* = maximum AP diameter of the body of the pancreas; *PV* = portal vein; *SMA* = superior mesenteric artery; *IVC* = inferior vena cava; *A* = aorta. The portal and splenic veins, which represent the posterior (dorsal) boundaries of the pancreas, are not included. (From Niederau C, et al: Radiology 1983; 149:537–540. Used by permission.)

In the midclavicular line, the upper portion of the liver was partly masked by the air inside the lung, and the margin between the lung and liver was used as the upper limit of the longitudinal diameter. In the midline, the upper margin of the liver under the dome of the diaphragm served as the upper limit of the longitudinal diameter. The AP diameters were measured at the midpoint of the longitudinal diameters. Both the liver and spleen were measured during deep inspiration. The cross-sectional area of the liver was calculated from the longitudinal and AP diameters using the equation:

$$(Longitudinal\ diameter \times AP\ diameter)/2 = cross\text{-}sectional\ area$$

The spleen was viewed along its longitudinal axis. Transverse, longitudinal, and diagonal diameters were measured from the image showing the maximum cross-sectional areas. The margin between lung and spleen served as both the transverse diameter and the limit of the longitudinal diameter. The cross-sectional diameter was calculated using all three diameters:

$$\frac{Diagonal\ X}{\sqrt{(Transverse^2 + longitudinal^2)/2}} = area$$

The maximum AP diameter of the pancreas was measured on a transverse/oblique scan, using the upper abdominal blood vessels as landmarks. The portal and splenic veins, which comprise the regular posterior (dorsal) boundaries of the body of the pancreas, were not included, nor was the tail of the pancreas measured since it is not often visible and varies widely in shape. The maximum diameter of the portal vein and the diameter at the porta hepatis were measured, with the inner dimensions being used for sonographic assessment.

Statistics

Statistical calculations were performed on a Telefunken TR 440 computer using a routine program. Linear regression analysis was carried out for age, gender, weight, height, surface area, and all diameters. The 95th percentile was considered the upper limit of normal, i.e., 95% of all measurements were below this point. Results of the χ^2 test were evaluated using Yates' correction.

Mean organ diameters are given in Table 1.

Source ▪

Data are based on a study of 1000 healthy subjects, 160 women and 840 men between the ages of 18 and 65 years. Eighty-five subjects were excluded.

REFERENCE

1. Niederau C, Sonnenberg A, et al: Sonographic measurements of the normal liver, spleen, pancreas, and portal vein. Radiology 1983; 149:537–540.

Table 1 ▪ Mean Organ Diameters

	DIAMETER (cm) (Mean ± SD)	95th PERCENTILE (cm)
Midclavicular longitudinal diameter of the liver (1)	10.5 ± 1.5	12.6
Midclavicular AP diameter of the liver (2)	8.1 ± 1.9	11.3
Midline longitudinal diameter of the liver (3)	8.3 ± 1.7	10.9
Midline AP diameter of the liver	5.7 ± 1.5	8.2
Transverse diameter of the spleen (5)	5.5 ± 1.4	7.8
Longitudinal diameter of the spleen (6)	5.8 ± 1.8	8.7
Diagonal diameter of the spleen (7)	3.7 ± 1.0	5.4
Maximum diameter of the head of the pancreas (8)	2.2 ± 0.3	2.6
Maximum diameter of the body of the pancreas (9)	1.8 ± 0.3	2.2
Maximum diameter of the portal vein	1.2 ± 0.2	1.4
Diameter of the portal vein at the porta hepatis	1.0 ± 0.2	1.2

Numbered as in Figures 1, 2, and 3.
From Niederau C, et al: Radiology 1983; 149:537–540. Used by permission.

▪: MEASUREMENT OF LIVER AND SPLEEN VOLUME BY CT[1]
▪ ACR Code: 761 (Liver)

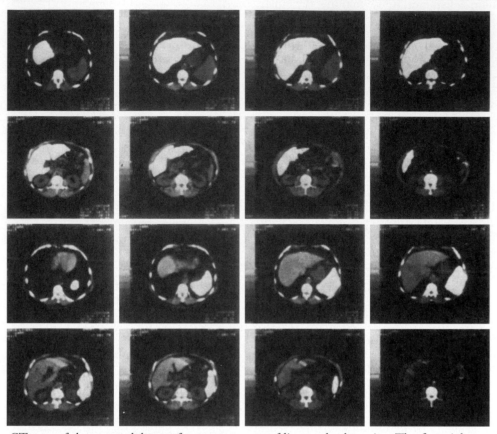

Figure 1 ▪ CT scan of the upper abdomen for measurement of liver and spleen size. The first eight panels show the liver blanked out with a light pen, while the next eight illustrate splenic measurement. (From Henderson JM, et al: Radiology 1981; 141:525. Used by permission.)

Table 1 ▪ Mean Liver and Spleen Volumes on Two Different Days as Read by Two Observers

	LIVER VOLUME (cm³)				SPLEEN VOLUME (cm³)			
	Observer 1		Observer 2		Observer 1		Observer 2	
	Scan 1	Scan 2	Scan 1	Scan 2	Scan 1	Scan 2	Scan 1	Scan 2
Mean	1445	1500	1468	1557	215	228	216	217
SD	±166	±295	±199	±270	±77	±85	±76	±72

From Henderson JM, et al: Radiology 1981; 141:525–527. Used by permission.

Technique ▪

1. A GE 8800 CT/T scanner was used to make 10-mm-thick slices at 2-cm intervals through the liver and spleen, beginning at the level of the diaphragm.
2. Breath holding was in comfortable inspiration. No intravenous contrast was used.

Measurements ▪ (Figure 1 and Table 1)

Each slice was displayed, the organ of interest outlined by the cursor, and the enclosed area calculated by the CT computer.

Areas of each organ were added and multiplied by 2 to estimate total organ volume.

Source ▪

Eleven normal subjects 20 to 30 years of age were studied on two occasions, 1 week apart.

REFERENCE

1. Henderson JM, Heymsfield SB, Horowitz J, et al: Measurement of liver and spleen volume by computed tomography: Assessment of reproducibility and changes found following a selective distal splenorenal shunt. Radiology 1981; 141:525–527.

▪: ESTIMATION OF LIVER VOLUME BY ULTRASOUND
- ACR Code: 761 (Liver)

Technique ▪

Ultrasound of the abdomen was done with an Ultramark 9 machine (ATL, Bothel, WA), and CT scans of the abdomen were done with a 2400 Elite unit (Elscint, Haifa, Israel) with 10-mm slices.[1]

Measurements ▪

The liver was measured in three dimensions (in centimeters) on ultrasound (longitudinal = LON, transverse at the maximal plane = TRV, and true anteroposterior = AP). Liver volume was derived from CT slices by tracing the area on all levels containing it and summing them.[1] Correlation between liver volume by CT and the product of linear ultrasound measurements yielded p = .0001, r = 0.7866, and the following equation:

$$\text{Liver volume by CT} = 320.86 + 0.317 \, (\text{LON} \times \text{TRV} \times \text{AP}).[1]$$

Source ▪

Liver volume was determined 79 times with both modalities in 33 patients (14 male, 19 female, age range 10 to 57 years) with Gaucher disease and varying degrees of splenomegaly.[1]

REFERENCE

1. Elstein D, Hadas-Halpern I, Azure Y, et al: Accuracy of ultrasonography in assessing spleen and liver size in patients with Gaucher disease: Comparison to computed tomographic measurements. J Ultrasound Med 1997; 16:209–211.

▪: MEASUREMENTS OF THE CAUDATE AND QUADRATE LOBES OF THE LIVER TO DIAGNOSE CIRRHOSIS
- ACR Code: 761 (Liver)

Technique ▪

Harbin and colleagues reviewed CT and/or ultrasound studies of the liver (machines and numbers of each not specified).[1] Giorgio and colleagues used an SSD-180 unit (Aloka, Japan), and Hess and group used a Sonoline-SL unit (Siemens, Erlangen, Germany).[2,3] In both studies, 3.5-MHz transducers were used to scan the liver. Lafortune and colleagues performed ultrasound of the liver with 3.5-MHz curved array, 3.5-MHz linear array, or 5-MHz sector transducers on a variety of machines.[4]

Measurements ▪

In three studies, measurements of the caudate and right lobes were made from transverse U/S (or axial CT, Harbin) images made through the level of the bifurcation of the portal vein.[1–3] Hess and group also measured the caudate lobe in the longitudinal plane, and Harbin and colleagues included measurement of the left lobe.[1, 3] Lafortune and colleagues used oblique scans to measure the quadrate lobe.[4] These measurements are shown in Figures 1 through 3. The results are listed in Table 1, and test performance statistics are given in Table 2.

Source ▪

Harbin and colleagues evaluated imaging studies of 55 patients who had died and undergone autopsy or had liver biopsy within 2 months of their scan as well as 20 healthy adult volunteers.[1] Giorgio's subjects consisted of 164 patients (113 male, 51 female, age range 15 to 73 years, mean age 42 years), who had liver biopsy within 3 weeks of ultrasound, and 25 age- and gender-matched controls. Of the biopsy patients, 156 had scans from which measurements could be made.[2] Hess and coworkers studied 58 patients (35 male, 23 female, mean age 55 years) with biopsy-proved cirrhosis and 75 patients (43 male, 32 female, mean age 50 years) with no clinical history of liver disease.[3] Lafortune's subjects were 167 patients (93 men, 74 women, age range 22 to 81 years, mean age 56 years) with clinical/histologic findings of cirrhosis and 125 patients (51 men, 74 women, age range 22 to 71, mean age 44 years) with no clinical/imaging evidence of liver disease.[4] Table 1 lists the numbers of patients having cirrhosis, non-cirrhotic liver disease (usually hepatitis), and normal livers from each series.

Comments ▪

The ratio of the transverse diameters of the caudate to right lobes has had the most study. Depending on the desired level of specificity, one may choose cut-offs between 0.45 and 0.65. Harbin and group suggest that 0.6 to 0.65 be considered borderline whereas Giorgio and group cite 0.50 to 0.60 as borderline (both working at 100% specificity).[1, 2] A ratio of the product of three caudate dimensions to transverse right lobe dimension performs well at a cut-off of 5.4 cm², and quadrate transverse dimension alone performs about as well.[3, 4] The caudate lobe measurements can be made from ultrasound or CT scans, though the longitudinal caudate dimension would be less accurate at

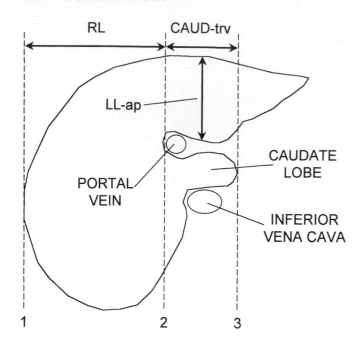

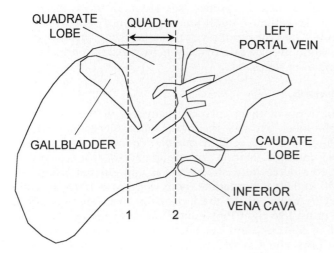

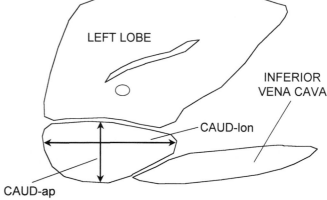

Figure 1 ▪ Measurements of caudate, right, and left lobes of the liver. Axial/transverse CT or ultrasound scan at the level of the bifurcation of the portal vein. The transverse dimension of the right lobe *(RL)* was measured between its lateral border *(line 1)* and the right wall of the portal vein *(line 2)*. The transverse dimension of the caudate lobe *(CAUD-trv)* was measured between the right wall of the portal vein *(line 2)* and the left border of the caudate lobe *(line 3)*. The anteroposterior dimension of the left lobe *(LL-ap)* was measured between lines 2 and 3.

Figure 2 ▪ Measurement of the caudate lobe. Longitudinal ultrasound scan through the caudate lobe through its maximal cephalocaudal extent. The anterior posterior *(CAUD-ap)* and longitudinal *(CAUD-lon)* dimensions were measured:
CAUD-product = CAUD-trv × CAUD-ap × CAUD-lon.

Figure 3 ▪ Measurement of the quadrate lobe. Oblique subcostal ultrasound scan through the gallbladder and left portal veins. The transverse dimension of the quadrate lobe *(QUAD-trv)* was measured between the left wall of the gallbladder *(line 1)* and the left wall of the ascending left portal vein where the vessel to the quadrate lobe originates *(line 2)*. If the gallbladder was absent, the main fissure was used.

Table 1 ▪ Measurements of the Caudate, Quadrate, and Right Lobes of the Liver

AUTHOR (NUMBERS) MEASUREMENT	NORMAL		CIRRHOSIS		ABNORMAL (NOT CIRRHOSIS)	
	Mean ± SD	Range	Mean ± SD	Range	Mean ± SD	Range
Harbin (25/25/15)						
CAUD-trv/RL	0.37 ± 0.16	0.0–0.59	0.83 ± 0.20	0.40–1.29	0.46 ± 0.48	0.20–0.59
LL-ap/RL	0.57 ± 0.20	0.0–1.20	0.81 ± 0.29	0.43–1.58		
Giorgio (25/103/53)						
CAUD-trv/RL	0.25 ± 0.05	0.15–0.32	0.62 ± 0.18	0.30–1.20	0.42 ± 0.15	0.18–0.50
Hess (58/75/0)						
CAUD-trv/RL	0.61 ± 0.25	0.3–1.8	0.31 ± 0.07	0.2–0.5		
CAUD-product/RL	16.7 ± 14.3	4.0–98.3	3.2 + 1.3	1.3–6.0		
CAUD-trv	4.7 ± 1.1	2.7–8.3	3.1 ± 0.6	1.8–4.4		
CAUD-ap	3.9 ± 1.2	1.7–8.3	2.2 ± 0.6	1.1–3.7		
CAUD-lon	6.2 ± 1.4	3.8–12.4	4.6 ± 0.6	3.0–6.0		
RL-trv	8.3 ± 1.8	3.5–12.5	10.3 ± 1.5	8.0–14.0		
Lafortune (125/167/0)						
QUAD-trv	4.3 ± 0.8		2.8 ± 0.9			

Numbers after authors indicate (normal/cirrhosis/abnormal). Measurements are in centimeters except CAUD-product/RL (square centimeters). Other ratios have no units. All other abbreviations as in Figures 1 through 3.

Table 2 ▪ Performance of Various Measurements/Ratios in Diagnosing Cirrhosis of the Liver

REFERENCE	MEASUREMENT	NO. +CIRRHOSIS	NO. −CIRRHOSIS	CRITERION FOR CIRRHOSIS	SENSITIVITY (%)	SPECIFICITY (%)
Harbin	CAUD-trv/RL	25	40	>0.65	84	100
Giorgio	CAUD-trv/RL	25	55	>0.60	54	100
Hess	CAUD-trv/RL	58	75	>0.43	73.3	95
	CAUD-product/RL	58	75	>5.4 sq cm	94.7	95
	CAUD-trv	58	75	>4.2 cm	67.2	95
	CAUD-ap	58	75	>3.2 cm	72.4	95
	CAUD-lon	58	75	>5.9 cm	55.2	95
	RL-trv	58	75	<8.3 cm	45.6	95
Lafortune	QUAD-trv	125	167	<3.0 cm	74	100

+Cirrhosis/−cirrhosis = with or without cirrhosis; other abbreviations as in Figures 1 through 3.

CT whereas the quadrate measurement can be done only from oblique U/S.

REFERENCES

1. Harbin WP, Robert NJ, Ferrucci JT: Diagnosis of cirrhosis based on regional changes in hepatic morphology. Radiology 1980; 135:273–283.
2. Giorgio A, Amoroso P, Lettieri G, et al: Cirrhosis: Value of caudate to right lobe ratio in diagnosis with US. Radiology 1986; 161:443–445.
3. Hess CF, Schmiedl U, Koelbel G, et al: Diagnosis of liver cirrhosis with US: Receiver-operating characteristic analysis of multidimensional caudate lobe indexes. Radiology 1989; 171:349–351.
4. Lafortune M, Matricardi L, Denys A, et al: Segment 4 (the quadrate lobe): A barometer of cirrhotic liver disease at US. Radiology 1998; 206:157–160.

▪: CT ATTENUATION VALUES OF LIVER
▪ ACR Code: 761 (Liver)

Technique ▪

Piekarski and colleagues performed CT of the abdomen with a CT/T-7800 machine (GE, Milwaukee, WI), with 4.8-sec scan time, 120 kVp, 200 mA, and no contrast.[1] Alpern and colleagues used a CT/T-9800 (GE) unit to scan the abdomen, with 10-mm-thick sections, 2.0-sec scan time, 140 kVp, and 120 mA. These were done without contrast and during administration of 50 gm of urographic contrast over 2 minutes. Dynamic technique (7.5 scans/minute) was used beginning 60 seconds after contrast.[2]

Jacobs and colleagues performed CT through the liver and spleen with a Hi Speed Advantage (GE) machine at 120 kVp and 280 to 320 mA. Three unenhanced scans at 7-mm slice thickness were initially made through the liver and spleen, followed by dynamic, spiral scans through the upper abdomen during injection of 150 ml of iodothalamate (Conray 60) at 2 ml/sec. Scans were begun either 80 or 90 seconds after the start of injection to allow evaluation of two time periods (80 to 100 and 101 to 120 sec) after injection.[3] Raptopolous used a CT/T 9800 (GE) scanner to perform single-level dual energy unenhanced scans

Table 1 ▪ Liver and Spleen Attenuation with Normal and Fatty Livers

SCAN PARAMETER	ATTENUATION VALUES (HU)	
	Normal Liver (n = 103)	Fatty Infiltration (n = 23)
Unenhanced		
Liver	55.2 ± 8.1	18.5 ± 21.8
Spleen	48.2 ± 74	46.0 ± 8.0
Liver-spleen	7.0 ± 5.8	−27.5 ± 19.3
Enhanced		
Liver	97.4 ± 16.4	45.4 ± 27.9
Spleen	109.4 ± 22.5	95.5 ± 14.6
Liver-spleen	−12.0 ± 11.7	−50.1 ± 26.0

Measurements given as mean ± standard deviation. HU = Hounsfield units.
From Alpern MB, Lawson TL, Foley WD, et al: Radiology 1986; 158:45–49.
Used by permission.

Table 2 ▪ Diagnostic Performance of CT Attenuation Values for Detecting Fatty Liver

PARAMETER	DISCRIMINATORY VALUE (HU)	SENSITIVITY (%)	SPECIFICITY (%)
Enhanced			
Liver-spleen	−30	79	94
Liver-spleen	−25	84	86
Liver-spleen	−20	87	75
Liver-spleen	−15	91	60
Unenhanced			
Liver-spleen	−10	84	99
Liver-spleen	−5	89	97
Liver-spleen	0	93	88
Unenhanced			
Liver	60	71	99
Liver	65	77	97
Liver	70	82	95
Liver	75	86	91
Liver	80	89	85

From Alpern MB, Lawson TL, Foley WD, et al: Radiology 1986; 158:45–49.
Used by permission.

through the midliver and spleen with 10-mm slice thickness at 140 kVp/120 mA and 80 kVp/170 mA.[4]

Measurements ▪

In all studies, CT attenuation values in HU were obtained from regions of interest (ROI) placed over the liver and spleen so as to avoid vessels, liver fissures, and the edges of the organs. The ROI sizes and number of samples obtained from each slice varied among studies. For the most part, values from two or more ROI (sometimes from multiple slices) were averaged to obtain representative measurements of the organ.[1–4] Raptopoulos and group placed one ROI over the biopsy site when possible. They also measured the aorta and adipose tissue as control substances.[4]

Piekarski and colleagues found an average liver attenuation of 24.8 HU (SD = 4.6, range 16.7 to 37.2), whereas that of the spleen was 21.1 HU (SD = 4.1, range 14.9 to 34.3). The average liver-spleen difference was 3.8 HU (SD = 2.1, range −0.04 to 9.7), and the difference was correlated with absolute liver attenuation (r = 0.33, p <.001).[1] Table 1 lists the attenuation values obtained by Alpern and group for normal and fatty livers at unenhanced and contrasted CT; Table 2 gives sensitivities and specificities of three parameters at various levels for diagnosis of fatty liver.[2] Table 3 shows test performance of various liver-spleen values from Jacobs' data.[3] Table 4 lists dual-energy CT attenuation values and differences for various tissues.[4]

Source ▪

Piekarski's subjects included 100 patients (gender and age not given) with no history or imaging findings to suggest liver or spleen abnormality.[1] Alpern and group studied a total of 185 patients, of whom 23 (gender and age not given) had fatty infiltration of the liver based on biopsy (n = 2), predisposing history, typical appearance, and clinical/imaging findings on follow-up.[2] Jacobs' subjects included 76 patients (46 men, 30 women, age range 18 to 85 years, mean age 55 years) without disease or condition that would affect the liver (other than possible fatty change) or spleen. Of these, 18 were found to have fatty change by unenhanced CT based on liver-spleen differences of >10 Hounsfield units.[3] Raptopoulos and associates studied 8 patients (5 men, 3 women, mean age 42 years) who had liver biopsy for hepatocellular disease, 6 (3 men, 3 women, mean age 56 years) who had liver biopsy of focal lesions,

Table 3 ▪ Diagnostic Performance of Enhanced CT Attenuation Values in Detecting Fatty Liver

80–100 SEC AFTER INJECTION			101–120 SEC AFTER INJECTION		
Discriminatory Value (HU)	Sensitivity (%)	Specificity (%)	Discriminatory Value (HU)	Sensitivity (%)	Specificity (%)
−68.5	17	99.9	−64.0	18	99.9
−48.5	40	99.3	−44.5	37	99.7
−35.0	62	97	−34.0	55	99.3
−28.0	74	94	−21.5	79	97
−20.5*	86*	87*	−18.5*	93*	93*
−16.5	96	69	−9.5	99.3	78
−13.0	98	59	−5.5	99.9	59
−5.5	99.5	37	−0.5	100	39
2.0	99.9	20	5.0	100	19

Asterisks indicate row chosen as having best discriminatory values by the investigators.
From Jacobs JE, Birnbaum BA, Shapiro MA, et al: AJR Am J Roentgenol 1998; 171:659–664. Used by permission.

Table 4 ▪ Dual-Energy CT Attenuation Values for Liver, Spleen, and Control Regions

| SUBSTANCE | NO. | MEAN ATTENUATION (HU) | | | |
		140 kVp	80 kVp	Difference	p VALUE
Normal liver	7	52.0	48.5	3.5	0.014
Spleen	18	40.5	38.5	2.0	0.005
Aorta	21	38.0	36.5	1.5	NS
Liver mass	6	34.5	32.0	2.5	0.081
Fatty liver + iron	3	49.3	49.0	0.3	NS
Fatty liver (% fat)	5	23.0	10.0	13.0	0.04
<25		47.5	41.0	6.5	—
25–50		33.5	22.0	11.5	—
25–50		41.0	30.0	11.0	—
50–75		− 8.5	− 22.5	14.0	—
<75		0.5	− 20.0	20.5	—
Adipose tissue	21	− 104.0	− 131.0	27.0	0.0001

NS = no significant difference, kVp = kilovolts; liver mass = 5 metastases, 1 hemangioma; + iron = iron deposition in combination with fatty liver on biopsy; % fat = as determined at liver biopsy

From Raptopoulos V, Karellas A, Bernstein J, et al: AJR Am J Roentgenol 1991; 157(4):721–725. Used by permission.

and 7 normal volunteers (4 men, 3 women, mean age 34 years). At least one of the scans of the patients having biopsies was done through the area sampled.[4]

Comments ▪

Piekarski's data show that the normal liver is slightly higher in attenuation than spleen.[1] Alpern and group found that fatty liver may be confidently diagnosed when the liver is 25 HU less than spleen on enhanced scans and 10 HU less than spleen on unenhanced scans.[2] Jacobs and associates showed that the postcontrast images made later into the injection discriminated fatty liver better than those made earlier. A liver-spleen attenuation difference of − 18.5 HU between 101 and 121 sec was the best cut-off value.[3] The

dual-energy data are promising in that the technique may be able to quantify the severity of fatty change.

REFERENCES

1. Piekarski J, Goldberg HI, Royal SA, Axel L, Moss AA: Difference between liver and spleen CT numbers in the normal adult: Its usefulness in predicting the presence of diffuse liver disease. Radiology 1980; 137:727–729.
2. Alpern MB, Lawson TL, Foley WD, et al: Focal hepatic masses and fatty infiltration detected by enhanced dynamic CT. Radiology 1986; 158:45–49.
3. Jacobs JE, Birnbaum BA, Shapiro MA, et al: Diagnostic criteria for fatty infiltration of the liver on contrast-enhanced helical CT. AJR Am J Roentgenol 1998; 171:659–664.
4. Raptopoulos V, Karellas A, Bernstein J, et al: Value of dual-energy CT in differentiating focal fatty infiltration of the liver from low-density masses. AJR Am J Roentgenol 1991; 157(4):721–725.

▪: RELAXATION TIMES OF THE NORMAL LIVER AT MRI
▪ ACR Code: 761 (Liver)

Technique ▪

The studies briefly abstracted here were done on various MRI units from 0.4 to 1.5 T, and there are numerous protocols for obtaining T1 and T2 relaxation times from liver parenchyma. Thomsen has reviewed the subject extensively.[1]

Measurements ▪

There have been attempts to standardize protocols and measurements for multicenter trials.[2–4] T1 and T2 relaxation times from normal liver obtained at 0.4 to 0.3 T (Table 1) and from 0.35 to 1.5 T (Table 2) are listed.[1, 5] Figure 1 is a plot of T1 and T2 relaxation times from all the series listed in the tables versus field strength. Linear regression of T1 and field strength yields the following equation:

$$T1/msec = 246 + 282 \times \text{field strength (T). (r = 0.79).}$$

Source ▪

The studies were done on healthy volunteers and/or patients who, for the most part, had no liver disease or were control subjects in studies of specific liver pathology.

Comments ▪

There is a wide variation in values for both T1 and T2, with T1 being strongly dependent on field strength. A considerable fraction of the remaining variation relates to differences in techniques used, with some superimposed biologic variation. Low field strength systems might be more useful for tissue characterization because of greater variation in T1 values of different tissues.[5]

Table 1 ▪ T1 and T2 of the Normal Liver at Low Field Strength

FIRST AUTHOR	JOURNAL	CITATION	FIELD (T)	T1/msec	T2/msec	NO.
Smith	Lancet	1981; 2:963–966	0.04	140–170	—	20
Runge	AJR	1983; 141:943–948	0.04	154±11	—	14
NMR Group	Clin Radiol	1987; 38:495–502	0.08	192±14	—	35
Richards	Br J Radiol	1988; 61:34–37	0.08	191±13	—	61
Keevil	Clin Radiol	1992; 45:302–306	0.08	213±14	66±5	42
de Certaines	Magn Res Imaging	1993; 11:841–850	0.08	227±13	68±4	—
Ebara	Radiology	1986; 159:371–377	0.10	230±21		12
de Certaines	Magn Res Imaging	1993; 11:841–850	0.10	222±21	59±3	—
Doyle	AJR	1982; 138:193–200	0.15	210–270	—	12
Bounocore	AJR	1983; 141:1171–1178	0.15	177±61	20±10	10
Leung	AJR	1984; 143:1215–1227	0.15	320–380	—	1
Brown	Magn Res Imaging	1985; 3:275–282	0.15	271±30	39±9	14
Flak	J Can Assoc Rad	1989; 40:135–138	0.15	237±39	54±11	19
Rupp	Eur J Radiol	1983; 3:68–76	0.20	380±20	40±20	>10
Rodl	RoFO	1985; 142:505–510	0.20	311±21	56±13	4
Ebara	Radiology	1986; 159:371–377	0.26	211±44	59±9	17
Fletcher	Radiology	1985; 155:699–703	0.30	317±47	37±10	8

Mean ± standard deviation or range is listed as reported.

Table 2 ▪ T1 and T2 Values in Normal Liver at Higher Field Strength

FIRST AUTHOR	JOURNAL	CITATION	FIELD (T)	T1/msec	T2/msec	NUMBER
Wesby	Soc Magn Res Med, Abstracts	1983; 373–374	0.35	—	49±15	11
Weinreb	AJR	1984; 143:1211–1214	0.35	505±172	54±11	13
Moss	Radiology	1984; 150:141–147	0.35	533±136	56±8	28
Ehman	AJR	1984; 143:1175–1182	0.35	267±51	—	5
Brash	Radiology	1984; 150:767–771	0.35	505	51	7
Ehman	JCAT	1985; 9:315–319	0.35	377±76	45±8	35/39
Glazer	Radiology	1985; 155:417–420	0.35	366±137	49±9	25
Heiken	Radiology	1985; 157:707–710	0.35	—	40±11	6
Nyman	Acta Radiol	1987; 28:527–533	0.35	442±67	51±5	14
Benson	Acta Radiol	1987; 28:13–15	0.35/0.50	425±53	54±3	12
Andersson	Acta Radiol	1988; 29:21–25	0.35/0.50	559±146	59±12	8
Nyman	Acta Radiol	1987; 28:527–533	0.50	651±117	42±4	7
Kinami	Gastroenterol Japonica	1988; 23:139–146	0.50	474±93	53±9	17
Bernardino	Magn Res Imaging	1989; 7:363–367	0.50	—	56±9	23
Andersson	Br J Radiol	1989; 62:433–437	0.50	488±30	51±3	8
de Certaines	Magn Res Imaging	1993; 11:841–850	0.50	358±18	67±4	—
Hardy	Magn Res Imaging	1985; 3:107–116	1.5	498±32	—	1?
Foley	AJR	1987; 149:1155–1160	1.5	800±450	34±8	31
Thomsen	Magn Res Imaging	1988; 6:431–436	1.5	445–920	42–65	4
Bernardino	Magn Res Imaging	1989; 7:363–367	1.5	—	44±10	23
Van Lorn	Magn Res Imaging	1991; 9:165–171	1.5	568±9	56±11	14
Bluml	Magn Res Imaging	1993; 30:289–295	1.5	570±43	—	11

Mean ± standard deviation or range is listed as reported.

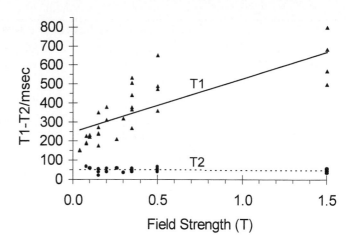

Figure 1 ▪ T1 and T2 values of normal liver versus field strength. T1 *(triangles)* is strongly dependent on field strength whereas T2 *(circles)* is constant. Linear regression lines *(T1 = solid, T2 = dotted)* are shown. T = tesla.

REFERENCES

1. Thomsen C: Quantitative magnetic resonance methods for in vivo investigation of the human liver and spleen. Technical aspects and preliminary clinical results. Acta Radiol (Suppl)1996; 401:1–34.
2. Lerski RA, McRobbie DW, Straughan K, et al: Multi-center trial with protocols and prototype test objects for the assessment of MRI equipment. Magn Reson Imaging 1988; 6:201–214.
3. Lerski RA, de Certaines JD: Performance assessment and quality control in MRI by eurospin test objects and protocols. Magn Reson Imaging 1993; 11:817–833.
4. Podo F: Tissue characterization by MRI. A multidisciplinary and multi-centre challenge today. Magn Reson Imaging 1988; 6:173–174.
5. Keevil SF, Dolke G, Brooks AP, et al: Proton NMR relaxation times in the normal human liver at 0.08 T. Clin Radiol 1992; 45(5):302–306.

▪: LIVER IRON CONCENTRATION DETERMINED BY MRI
▪ ACR Code: 761 (Liver)

Technique ▪

Three of the studies described herein were done with 0.5-T MR-max machines (General Electric, Milwaukee, WI) to perform imaging of the liver and upper abdomen.[1-3] Gandon and colleagues used multiple sequences, including spin-echo T1 and T2, inversion recovery for relaxation time determination, and several gradient echo (GRE) sequences done during breath holding.[1] Ernst performed two GRE sequences weighted for T1 and T2* during quiet breathing, with an abdominal belt to reduce motion.[2] Papakonstantinou and colleagues used a multislice double-echo technique (2500/12,80) for proton density (PD) and T2 weighting and a single-slice multiple echo scan (2500/12, X20 echoes) for calculation of T2 relaxation time.[3] Bonkovsky used a 1.5 T Signa scanner (General Electric, Milwau-

kee, WI) to perform spin echo T1- and T2-weighted sequences, as well as six different GRE sequences.[4] Relevant slice parameters are shown in Tables 1 and 2.

Measurements ▪

Gandon and colleagues placed regions of interest (ROI) of greater than 50 pixels over the right lobe of the liver (near a typical biopsy site), paraspinous muscle, fat, and the air outside the patient (noise). Signal intensity (SI) was measured in each ROI, and T2 relaxation time was calculated for the liver ROI from the inversion recovery data set.[1] Ernst and colleagues placed ROI (about 30 pixels) over the right lobe of the liver and paraspinous muscles for SI measurement.[2] Papakonstantinou and colleagues placed ROI (157 pixels) over liver, muscle, and fat for SI measure-

Table 1 ▪ Quantification of Liver Iron Concentration with MRI

AUTHOR/SEQUENCE	PARAMETERS (TR/TE/Flip)	USABLE RANGE OF LIC (µmol/gm)	EQUATION FOR LIC (µmol/gm)	CORRELATION COEFFICIENT (r)
Ernst[2]				
GRE T1	400/12/90°	<100	351 − 195(SI liver/SI muscle)	−0.67
GRE T2*	700/30/30°	100–300	104 − 60(SI liver/SI muscle)	−0.71
Gandon[1]				
GRE short TE	120/14/90°	150–300	277 − 248(SI liver/SI fat)	−0.66
GRE long TE	120/30/20°	<150	141 − 95(SI liver/SI fat)	−0.87
Bonkovsky[4]				
GRE (best)	18/5/10°	<180	356 − 89 × ln(SI liver/SD air)	−0.94
		180–350 Less Precise		

LIC = liver iron concentration, µmol/gm = micromole per gram, SI = signal intensity, SD = standard deviation, ln = natural logarithm. MR sequence and relaxation time abbreviations are standard.[1, 2, 4]

Table 2 ▪ Relationship Between Liver MRI Parameters and Histologic Grade of Siderosis

PARAMETER/ SEQUENCE USED	CONTROLS (n = 11)	GRADE 1 (n = 8)	GRADE 2 (n = 5)	GRADE 3 (n = 10)	GRADE 4 (n = 8)
Calculated T2 (ms)					
Multi 2500/12 (×20)	45.5±2.5	36.9±5.4	26.6±1.5	22.9±3.6	15.6±2.7
Liver/muscle SIR					
SE 2500/12 (PD)	1.31±0.22	1.2±0.16	0.98±0.2	0.66±0.2	0.45±0.25
SE 2500/80 (T2)	1.35±0.41	1.1±0.2	0.73±0.3	0.58±0.2	0.42±0.3
Liver/fat SIR					
SE 2500/12 (PD)	0.82±0.32	0.67±0.09	0.65±0.3	0.43±0.13	0.31±0.17
SE 2500/80 (T2)	0.45±0.53	0.49±0.32	0.48±0.2	0.26±0.15	0.07±0.02

All measurements are given as mean ± standard deviation. SIR = signal intensity ratio. MR sequence and relaxation time abbreviations are standard.
From Papakonstantinou OG, Maris TG, Kostaridou V, et al: Magn Reson Imaging 1995; 13:967–977. Used by permission.

ment. T2 relaxation time was calculated from liver using the multiple echo sequence.[3] Liver signal intensity ratios (SIR) were formed by dividing liver SI by that in muscle (L/M) or fat (L/F).[1–3] Bonkovsky measured SI from five ROI (50 pixels) from within the liver and from the surrounding air, and these were averaged and a ratio calculated by dividing the SI in the liver by the standard deviation (SD) of the surrounding air, and took the natural logarithm.[4]

Gandon and Ernst and their colleagues correlated SIR on the various MRI sequences with liver iron concentration (LIC) obtained from core biopsy specimens from the right lobe of the liver.[1, 2] Gandon and group also correlated T2 with LIC.[1] Papakonstantinou and colleagues correlated SIR and calculated T2 with a four-step histologic grade (Grade 1 = minimal through Grade 4 = heavy) for hemosiderosis[4, 5] applied to liver biopsy specimens.[3] Bonkovsky correlated their ln(SI liver/SD air) with LIC obtained from core biopsy of the right lobe of the liver.[4]

Figure 1 is a scatterplot from Gandon and group, showing LIC versus L/F SIR obtained from the GRE technique (120/30/20 degrees) found to work best for lower LIC concentrations. Figures 2 and 3 are scatterplots from Ernst and colleagues, showing LIC versus L/M SIR from both sequences used in their study.[2] Table 1 lists both of the sequences used by Ernst and associates, the two best GRE sequences as determined by Gandon and associates, and the best GRE sequence found by Bonkovsky, along with equations for calculating LIC from SIR measurements.[1, 2] Table 2 lists correlation between T2 relaxation times in the liver, as well as SIR measurements and histologic siderosis grades.[3] Figure 4 is a scatterplot of the LIC versus ln(SI liver/SD air) as determined by Bonkovksy.[4]

Source ▪

Gandon and colleagues evaluated 77 patients (56 men, 21 women, mean age 51 years) who underwent liver biopsy because of suspected iron overload. Of these, 67 did have iron overload by histologic examination (LIC >36 μmol/gm).[1] Ernst and associates studied 58 patients (46 men, 12 women, mean age 46 years) who had liver biopsy for suspected iron overload. Of these, 49 had LIC >36 μmol/gm.[2] Papakonstantinou's subjects included 40 patients with beta-major thalassemia (age range 13 to 35 years, mean age 21 years) and 11 healthy controls. Of the 40 thalassemic

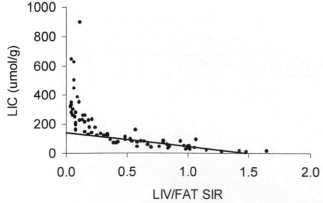

Figure 1 ▪ Plot of liver iron concentration (LIC) versus liver to fat (L/F) signal intensity ratio (SIR) from gradient echo (120/30/20 degrees) sequences. The regression line, LIC = 141 − (95 × L/F), is shown. (From Gandon Y, Guyader D, Heautot JF, et al: Radiology 1994; 193(2):533–538. Used by permission.)

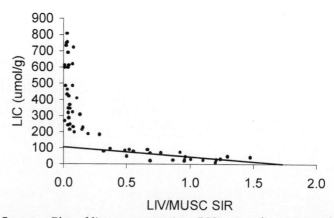

Figure 2 ▪ Plot of liver concentration (LIC) versus liver to muscle (L/M) signal intensity ratio (SIR) from gradient echo (700/30/30 degrees) sequences. The regression line, LIC = 104 − (60 × L/M), is shown. (From Ernst O, Sergent G, Bonvariet P, et al: AJR Am J Roentgenol 1997; 168:1205–1208. Used by permission.)

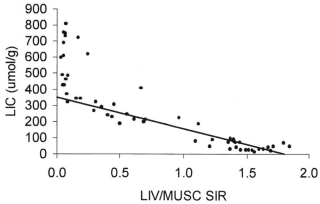

Figure 3 ▪ Plot of liver iron concentration *(LIC)* versus liver to muscle *(L/M)* signal intensity ratio *(SIR)* from gradient echo (400/12/90 degrees) sequences. The regression line, LIC = 351 − (195 × L/M), is shown. (From Ernst O, Sergent G, Bonvariet P, et al: AJR Am J Roentgenol 1997; 168:1205–1208. Used by permission.)

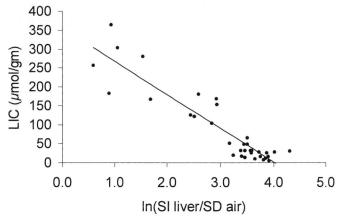

Figure 4 ▪ Scatterplot of liver iron concentration (LIC) versus the natural log of liver signal intensity over standard deviation of signal intensity from the surrounding air from gradient echo (18/5/10 degrees) sequences. The regression line, 356 − (89 × ln[SI liver/SD air]), is shown. (From Bonkovsky HL, Rubin RB, Cable EE, et al: Radiology 1999; 212:227–234. Used by permission.)

patients, 31 had liver biopsy.[3] Bonkovsky evaluated 38 patients (30 men, 8 women, median age 44 years, age range 28 to 68 years) who had various causes of possible iron overload within 1 month of liver biopsy.[4]

Comments ▪

There is some disagreement about whether T2 relaxation times or SIR determinations are more accurate to quantify LIC, with Gandon and group finding SIR to be superior and Papakonstantinou and colleagues finding better correlation between LIC and calculated T2.[1, 3] There have been several studies by others of either SIR[7–9] or calculated T2[10–14] to quantify LIC. Using SIR measurements may be somewhat easier to perform than calculating T2 relaxation times. The various methods seem to have adequate performance in detecting and quantifying mild-moderate overload.[1, 2, 4] Using a threshold of L/F SIR of 1.0 on GRE (120/30/20 degrees) sequences, Gandon and group found sensitivity 94% and specificity 90% for LIC >36 μmol/gm.[1] Similarly, Ernst and associates used an L/M SIR threshold of 0.8 on GRE (700/30/30 degrees) sequences and found sensitivity 91% and specificity 88% for LIC >36 μmol/gm.[2] Ernst and group found that the estimated LIC by MRI (formulas in Table 1) was accurate to within 22% when compared with histologically determined LIC.[2] Using SI measurements to calculate LIC >200 μmol/gm became more prone to error because measurements of SI give lower numbers, though variability remained constant, yielding increased coefficients of variation. For example, Bonkovsky found that the coefficients of variation ranged from 8% to 13% below 180 μmol/gm and 13% to 20% above.[4] Most investigators agree that accurate quantification of LIC >300 μmol/gm by MRI (either calculated T2 or SIR measurements) is not possible, though probably not clinically relevant.

To convert between μmol/gm and mg/gm, the following equations may be used:

$$mg/gm = 0.0557 \ \mu mol/gm.$$
$$\mu mol/gm = 17.96 \ mg/gm.$$

REFERENCES

1. Gandon Y, Guyader D, Heautot JF, et al: Hemochromatosis: Diagnosis and quantification of liver iron with gradient-echo MR imaging. Radiology 1994; 193(2):533–538.
2. Ernst O, Sergent G, Bonvariet P, et al: Hepatic iron overload: Diagnosis and quantification with MR imaging. AJR Am J Roentgenol 1997; 168:1205–1208.
3. Papakonstantinou OG, Maris TG, Kostaridou V, et al: Assessment of liver iron overload by T2-quantitative magnetic resonance imaging: Correlation of T2-QMRI measurements with serum ferritin concentration and histologic grading of siderosis. Magn Reson Imaging 1995; 13:967–977.
4. Bonkovsky HL, Rubin RB, Cable EE, et al: Hepatic iron concentration: Noninvasive estimation by means of MR imaging techniques. Radiology 1999; 212:227–234.
5. Rowe JW, Wands JR, Mesey G, et al: Familial hemochromatosis: Characteristics of the precirrhotic stage in a large kindred. Medicine 1977; 56:197–211.
6. Searle JW, Kerr FR, Halliday JW, Powell LW: Iron storage disease. In MacSween RM, Schuer P (eds): Pathology of the Liver. Churchill Livingstone, London, 1987, pp. 181–201.
7. Hernandez RJ, Sarnaik SA, Lande I, et al: MR evaluation of liver iron overload. J Comput Assist Tomogr 1988; 12:91–94.
8. Bonkovsky HL, Slaker DB, Bills EB, Wolf DC: Usefulness and limitations of laboratory and hepatic imaging studies in iron-storage disease. Gastroenterology 1990; 99:1079–1091.
9. Guyander D, Gandon Y, Robert JY, et al: Magnetic resonance imaging and assessment of liver iron content in genetic hemochromatosis. J Hepatol 1992; 15:304–308.
10. Chezmar JL, Nelson RC, Malko JA, Bernardino ME: Hepatic iron overload: Diagnosis and quantification by noninvasive imaging. Gastrointest Radiol 1990; 15:27–31.
11. Kaltwasser JP, Gottschalk R, Schalk KP, Hartl W: Non-invasive quantitation of liver iron-overload by magnetic resonance imaging. Br J Haematol 1990; 74:360–363.
12. Gomori JM, Horev G, Tamary H, et al: Hepatic iron overload: Quantitative MR imaging. Radiology 1991; 179:367–369.
13. Villari N, Caramella D, Lippi A, Guazelli C: Assessment of liver iron overload in thalassemic patients by MR imaging. Acta Radiol 1992; 4:347–350.
14. Rocchi E, Cassanelli M, Borghi A, et al: Magnetic resonance imaging and different levels of iron overload in chronic liver disease. Hepatology 1993; 17:997–1002.

▪: MEASUREMENT OF NEONATAL GALLBLADDER BY REAL-TIME ULTRASOUND[1]

▪ ACR Code: 762 (Gallbladder)

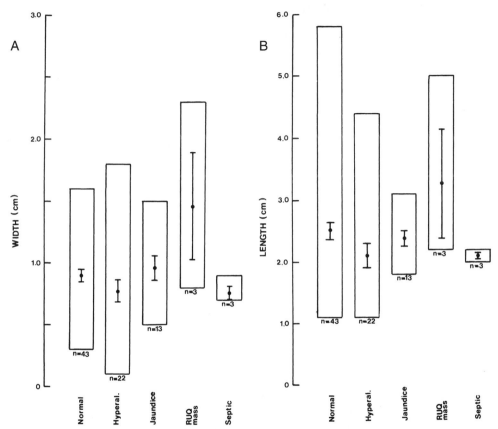

Figure 1 ▪ Graphs display the range of neonatal gallbladder measurements and the mean ± SEM. *A*, Width; *B*, length. (From Carroll BA, et al: Radiology 1982; 145:437. Used by permission.)

Table 1 ▪ Infant Ages	
AGE (WK GESTATION OR POSTPARTUM)	NO. OF INFANTS
25–29	6
30–34	25
35–39	16
40–42	23
1–2 wk	8
3 wk–3 mon	7
TOTAL	85

From Carroll BA, et al: Radiology 1982; 145:437–440. Used by permission.

Table 2 ▪ Sludge in Infant Gallbladders*		
MEDICAL STATUS OF NEONATE		NO. OF NEONATES INVOLVED
Hyperalimented	(HA)	6
HA only	(2)	
HA + jaundice	(2)	
HA + sepsis	(1)	
HA + sepsis + jaundiced	(1)*	
Jaundiced only		1
Prior history of HA, sepsis, and jaundice. Now clinically normal at discharge		1
Never HA, no sepsis or jaundice		4
Congenital heart disease	(1)	
Meconium aspiration	(2)	
Severe hypotension	(1)	
TOTAL		12 (14%)

*Sludge persisted after hyperalimentation ceased and jaundice and sepsis resolved.

From Carroll BA, et al: Radiology 1982; 145:437. Used by permission.

Technique ▪

1. A 6.0- or 7.5-MHz transducer and a mechanical sector real-time scanner were used and images recorded on Polaroid or multiformat transparencies.
2. Scans were in the transverse and sagittal projections and in the supine and left lateral decubitus positions.
3. Subjects were scanned immediately prior to next feeding or fasting state.

Measurements ▪ (Figure 1; Tables 1 and 2)

Measurements were made from prints or film and corrected for magnification.

Source ▪

Eighty-five neonates were studied, 29 female and 56 males; 43 were normal and nonjaundiced; 42 had potential biliary tract abnormalities, including 22 on hyperalimentation, 14 with jaundice, 3 with right upper quadrant masses, and 3 with sepsis only.

REFERENCE

1. Carroll BA, Oppenheimer DA, Muller HH: High-frequency real-time ultrasound of the neonatal biliary system. Radiology 1982; 145:437–440.

▪: MEASUREMENT OF NORMAL AND ABNORMAL GALLBLADDER WALL THICKNESS BY ULTRASOUND[1]
▪ ACR Code: 762 (Gallbladder)

Technique ▪

1. All subjects were studied with an electronic sector scanner (Varian 3000) using a 2.25-MHz fixed focus transducer. Additional views optionally taken with a manual sector scanner (Searle Phosonic).
2. Standard viewing is via an intercostal transhepatic portal, but additional decubitus or upright views were used.

Measurements ▪ (Figure 1 and Table 1)

The gallbladder wall is measured between the fluid-filled lumen and the nearer subhepatic wall, with the ultrasound beam perpendicular to the wall. Measurements are rounded to the nearest millimeter as measured on the prints or transparencies.

Wall thickness greater than 2 mm was seen in only 3.5% of 368 patients with otherwise normal scans.

Wall thickness was greater than 2 mm in 21 of 40 pathologically confirmed cholecystitis cases and 47 of 103 sonographically diagnosed cases of cholelithiasis.

Raghavendra and colleagues showed that 70% of patients with acute cholecystitis had gallbladder wall measurements of 5 mm or greater, gallbladder wall anechoicity, a gallbladder AP diameter of 4 cm or greater (external width), and cholelithiasis.[2]

Other causes of increased thickness of the gallbladder wall measurements include ascites, hypoalbuminemia, hepatitis, heart failure, renal disease, and multiple myeloma.

Source ▪

The data of Finberg and Birnholz are based on 47 surgical patients.

Raghavendra's data are based on 30 patients without biliary tract symptoms and 24 patients with proved acute cholecystitis.

Lewandowski and Winsberg's data are based on 8 pa-

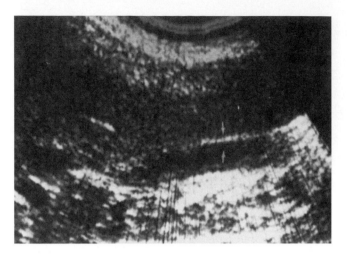

Figure 1 ▪ Measurement of the gallbladder wall *(arrows)* made along the axis of the ultrasound beam using the portion of the gallbladder contiguous with the liver and including all identifiable layers. Note the distinguishable, less echodense zone adjacent to the lumen. (From Finberg HJ, et al: Radiology 1979; 133:693. Used by permission.)

Table 1 ▪ Pathologic Findings in 40 Patients: Type of Cholecystitis

ULTRASOUND WALL (mm)	CHRONIC	CHRONIC ACTIVE	CHRONIC AND ACUTE	SUBACUTE	ACUTE
1–2*	15	1	3	0	0
3	3	0	0	0	1
4	6	1	1	1	0
≥5	3	0	4	0	1

*1–2 different from ≥5 at $p < .05$.
From Finberg HJ, et al: Radiology 1979; 133:693–698. Used by permission.

tients with ascites. Ralls' data are based on 40 patients with hypoalbuminemia.

The data of Shlaer and colleagues are based on a study of 20 patients with thickened gallbladder walls. Only eight had cholecystitis.

REFERENCES

1. Finberg HJ, Birnholz JC: Ultrasound evaluation of the gallbladder wall. Radiology 1979; 133:693–698.

2. Raghavendra BN, Feiner HD, Subramanyam BR, et al: Acute cholecystitis; Sonographic-pathologic analysis. AJR Am J Roentgenol 1981; 137:327–332.
3. Lewandowski BJ, Winsberg F: Gallbladder wall thickness distortion by ascites. AJR Am J Roentgenol 1981; 137:519–521.
4. Ralls PW, Quinn MF, Juttner HU, et al: Gallbladder wall thickening; Patients without intrinsic gallbladder disease. AJR Am J Roentgenol 1981; 137:65–68.
5. Shlaer WJ, Leopold GR, Scheible FW: Sonography of the thickened gallbladder wall; A nonspecific finding. AJR Am J Roentgenol 1981; 136:337–339.

▪: METHODS OF GALLBLADDER VOLUME MEASUREMENT
▪ ACR Code: 762 (Gallbladder)

Technique ▪

Several models of commercially available ultrasound scanners with 3.5- to 7.0-MHz real-time sector or curved array transducers were used in the studies described here.[1–4] Pauletzki and colleagues used an EchoScan 3D reconstruction system (TomTec Imaging, Unterschleissheim, Germany), which consists of a stepping motor and a special sledge to hold and translate the transducer.[3] A balloon or condom filled with water and suspended in a water bath was used in three in vitro studies.[1–3] Two studies also utilized an excised gallbladder suspended in a water bath.[1–2] Various known volumes of water were instilled into the phantoms and they were scanned for volume measurements.

Measurements ▪

There are basically two commonly available methods for measuring gallbladder volume. The sum of cylinders (SOC) is performed using a longitudinal scan through the long axis of the gallbladder, with a correction factor for off-axis scanning calculated from a transverse image through the midportion; this is shown in Figure 1.[5] The SOC method is time consuming to do by hand, and a computed method has been developed that is contained in the measurement software package of many modern ultrasound units.[6] The ellipsoid (ELIP) method also uses longitudinal and transverse images and is simply the product of three axis measurements multiplied by a constant.[1] This is shown in Figure 2. Anderson's modification of the SOC method (SOC-MOD) involves calculating the SOC without correction from two roughly perpendicular (parasagittal/coronal) longitudinal images and averaging the derived volumes.[2] Pauletzki's 3D method produces a series of parallel transverse images, and this data set was transferred to a 3D workstation where prototype software was used to calculate

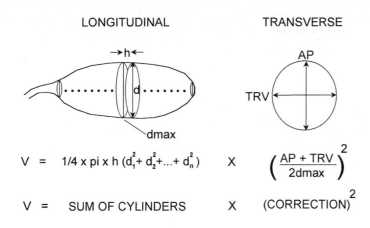

LONGITUDINAL   TRANSVERSE

$$V = 1/4 \times pi \times h\,(d_1^2 + d_2^2 + \ldots + d_n^2) \quad X \quad \left(\frac{AP + TRV}{2dmax}\right)^2$$

$$V = \text{SUM OF CYLINDERS} \quad X \quad (\text{CORRECTION})^2$$

$$1/4 \times pi = 0.785$$

Figure 1 ▪ The sum of cylinders method of gallbladder volume measurement. The anteroposterior diameter *(d)* is measured at interval *(h)* from the cystic duct insertion to the gallbladder tip on a longitudinal image through its middle. The diameters are squared, summed, and multiplied by *h* and a constant as shown. The correction factor compensates for off-axis error in the longitudinal scan. It combines anteroposterior diameter *(AP)* and width *(TRV)* measured from a transverse image combined with the maximum diameter *(dmax)* from the longitudinal image, as shown.

the volume.[3] Hurrell's study was designed to assess variability of the SOC method and was not validated against known volumes.[4]

Figure 3 shows measured versus actual volumes from Dodds' balloon study for SOC and ELIP methods. Figure 4 shows percent errors versus volumes for the two methods as calculated by us from Figure 3. These are fairly typical representations of such experiments. Note that the percent errors are rather high for low volumes, though the absolute magnitudes of error are actually greater at larger volumes. Table 1 lists the results from the cited studies in tabular form.

Source ▪

Anderson and colleagues measured gallbladder volumes in 11 patients prior to percutaneous cholecystostomy and correlated them with aspirated bile volume.[2] Hurrell and asso-

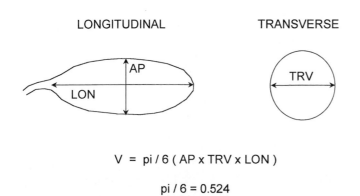

LONGITUDINAL   TRANSVERSE

$$V = pi / 6\,(AP \times TRV \times LON)$$

$$pi / 6 = 0.524$$

Figure 2 ▪ Ellipsoid method of gallbladder volume measurement. The product of longitudinal *(LON)*, anteroposterior *(AP)*, and transverse *(TRV)* dimensions is multiplied by a constant as shown.

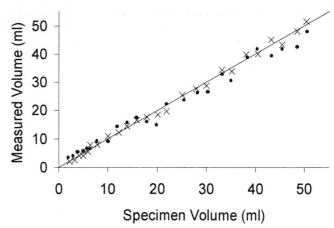

Figure 3 ▪ In vitro measurement of excised gallbladder volumes with sum of cylinders *(dots)* and ellipsoid *(crosses)* ultrasound methods. The line depicts unity between measured and actual volumes. (From Dodds WJ, Groh WJ, Darweesh RM, et al: AJR Am J Roentgenol 1985; 145:1009–1011. Used by permission.)

ciates evaluated 17 patients (age range 30 to 69 years, mean age 54 years) before and after intravenous cholecystokinin and Lundh meal to stimulate gallbladder contraction. This was done on two separate occasions for each patient, providing a total of 136 separate examinations. During each examination the gallbladder was scanned for volume measurements with the patient in the decubitus and left posterior oblique (LPO) positions.[4]

Comments ▪

Volume measurement is vital in studying the kinetics of gallbladder contraction and to determine ejection fraction. Therefore, a method that is accurate, precise, reproducible, and easy to perform has been sought. Dodds and colleagues concluded that the difference in measured volumes between SOC and ELIP methods was negligible.[1] Wedmann and associates performed similar in vivo and in vitro experiments testing the SOC and ELIP methods, and the results agreed with Dodds'. Wedmann and group also evaluated

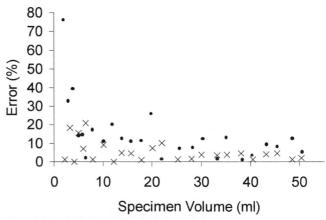

Figure 4 ▪ Percentage errors (absolute values) of in vitro measurement of excised gallbladder volumes with sum of cylinders *(dots)* and ellipsoid *(crosses)* ultrasound methods. (From Dodds WJ, Groh WJ, Darweesh RM, et al: AJR Am J Roentgenol 1985; 145:1009–1011. Used by permission.)

Table 1 ▪ Performance of Ultrasound Measurement Methods of Gallbladder Volume

REFERENCE	METHOD	TEST MODEL	AVERAGE ERROR, MEAN ± SD OR MEAN (RANGE) (ml)	(%)	COMMENTS
Dodds[1]	SOC	Excised GB	2.1 ± 1.6	14.8 ± 15.7	
	ELIP	Excised GB	0.8 ± 0.7	5.3 ± 5.6	
Anderson[2]	SOC	Balloon	0.6 ± 4.2	8–10	Underestimate small, overestimate large
	SOC	Excised GB	3.7 ± 3.2		Overestimate
	SOC (modified)	Balloon	0.3 ± 1.7	2–3	Underestimate small, overestimate large
	SOC (modified)	Excised GB	4.3 ± 1.2		Overestimate
	SOC (modified)	In vivo (perc drain)	1.5 ± 10.4		
Pauletzki[3]	3D	Balloon (condom)	0.7 (−4.0–2.6)	1.9	Underestimate
	SOC	″	1.4 (−4.7–7.5)	4.2	Overestimate
	ELIP	″	4.3 (−8.4–16.9)	12.5	Overestimate
Hurrell[4]	SOC	In vivo	—	—	Variation between supine and LPO measurements = 20.66%

SD = standard deviation, SOC = sum of cylinders, ELIP = ellipsoid method, SOC-MOD = modified sum of cylinders, 3D = 3 dimensional, perc drain = percutaneous gallbladder drainage, GB = gallbladder.

other methods (transverse planimetry, longitudinal planimetry, and width) and found them to be unsatisfactory.[7] Stolk and colleagues found that the SOC method was superior to ELIP and area-length methods in vivo.[8] Hurrell's finding of an average 21% variation of measured volumes between supine and LPO positions in the same patient illustrates an additional significant source of error.[4]

REFERENCES

1. Dodds WJ, Groh WJ, Darweesh RM, et al: Sonographic measurement of gallbladder volume. AJR Am J Roentgenol 1985; 145:1009–1011.
2. Anderson I, Monrad H, Gronvall S, Hojgaard L: In vitro and in vivo accuracy of sonographic gallbladder volume determinations. J Clin Ultrasound 1993; 21:157–162.
3. Pauletzki J, Sackmann M, Holl J, Paumgartner G: Evaluation of gallbladder volume and emptying with a novel three-dimentional ultrasound system: Comparison with the sum-of-cylinders and the ellipsoid methods. J Clin Ultrasound 1996; 24:277–285.
4. Hurrell MA, Chapman BA, Wilson IR: Variation in the estimation of gallbladder volume using the sum-of-cylinders method. Invest Radiol 1994; 29:536–539.
5. Everson GT, Braverman DZ, Johnson ML, et al: A critical evaluation of real-time ultrasonography for the study of gallbladder volume and contraction. Gastroenterology 1980; 79:40–46.
6. Hopman WPM, Brouwer WFM, Rosenbusch G, et al: A computerized method for rapid quantification of gallbladder volume from real-time sonograms. Radiology 1985; 154:236–237.
7. Wedmann B, Schmidt G, Wegener M, et al: Sonographic evaluation of gallbladder kinetics: In vitro and in vivo comparison of different methods to assess gallbladder emptying. J Clin Ultrasound 1991; 19:341–349.
8. Stolk MF, Van Erpecum KJ, Van Berge Henegouwen GP, et al: Gallbladder volume and contraction measured by sum-of-cylinders method compared to ellipsoid and area-length methods. Acta Radiol 1990; 31:591–596.

▪: GALLBLADDER EMPTYING STUDIED WITH ULTRASOUND
▪ ACR Code: 762 (Gallbladder)

Technique ▪

Strict overnight fasting (including water and cigarettes) was usually done before testing. Real-time ultrasound was performed to evaluate fasting gallbladder volume (FV) and morphology. Intravenous contraction stimuli consisted of cholecystokinin (CCK, Kabi) or cholecystokinin-octapeptide (sincalide, Squibb or Bracco) diluted in saline. Oral stimulus preparations usually contained a mixture of protein, fat, and carbohydrate in various proportions and were in liquid form, as powder reconstituted with water, or in the form of a candy bar. After the stimulus was administered, continuous or intermittent ultrasound of the gallbladder was done for from 30 to 90 minutes. Gallbladder volumes were measured at various intervals during the poststimulus period. The minimal volume (MV) and the time to reach MV, sometimes called ejection time (ET), were recorded.

Measurements ▪

Study details are listed in Table 1, including stimulus material, dosage of CCK/sincalide, form of oral material, observation interval after stimulus (study time), and method of gallbladder volume determination. The measurement of gallbladder volume was done with either the ellipsoid or the sum of cylinders methods (covered in the previous section). Table 2 lists the FV, ejection fraction (EF = [FV − MV]/FV × 100), and ET for each study (grouped by type of stimulus).

Source ▪

The studies abstracted here were done to test the method using healthy volunteers[1,2] or were normal control subjects in studies of acalculous symptomatic patients,[3,4] patients

Table 1 ▪ Details of Sonographic Studies of Gallbladder Emptying

REFERENCE	STIMULUS MATERIAL	DOSE/FORM	GB VOLUME METHOD	STUDY TIME (min)	AGES (Yr)	MALE/FEMALE	NO. OF SUBJECTS
Barr[3]	Sincalide	0.12 µg/kg over 30 min	Ellipsoid	60	16–69	24/36	60
Davis[4]	Sincalide	20 ng/kg over 3 min	Ellipsoid	30	Adults	—	10
Hopman[1]	CCK	1 U/kg over 1 min	Sum of cylinders	75	22–31	4/2	6
Donald[2]	Neocholex	Liquid meal	Ellipsoid	60	22–65	15/15	30
Hopman[1]	Biloptin	Liquid meal	Sum of cylinders	75	22–31	4/2	6
Kishk[5]	Lipomul	Liquid meal	Ellipsoid	60	24–66	11/9	20
Pauletzki[6]	Specified as "standard"	Liquid meal	Sum of cylinders	90	Mean = 41	8/11	19
Hopman[1]	Sorbitract	Chocolate bar	Sum of cylinders	75	22–31	4/2	6
Nino-Murcia[7]	Commercially available	Chocolate bar	Ellipsoid	60	24–71	—	28

GB = gallbladder, CCK = cholecystokinin, µg = micrograms, ng = nanograms, kg = kilograms, U = Ivy Dog Unit, min = minutes.

Table 2 ▪ Gallbladder Emptying in Normal Adults as Studied by Ultrasound

REFERENCE	STIMULUS	FASTING VOLUME (ml)	EJECTION FRACTION (%)	EJECTION TIME (min)	COMMENTS
Barr[3]	Sincalide, 30 min	23.0	80.7 ± 16.1*	30	Suggested >60% = normal, 50–59% = borderline, <50% = abnormal
Davis[4]	Sincalide, 3 min		61 ± 28* (15–75)	10	High correlation with nuclear medicine but large intersubject variability with both methods
Hopman[1]	CCK, 1 min	25.0 ± 4.5	48 ± 10	20	Sincalide offers no advantage over solid or liquid fatty meal
Donald[2]	Liquid meal	19 ± 9* (1.9–46)	69 ± 19* (−10–99)	45	Large intrasubject day-to-day variations: (FV = 1.5–26.2 ml, EF = 6–87%)
Hopman[1]	Liquid meal	27.0 ± 4.9	62 ± 7	25	
Kishk[5]	Liquid meal	28 ± 12 (11–51)	67 ± 3 (47–91)	45–60	Separate group with gallstones: (FV = 56 ± 10 ml, EF = 36 ± 4%, ET = 60 min)
Pauletzki[6]	Liquid meal	15.3 ± 1.2	70 ± 8.7	30	Separate group with gallstones: (FV = 23.6 ± 1.5 ml, EF = 62 ± 9.0%, ET = 60 min)
Hopman[1]	Chocolate bar	26 ± 4.2	55 ± 6	40	
Nino-Murcia[7]	Chocolate bar	28 ± 2.3	62 + 2.1	48 ± 2.6	Separate group with spinal cord injury: (FV = 21 ± 1.4 ml, EF = 49 ± 3.6%, ET = 43 ± 2.9 min)

Measurements are given as mean ± standard error, mean ± standard deviation (asterisk), and ranges where available (in parentheses). CCK = cholecystokinin, ml = milliliters, min = minutes, FV = fasting volume, EF = ejection fraction, ET = ejection time.

with gallstones,[5, 6] or spinal cord injury patients.[7] Subject ages, genders, and numbers are listed in Table 1.

Comments ▪

Several factors contribute to variability in normal gallbladder contraction measured by ultrasound: measurement errors related to the method of volume determination by ultrasound as well as inter- and intraobserver variability, type of contraction stimulus used, day-to-day variation in gallbladder kinetics in the same subject, biologic intersubject variability, gender, and habitus. Intravenous infusion of sincalide over 30 minutes yielded the largest EF, and less than 50% was given as the lower limit of normal.[3] Bolus infusions of sincalide or CCK have variable results.[1, 4] Combining the results of studies done with oral stimuli gives an EF of (mean ± 1 SD, 67 ± 11%) and mean −2 SD = 45%.[2, 5–7] It would seem reasonable to use 40% to 50% as borderline and 40% as the lower limit of normal for studies done with oral stimuli.

REFERENCES

1. Hopman WP, Rosenbusch G, Jansen JB, et al: Gallbladder contraction: Effects of fatty meals and cholecystokinin. Radiology 1985; 157:37–39.
2. Donald JJ, Fache JS, Buckley AR, Burhenne HJ: Gallbladder contractility: Variation in normal subjects. AJR Am J Roentgenol 1991; 157:753–756.
3. Barr RG, Agnesi JN, Schaub CR: Acalculous gallbladder disease: US evaluation after slow-infusion cholecystokinin stimulation in symptomatic and asymptomatic adults. Radiology 1997; 204:105–111.
4. Davis GB, Berk RN, Scheible FW, et al: Cholecystokinin cholecystography, sonography, and scintigraphy: Detection of chronic acalculous cholecystitis. AJR Am J Roentgenol 1982; 139:1117–1121.
5. Kishk SMA, Darweesh RMA, Dodds WJ, et al: Sonographic evaluation of the resting gallbladder volume and postprandial emptying in patients with gallstones. AJR Am J Roentgenol 1987; 148:875–879.
6. Pauletzki J, Cicala M, Holl J, et al: Correlation between gallbladder fasting volume and postprandial emptying in patients with gallstones and healthy controls. Gut 1993; 34:1443–1447.
7. Nino-Murcia M, Burton D, Chang P, et al: Gallbladder contractility in patients with spinal cord injuries: A sonographic investigation [see comments]. AJR Am J Roentgenol 1990; 154(3):521–524.

▪: MEASUREMENT OF NORMAL PEDIATRIC GALLBLADDER AND BILIARY TRACT BY ULTRASOUND[1]
- ▪ ACR Code: 762 (Gallbladder); 764 (Hepatic Duct)

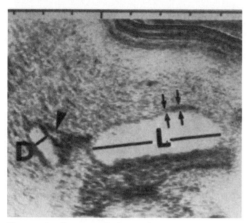

Figure 1 ▪ Parasagittal scan of the right upper quadrant, showing the common hepatic duct (*arrowhead*), right portal vein (*D*), and gallbladder. The length (*L*), AP dimension, and wall thickness of the gallbladder (*arrows*) were measured on this scan. (From McGahan JP, et al: Radiology 1982; 144:873. Used by permission.)

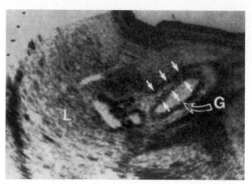

Figure 2 ▪ Longitudinal scan of the right upper quadrant in an 8-year-old boy with serum hepatitis. Note increased thickness (*arrows*) giving a "tram-track" appearance to the gallbladder wall. *G* = gallbladder lumen; *L* = liver. (From McGahan JP, et al: Radiology 1982; 144:873. Used by permission.)

Table 1 ▪ Sonographic Measurements of the Normal Pediatric Gallbladder and Biliary Tract

AGE RANGE (yr)	AP DIAMETER (cm)		CORONAL DIAMETER (cm)		LENGTH (cm)		WALL THICKNESS (mm)		COMMON HEPATIC DUCT SIZE (mm)		RIGHT PORTAL VEIN SIZE (mm)	
	Mean	Range	Mean	Range	Mean	Range	Mean	Range	Mean	Range	Mean	Range
0–1 (8 patients)	9.9	0.5–1.2	0.9	0.7–1.4	2.5	1.3–3.4	1.7	1.0–3.0	1.3	1.0–2.0	3.8	3.0–5.0
2–5 (10 patients)	1.7	1.4–2.3	1.8	1.0–3.9	4.2	2.9–5.2	2.0	None	1.7	1.0–3.0	4.8	3.0–7.0
6–8 (11 patients)	1.8	1.0–2.4	2.0	1.2–3.0	5.6	4.4–7.4	2.2	2.0–3.0	2.0	None	5.7	6.0–9.0
9–11 (12 patients)	1.9	1.2–3.2	2.0	1.0–3.6	5.5	3.4–6.5	2.0	1.0–3.0	1.8	1.0–3.0	6.8	4.0–9.0
12–16 (10 patients)	2.0	1.3–2.8	2.1	1.6–3.0	6.1	3.8–8.0	2.0	1.0–3.0	2.2	1.0–4.0	7.8	6.0–10.0

From McGahan JP, et al: Radiology 1982; 144:873. Used by permission.

Technique ▪
1. Either static sector or linear array real-time scanners with 3.5- or 5-MHz transducers were used.
2. Younger subjects fasted about 3 hours and older ones 8 hours or more.
3. Sagittal, transverse, and oblique images were used to outline the gallbladder and ducts optimally.

Measurements ▪ (Figures 1 and 2)
Length, AP diameter, and width (coronal size) of the gallbladder were measured on images that gave greatest dimensions. All measurements were made intraluminally, except gallbladder wall thickness (Table 1).

Portal vein and common hepatic duct were measured as internal diameters.

Source ▪
Fifty-one patients aged 1 month to 16 years were evaluated. None had signs, symptoms, or laboratory evidence of gallbladder or biliary tract disease.

REFERENCE
1. McGahan JP, Phillips HE, Cox KL: Sonography of the normal pediatric gallbladder and biliary tract. Radiology 1982; 144:873.

▪: MEASUREMENT OF THE COMMON BILE DUCT IN CHILDREN[1]
▪ ACR Code: 766 (Common Bile Duct)

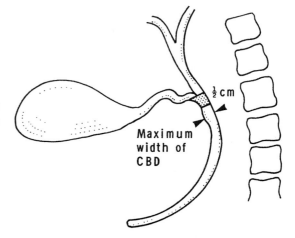

Figure 1 ▪ The duct is measured at its widest diameter, ignoring the proximal 5 mm. (From Witcombe JB, Cremin BJ: Pediatr Radiol 1978; 7:147. Used by permission.)

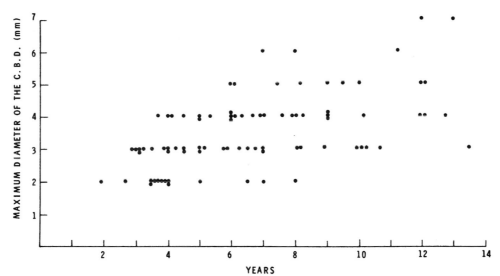

Figure 2 ▪ Normal range of measurements of the common bile duct. (From Witcombe JB, Cremin BJ: Pediatr Radiol 1978; 7:147. Used by permission.)

Technique ▪

Intravenous cholangiography by drip infusion of 20 ml of 50% meglumine iodipamide.

Central ray: Perpendicular to plane of film centered over right upper abdomen.
Position: 15° prone oblique.
Target-film distance: 100 cm.

Measurements ▪ (Figure 1)

The widest diameter of the common bile duct was measured to the nearest millimeter. Measurements were not taken within 5 mm because of overlapping of the cystic duct and common hepatic duct near their junction.

Normal measurements are given in Figure 2.

Source ▪

Data based on study of 44 girls and 41 boys of African, European, and mixed parentage.

REFERENCE

1. Witcombe JB, Cremin BJ: The width of the common bile duct in childhood. Pediatr Radiol 1978; 26:147–149.

⁎⁝ MEASUREMENT OF THE BILIARY DUCTS BY ENDOSCOPIC RETROGRADE CHOLANGIOGRAPHY[1]
- ACR Code: 768 (Bile Ducts)

Technique ▪

Endoscopic retrograde cholangiopancreatography with Olympus JF-B endoscope.

Central ray: Perpendicular to plane of film.
Position: Anteroposterior supine.
Target-film distance: Immaterial. Measurements were corrected for magnification relative to the size of the endoscope.

Measurements ▪ (Figure 1)

The widest diameter of the intrapancreatic portion of the common duct was measured. This is defined as the portion of the common bile duct that runs parallel to the ascending part of the pancreatic duct. The widest part of the prepancreatic portion of the common bile duct was also measured. This region started at the upper border of the intrapancreatic common bile duct and ended at the origin of the cystic duct. The common hepatic duct that extends from the end of the cystic duct to the bifurcation of the common hepatic duct was also measured.

Normal measurements were as follows:

1. The common hepatic duct: 4.6 mm (range, 2.1 to 9.2 mm).
2. The prepancreatic portion of the common bile duct: 4.9 mm (range, 2.3 to 8.5 mm).
3. The intrahepatic portion of the common bile duct: 4.3 mm (range, 2.3 to 6.9 mm).

Source ▪

Data based on study of 49 normal patients, 36 men and 13 women, aged 18 to 72 years. The mean age was 50.5 years.

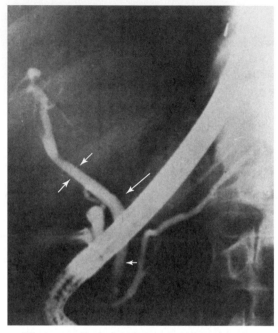

Figure 1 ▪ The normal cholangiogram and pancreatogram. The *short arrow* points to the intrapancreatic portion of the common bile duct. The *long arrow* points to the prepancreatic portion of the common bile duct, and the *double arrows* point to the common hepatic duct. These are the areas measured. (From Lasser RB, et al: Am J Dig Dis 1978; 23:586–590. Used by permission.)

REFERENCE

1. Lasser RB, Silvis SE, Vennes GA: The normal cholangiogram. Am J Dig Dis 1978; 23:586–590.

⁎⁝ COMMON BILE DUCT DIAMETER THROUGHOUT LIFE WITH ULTRASOUND
- ACR Code: 766 (Common Duct)

Technique ▪

Hernanz-Schulman and colleagues performed upper abdominal ultrasound with 270 (Toshiba, Tustin, CA) or 128 (Acuson, Mountain View, CA) machines and 5-MHz sector or linear transducers, with attention to the extrahepatic bile ducts and gallbladder. Prandial status was not controlled.[1] Wu and colleagues used a SAL-22A machine (Toshiba), with a 3.5-MHz linear array transducer, to scan the upper abdomen. Patients had been fasting for at least 4 hours.[2] In both studies, scanning through the porta hepatis region was done in appropriate obliquity to best visualize the extrahepatic part of the common bile duct (CBD).

Measurements ▪

Both investigators measured the extrahepatic CBD (in millimeters) between the cystic duct and the pancreas, with Hernanz-Schulman and group describing the measurement as being done from inner wall to inner wall and Wu and group stating that the maximal anteroposterior (AP) inner diameter was recorded.[1, 2] Figure 1 shows the CBD diameter for children through 13 years.[1] Table 1 lists CBD diameter for adults by age and gender.[2] Figure 2 graphically depicts data from both studies. Neither study documented any gender differences and both found a slight increase in CBD diameter with age (0.08 mm/year in children and

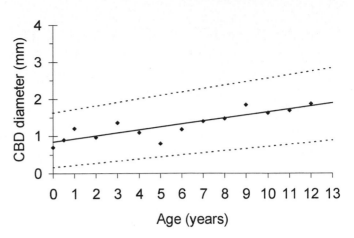

Figure 1 ▪ Common bile duct (CBD) size in children. Diamonds = mean for age group. *Solid line* = linear regression of CBD diameter versus age. *Dotted lines* = 95% confidence intervals. (From Hernanz-Schulman M, Ambrosino MM, Freeman PC, Quinn CB: Radiology 1995;195(1):193–195. Used by permission.)

Table 1 ▪ Common Duct Size in Adults

Gender	Age (years) →	<21	21–30	31–40	41–50	51–60	>60
Men	Number	9	12	14	13	15	7
	CBD (mm)	3.3 ± 1.1	4.7 ± 1.3	5.0 ± 1.5	5.4 ± 1.4	6.2 ± 1.9	6.1 ± 2.0
Women	Number	9	28	38	21	15	22
	CBD (mm)	3.3 ± 1.1	4.7 ± 1.2	4.6 ± 1.4	5.3 ± 1.2	5.3 ± 1.8	6.8 ± 1.7
	p value	>0.05	>0.05	>0.05	>0.05	>0.05	>0.05
Combined	Number	18	40	52	34	30	29
	CBD (mm)	3.3 ± 1.2	4.7 ± 1.3	4.7 ± 1.5	5.5 ± 1.3	5.8 ± 1.9	6.6 ± 1.8

All measurements in millimeters (mean ± standard deviation). CBD = common bile duct, p value = difference between male and female means. Combined diameters calculated from male and female data.

From Wu CC, Ho YH, Chen CY: J Clin Ultrasound 1984; 12:473–478. Used by permission.

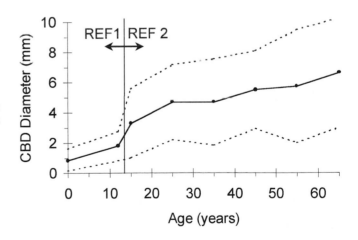

Figure 2 ▪ Common duct size throughout life. Combined data from both Hernanz-Schulman and Wu and their associates. Vertical line shows from which reference the data were obtained. *Solid line* = mean diameter; dotted lines = 95% confidence intervals.[1, 2]

0.06 mm/year in adults). Wu and associates gave a linear regression formula for CBD size versus age as follows:

$$\text{CBD (maximum, mm)} = 2.72 + 0.06 \times \text{Age (years). } r = 0.60, p < .001.[2]$$

Source ▪

Hernanz-Schulman and colleagues studied 173 children who ranged in age from neonate to 13 years. There were 10 or more patients in each 1-year interval (25 <1 year). The patients were having ultrasound for problems not related to the biliary system.[1] Wu and colleagues evaluated 203 subjects ranging in age from infancy to over 80 years (gender and age distribution in Table 1) with no history or imaging findings to suggest biliary disease.[2]

REFERENCES

1. Hernanz-Schulman M, Ambrosino MM, Freeman PC, Quinn CB: Common bile duct in children: Sonographic dimensions. Radiology 1995; 195(1):193–195.
2. Wu CC, Ho YH, Chen CY: Effect of aging on common duct diameter: A real-time ultrasonographic study. J Clin Ultrasound 1984; 12:473–478.

": MEASUREMENT OF EXTRAHEPATIC BILE DUCTS IN HEALTHY SUBJECTS, PATIENTS WITH GALLSTONES, AND POSTCHOLECYSTECTOMY PATIENTS BY ULTRASOUND[1]
- ACR Code: 766 (Common Bile Duct)

Technique •

1. Patients were imaged with a 3.5-MHz real-time or static scanner.
2. Supine or right-side elevated position. All subjects were imaged after an overnight fast. The lumen of the duct was measured in the porta hepatis where it parallels the main portal vein, and at the widest point, generally more distal than the first measurement. Electronic cursors were used.

Measurement • (Table 1)

Healthy subjects had common duct diameters of 4 mm or less, whereas patients with gallstones or postcholecystectomy had significantly larger diameters.

Source •

Eight hundred thirty normal volunteers were recruited from blood donors. In addition, 73 patients with gallstones and 55 who had undergone cholecystectomy were studied. Patients with jaundice or stones in the extrahepatic ducts were excluded.

An ultrasonographic study by Mueller and colleagues[2] of pre- and postcholecystectomy patients has indicated that postcholecystectomy dilatation of the common bile duct does not occur in most normal patients.

Table 1 • Diameter of Common Duct Size (mm) in 830 Normal Subjects, 73 Patients with Gallstones, and 55 Patients After Cholecystectomy Without Signs of Biliary Obstruction

	MEAN ± SD	RANGE	95th PERCENTILE
Normal subjects			
Porta hepatis	2.5 ± 1.1	1–7	4
Widest point	2.8 ± 1.2	1–7	4
Patients with gallstones			
Porta hepatis	3.8 ± 2.0	1–10	8
Widest point	4.8 ± 2.2	2–12	9
Patients after cholecystectomy			
Porta hepatis	5.2 ± 2.3	1–11	10
Widest point	6.2 ± 2.5	3–13	11

From Niederau D, et al: J Clin Ultrasound 1983; 11:23–27. Used by permission.

References

1. Niederau C, Muller HH, Sonnenberg A, et al: Extrahepatic bile ducts in healthy subjects, in patients with cholelithiasis, and in postcholecystectomy patients. J Clin Ultrasound 1983; 11:23–27.
2. Mueller PR, Ferrucci JT, Simeone JF, et al: Postcholecystectomy bile duct dilation: Myth or reality? AJR Am J Roentgenol 1981; 136:355–358.

": CHANGES IN THE EXTRAHEPATIC BILE DUCT AFTER CHOLECYSTECTOMY
- ACR Code: 766 (Common Duct)

Technique •

Real-time gray scale ultrasound (machine and transducers not described) was performed of the abdomen with attention to the biliary system.[1, 2]

Measurements •

Hunt and Scott measured the common hepatic duct (CHD) diameter just beyond the confluence of ducts multiple times and averaged the measurements. The common bile duct (CBD) diameter was measured at its widest point when possible.[1] Feng and Song measured the CBD at its widest point in the proximal segment.[2] Table 1 lists the reported results from both studies as mean ± SD at different time intervals after cholecystectomy and preoperatively. Feng and Song excluded 37 patients with a CBD greater than 6 mm from these figures. Table 2 gives the distribution in duct diameters before and after cholecystectomy.[1, 2]

Source •

Hunt and Scott evaluated 21 patients (ages and genders not given) in a prospective study of bile duct diameters before and after cholecystectomy. All had open cholecystectomy, and five had bile duct exploration and T-tube placement (all removed by the 9th postoperative day with no stones on T-tube studies). Preoperative scans were done within 1 month of operation, and postoperative scans were done in the first postoperative year, at 1 year, and at 5 years in 13 while 8 had only postoperative scans at 5 years.[1] Feng and Song performed retrospective analysis of 234 patients (49 men, 185 women, age range 28 to 68 years, mean age 49 years) who had ultrasound 4 to 15 days prior to simple cholecystectomy and repeat scans from 1 week to 6 years postoperatively.[2] In both series, none of the patients experienced significant postoperative symptoms related to the biliary tract.[1, 2]

Comments •

Hunt and Scott found no statistically significant increase in duct size, and Feng and Song found a slight generalized increase in CBD of less than 1 mm.[1, 2] Hunt and Scott observed that 2 of 21 patients (10%) had significant increases (3 to 4 mm) in CHD size, and Feng and Song

Table 1 • Changes in Bile Duct Diameter After Cholecystectomy

AUTHOR (Study Type)	NO.	EXAM TIME	CBD (mm) Mean ± SD	CHD (mm) Mean ± SD
Hunt and Scott (prospective)	13	preop		3.54 ± 0.55
	13	<1 yr		3.50 ± 0.59
	13	1 yr	4.77 ± 0.69	3.81 ± 0.36
	13	5 yr	5.92 ± 0.56	4.69 ± 0.64
	21	preop		3.95 ± 0.46
	21	5 yr		4.48 ± 0.47

			CBD (mm) MEAN ± SD	
			Preop	Postop
Feng and Song (retrospective)	50	7–30 days	5.0 ± 0.9	5.5 ± 0.9
	51	2–6 mon	5.4 ± 0.5	6.1 ± 1.6
	33	7–12 mon	5.3 ± 0.6	5.9 ± 1.2
	41	2–3 yr	5.7 ± 0.5	6.6 ± 1.8
	22	4–6 yr	5.6 ± 0.5	6.2 ± 1.4
	197	Total	5.4 ± 0.7	6.0 ± 1.4

Preop = preoperative scan, postop = postoperative scan, CBD = common bile duct (maximum), CHD = common hepatic duct (average).[1,2]

Table 2 • Bile Duct Size Distribution Before and After Cholecystectomy

REFERENCE	STRUCTURE	EXAM TIME	DUCT DIAMETER (mm) ≤4 (%)	5–6 (%)	7–8 (%)	≥9 (%)
Hunt	CHD	preop	13 (62)	6 (28)	1 (5)	1 (5)
	(n = 21)	5 yr	14 (67)	3 (13)	2 (10)	2 (10)
	CBD	1 yr	6 (46)	4 (31)	2 (15)	1 (8)
	(n = 13)	5 yr	3 (23)	4 (31)	5 (38)	1 (8)
Feng	CBD	preop	17 (7)	180 (77)	26 (11)	11 (5)
	(n = 234)	postop	22 (9)	145 (62)	51 (22)	16 (7)

Preop = preoperative, postop = postoperative, CBD = common bile duct (maximum), CHD = common hepatic duct (average).[1,2]

found 67 of 234 (29%) with a dilated CBD (>7 mm) postoperatively. Using Feng's postoperative mean +2 SD for CBD yields 8.8 mm, and it seems reasonable to consider 9 to 10 mm as a borderline value. Other studies of asymptomatic postcholecystectomy patients present a somewhat confusing picture, with Niederau and colleagues[3] finding a significant increase in mean CBD size of up to 3 mm, and others[4-6] finding no generalized increase. Many series describe a fraction (<10 to 20%) of patients with a CBD diameter of 10 mm or more and no apparent obstruction.[3-7]

REFERENCES

1. Hunt DR, Scott AJ: Changes in bile duct diameter after cholecystectomy: A 5-year prospective study. Gastroenterology 1989; 97(6):1485–1488.

2. Feng B, Song Q: Does the common bile duct dilate after cholecystectomy? Sonographic evaluation in 234 patients. AJR Am J Roentgenol. 1995; 165:859–861.

3. Niederau C, Muller HH, Sonnenberg A, et al: Extrahepatic bile ducts in healthy subjects, in patients with cholelithiasis and in postcholecystectomy patients. J Clin Ultrasound 1983; 11:23–27.

4. Edmunds R, Katz S, Garciano V, Finby N: The common duct after cholecystectomy. Interval report. Arch Surg 1971; 103(1):79–81.

5. Graham MF, Cooperberg PL, Cohen MM, Burhenne HJ: The size of the normal common hepatic duct following cholecystectomy: An ultrasonographic study. Radiology 1980; 135:137–139.

6. Mueller PR, Ferrucci JT, Simeone JF, et al: Postcholecystectomy bile duct dilation: Myth or reality? AJR Am J Roentgenol 1981; 136:355–358.

7. Graham MF, Cooperberg PL, Cohen MM, et al: Ultrasonographic screening of the common hepatic duct in symptomatic patients after cholecystectomy. Radiology 1981; 138:137–139.

▪: MEASUREMENT OF THE DUODENAL MAJOR PAPILLA OF VATER[1]
▪ ACR Code: 767 (Papilla, Ampulla of Vater)

Table 1 ▪ Normal Measurements of the Papilla of Vater

	LENGTH (cm)	WIDTH (cm)	HEIGHT (cm)
Measurements of major papilla from anatomic specimens			
Average size	1.5	0.5	0.5
Minimum size	0.1	0.1	0.1
Maximum size	3.0	1.2	1.2
Measurements from series of gastrointestinal films			
Average size (cm)	1.5	0.7	

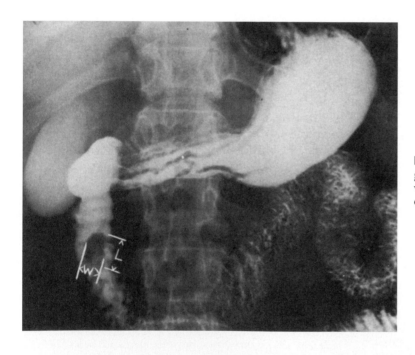

Figure 1 ▪ Measurement of the papilla of Vater from radiographs of the barium-filled duodenum. The transverse width (*W*) and cephalocaudal length (*L*) were measured directly from the film.

Technique ▪

Central ray: To second lumbar vertebra.
Position: Posteroanterior abdomen for stomach and duodenum.
Target-film distance: 36 inches.

Measurements ▪ (Figure 1 and Table 1)

The papilla position is most frequently on the medial duodenal wall toward the posterior portion of the mid-descending duodenum.

Source ▪

The anatomic measurements were made on 100 specimens described as normal, fresh, and unassociated with any history, symptoms, or gross evidence of disease referable to the biliary tract, pancreas, or duodenum.

The measurements of papilla size from the films correspond well to the anatomic measurements.

REFERENCE

1. Poppel MH, Jacobsen HG, Smith RW: The Roentgen Aspects of the Papilla and Ampulla of Vater. Charles C Thomas, Springfield, IL, 1953.

▪: MEASUREMENT OF DISTAL COMMON BILE DUCT AND PANCREATIC HEAD BY CT CHOLANGIOGRAPHY[1]
▪ ACR Code: 770 (Pancreas); 766 (Common Bile Duct)

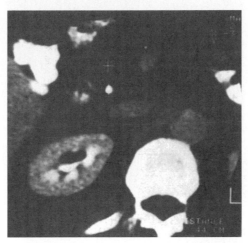

Figure 1 ▪ Magnified view (×2) of the distal common bile duct, illustrating its measurement (0.44 cm) using electronic cursors. (From Greenberg M: Radiology 1982; 144:363. Used by permission.)

Technique ▪

1. A GE CT/T 8800 scanner was used to scan 5- or 10-mm sections at a scan speed of 9.6 seconds. Sections were usually at 1-cm intervals, with 5-mm sections through the pancreas.
2. The night before the scan, the patient was given 3 gm of iopanoic acid (Telepaque) and kept on a clear liquid diet. The next morning the patient was given calcium ipodate granules (Oragrafin, 2 packages) and scanned about 1.5 hours later, after oral administration of dilute Gastrografin or barium.
3. Opacification of the biliary tree is better seen if intravenous contrast is not given. Repeat studies with intravenous contrast may be used to show vascular structures better.

Measurements ▪ (Figures 1, 2, and 3)

In 84 of 97 patients, the gallbladder and/or biliary tree was visualized well.

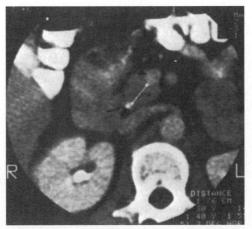

Figure 2 ▪ Typical case illustrating measurements for the uncinate process. Line drawn between the common bile duct (*arrow*) and superior mesenteric vein (*arrowhead*) represents true transverse diameter of the uncinate process (1.76 cm). (From Greenberg M: Radiology 1982; 144:363.)

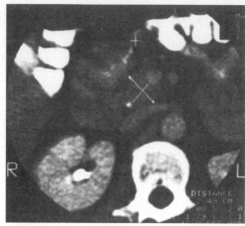

Figure 3 ▪ Line drawn perpendicular to figure on left represents true ventral-dorsal measurement of the uncinate process (2.49 cm). (From Greenberg M: Radiology 1982; 144:363. Used by permission.)

The distal common bile duct measured 4.7 ± 1.2 mm in 56 normal patients and 6.8 ± 1.1 mm in 10 patients postcholecystectomy (p <.001). The distal common bile duct was anterior to the inferior vena cava in 55 patients, lateral in 8, and medial in 5.

The transverse measurement of the uncinate process in 44 patients was 2.06 ± 0.53 cm. The AP diameter was 2.34 ± 0.51 cm in 28 patients.

Source ▪

Data are based on a study of 97 patients.

REFERENCE

1. Greenberg M, Greenberg BM, Rubin JM, Greenberg IM: Computer-tomographic cholangiography; A new technique for evaluating the head of the pancreas and distal biliary tree. Radiology 1982; 144:363–368.

▪: MEASUREMENT OF THE NORMAL PANCREAS BY CT[1]
▪ ACR Code: 770 (Pancreas)

Technique ▪

1. The measurements are based on 15 postmortem pancreas studies and 50 patients studied on a prototype EMI scanner using 15-mm slices generated in 20 seconds. The postmortem measurements were made on radiographs of formalin-fixed glands injected with a barium suspension in the pancreatic duct.
2. An anticholinergic drug was used to reduce artifact from bowel movement. Dilute oral contrast helped identify bowel.

Measurements ▪ See Figure 1.

Radiographs and hard-copy images of CT were measured to determine the ventrodorsal diameter of the head, neck, body, and tail. The autopsy specimens were also measured in the craniocaudal diameter. Comparison of the in vivo and postmortem studies demonstrated close correlation of measurements. See Table 1.

Table 1 ▪ Normal Pancreas (Postmortem) in 15 Patients (5 Men and 10 Women) Aged 25 to 65 Years (Mean 45.4 Yr)		
LOCALIZATION IN PANCREAS	MEAN VENTRODORSAL DIAMETER (mm)	MEAN CRANIOCAUDAL DIAMETER (mm)
Head	24	44
Neck	17	34
Body	20	35
Tail	15	30

From Kreel L, et al: J Comput Assist Tomogr 1977; 1:290–299. Used by permission.

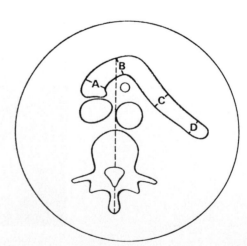

Figure 1 ▪ Schematic representation of a section showing normal values (mean ± SD) as seen on CT. (A = 23 ± 3.0 mm, B = 19 ± 2.5 mm, C = 20 ± 3.0 mm, D = 15 ± 2.5 mm.) (From Kreel L, et al: J Comput Assist Tomogr 1977; 1:290. Used by permission.)

Source ▪

Fifty patients without evidence of pancreatic disease, aged 25 to 65 years (mean 45.8), and 15 patients with normal pancreases, aged 25 to 65 years (mean 45.4), studied at autopsy.

REFERENCE

1. Kreel L, Haertel H, Katz D: Computed tomography of the normal pancreas. J Comput Assist Tomogr 1977; 1:290–299.

▪: CHANGES IN PANCREATIC SIZE AND MORPHOLOGY WITH AGING
▪ ACR Code: 770 (Pancreas)

Technique ▪

Heuck and colleagues used a Somotom SD unit (Siemens, Erlangen, Germany) to perform abdominal CT. Scan times were 4.5 sec, and slice thickness was 4 to 8 mm; scanning was done at inspiration. Oral contrast (100 to 150 ml of dilute Gastrografin) was given to 82% of subjects prior to scanning, intravenous contrast (100 ml of Telebrix 30) was used in 65%, and 58% had both types of contrast.[1] Matsumoto and colleagues reviewed abdominal CT scans done on several machines, with scan times ranging from 1.9 to 4.5 sec and slice thickness of 10 mm. Oral contrast was not used, and intravenous contrast was used in most patients.[2]

Measurements ▪

Heuck and colleagues measured the diameter of the head, body, and tail of the pancreas, as well as the transverse diameter of the adjacent vertebral body, as shown in Figure 1. They also noted the contour (smooth versus lobular) of the pancreas and its internal structure (homogeneous versus heterogeneous). Table 1 lists the pancreatic diameters as raw values and vertebral body–pancreas ratios (vertebral body = 100%) by decade.[1] Matsumoto and colleagues divided patients into four groups based on the location and extent of uneven fatty replacement of the pancreas. These are shown in Figure 2, along with percentages of occurrence (of 1000 patients). Table 2 lists the percentages of patients showing lobular pancreatic contour, heterogene-

Table 1 ▪ Pancreatic Diameters Versus Age in 360 Normal Adults			
AGE RANGE (n = 60 Each)	**DIAMETER (mm)**		
	Head	Body	Tail
20–30	28.6 ± 3.8	19.1 ± 2.1	18.0 ± 1.6
31–40	26.0 ± 3.4	18.2 ± 2.4	16.5 ± 1.8
41–50	25.2 ± 3.6	17.8 ± 2.2	15.8 ± 1.7
51–60	24.0 ± 3.6	16.0 ± 2.0	15.1 ± 1.9
61–70	23.4 ± 3.5	15.8 ± 2.4	14.7 ± 1.8
71–80	21.2 ± 4.3	14.4 ± 2.7	13.0 ± 2.1
	PANCREAS/VERTEBRAL BODY × 100		
20–30	68.2 ± 8.5	47.0 ± 5.6	45.1 ± 4.4
31–40	62.1 ± 9.3	43.2 ± 6.0	38.9 ± 5.9
41–50	58.0 ± 7.8	41.6 ± 6.0	36.1 ± 4.3
51–60	55.0 ± 9.7	37.2 ± 6.4	35.6 ± 5.7
61–70	53.4 ± 7.8	36.1 ± 6.2	33.6 ± 4.7
71–80	48.2 ± 12.2	32.4 ± 6.1	29.4 ± 5.1

Measurements are given as mean ± standard deviation
From Heuck A, Maubach PA, Reiser M, et al: Gastrointest Radiol 1987; 12:18–22. Used by permission.

ous internal structure, and uneven fatty replacement by decade.[1, 2]

Source ▪

Heuck's subjects were 360 adults (187 men, 173 women, age range 20 to 80 years, 60 patients in each decade) with no biliary, pancreatic, gastrointestinal, or abdominal

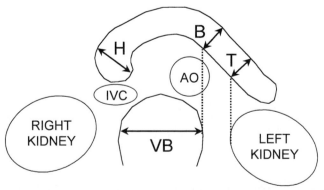

Figure 1 ▪ Measurements of pancreatic diameter from CT scans. All measurements were made perpendicular to the long axis of the gland. The head *(H)*, body *(B)*, and tail *(T)*, and transverse vertebral body *(VB)* were measured as shown. The left margin of the vertebra marked the body, and the medial margin of the left kidney marked the tail *(dotted lines)*. *IVC* = inferior vena cava, *AO* = aorta. (From Heuck A, et al: Gastrointest Radiol 1987;12:18–22. Used by permission.)

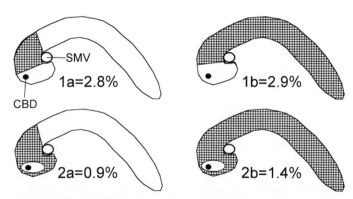

Figure 2 ▪ Patterns of uneven fatty replacement of the pancreas. Fatty change is shown by shaded portions. The percentages are from a group of 1000 abdominal CT scans initially reviewed. *CBD* = common bile duct, *SMV* = superior mesenteric vein. (From Matsumoto S, Mori H, Miyake H, et al: Radiology 1995;194:453–458. Used by permission.)

Table 2 ▪ Morphologic Changes in the Aging Pancreas by Decade

DECADE	LOBULAR CONTOUR (%)	INHOMOGENEOUS DENSITY (%)	UNEVEN FATTY REPLACEMENT (%)
3rd	10.6	3.7	—
4th	33.6	30.9	0.3
5th	41.1	44.9	1.0
6th	44.9	49.5	1.9
7th	56.2	55.2	3.1
8th	70.1	71.1	1.5
>80 years	—	—	0.2

Numbers given are percentages from 360 scans for contour/density and from 1000 scans for uneven replacement.[1, 2]

lymphatic disease.[1] Matsumoto and colleagues reviewed 1000 CT scans and selected for further review 80 subjects (42 men, 38 women, age range 34 to 84 years, mean age 61 years) who exhibited uneven fatty replacement of the pancreas. Patients with peripancreatic or pancreatic disease and those with complete fatty replacement were not studied.[2]

Comments ▪

The pancreas decreases in size with age, and this would seem to be a real change since it persists after correction for vertebral body size.[1] There is a gradual tendency toward increasing lobulation of contour and heterogeneous density on CT, which Heuck and group ascribe to lipomatosis, fibrosis, and sclerosis.[1] In a small fraction of patients (8%), there is uneven fatty replacement of the pancreas at CT, which might be confused with focal disease. This may be related to differences in histomorphologic structure of the ventral and dorsal portions of the gland.[2]

REFERENCES

1. Heuck A, Maubach PA, Reiser M, et al: Age-related morphology of the normal pancreas on computed tomography. Gastrointest Radiol 1987; 12:18–22.
2. Matsumoto S, Mori H, Miyake H, et al: Uneven fatty replacement of the pancreas: Evaluation with CT. Radiology 1995; 194:453–458.

▪▪ PANCREATIC DIMENSIONS IN NORMAL HEALTH AND VARIOUS DISEASE STATES
▪ ACR Code: 770 (Pancreas)

Technique ▪

Ultrasound scanning was done over the pancreas, mostly in the transverse plane, with real-time sector or curved-array transducers ranging in frequency from 3.5 to 7.5 MHz.[1, 4, 7–9] Two of the earlier ultrasound studies used B-mode articulated arm scanners.[2, 3] CT of the pancreas was done with a prototype EMI scanner, with 13-mm section thickness and 10-mm increments.[5] Another study used a CR CT scanner (Siemens, Erlangen, Germany) and contiguous 8-mm slices.[6] All patients were fasting, and oral but not intravenous contrast was given for the CT studies.

Measurements ▪

Measurements were made from the operator's console of the machine being used or with calipers from hard copies of the images through the middle of the pancreatic portion (head, body, tail) being studied. For the most part, anteroposterior (AP) measurements of the body and tail thickness perpendicular to the long axis of the organ were made in centimeters. Measurements of the AP thickness of the pancreatic head were typically performed in the true AP dimension.[1–9] These measurement locations are shown in Figure 1. Two investigators also measured the pancreas in the cephalocaudal or longitudinal (LON) dimension.[3, 7] Tables 1 and 2 list reported measurements of the pancreatic head, body, and tail in AP and LON dimensions, respectively.

Source ▪

Patient ages, numbers of subjects, and type of group (normal, disease entity) are listed in Tables 1 and 2.

Comments ▪

The pancreas is smaller in patients with insulin-dependent diabetes and in adults with cystic fibrosis.[6, 7, 9] Coleman and colleagues found that in children with acute pancreatitis the gland was focally enlarged in 15 of 25, mostly involving the head.[8] Siegel and colleagues found enlargement of the

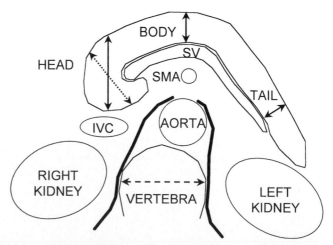

Figure 1 ▪ Measurements of the AP dimensions of the pancreas from axial/transverse images. The body and tail typically were measured as shown (*solid lines with arrows*). The head usually was measured in the true AP dimension on ultrasound (*solid line with arrows*) and perpendicular to the long axis on CT (*dotted line with arrows*). The transverse diameter of the adjacent vertebral body was measured (*dashed line with arrows*) and used as a reference by Fleischer.[10] *SMA* = superior mesenteric artery, *SV* = splenic vein, *IVC* = inferior vena cava.

Table 1 ▪ Anteroposterior Dimensions of the Pancreas

REFERENCE	GROUP	AGE	NO.	HEAD	BODY	TAIL
Siegel—U/S[1]	Normal	<1 mon	15	1.0±0.4	0.6±0.2	1.0±0.4
	Normal	1 mon–1 yr	23	1.5±0.5	0.8±0.3	1.2±0.4
	Normal	1–5 yr	49	1.7±0.3	1.0±0.2	1.8±0.4
	Normal	5–10 yr	69	1.6±0.4	1.0±0.3	1.8±0.4
	Normal	10–19 yr	117	2.0±0.5	1.1±0.3	2.0±0.4
Weill—U/S[2]	Normal	17–85 yr	135	1.7±0.5	1.0±0.3	1.5±0.7
Haber—U/S[3]	Normal	Adult	382	2.7±0.7	2.2±0.7	2.4±0.4
Niederau—U/S[4]	Normal	18–68 yr	1000	2.2±0.3	1.8±0.3	—
Kreel—CT[5]	Normal	25–65 yr	50	2.3±0.3	2.0±0.3	1.5±0.3
Gilbeau—CT[6]	Control	27–83 yr	57	1.6	1.6	1.6
	IDDM	23–72 yr	20	1.2	1.1	1.2
	NIDDM-D	44–86 yr	25	1.5	1.4	1.4
	NIDDM-I	51–83 yr	12	1.2	1.2	1.3
Altobelli—U/S[7]	Normal	3–7 yr	20	2.0±0.4	1.2±0.3	1.4±0.3
	Normal	8–12 yr	20	2.3±0.4	1.1±0.3	1.8±0.5
	Normal	13–15 yr	20	2.4±0.4	1.3±0.3	2.0±0.4
	IDDM	3–7 yr	20	1.7±0.4	0.9±0.3	1.3±0.3
	IDDM	8–12 yr	20	1.9±0.3	0.8±0.3	1.3±0.3
	IDDM	13–15 yr	20	2.0±0.4	0.8±0.2	1.4±0.4
Coleman—U/S[8]	Normal	0–18 yr	75	(1.0–2.2)	(0.4–1.0)	(0.8–1.8)
	Pancreatitis	0–18 yr	25	(2.2–4.0)	(0.8–2.0)	(1.4–3.5)
Phillips—U/S[9]	CF	3–16 yr	12	1.2 (0.8–1.5)	1.2 (0.7–1.0)	1.6 (0.8–2.0)
	CF	17–41 yr	8	1.3 (1.0–1.5)	1.1 (0.7–1.5)	1.5 (1.1–2.1)

All measurements in centimeters. When reported, mean ± standard deviations are given. Reported ranges are in parentheses. IDDM = insulin-dependent diabetes mellitus, NIDDM-D = noninsulin-dependent diabetes mellitus—diet controlled, NIDDM-I = noninsulin-dependent diabetes mellitus—insulin requiring, CF = cystic fibrosis.

Table 2 ▪ Cephalocaudal (Longitudinal) Measurements of the Pancreas

REFERENCE	GROUP	AGE (Yr)	NUMBER	HEAD	BODY	TAIL
Haber—U/S[3]	Normal	Adult	382	3.6±1.2	3.0±0.6	2.9±0.4
Altobelli—U/S[7]	Normal	3–7	20	2.7±0.4	1.9+0.3	1.8±0.3
	Normal	8–12	20	3.1±0.6	2.3±0.5	2.0±0.5
	Normal	13–15	20	3.4±0.4	2.8±0.4	2.3±0.4
	IDDM	3–7	20	2.3±0.6	1.8±0.3	1.5±0.3
	IDDM	8–12	20	2.2±0.4	0.9±0.3	1.7±0.4
	IDDM	13–15	20	2.5±0.8	0.9±0.6	1.7±0.5

All measurements in centimeters (mean ± standard deviation). IDDM = insulin-dependent diabetes mellitus.

gland in 5 of 13 children with acute pancreatitis, mostly involving the head and body.[1]

Fleischer and colleagues used the transverse dimension of the adjacent vertebral body (TVB) as a reference in their ultrasound study of children with acute pancreatitis (n = 19) compared with normals (n = 17). They evaluated the AP dimension of the body (PB) and found that PB/TVB was 0.3 ± 0.06 cm in normal children and 0.58 ± 0.24 cm in those with pancreatitis and suggested a cut-off of 0.3 cm.[10]

REFERENCES

1. Siegel MJ, Martin KW, Worthington JL: Normal and abnormal pancreas in children: US studies. Radiology 1987; 165:15–18.
2. Weill F, Schraub A, Eisenscher A, et al: Ultrasonography of the normal pancreas: Success rate and criteria for normality. Radiology 1977; 123:417–423.
3. Haber K, Freimanis AK, Asher WM: Demonstration and dimensional analysis of normal pancreas with gray-scale echography. AJR Am J Roentgenol 1976; 126:624–628.
4. Niederau C, Sonnenberg A, et al: Sonographic measurements of the normal liver, spleen, pancreas, and portal vein. Radiology 1983; 149:537–540.
5. Kreel L, Haertel M, Katz D: Computed tomography of the normal pancreas. J Comput Assist Tomogr 1977; 1:290–299.
6. Gilbeau JP, Poncelet V, Libon E, et al: The density, contour, and thickness of the pancreas in diabetics: CT findings in 57 patients. AJR Am J Roentgenol 1992; 159(3):527–531.
7. Altobelli E, Blasetti A, Verrotti A, et al: Size of pancreas in children and adolescents with type I (insulin-dependent) diabetes. J Clin Ultrasound 1998; 26:391–395.
8. Coleman BG, Arger PH, Rosenberg HK, et al: Gray-scale sonographic assessment of pancreatitis in children. Radiology 1983; 146:145–150.
9. Phillips HE, Cox KL, Reid MH, McGahan JP: Pancreatic sonography in cystic fibrosis. AJR Am J Roentgenol 1981; 137:69–72.
10. Fleischer AC, Parker P, Kirchner SG, James AE: Sonographic findings of pancreatitis in children. Radiology 1983; 146:151–155.

▪: DOPPLER ULTRASOUND OF PANCREATIC TRANSPLANTS
▪ ACR Code: 770 (Pancreas)

Table 1 ▪ Resistive Index (RI) of Small Arteries in Pancreatic Allografts

REFERENCE	PATHOLOGIC DIAGNOSIS	NO. PATIENTS	MEAN ± SD	RANGE
Patel[1]	Normal	52	0.59 ± 0.06	0.55–0.69
	Rejection	29	0.79 ± 0.08	0.55–0.94
	Cyclosporine toxicity	2	—	0.60–0.69
	Pancreatitis	10	—	0.55–0.64
Aideyan[2]	No rejection	9	0.64 ± 0.10	0.49–0.80
	Acute mild rejection	1	0.66	0.66
	Acute moderate rejection	5	0.67 ± 0.06	0.56–0.73
	Acute severe rejection	2	0.85 ± 0.07	0.80–0.90
Combined	Normal/no rejection	61	0.60 ± 0.07	0.49–0.80
	Rejection	37	0.77 ± 0.08	0.55–0.94

Technique ▪

Patel and colleagues used a 128 model scanner (Acuson, Mountain View, CA) with a 3.28-MHz phased-array transducer to perform duplex sonography of pancreatic transplants.[1] Aideyan and colleagues performed pancreatic transplant ultrasound with 128-XP10 (Acuson) or Ultramark 9 (Advanced Technology Laboratories, Bothell, WA) machines with 2- to 4-MHz sector or curved-array transducers.[2] Doppler signals were obtained from the main splenic artery[1] and from small intraparenchymal arteries within the graft.[1, 2]

Measurements ▪

Resistive index (RI) was calculated from duplex Doppler examinations using the following formula:

$$RI = (\text{peak systolic velocity} - \text{end-diastolic velocity})/\text{peak systolic velocity}.$$

Patel and group averaged the RI from up to three different locations within the grafts.[1] Table 1 lists the RI values from each study by clinical/pathologic diagnosis. The RI from the main splenic artery had a range of 0.70 to 0.74 and was not used to detect rejection.[1] Table 2 lists test performance of RI in diagnosing transplant rejection as calculated by Patel.[1]

Source ▪

Patel's subjects were 22 patients (16 male, 6 female, ages not given) who had undergone pancreatic transplant. A total of 98 separate examinations was done, ranging in time after transplant from 3 days to 1.5 years. Clinical status, laboratory data, and status of the corresponding renal transplant were used to establish the status of the pancreatic transplant. Biopsies of the pancreatic transplants were not done.[1] Aideyan and group evaluated 17 patients (6 men, 11 women, age range 24 to 60 years, mean age 41 years) who had undergone pancreatic transplantation and had biopsy of the graft up to 8 days after ultrasound examination. Histopathologic diagnoses from the biopsies were correlated with ultrasound findings.[2]

Table 2 ▪ Test Performance of Doppler Ultrasound in Detecting Pancreatic Transplant Rejection

RI	SENS.	SPEC.	PPV	NPV
≥0.50	100	0	31	100
≥0.55	100	22	37	100
≥0.60	97	41	42	96
≥0.65	97	66	48	98
≥0.70	76	100	100	90
≥0.75	66	100	100	86
≥0.80	45	100	100	80
≥0.85	17	100	100	73
≥0.90	17	100	100	70
≥0.95	0	100	100	69

RI = resistive index from small parenchymal arteries, Sens. = sensitivity, Spec. = specificity, PPV = positive predictive value, NPV = negative predictive value.
From Patel B, Wolverson MK, Mahanta B: Radiology 1989; 173:131–135. Used by permission.

Comments ▪

Patel and group found an RI of more than 0.70 in 7 of 8 (88%) episodes of rejection and suggest using this value for a cut-off.[1] Aideyan and associates found a significant difference in RI only between the no rejection and severe acute rejection groups and felt that there was too great an overlap of values for RI to be useful in predicting rejection.[2] This is supported by Kubota and colleagues, who reported acute rejection in some grafts with an RI of less than 0.70.[3] Gilabert and colleagues found that all patients having rejection fell above an RI of 0.80.[4]

REFERENCES

1. Patel B, Wolverson MK, Mahanta B: Pancreatic transplant rejection: Assessment with duplex US. Radiology 1989; 173:131–135.
2. Aideyan OA, Foshager MC, Beneditte E, et al: Correlation of the arterial resistive index in pancreas transplants of patients with transplant rejection. AJR Am J Roentgenol 1997; 168:1445–1447.
3. Kubota K, Billing H, Kelter U, et al: Duplex-Doppler ultrasonography for evaluating pancreatic grafts. Transpl Proc 1990; 22:183.
4. Gilabert R, Fernandez-Cruz L, Bru C, et al: Duplex-Doppler ultrasonography in monitering clinical pancreas transplantation. Transpl Int 1988; 1:172–177.

▪: THE NORMAL ENDOSCOPIC PANCREATOGRAMS[1]
▪ ACR Code: 774 (Pancreatic Ducts)

Table 1 ▪ Main Pancreatic Ductal Dimensions (mm)*				
	NO.	MEAN	RANGE	SD
Diameter				
Head	93	3.1	1.5–6.9	±0.9
Body	88	2.0	1.3–3.6	±0.7
Tail	83	0.9	0.6–2.3	±0.4
Length	80	169	107–223	±27

*Corrected for magnification.
From Varley PF, et al: Radiology 1976; 118:295–300. Used by permission.

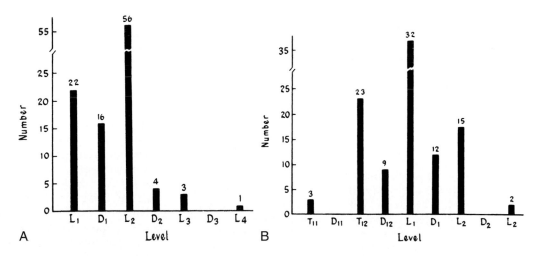

Figure 1 ▪ *A*, Level of the ampulla with respect to the lumbar spine. *L* = lumbar vertebra; *D* = intervening disc space. *B*, Level at which the main pancreatic duct crosses the spine. (From Varley PF, et al: Radiology 1976; 118:295. Used by permission.)

Technique ▪

Central ray: Perpendicular to plane of film.
Position: Anteroposterior supine.
Target-film distance: Immaterial. Magnification corrected using the dimension of the endoscope as a standard.

Measurements ▪

See Figure 1 and Table 1 for normal position and caliber of ducts.

The ampulla was found at the level of L2 in 75% of cases; the pancreatic duct crossed the spine at L1 in most cases. Mean ductal diameters were 3.1, 2.0, and 0.9 mm in the head, body, and tail, respectively.

Source ▪

Based on a study of 102 normal endoscopic pancreatograms in 68 men and 34 women from 11 to 81 years of age; 47% of the patients were between 40 and 60 years of age.

REFERENCE

1. Varley PF, Rohrmann CA Jr, Silvis SE, Vennes JA: The normal endoscopic pancreatogram. Radiology 1976; 118:295–300.

¨: PANCREATIC DUCT DIAMETER AT ERCP IN OLDER ADULTS
▪ ACR Code: 774 (Pancreatic Ducts)

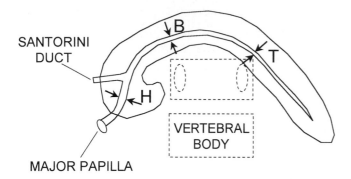

Figure 1 ▪ Measurement of the main pancreatic duct. Hastier and associates measured the diameter in three locations from pancreatograms; the greatest diameter in the head *(H)* between the papilla and the Santorini duct junction; in the body *(B)* adjacent to the right vertebral margin; and in the tail *(T)* adjacent to the left vertebral margin.[1] Measurement positions were not specified by Ladas et al.[2]

Table 1 ▪ Pancreatic Duct Diameter Through the 9th Decade

REFERENCE/GROUP	AGES (yr)	NO.	HEAD (mm) MEAN ± SD	BODY (mm) MEAN ± SD	TAIL (mm) MEAN ± SD
Hastier					
Normal	≤50	50	3.3 ± 1.2	2.3 ± 0.7	1.6 ± 0.4
Normal	70–79	47	4.8 ± 1.3	3.2 ± 1.1	2.1 ± 0.8
Normal	80–89	42	5.4 ± 2.1	4.1 ± 1.7	2.9 ± 1.4
Normal	90–99	16	6.4 ± 1.6	4.2 ± 1.4	3.0 ± 1.2
Ladas	≤40	17	2.82 ± 0.65	2.04 ± 0.51	1.09 ± 0.56
Normal	41–50	17	2.47 ± 0.60	2.20 ± 0.73	1.19 ± 0.40
Normal	51–60	58	2.92 ± 1.01	2.06 ± 0.55	1.16 ± 0.29
Normal	61–70	78	3.21 ± 1.21	2.38 ± 0.81	1.19 ± 0.38
Normal	71–80	56	3.70 ± 1.08	2.50 ± 0.64	1.91 ± 0.33
Normal	≥80	14	3.71 ± 0.93	2.74 ± 0.47	1.49 ± 0.19
Pancreatic cancer	mean = 64	60	5.28 ± 3.26	6.28 ± 3.36	5.17 ± 4.30
Chronic pancreatitis	mean = 61	38	5.21 ± 2.43	5.56 ± 3.66	3.29 ± 2.09

Technique ▪

Endoscopic retrograde cholangiopancreatography (ERCP) was done with standard techniques.[1, 2]

Measurements ▪

The pancreatic duct diameter was measured with calipers from pancreatograms obtained during ERCP in the head, body, and tail.[1, 2] Ladas and colleagues measured the length of the duct as well.[2] These measurements were corrected for radiographic magnification by using the apparent diameter of the endoscope tip. Figure 1 shows the measurement positions. Table 1 lists the results for duct diameters. The duct length (when filled) was 16.8 ± 2.3 cm in males, 15.9 ± 2.3 cm in females, and 16.4 ± 2.3 in those with normal pancreatograms.[2] The pancreatic duct (especially proximally) gradually increases in diameter by 1 to 3 mm from the 4th through 9th decades. Ladas and colleagues cited upper limits of normal of 8.0 mm, 4.0 mm, and 2.4 mm in the head, body, and tail, respectively, and found that distal measurements were more sensitive for pathologic dilation.[2]

Source ▪

Hastier and colleagues evaluated 155 adults with no evidence of pancreatic or biliary pathology on the ERCP.[1] Ladas and group evaluated 240 patients with morphologically normal pancreatograms and no history of pancreatic disease.[2] Age distributions for both these normal populations are listed in the data table. Ladas also reviewed pancreatograms from 60 patients (35 men, 25 women, mean age 64 years) with pancreatic cancer confirmed at surgery and 38 patients (24 men, 14 women, mean age 61 years) with chronic or relapsing pancreatitis.[2]

REFERENCES

1. Hastier P, Buckley MJ, Dumas R, et al: A study of the effect of age on pancreatic duct morphology. Gastrointest Endosc 1998; 48:53–57.
2. Ladas SD, Tassios PS, Giorgiotis K, et al: Pancreatic duct width: Its significance as a diagnostic criterion for pancreatic disease. Hepatogastroenterology 1993; 40:52–55.

▪: NORMAL PANCREATIC DUCT DIMENSIONS AT ULTRASOUND AND ERCP

▪ ACR Code: 774 (Pancreatic Ducts)

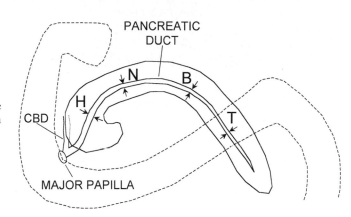

Figure 1 ▪ Measurements of the pancreatic duct diameter were done in the head *(H)*, neck *(N)*, body *(B)*, or tail *(T)*. CBD = common bile duct.

Technique ▪

Real-time ultrasound with 3- to 5-MHz linear,[1] B-mode static,[2, 4, 5] or sector[3, 5] transducers was done of the pancreas in fasting patients. Endoscopic retrograde cholangiopancreatography (ERCP) was performed with standard techniques.[5, 6]

Measurements ▪

Ultrasound measurements were made at the operator's console with electronic calipers or from hard copy images with manual calipers calibrated to distance scales on the images.[1-4] Ductal diameter measurements from ERCP films were made with calipers or ruler. The total duct length was measured from head to last visible portion in the tail. The measurements were corrected for magnification by comparison with the known diameter of the endoscope.[5, 6] Figure 1 shows diameter measurement locations of the duct in the head, body, and tail. Table 1 lists the reported measurements of the pancreatic duct diameter and length. The percentage of cases in which the normal duct lumen was visualized at ultrasound ranged from 45% to 84%.[1-3]

Didier and colleagues compared ultrasound and ERCP in a second group of 80 patients of whom 55 had duct dilation at ERCP. Ultrasound had a sensitivity of 65% and specificity of 95% in detecting dilation seen on ERCP, with 8 false-negatives and 2 false-positives.[6]

Source ▪

Patient age ranges and numbers of subjects are shown in Table 1. All subjects were considered to have normal ultrasound and ERCP studies and had no history of pancreatitis or other pancreatic disease. Often patients with pancreatic problems were described in the papers, and only the normal or control patients are listed in Table 1.[1-6]

REFERENCE	AGE RANGE (Yr)	NO.	PORTION	MEAN ± SD	RANGE	LUMEN SEEN WITH U/S (%)
Ohto—U/S[1]	Adults	25	Body		0.0–0.8	84
Parulekar—U/S[2]	20–65	100	Body	1.3 ± 0.3	0.6–2.6	82
Lawson—U/S[3]	Adults	31	Body	1.3 ± 0.4	0.0–2.0	45
Hadidi–U/S[4]	22–59	45	Head	3.0	2.8–3.3	NR
	22–59	45	Neck	2.1	2.0–4.0	NR
	22–59	45	Body	1.6	1.0–1.7	NR
Varley—ERCP[5]	11–81	93	Head	3.1 ± 0.9	1.5–6.9	—
	11–81	88	Body	2.0 ± 0.7	1.3–3.6	—
	11–81	83	Tail	0.9 ± 0.4	0.6–2.3	—
		80	Length	169 ± 27	107–223	—
Didier—ERCP[6]	21–85	37	Head	3.4 ± 0.9	1.5–5.0	—
	21–85	37	Body	2.6 ± 0.7	1.5–4.0	—
	21–85	37	Tail	1.6 ± 0.45	1.5–2.5	—
	21–85	37	Length	180 ± 24	170–230	—

Table 1 ▪ Normal Pancreatic Duct Diameters

All measurements are in millimeters. ERCP = endoscopic retrograde cholangio-pancreatography. NR = not reported.

REFERENCES

1. Ohto M, Saotome N, Saisho H, et al: Real-time sonography of the pancreatic duct: Application to percutaneous pancreatic ductography. AJR Am J Roentgenol 1980; 134:647–652.
2. Parulekar SG: Ultrasonic evaluation of the pancreatic duct. J Clin Ultrasound 1980; 8:457–463.
3. Lawson TL, Berland LL, Foley WD, et al: Ultrasound visualization of the pancreatic duct. Radiology 1982; 144:865–871.
4. Hadidi A: Pancreatic duct diameter: Sonographic measurement in normal subjects. J Clin Ultrasound 1983; 11:17–22.
5. Varley PF, Rohrmann CA Jr, Silvis SE, Vennes JA: The normal endoscopic pancreatogram. Radiology 1976; 118(2):295–300.
6. Didier D, Deschamps JP, Rhomer P, et al: Evaluation of the pancreatic duct: A reappraisal based on a retrospective correlative study by sonography and pancreatography in 117 normal and pathologic subjects. Ultrasound Med Biol 1983; 9:509–518.

▪: MEASUREMENT OF NORMAL PANCREATIC DUCT USING REAL-TIME ULTRASOUND[1]

▪ ACR Code: 774 (Pancreatic Ducts)

Technique ▪

1. Patients were imaged with a linear array real-time scanner using a 3.5-MHz focused transducer.
2. Images were stored on an analogue freeze-frame device.
3. Most patients fasted overnight and received a laxative the previous day. If the pancreas was nonvisualized because of overlying bowel gas, the patient was given water to drink and rescanned in the erect position.

Measurements ▪ (Tables 1 and 2)

In 65 patients, the pancreatic duct was identified as a tubular structure. Only a single line could be identified in 21 patients.

There was a tendency for younger patients to have smaller ducts, but this was not statistically significant.

Source ▪

One hundred patients who were having abdominal sonograms for reasons other than biliary or pancreatic disease, in whom at least a portion of the pancreas was seen.

Table 1 ▪ Appearance of the Pancreatic Duct

Single line	21
1 mm	47
2 mm	17
3 mm	1
Not seen	14
TOTAL	100

From Bryan PJ: J Clin Ultrasound 1982; 10:63–66. Used by permission.

Table 2 ▪ Segment of the Pancreatic Duct Seen

Body alone	64
Head and body	20
Head alone	2
Not seen	14

From Bryan PJ: J Clin Ultrasound 1982; 10:63–66. Used by permission.

REFERENCE

1. Bryan PJ: Appearance of normal pancreatic duct: A study using real-time ultrasound. J Clin Ultrasound 1982; 10:63–66.

▪: EFFECTS OF AGING AND SECRETIN ON PANCREATIC DUCT DIAMETER AT ULTRASOUND

▪ ACR Code: 774 (Pancreatic Ducts)

Technique ▪

Ultrasound of the pancreas was done with a real-time ultrasound scanner (type not specified) and a 3.5-MHz curved-array transducer. In a separate group of patients, scanning was repeated several times during the 10 minutes after intravenous injection of 1.0 CU/kg of Secretin (Kabi Vitrum or Hoechst).[1]

Measurements ▪

The pancreatic duct was measured with electronic calipers above the aorta, including the echogenic walls, from frozen images.[1] Figure 1 shows the measurement position. Table 1 lists the results.

Source ▪

Subjects included 84 patients who had no history, laboratory findings, or imaging findings of pancreatic or biliary disease, to determine the effect of aging on duct size. Three additional subsets of patients (n = 9 each) were scanned before and after Secretin stimulation. These consisted of normal young adults, normal elderly adults, and patients with chronic pancreatitis.[1] Age ranges and numbers of the 84 normals are given in Table 1.

Comments ▪

These data show that the pancreatic duct measured by U/S increases by about 33% in size with aging (p <.01). The upper limit of normal at ultrasound (mean + 2 SD), even for the most elderly, is still 3.0 mm. In 18 normal patients, the duct almost doubled in size after Secretin stimulation (1.8 mm to 3.4 mm), whereas in those with chronic pancreatitis there was no significant change (2.9 mm to 3.0 mm). Secretin stimulation may be helpful in

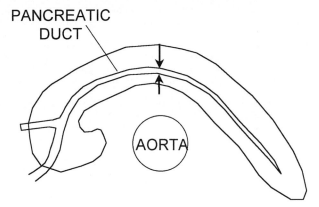

Figure 1 ▪ Measurement of the main pancreatic duct. Measurement from transverse ultrasound was done in the body adjacent to the aorta.

AGE RANGE (Yr)	NO.	PANCREATIC DUCT DIAMETER (mm)		
		Men	Women	Total
18–29	16	1.7 ± 0.5	1.4 ± 0.5	1.5 ± 0.5
30–39	15	1.7 ± 0.6	1.5 ± 0.4	1.6 ± 0.5
40–49	13	1.8 ± 0.4	2.0 ± 0.3	1.9 ± 0.3
50–59	16	2.0 ± 0.6	2.1 ± 0.3	2.0 ± 0.5
60–69	11	2.0 ± 0.3	2.2 ± 0.5	2.1 ± 0.4
70–81	13	2.2 ± 0.5	1.9 ± 0.5	2.0 ± 0.5

Table 1 ▪ Pancreatic Duct Diameters with Aging and Secretin Stimulation

Measurements are given as mean ± standard deviation.
From Glaser J, Hogemann B, Krummenerl T, et al: Dig Dis Sci 1987; 32:1075–1081. Used by permission.

distinguishing age-related pancreatic duct dilation from that caused by chronic pancreatitis by virtue of the fact that normal subjects show increased diameters and those with chronic pancreatitis do not.[1] *Note*: Abnormally increased duct size after Secretin stimulation has been noted in patients with sphincter of Oddi dysfunction and pancreas divisum.[2–5]

REFERENCES

1. Glaser J, Hogemann B, Krummenerl T, et al: Sonographic imaging of the pancreatic duct: New diagnostic possibilities using secretin stimulation. Dig Dis Sci 1987; 32:1075–1081.
2. Warshaw AL, Simeone J, Schapiro RH, et al: Objective evaluation of ampullary stenosis with ultrasonography and pancreatic stimulation. Am J Surg 1985; 149:65–72.
3. Lowes JR, Lees JR, Cotton PB: Pancreatic duct dilatation after secretin stimulation in patients with pancreas divisum. Pancreas 1989; 4.371–374.
4. Cavallini G, Rigo L, Bovo P, et al: Abnormal US response of main pancreatic duct after secretin stimulation in patients with acute pancreatitis of different etiology. Clin Gastroenterol 1994; 18:298–303.
5. Matos C, Metens T, Deviere J, et al: Pancreatic duct: Morphologic and functional evaluation with dynamic MR pancreatography after secretin stimulation. Radiology 1997; 203:335–341.

▪: MEASUREMENT OF SPLEEN POSITION AND SIZE[1]
▪ ACR Code: 775 (Spleen)

Technique ▪

Central ray: At the level of the iliac crests on the median plane.
Position: Anteroposterior.
Target-film distance: 36 inches.

Measurements ▪ (Figure 1 and Table 1)

The transverse diameter of the lower pole of the spleen was determined at a point 2 cm above the tip of the lower pole.

Enlargement of the splenic shadow occurs in a signifi-

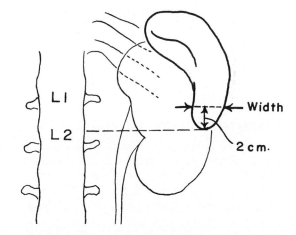

Figure 1 ▪ Measurement of the spleen from abdominal radiographs. The position of the inferior tip was related to the adjacent vertebral level. Its width was measured 2 centimeters above the tip.

Table 1 ▪ Normal Spleen Position and Width on Abdominal Radiographs

NO. CASES (288 Total)	AGE (Yr)	LEVEL OF LOWER POLE TIP	WIDTH (cm) AT 2 cm ABOVE TIP OF SPLEEN
16	Under 5	L1–L3 (usually L2)	2.0–3.6 (avg. 3.0)
37	5–10	L1–L3 (usually L1–L2)	2.5–3.8 (avg. 3.3)
36	11–20	L1–L3 (usually L1–L2)	2.5–3.8 (avg. 3.2)
82	21–30	T12–L2 (usually L1)	2.0–4.2 (avg. 3.5)
117	Over 30	T12–L2 (usually L1)	2.0–4.6 (avg. 3.5)

cantly large number of cases of ruptured spleen. Because the spleen outline is not demonstrated in 58% of abdominal roentgenograms, absence of this sign does not exclude the diagnosis of ruptured spleen.

Source ▪

Five hundred consecutive cases with films of the abdomen were evaluated regardless of the diagnostic problem.

REFERENCE

1. Wyman AC: AJR Am J Roentgenol 1954; 72:51.

▪▪ MEASUREMENT OF SPLEEN LENGTH[1]
▪ ACR Code: 775 (Spleen)

Technique ▪

Central ray: Centered over spleen.
Position: Anteroposterior abdomen.
Target-film distance: 100 cm.

Film taken in deep inspiration.

Measurements ▪

The spleen length is the distance between the level of the most cranial part of the diaphragmatic arch and the lower pole of the spleen.

Mean length = 12.4 ± 2.2 cm (range, 8–19 cm). If the spleen length exceeds 16 cm, there is 97% probability that the spleen is enlarged.

Source ▪

Studies were made of 50 adults (23 men, 27 women) without known symptoms or signs of liver or spleen disease.

REFERENCE

1. Bergstrand I, Eckman C-A: Acta Radiol 1957; 47:1.

▪▪ SPLEEN LENGTH RELATED TO VERTEBRAL HEIGHT[1]
▪ ACR Code: 775 (Spleen)

Technique ▪

Central ray: Perpendicular to the plane of the film.
Position: Anteroposterior upright.
Target-film distance: Immaterial.

Measurements ▪ (Figure 1)

The spleen is measured from its most superior extent under the diaphragm to its caudal tip. This is compared with the distance from the upper margin of T12 to the lower margin of L3. Normal values are given in Figure 2. The normal ratio of spleen length to the vertebral height T12–L3 is

0.82 ± 0.09. Two standard deviations are represented by ratios from 0.64 to 1.0. Spleen length greater than vertebral height T12–L3 indicates pathologic enlargement of the spleen.

Source ▪

Based on a study of 97 healthy adult patients.

REFERENCE

1. Schindler G, Longin F, Helmschrott M: [The individual limit of normal spleen size in routine x-ray film (author's translation)] [German]. Radiologe 1976; 16:166–171.

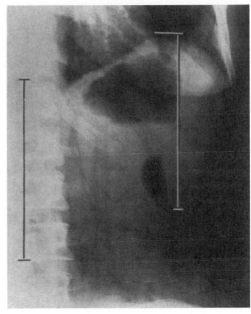

Figure 1 ▪ Measurement of the spleen. (From Schindler G, et al: Radiologe 1976;16:166. Used by permission.)

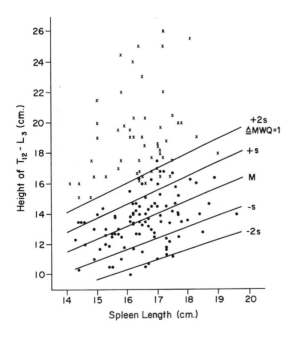

Figure 2 ▪ Normal range of the measurements of the spleen related to the height of T12–L3. The *dots* are normals. The *x's* are patients with splenomegaly. (From Schindler G, et al: Radiologe 1976;16:166. Used by permission.)

▪⫶ SPLEEN LENGTH IN CHILDREN AND ADOLESCENTS
▪ ACR Code: 775 (Spleen)

Table 1 ▪ Length of Spleen in Children Versus Body Height and Age

BODY HEIGHT (cm)	NO.	AGE RANGE (mon)	MEAN ± SD	RANGE	NORMAL LIMITS
48–64	52	1–3	53 ± 7.8	33–71	30–70
54–73	39	4–6	59 ± 6.3	45–71	40–75
65–78	18	7–8	63 ± 7.6	50–77	45–80
71–92	18	12–30	70 ± 9.6	54–86	54–85
85–109	27	36–59	75 ± 8.4	60–91	55–95
100–130	30	60–83	84 ± 9.0	61–100	60–105
110–131	36	84–107	85 ± 10.5	65–102	65–105
125–149	29	108–131	86 ± 10.7	64–114	65–110
137–153	17	132–155	97 ± 9.7	72–100	75–115
143–168	21	156–179	101 ± 11.7	84–120	80–120
152–175	12	180–200	101 ± 10.3	88–120	85–120

All measurements are in centimeters.
From Konus OL, Ozdemir A, Akkaya A, et al: AJR Am J Roentgenol 1998; 171:1693–1698. Used by permission.

Table 2 ▪ Spleen Length in Children and Adolescents

GROUP	NO.	10TH CENTILE	MEDIAN	90TH CENTILE	UPPER LIMIT
0–3 mon	28	3.3	4.5	5.8	6.0
3–6 mon	13	4.9	5.3	6.4	6.5
6–12 mon	17	5.2	6.2	6.8	7.0
1–2 yr	12	5.4	6.9	7.5	8.0
2–4 yr	24	6.4	7.4	8.6	9.0
4–6 yr	39	6.9	7.8	8.8	9.5
6–8 yr	21	7.0	8.2	9.6	10.0
8–10 yr	16	7.9	9.2	10.5	11.0
10–12 yr	17	8.6	9.9	10.9	11.5
12–15 yr	26	8.7	10.1	11.4	12.0
15–20 yr (male)	5	9.0	10.0	11.7	12.0
15–20 yr (female)	12	10.1	11.2	12.6	13.0

All measurements are in centimeters. Upper limits are the next highest whole integer over the 90th percentile.
From Rosenberg HK, Markowitz RI, Kolberg H, et al: AJR Am J Roentgenol 1991; 157:119–121. Used by permission.

Technique ▪

Konus and colleagues performed ultrasound of the abdomen with SSA 27A (Toshiba, Tokyo, Japan) and EUB-515 (Hitachi, Tokyo, Japan) machines and 3.5-MHz transducers.[1] Rosenberg and colleagues also did abdominal ultrasound (machine and transducer types not reported).[2] Patients were supine, breathing quietly, and unsedated.[1, 2] Occasionally, right-side-down oblique scanning was done to visualize the spleen better.[2]

Measurements ▪

From frozen images of coronally oriented scans, the cephalocaudal dimension (length) was measured from the most superomedial to the most inferolateral points. Table 1 lists spleen lengths by age and body height of the patients.[1] Table 2 lists spleen lengths by age and by gender for 15 to 20 year olds.[2]

Source ▪

Konus' subjects were 307 children (138 boys, 169 girls, age range neonate to 16 years) with no history, clinical findings, or sonographic evidence of disease affecting the spleen.[1] Rosenberg studied 230 patients (89 boys, 141 girls, age range neonate to 20 years), with no splenic abnormalities, scanned for unrelated reasons.[2]

Comments ▪

There were no significant differences between genders at any age except between 15 and 20 years in Rosenberg's study.[1, 2] The best correlation between splenic measurements and patient parameters was for spleen length versus body height.[1]

REFERENCES

1. Konus OL, Ozdemir A, Akkaya A, et al: Normal liver, spleen, and kidney dimensions in neonates, infants and children: Evaluation with sonography. AJR Am J Roentgenol 1998; 171:1693–1698.
2. Rosenberg HK, Markowitz RI, Kolberg H, et al: Normal splenic size in infants and children: Sonographic measurements. AJR Am J Roentgenol 1991; 157:119–121.

•: SPLEEN LENGTH THROUGHOUT LIFE
■ ACR Code: 775 (Spleen)

Table 1 • Normal Spleen Length from Birth Through the
9th Decade in 783 Subjects

AGE RANGE (Yr)	NUMBER MALES	MALE MEAN ± SD	NUMBER FEMALES	FEMALE MEAN ± SD
0–4	65	5.94 ± 1.18	38	5.77 ± 1.21
5–9	40	7.81 ± 1.28	25	7.48 ± 1.21
10–14	27	9.10 ± 1.41	28	8.76 ± 1.10
15–19	10	10.04 ± 1.29	21	8.61 ± 1.03
20–29	25	9.57 ± 1.05	40	9.08 ± 1.26
30–39	40	9.52 ± 1.29	41	8.88 ± 1.28
40–49	41	9.38 ± 1.48	44	8.92 ± 1.54
50–59	40	8.83 ± 1.33	39	8.25 ± 1.39
60–69	43	8.99 ± 1.61	40	8.66 ± 1.50
70–79	44	8.60 ± 1.62	42	8.25 ± 1.54
80–89	25	7.90 ± 1.85	25	7.59 ± 1.53

All measurements are in centimeters.
From Loftus WK, Metrewili C: J Ultrasound Med 1997; 16:345–347. Used by permission.

Technique ■

Ultrasound of the left abdomen was done (machine and transducer parameters not given).[1]

Measurements ■

The maximum cephalocaudal length of the spleen was measured from oblique sagittal scans through the hilum.[1] Results are listed in Table 1. Gender differences were significant (p <.05) only from ages 15 to 39 years.[1]

Source ■

Subjects consisted of 783 Hong Kong Chinese patients (age and gender distribution given in Table 1) with no known splenic disease.[1]

REFERENCE

1. Loftus WK, Metrewili C: Normal splenic size in a Chinese population. J Ultrasound Med 1997; 16:345–347.

•: VOLUME OF THE SPLEEN IN CHILDREN AT CT
■ ACR Code: 775 (Spleen)

Technique ■

Prassopoulos and Schlesinger and their colleagues performed CT of the abdomen (machine type and parameters not given).[1, 2] Younger children were sedated with chloral hydrate, and older children were examined in quiet expiration.[1]

Measurements ■

Both groups measured the volume of the spleen by summing traced areas of the spleen on all sections containing it and correcting for slice interval.[1, 2] Prassopoulos measured the splenic width and thickness from the scan through the hilum. The largest area was traced and recorded and the cephalocaudal length determined by the difference in table positions between the top and bottom. The transverse diameter of L1 was measured and noted.[1] Figure 1 shows measurements made at the hilar level. Table 1 lists the splenic dimensions and volumes by age.[1] Figure 2 depicts splenic volume by patient weight.[2]

Prassopoulos performed linear regression between linear dimensions and volume and found that the product of length, width, and thickness correlated best (r = 0.91, p <.001) with volume.[1] Schlesinger regressed volume on weight and produced the following equation:

$$\text{Volume} = 0.7 + 4.6 \times \text{weight (kg)}.$$
$$(r = 0.85 \text{ for } 0 \text{ to } 75 \text{ kg}).$$

This equation may be simplified to obtain a "rule of thumb" for this weight range:

$$\text{Volume} = 4.5 \times \text{weight (kg)}.$$
$$\text{Upper limit (95\%) of volume} =$$
$$150 + 4.5 \times \text{weight (kg)}.$$

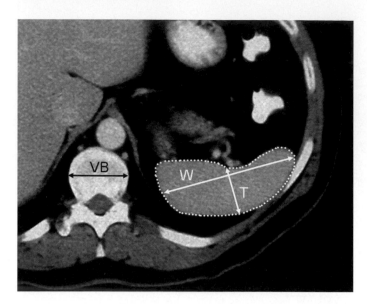

Figure 1 ▪ Measurements of the spleen from CT. The width *(W)* and thickness *(T)* were measured on the slice through the hilum. The perimeter *(dotted line)* was traced on all slices and the area obtained from software on the scanner. Areas were summed to obtain volume (with correction for slice interval). The width of L1 *(VB)* was also measured (L1 was on a different slice of the scan depicted here).

Table 1 ▪ Normal Spleen Dimensions and Volumes in 153 Children

AGE (Yr)	NO.	LENGTH (cm)	THICKNESS (cm)	WIDTH (cm)	AREA (max) (sq cm)	VOLUME (ml)	THICKNESS/ L1 DIAMETER
0.5–1	6	4.0 ± 0.8	1.9 ± 0.3	4.6 ± 1.0	7 ± 2	23 ± 6	0.9 ± 0.2
1–2	7	4.4 ± 0.7	2.0 ± 0.4	5.0 ± 0.9	9 ± 2	24 ± 7	0.8 ± 0.2
2–3	7	6.0 ± 1.0	2.8 ± 0.3	6.8 ± 1.2	17 ± 4	79 ± 25	1.0 ± 0.2
3–4	14	6.2 ± 1.1	3.0 ± 0.5	7.2 ± 1.4	22 ± 4	108 ± 29	1.1 ± 0.1
4–5	16	6.2 ± 0.9	3.3 ± 0.2	7.3 ± 1.0	23 ± 3	121 ± 32	1.2 ± 0.1
5–6	11	6.5 ± 1.0	3.3 ± 0.4	8.1 ± 1.1	26 ± 4	130 ± 34	1.0 ± 0.2
6–7	12	7.0 ± 1.4	3.3 ± 0.5	8.2 ± 1.5	25 ± 5	134 ± 34	1.1 ± 0.1
7–8	9	7.1 ± 1.1	3.8 ± 0.6	7.6 ± 1.7	26 ± 4	135 ± 39	1.2 ± 0.2
8–9	8	7.0 ± 0.9	3.5 ± 0.6	8.8 ± 2.1	25 ± 7	132 ± 44	1.1 ± 0.1
9–10	9	8.0 ± 1.1	4.0 ± 0.5	8.9 ± 2.0	28 ± 6	134 ± 38	1.2 ± 0.1
10–11	10	7.1 ± 0.8	4.1 ± 0.7	10.3 ± 2.1	30 ± 7	145 ± 41	1.1 ± 0.2
11–12	11	7.7 ± 0.9	3.9 ± 0.5	9.2 ± 2.2	29 ± 8	142 ± 39	1.1 ± 0.1
12–13	7	8.6 ± 1.3	4.3 ± 0.7	10.2 ± 1.9	25 ± 8	155 ± 37	1.2 ± 0.3
13–14	12	8.7 ± 1.1	4.4 ± 0.8	10.8 ± 2.1	35 ± 7	185 ± 48	1.3 ± 0.2
14–15	14	9.4 ± 1.7	4.1 ± 0.5	8.8 ± 2.4	32 ± 8	170 ± 41	1.1 ± 0.3

All measurements given as mean ± standard deviation. L1 = 1st lumbar vertebra.
From Prassopoulos P, Cavouras D: Acta Radiol 1994; 35(2):152–154. Used by permission.

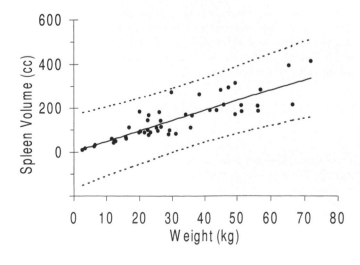

Figure 2 ▪ Splenic volume versus weight (0–75 kg) in 48 children. Individual measurements *(circles)*, linear regression *(solid line)*, and 95% tolerance intervals *(dotted lines)* are shown. (From Schlesinger AE, Edgar KA, Boxer LA: AJR Am J Roentgenol 1993;160(5):1107–1109. Used by permission.)

Source ▪

Prassopoulos studied 153 children (87 boys, 66 girls, age range 5 months to 15 years) with no clinical or imaging evidence of splenic abnormality.[1] Schlesinger evaluated 48 children (30 boys, 18 girls, age range neonate to 18 years) with normal spleens on CT and no diseases that might be expected to cause splenic enlargement.[2]

REFERENCES

1. Prassopoulos P, Cavouras D: CT assessment of normal splenic size in children. Acta Radiol 1994; 35(2):152–154.
2. Schlesinger AE, Edgar KA, Boxer LA: Volume of the spleen in children as measured on CT scans: Normal standards as a function of body weight. AJR Am J Roentgenol 1993; 160(5):1107–1109.

▪▪ PREDICTION OF SPLENIC VOLUME BY LINEAR MEASUREMENTS AT CT

▪ ACR Code: 775 (Spleen)

Technique ▪

Schlesinger and colleagues performed CT of the abdomen with a Somatom Plus S (Siemens, Erlangen, Germany), with 33 of 50 scans done conventionally and 17 of 50 scans using spiral technique.[1] Cools and colleagues used a Somatom SF CT scanner (Siemens) to perform abdominal studies with 5-sec scan time, slice thickness of 8 mm, and 230 mAs.[2]

Measurements ▪

Both groups traced the perimeter of the spleen on all sections containing it and summed the areas with correction for slice interval to obtain the volume, and this was used as the true volume.[1, 2] Both groups measured the length (L) of the spleen by taking the difference between table positions of the top and bottom slices. The width (W) was measured at its widest point and the thickness (T) was measured at two places on 2 slices (total of 4 measurements = T1–T4). The positions of W and T1–T4 measurements are shown in Figure 1. Linear regression was done between various combinations of single and mul-

tiple linear measurements, and these results are shown in Table 1. Cools and colleagues found the best correlation between the product $L \times W \times T2$.[2] Schlesinger and group found nearly equal correlations between the $L \times W \times T2$ and $L \times W \times T3$ products and concluded that the former was preferable because it could be done from one slice (maximal width).[1]

The equations for spleen volume cited by each investigator are:

Spleen volume (ml) =
$$(0.7664 \times [L \times W \times T2]) + 10.97 \text{ (Cools)}.$$

Spleen volume (ml) =
$$(0.67 \times [L \times W \times T2]) + 7.52 \text{ (Schlesinger)}.$$

These relationships are depicted in Figure 2. Considering the similarity of the studies, it might be reasonable to use an equation containing the average values for slope and constant:

Spleen volume (ml) =
$$(0.7182 \times [L \times W \times T2]) + 9.25.$$

Source ▪

Schlesinger and colleagues evaluated 50 consecutive children (26 boys, 24 girls, age range 8 days to 19 years, mean

SECTION WITH MAXIMUM WIDTH

SECTION WITH MAXIMUM THICKNESS

Figure 1 ▪ Linear measurements of the spleen for CT volume estimation. The width (W) was measured along the long axis on the slice at which it was widest. Thickness was measured perpendicular to the long axis on the same slice, at its maximum (T1) and at the midpoint (T2). The thickness was also measured on the slice where it was maximal (T3) and at the midpoint (T4) on the same slice.

Table 1 ▪ Regression of Linear Measurement Combinations and Spleen Volume by Summing Areas

REFERENCE	NO.	LINEAR PARAMETERS (x)	SLOPE (a)	INTERCEPT (b)	r VALUE
Cools	50	L	67.98	−271.9	0.811
	50	W	93.68	−651.9	0.858
	50	L × W	4.787	−130.7	0.954
	50	L × W × T1			0.982
	50	L × W × T2	0.7664	+10.97	0.991
	50	L × W × T3			0.988
	50	L × W × T4			0.979
Schlesinger	50	L × W × T1			0.96
	50	L × W × T2	0.67	+7.52	0.97
	50	L × W × T3			0.99
	50	L × W × T4			0.95

Values of slope (a) and intercept (b) are given for equations of the form: volume = ax + b (x = linear measurement or product). L = length, W and T1–T4 as in Figure 1.[1, 2]

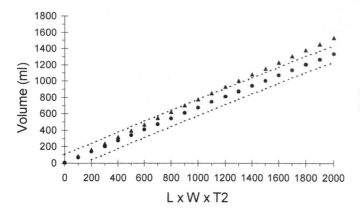

Figure 2 ▪ Linear regression of the product *(L × W × T2)* plotted against volume derived by summing traced areas from Schlesinger *(circles)* and Cools *(triangles)*. Schlesinger's 95% prediction intervals *(dotted lines)* are also shown.[1, 2]

age 8 years and 10 months) referred for abdominal CT scanning.[1] Cools and associates studied 50 subjects (age and sex not given) with both normal and pathologically enlarged spleens.[2]

Comments ▪

Lackner and colleagues found the simple product of L × W × T of the spleen at CT to lie between 120 and 480 in normal adults.[3] Strijk recorded L × W × T products ranging between 153 and 690 in adult lymphoma patients with histologically normal spleens and derived an equation to predict splenic weight: Weight (gm) = 0.55 (L × W × T).[4] Cools and group reported the values for each splenic dimension: L = 7.56 ± 3.32 (range 3.2 to 17.8), W = 9.95 ± 2.55 (range 3.2 to 18.2), T2 = 3.26 ± 1.14 (1.8 to 6.4), though it should be noted that some of the

subjects had varying amounts of enlargement.[2] Henderson (detailed in a separate section) found the normal splenic volume by summation of areas on CT to be 219 ± 76 ml.[5]

REFERENCES

1. Schlesinger AE, Hildebolt CF, Siegel MJ, Pilgrim TK: Splenic volume in children: Simplified estimation at CT. Radiology 1994; 193:578–580.
2. Cools L, Osteaux M, Divano L, et al: Prediction of splenic volume by a simple CT measurement: A statistical study. J Comput Assist Tomogr 1983; 7:426–430.
3. Lackner K, Brecht G, Janson R, et al: Wertigkeit der computertomographie brei der stadieneinteilung primarer lymphoknotenneoplasien. Fortschr Rontgenstr 1980; 132:21–30.
4. Strijk SP, Wagener DJT, Bogman MJJT, et al: The spleen in Hodgkin disease: Diagnostic value of CT. Radiology 1985; 154:753–757.
5. Henderson JM, Heymsfield SB, Horowitz J, et al: Measurement of liver and spleen volume by computed tomography: Assessment of reproducibility and changes found following a selective distal splenorenal shunt. Radiology 1981; 141:525–527.

▪: ESTIMATION OF SPLEEN VOLUME BY ULTRASOUND
▪ ACR Code: 775 (Spleen)

Technique ▪

Ultrasound of the abdomen was done with an Ultramark 9 machine (ATL, Bothel, WA), and CT scans of the abdomen were done with a 2400 Elite unit (Elscint, Haifa, Israel) with 10-mm slices.[1]

Measurements ▪

The spleen was measured in three dimensions (in centimeters) on ultrasound (longitudinal = LON, transverse at the maximal plane = TRV, and true anteroposterior = AP). Spleen volume was derived from CT slices by tracing the area on all levels containing it and summing them.[1] Correlation between spleen volume by CT and the product of linear ultrasound measurements yielded p = .0001, r = 0.8656, and the following equation:

Spleen volume by CT (ml) =
$$539.5 + 0.344 \ (LON \times TRV \times AP).[1]$$

Source ▪

Spleen volume was determined 69 times with both modalities in 33 patients (14 male, 19 female, age range 10 to 57 years) with Gaucher disease and varying degrees of splenomegaly.[1]

REFERENCE

1. Elstein D, Hadas-Halpern I, Azure Y, et al: Accuracy of ultrasonography in assessing spleen and liver size in patients with Gaucher disease: Comparison to computed tomographic measurements. J Ultrasound Med 1997; 16:209–211.

▪ THICKNESS OF THE LESSER OMENTUM FOR DETECTION OF PORTAL HYPERTENSION

▪ ACR Code: 799 (Lesser Omentum)

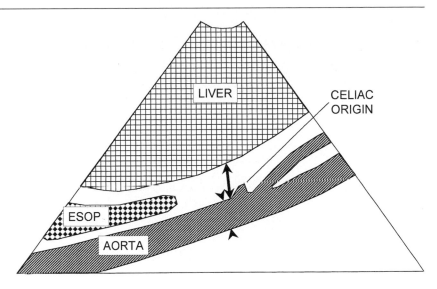

Figure 1 ▪ Measurement of the lesser omentum (LO) from paramedian longitudinal ultrasound. The LO was measured between the posterior liver and anterior aorta (Ao) at the level of the celiac origin *(line with arrowheads)*. The AP diameter of the aorta was measured at the same level *(arrowheads)*. A ratio was formed (LO/Ao) that had an average value of 1.7 in normals and often exceeds 2.0 in patients with varices. ESOP = esophagus.

Technique ▪

Longitudinal paramedian real-time ultrasound of the upper abdomen was performed, centered over the aorta and the origins of the celiac axis and superior mesenteric artery.[1]

Measurements ▪

The anteroposterior (AP) distance between the anterior wall of the aorta and the posterior border of the liver was measured at the origin of the celiac artery. This was taken to be the thickness of the lesser omentum (LO). The AP diameter of the aorta (Ao) was measured at the same level. A ratio was formed (LO/Ao), which was compared in the normal and portal hypertension groups. Change in normal subjects with age was also evaluated. Figure 1 shows the measurement. Figure 2 is a scatterplot of the LO/Ao ratios versus age for both groups. There was no change in LO/Ao with age in the normal subjects. The normal mean and standard deviations were 1.1 ± 0.27, and the range was 0.57 to 1.70. In the patients with portal hypertension and varices, LO/Ao exceeded 2.0 in all cases, the mean and

standard deviations were 2.65 ± 0.55, and the range was 1.94 to 3.40.[1]

Source ▪

Children and adolescents were scanned ranging in age from 1 week to 20 years of age, with no history, clinical evidence, or imaging findings to suggest portal hypertension or other abnormality that might distort the lesser omentum. A second group of 10 children was studied, ranging in age from 1 to 20 years, with portal hypertension and esophageal varices.[1]

Comments ▪

An LO/Ao ratio of 2.0 or greater in children and adolescents is highly suggestive of esophageal varices in the appropriate clinical setting.[1, 2] Possible causes of false-positives are obesity, steroid therapy, and interposition of the pancreas.[1] In a study of adults with varices, Subramanyam found that 5 of 32 had a somewhat thickened lesser omentum, and it was not seen in 27.[3]

Figure 2 ▪ Scatterplot of lesser omentum thickness to aorta diameter ratio *(LO/Ao)* in 150 normal children and adolescents *(dots)* and in 10 with portal hypertension and varices *(triangles)*. (From Patriquin H, Tessier G, Grignon A, Boisvert J: AJR Am J Roentgenol 1985;145:693–696. Used by permission.)

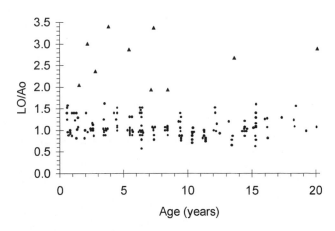

REFERENCES

1. Patriquin H, Tessier G, Grignon A, Boisvert J: Lesser omental thickness in normal children: Baseline for detection of portal hypertension. AJR Am J Roentgenol 1985; 145:693–696.

2. Brunelle F, Alagille D, Pariente D, Chaumont P: Étude echographique de l'hypertension portale chez l'enfant. Ann Radiol 1981; 24:121–130.

3. Subramanyam BR, Balthazar EJ, Madamba MR, et al: Sonography of portosystemic venous collaterals in portal hypertension. Radiology 1983; 146:161–166.

⁚ DENSITY OF LIVER, SPLEEN, AND KIDNEYS FOR MASS DETERMINATION

- ACR Code: 78 (Organ Density)

Technique ▪

Excised liver, spleen, and kidneys from 12 cadavers were weighed and the volume determined by water displacement.

Measurements ▪

The densities (grams, milliliters, mean ± standard error) were liver, 1.058 ± 0.011; spleen, 1.043 ± 0.011; and kidney, 1.037 ± 0.006. To calculate mass from volume derived by imaging, simply multiply by the appropriate density. This was validated using CT volumes obtained by summing areas with the same organs. The differences between calculated and true mass expressed as percentage of true mass averaged 5.6%, with a range of 3% to 13%.

REFERENCE

1. Heymsfield SB, Fulenwider T, Nordlinger B: Accurate measurement of liver, kidney, and spleen volume and mass by computerized tomography. Ann Intern Med 1979; 90:185–187.

CHAPTER 12

Genitourinary System

': KIDNEY LENGTH CORRELATED WITH AGE IN CHILDREN[1]
- ACR Code: 81 (Kidney)

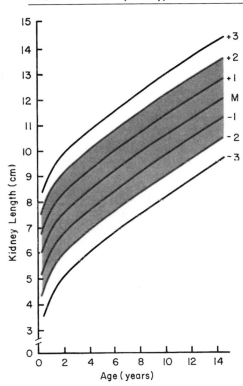

Figure 1 ▪ Graph of kidney length versus age, including 3 SD above and below the mean: 1 SD = 0.785 cm. (From Currarino G, et al: Radiology 1984; 150:703. Used by permission.)

Technique ▪

Central ray: Centered over midabdomen.
Position: Anteroposterior supine.
Target-film distance: 40 inches.

Measurements ▪

The length of the kidney was determined by measuring the maximum distance from the cephalad to the caudad margin. The measurements of length versus age with 3 standard deviations are shown in Figure 1.

Source ▪

Data were obtained from excretory urograms of 262 children ranging in age from birth to 14.5 years. Four hundred twenty-two kidneys were measured.

REFERENCE

1. Currarino G, Williams B, Dana K: Kidney length correlated with age: Normal values in children. Radiology 1984; 150:703–704.

▪: SIZE OF NORMAL KIDNEYS RELATED TO VERTEBRAL HEIGHT
- ▪ ACR Code: 81 (Kidney)

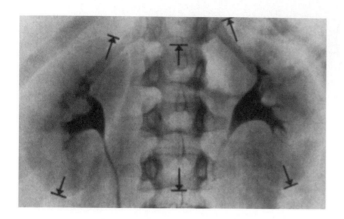

Figure 1 ▪ Supine films demonstrating technique of measurement. (From Eklöf O, Ringertz H: Acta Radiol Diagn 1976; 17:617. Used by permission.)

In Children[1] ▪

Technique

Central ray: Perpendicular to plane of film centered over midabdomen.
Position: Anteroposterior with patient supine.
Target-film distance: Immaterial.

Measurements

A linear correlation exists between the length of the kidney and that of the lumbar vertebrae L1–L3, including the intervertebral spaces comprised by these vertebrae. The left kidney, as a rule, appears approximately 2% longer than the right one. The procedure of measurement is shown in Figure 1. A nomogram (Figure 2A) is used to determine the mean of the kidney at any length of the lumbar spine. Figure 2B illustrates the method applied in practice. The kidney in the example given has a length of about − 5 SD.

The right-to-left kidney length ratio may be determined to make comparison of consecutive examinations easier. This ratio has a 96% probability interval between 1.12 and 0.84. It is independent of the length of the lumbar segment L1–L3.

Source

Based on a series of 135 patients in the pediatric age group. The material comprised 15 patients for every centimeter of lumbar length. The sexes were equally represented.

In Adults ▪

Technique

Central ray: Perpendicular to plane of film centered over midabdomen.

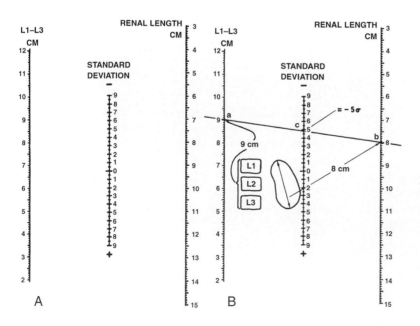

Figure 2 ▪ *A*, Nomogram for length of any given kidney in standard deviations. *B*, The method in practice. The length of the selected kidney is at the level of − 5 SD. (From Eklöf O, Ringertz H: Acta Radiol Diagn 1976; 17:617. Used by permission.)

In Adults

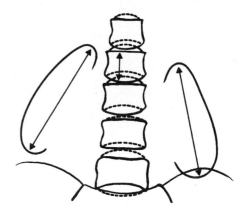

Figure 3 ▪ Measurement of kidney lengths and the height of L2 (see text for details). (Adapted from Simon AL: AJR Am J Roentgenol 1964; 92:270. Used by permission.)

Position: Anteroposterior supine.
Target-film distance: Immaterial.

Measurements (Figure 3)

The length of each kidney was determined in its longest axis. The height of the second lumbar vertebral body was determined with and without the L2–L3 disc. The measurements were made at the posterior margins of the body. These are then used to create two sets of ratios: kidney length/height of L2 and kidney length/height of L2 plus disc. The normal values are given in Table 1.

Source

The data were derived from a study of roentgenograms of 100 consecutive patients with autopsy-proved kidneys of normal weight and normal gross and microscopic appearance. There were 55 women and 45 men, ranging in age from 23 to 86 years. About half the patients were in the sixth and seventh decades.

AGE (Decade)	MEAN WEIGHT (gm)	MEAN LENGTH (cm)	MEAN RATIO (Kidney Length/Height of L2)	MEAN RATIO (Kidney Length/Height of L2 Plus Disc)
2nd	210	12.4	4.1	3.6
3rd	170	12.2	3.5	3.0
4th	155	11.2	3.5	3.0
5th	135	12.2	3.8	3.1
6th	145	11.8	3.7	3.1
7th	125	11.5	3.6	3.1
8th	120	11.3	3.7	3.1
9th	100	11.4	3.7	3.1

Table 1 ▪ **Normal Values**

From Simon AL: AJR Am J Roentgenol 1964; 92:270. Used by permission.

REFERENCES

1. Eklöf O, Ringertz H: Kidney size in children. A method of assessment. Acta Radiol Diagn 1976; 17(5A):617–625.
2. Simon AL: AJR Am J Roentgenol 1964; 92:270.

▪▪ MEASUREMENT OF THE NORMAL POSITION OF THE KIDNEYS IN RELATION TO THE CORONAL PLANES OF THE BODY FOR DETERMINATION OF TOMOGRAPHIC PLANE[1]

▪ ACR Code: 81 (Kidney)

Technique ▪

Central ray: Perpendicular to plane of film.
Position: Center posterior supine, expiratory phase of respiration without compression.
Target-film distance: 40 inches.

Measurements ▪

This study shows that the distance from the tabletop to the kidneys in the supine position varies greatly. A 2-cm-thick tomographic cut at 8 cm will include only 41% of the kidneys. A 3-cm cut at 8.5 cm will include 56% of the kidneys. The study also shows that the depth of the kidneys can be predicted with greater accuracy in relation to one third of the body thickness. One third of the body thickness in this study is the plane that is one third of the distance from the tabletop to the anterior abdominal wall at the inferior margin of the rib cage. The kidneys usually lie anterior to this plane, and a 2-cm-thick tomographic cut

1.5 cm anterior to the one-third plane will include 61% of the kidneys, whereas a 3-cm-thick cut 1 cm anterior to the one-third plane will include 79% of the kidneys. Of the few kidneys not included in these cuts, approximately half will be found farther anterior and half farther posterior.

The left kidney usually lies in the plane anterior to the right. As a general rule, therefore, if one kidney is in a tomographic cut and the other is not, the left will be found in a more anterior plane, and the right will be found in a more posterior plane. The difference in level is not great, and a 2-cm-thick tomographic cut will include both kidneys in 81% of persons.

Source ▪

Data were obtained from measurement of 61 kidneys.

REFERENCES

1. McConnell F: Measurement of the normal position of the kidney in relation to the coronal planes of the body; A study of 35 adults. J Can Assoc Radiol 1972; 23(4):241–244.

▪: RENAL SIZE IN PREMATURE AND TERM INFANTS AT ULTRASOUND
▪ ACR Code: 81 (Kidney)

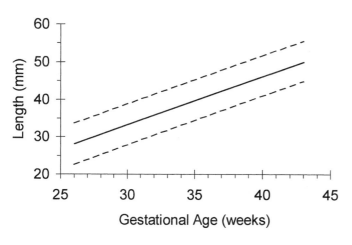

Figure 1 ▪ Renal length versus gestational age in newborn infants. Linear regression mean *(solid line)* and residual standard deviations *(dashed lines)* are shown. (From Chiara A, Chirico G, Barbarini M, et al: Eur J Pediatr 1989; 149:94–95. Used by permission.)

Technique ▪

Real-time sector[1,2] or articulated arm[3] ultrasound was done with 5- to 5.5-MHz transducers over the renal fossae. Transverse and longitudinal scans were obtained in the prone or lateral decubitus positions.

Measurements ▪

Renal length from longitudinal scans was measured in millimeters by Chiara and Schlesinger and their associates from frozen images with electronic calipers[1,2] or by Holloway and colleagues from hard copy images.[3] Holloway and group determined renal volume by tracing the area of serial transverse sections and summing or by the prolate ellipse formula (product of three dimensions $\times$ $\pi/6$).[3] Measurements in premature infants[1,2] were correlated with birth weight, body length, and gestational age by maternal dates and Dubowitz assessment.[4] Figures 1 and 2 show results of linear regression of kidney length versus gestational age and birth weight from Chiara and colleagues.[1]

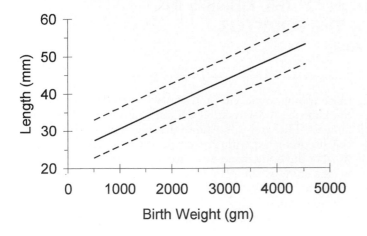

Figure 2 ▪ Renal length versus birth weight in newborn infants. Linear regression mean *(solid line)* and residual standard deviations *(dashed lines)* are shown. (From Chiara A, Chirico G, Barbarini M, et al: Eur J Pediatr 1989; 149:94–95. Used by permission.)

Table 1 ▪ Renal Length Versus Birth Weight in Newborn Infants

BODY WEIGHT (gm)	RENAL LENGTH (mm)	
	Lower Limit	Upper Limit
600	26.4	35.7
700	27.2	36.5
800	27.9	37.2
900	28.7	38.0
1000	29.4	38.7
1100	30.1	39.5
1200	30.9	40.2
1300	31.6	41.0
1400	32.4	41.7
1500	33.1	42.5
1600	33.9	43.2
1700	34.6	43.9
1800	35.4	44.7
1900	36.1	45.4
2000	36.9	46.2
2100	37.6	46.9
2200	38.4	47.7
2300	39.1	48.4
2400	39.9	49.2
2500	40.6	49.9
2600	41.3	50.7
2700	42.1	51.4
2800	42.8	52.2
2900	43.6	52.9
3000	44.3	53.7

Upper and lower limits are 95% confidence intervals from linear regression analysis.

From Schlesinger AE, Hedlund GL, Pierson WP, Null DM: Radiology 1987; 164:127–129. Used by permission.

Table 2 ▪ Renal Length and Volume in Term Newborn Infants

PARAMETER	GENDER	RIGHT KIDNEY		LEFT KIDNEY	
		Number	Mean ± SD	Number	Mean ± SD
Volume (cc) (serial area)	Male	36	9.9 ± 2.8	36	11.3 ± 3.8
	Female	25	9.2 ± 2.3	26	9.8 ± 2.7
Volume (cc) (prolate ellipse)	Male	35	10.4 ± 2.6	36	10.6 ± 3.2
	Female	26	8.4 ± 2.6	26	9.1 ± 2.1
Length (mm)	Male	36	41.2 ± 4.4	36	42.7 ± 4.8
	Female	24	41.8 ± 3.2	24	42.7 ± 3.7

From Holloway H, Jones JB, Robinson AE, et al: Pediatr Radiol 1983; 13:212–214. Used by permission.

Table 1 lists the upper and lower 95% confidence limits for kidney length versus birth weight calculated from linear regression by Schlesinger and associates.[2] Table 2 lists renal volumes and lengths by gender and side in term infants, as determined by Holloway and associates.[3]

Source ▪

Chiara and group evaluated 132 infants (63 boys, 69 girls; gestational age range, 27 to 42 weeks; birth weight range, 790 to 4200 gm) within 48 hours of birth.[1] Schlesinger and group studied 52 premature infants (28 boys, 24 girls; gestational age range, 23 to 37 weeks; birth weight range, 530 to 3680 gm) with 72 hours of birth.[2] Holloway's subjects were 62 term infants (36 boys, 26 girls) within 7 days of birth.[3]

Comments ▪

Chiara and Schlesinger and associates found no significant differences between left and right kidneys or with genders in renal length in premature infants, whereas there were strong correlations with gestational age and birth weight.[1,2]

REFERENCES

1. Chiara A, Chirico G, Barbarini M, et al: Ultrasonic evaluation of kidney length in term and preterm infants. Eur J Pediatr 1989; 149:94–95.
2. Schlesinger AE, Hedlund GL, Pierson WP, Null DM: Normal standards for kidney length in premature infants: Determination with US. Radiology 1987; 164:127–129.
3. Holloway H, Jones JB, Robinson AE, et al: Sonographic determination of renal volumes in normal neonates. Pediatr Radiol 1983; 13:212–214.
4. Dubowitz LMS, Dubowitz V, Goldberg C: Clinical assessment of gestational age in the newborn infant. J Pediatr 1970; 77:1–10.

⁗ MEASUREMENT OF RENAL LENGTH IN CHILDREN BY ULTRASOUND[1]
▪ ACR Code: 81 (Kidney)

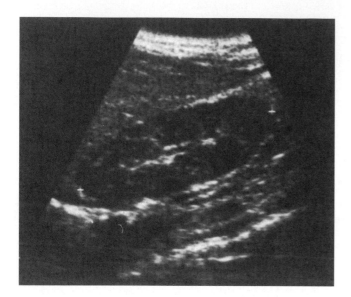

Figure 1 ▪ Length of the kidney can be measured with electronic calipers, as on this image of right kidney in a 5-month-old baby. For purpose of this study, measurements were done with mechanical calipers. (From Rosenbaum DM, et al: AJR Am J Roentgenol 1984; 142:467–469. Used by permission.)

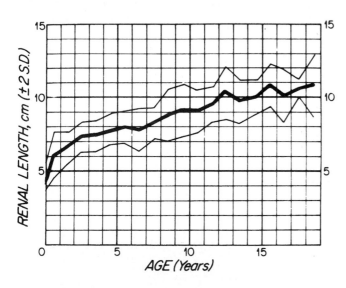

Figure 2 ▪ Sonographic renal length plotted against age. (From Rosenbaum DM, et al: AJR Am J Roentgenol 1984; 142:467–469. Used by permission.)

Technique ▪

Images obtained with a real-time mechanical sector scanner, either a Diasonics Wide-vue using a 3.5-, 5-, or 7.5-MHz transducer, or a Diasonics Neonatal unit using a 6-MHz transducer.

Measurements ▪ (Figure 1)

The transducer was positioned to image the kidney in its longest dimension, and the renal length was measured with mechanical calipers from the hard-copy transparencies. Sonographic renal length plotted against age is shown in Figure 2.

Source ▪

Data were derived from sonographic examination of 203 children ranging in age from several hours to 19 years.

REFERENCE

1. Rosenbaum DM, Korngold E, Teele RL: Sonographic assessment of renal length in normal children. AJR Am J Roentgenol 1984; 142:467–469.

▪: MEASUREMENT OF KIDNEY LENGTH AND VOLUME IN CHILDREN BY ULTRASOUND[1]
▪ ACR Code: 81 (Kidney)

Technique ▪

Sonographic examinations were performed with a 3.5-MHz mechanical Combison 100 scanner equipped with a freeze frame, calibration setting, and a water display. Examinations were performed with the patient in the prone position.

Measurements ▪ (Figure 1)

The normal lengths of the kidneys related to body height are shown in Figure 2.

The kidney volumes related to body weight are shown in Figure 3.

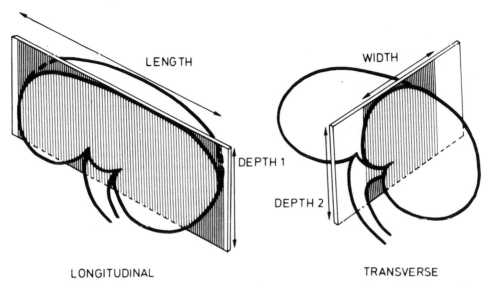

LONGITUDINAL   TRANSVERSE

Figure 1 ▪ Standardized planes in renal biometry. Sonographic measurements performed in the maximum longitudinal and transverse kidney section. The latter were obtained in the kidney hilar region. Volume formula for an ellipsoid:

$$\text{Kidney volume (ml)} = L \times W \times \frac{D1 + D2}{2} \times 0.523$$

L = maximum bipolar length; W = maximum width in the hilar region; D = maximum depth in the longitudinal *(depth 1)* and transverse section *(depth 2)*. (From Dinkel E, et al: Pediatr Radiol 1985; 15:38–43. Used by permission.)

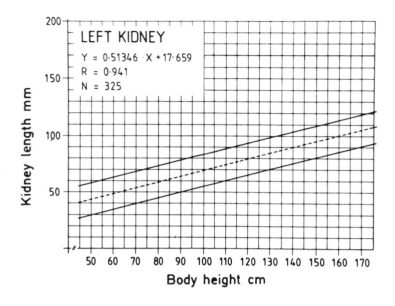

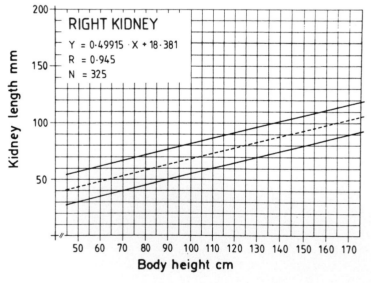

Figure 2 ▪ Length of both kidneys related to body height. Mean values and the 95% regions of tolerance are determined by routine statistical analysis of 325 children. (From Dinkel E, et al: Pediatr Radiol 1985; 15:38–43. Used by permission.)

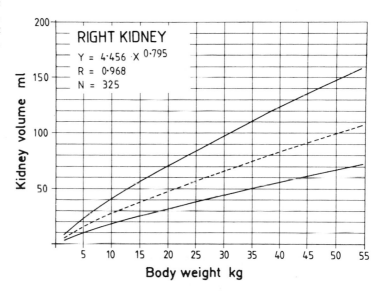

Figure 3 ▪ Volume of left and right kidney correlated to body weight. Median values and the 95% regions of tolerance were determined by statistical analysis of 325 children. Regression line and tolerance limits were computed after logarithmic transformation of volume and weight and then retransformed. There is only a slight difference between the left and right kidneys. (From Dinkel E, et al: Pediatr Radiol 1985; 15:38–43. Used by permission.)

Source ▪

Data were derived from sonographic study of 325 children without kidney disease, 188 boys and 137 girls aged between 3 days and 15 years 11 months.

REFERENCE

1. Dinkel E, Ertel M, Dittrich M, et al: Sonographical growth charts for kidney length and volume. Pediatr Radiol 1985; 15:38–43.

⁚ KIDNEY LENGTH VERSUS BODY HEIGHT IN CHILDREN
▪ ACR Code: 81 (Kidney)

Technique ▪

Ultrasound of the abdomen was done with SSA 27A (Toshiba, Tokyo, Japan) and EUB-515 (Hitachi, Tokyo, Japan) machines and 3.5-MHz transducers. Patients were supine without preparation or sedation.[1]

Measurements ▪

From frozen images of coronally oriented scans passing through the renal hilum, the cephalocaudal dimension (length) was measured. Tables 1 and 2 list right and left renal lengths by age and body height of the patients.[1]

Source ▪

Subjects were 307 children (138 boys, 169 girls; age range, newborn to 16 years) with no history, clinical findings, or sonographic evidence of disease affecting the kidney.[1]

Comments ▪

There were no significant differences between genders at any age. The best correlation between renal measurements and patient parameters was for kidney length versus body height.[1]

REFERENCE

1. Konus OL, Ozdemir A, Akkaya A, et al: Normal liver, spleen, and kidney dimensions in neonates, infants and children: Evaluation with sonography. AJR Am J Roentgenol 1998; 171:1693–1698.

Table 1 ▪ Length of Right Kidney in Children Versus Body Height and Age

BODY HEIGHT (cm)	NO.	AGE RANGE (mon)	MEAN ± SD	RANGE	NORMAL LIMITS
48–64	50	1–3	50 ± 5.8	38–66	35–65
54–73	39	4–6	53 ± 5.3	41–66	40–70
65–78	17	7–9	59 ± 5.2	50–70	45–70
71–92	18	12–30	61 ± 3.4	55–66	50–75
85–109	22	36–59	67 ± 5.1	57–77	55–80
100–130	26	60–83	74 ± 5.5	62–83	60–85
110–131	32	84–107	80 ± 6.6	68–93	65–95
124–149	27	108–131	80 ± 7.0	69–96	65–100
137–153	15	132–155	89 ± 6.2	81–102	70–105
143–168	22	156–179	94 ± 5.9	83–105	75–110
152–175	11	180–200	92 ± 7.0	80–107	75–110

From Konus OL, Ozdemir A, Akkaya A, et al: AJR Am J Roentgenol 1998; 171:1693–1698. Used by permission.

Table 2 ▪ Length of Left Kidney in Children Versus Body Height and Age

BODY HEIGHT (cm)	NO.	AGE RANGE (mon)	MEAN ± SD	RANGE	NORMAL LIMITS
48–64	50	1–3	50 ± 5.5	39–61	35–65
54–73	39	4–6	56 ± 5.5	44–68	40–70
65–78	17	7–9	61 ± 4.6	54–68	45–75
71–92	18	12–30	66 ± 5.3	54–75	50–80
85–109	22	36–59	71 ± 4.5	61–77	55–85
100–130	26	60–83	79 ± 5.9	66–90	60–95
110–131	32	84–107	84 ± 6.6	71–95	65–100
124–149	27	108–131	84 ± 7.4	71–99	65–105
137–153	15	132–155	91 ± 8.4	71–104	70–110
143–168	22	156–179	96 ± 8.9	83–113	75–115
152–175	11	180–200	99 ± 7.5	87–116	80–120

From Konus OL, Ozdemir A, Akkaya A, et al: AJR Am J Roentgenol 1998; 171:1693–1698. Used by permission.

▪: LENGTH OF A SINGLE FUNCTIONING KIDNEY IN CHILDREN
▪ ACR Code: 81 (Kidney)

Table 1 ▪ Renal Length in Single Functioning Kidneys and Controls

AGE RANGE (mon)	SINGLE KIDNEY		CONTROL KIDNEY	
	No.	Length	No.	Length
0.0–1.0	13	51.0 ± 5.8	10	44.8 ± 3.1
1.3–3.8	40	56.8 ± 6.3	54	52.8 ± 6.6
4.3–8.5	25	62.8 ± 5.6	20	61.5 ± 6.7
8.5–13.0	18	69.6 ± 6.8	8	62.3 ± 6.3
13.3–23.5	33	71.7 ± 7.9	28	66.5 ± 5.4
25.8–38.3	32	78.0 ± 8.0	12	73.8 ± 5.4
39.0–51.8	17	79.6 ± 8.2	30	73.6 ± 6.4
52.0–64.5	14	86.7 ± 9.5	26	78.7 ± 5.0
65.0–78.0	12	91.0 ± 7.9	10	80.9 ± 5.4

All measurements are in millimeters (mean ± standard deviation). Control data from Rosenbaum DM, Korngold E, Teele RL: AJR Am J Roentgenol 1984; 142:467–469.[2]

Technique ▪

Renal sonography was done with a 128 scanner (Acuson, Mountain View, CA) equipped with 5- to 7-MHz transducers, in the supine or prone positions depending on patient age.[1]

Measurements ▪

The length of the functioning kidney was measured from the largest longitudinal section.[1] Comparison was made with normative data from Rosenbaum and colleagues.[2] Table 1 lists renal length versus age from both studies, and Table 2 lists growth rate in the single kidneys from serial sonograms. Figure 1 depicts these relationships.

Source ▪

Retrospective review of 56 children with unilateral multicystic dysplastic kidney (MCDK) presenting between 0 and 48 weeks of age, with follow-up from 8 to 296 weeks after presentation, yielded 206 individual renal measurements (mean per patient, 3.66). The presence of a single functioning kidney was confirmed by nuclear renography, and none of the patients had reflux on the functioning side at voiding cystourethrogram.[1]

Comments ▪

These data are in agreement with others[3] in that compensatory renal growth of a single functioning kidney occurs in utero (significant difference in length compared with normal subjects at birth), and this relative size difference continues through infancy and childhood. This effect is not large (typically 1 to 2 standard deviations above mean norms for binephric individuals). The postnatal growth rate of single kidneys seems to be greater than that in binephric individuals until 18 months and parallel thereafter, al-

Table 2 ▪ Growth in Renal Length of Single Functioning Kidneys on Serial Sonograms

AGE RANGE (mon)	NO.	GROWTH RATE	
		Mean ± SD	Range
0–6	5	0.66 ± 0.24	0.28–0.94
6–12	18	0.297 ± 0.34	0–1.46
12–24	15	0.21 ± 0.97	0.05–0.34
24–36	8	0.14 ± 0.17	0.02–0.54
36–48	10	0.167 ± 0.11	0–0.21
48–60	6	0.105 ± 0.12	0–0.31

Growth rates are in millimeters per week. SD = standard deviation.
From Rottenberg GT, Bruyn RD, Gordon I: AJR Am J Roentgenol 1996; 167(5):1255–1259. Used by permission.

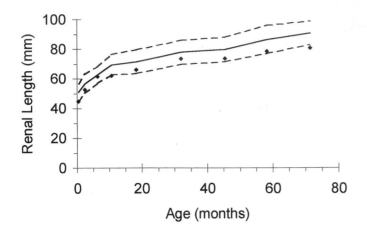

Figure 1 ▪ Renal length versus age for infants and young children with unilateral functioning kidneys (mean = *solid line*, ± 1 SD = *dashed lines*) from Rottenberg,[1] compared with binephric individuals (mean = *diamonds*) from Rosenbaum.[2] (From Rottenberg GT, Bruyn RD, Gordon I: AJR Am J Roentgenol 1996; 167(5):1255–1259. Used by permission.)

though an absolute size difference persists.[4] Fetal renal volumes show greater differences than length alone between the unaffected kidney with unilateral MCDK and kidneys of normal subjects.[5]

REFERENCES

1. Rottenberg GT, Bruyn RD, Gordon I: Sonographic standards for a single functioning kidney in children. AJR Am J Roentgenol 1996; 167(5):1255–1259.

2. Rosenbaum DM, Korngold E, Teele RL: Sonographic assessment of renal length in normal children. AJR Am J Roentgenol 1984; 142:467–469.
3. Glazebrook KN, McGrath FP, Steele BT: Prenatal compensatory renal growth: Documentation with US. Radiology 1993; 189:733–735.
4. Laufer I, Griscom NT: Compensatory renal hypertrophy: Absence in utero and development in early life. AJR Am J Roentgenol 1971; 113:464–467.
5. Gloor J, Sistrom CL, Chevalier RL, Feguson JE.: Compensatory renal hypertrophy in utero in fetuses with unilateral renal function (abstract). Southern Society for Pediatric Research, New Orleans, March, 1993.

▪▪ MEASUREMENT OF NORMAL RENAL DIMENSIONS BY ULTRASOUND[1]

▪ ACR Code: 81 (Kidney)

Technique ▪

1. All studies were performed with static-image scanners using 3.5-MHz or 5-MHz focused transducers. In many examinations, a 3-MHz mechanical real-time sector scanner was also used.
2. Kidneys were measured in longitudinal plane parallel to the longest renal axis. When possible, the height (ventral dorsal dimension) and transverse width were also measured.
3. Measurements were obtained in prone and oblique positions.

Table 1 ▪ Right Renal Dimensions in Sample Groups of Patients Examined Retrospectively

	MEAN (cm)	SD
Length		
Oblique (n = 52)	10.646	1.345
Prone (n = 51)	10.743	1.349
Width*		
Oblique (n = 35)	4.920	0.638
Prone (n = 32)	5.047	0.764
Depth*		
Oblique (n = 19)	3.947	0.812
Prone (n = 9)	4.167	0.507

*Approximate values.
From Brandt TD, et al: J Ultrasound Med 1982; 1:49. Used by permission.

Table 2 ▪ Left Renal Dimensions in Sample Groups of Patients Examined Retrospectively

	MEAN (cm)	SD
Length		
Oblique (n = 50)	10.130	1.165
Prone (n = 50)	11.096	1.152
Width*		
Oblique (n = 36)	5.303	0.744
Prone (n = 31)	5.300	0.802
Depth*		
Oblique (n = 18)	3.578	0.912
Prone (n = 10)	4.140	0.844

*Approximate values.
From Brandt TD, et al: I Ultrasound Med 1982; 1:49. Used by permission.

Measurement ▪ (Tables 1 and 2)

Source ▪

Fifty-two patients with normal renal function referred for nonrenal illnesses and 10 normal volunteers were studied. Sonographic renal dimensions are smaller than those obtained by radiography, because there is no geometric magnification or osmotic diuresis.

REFERENCE

1. Brandt TD, Neiman HL, Dragowski MJ, et al: Ultrasound assessment of normal renal dimension. J Ultrasound Med 1982; 1:49–52.

▪▪ SIZE OF THE ADULT KIDNEY WITH AGING
▪ ACR Code: 81 (Kidney)

Table 1 ▪ Renal Size in Adults Measured with Ultrasound

REFERENCE PARAMETER	DECADE						
	3	4	5	6	7	8	9
Emamian							
Number	121	144	168	162	70		
Length (left)	11.5	11.3	11.3	11.1	10.5		
	(10.4–12.8)	(10.3–12.3)	(10.2–12.5)	(10.0–12.2)	(9.4–12.0)		
Length (right)	11.1	11.2	11.0	10.8	10.4		
	(10.1–12.4)	(10.0–12.3)	(10.0–12.2)	(9.5–12.0)	(9.1–11.8)		
Width (left)	5.9	5.8	5.8	5.8	5.6		
	(5.1–6.6)	(5.0–6.5)	(5.3–6.5)	(5.1–6.5)	(4.9–6.2)		
Width (right)	5.8	5.8	5.8	5.7	5.5		
	(5.0–6.6)	(5.2–6.6)	(5.2–6.4)	(5.0–6.4)	(5.0–6.3)		
Miletic							
Number	32	32	42	28	22	11	8
Length (left)	11.5	11.5	11.4	11.3	10.9	10.2	9.8
	(10.1–13.0)	(9.9–13.1)	(9.5–13.4)	(10.2–12.4)	(9.2–12.5)	(9.4–11.0)	(8.7–10.9)
Length (right)	11.3	11.2	11.2	11.0	10.7	9.9	9.6
	(10.2–12.8)	(9.7–12.9)	(9.6–12.8)	(10.3–11.7)	(9.3–12.1)	(9.0–10.8)	(8.5–10.7)

All measurements are in centimeters. Emamian's data are median and 10th to 90th percentiles (in parentheses). Miletic's data are given as mean and ± 2 standard deviations (in parentheses).

Technique ▪

Emamian and colleagues performed real-time ultrasound of the kidneys with an LSC 7000/7000A machine (Picker, Frankfurt, Germany) and a 3.5-MHz curved array transducer with a wide (11 cm) contact surface.[1] Miletic and colleagues used an EUB 515 unit (Hitachi of America, Tarrytown, NY) with a 3.5-MHz transducer to perform real-time ultrasound of the kidneys.[2]

Measurements ▪

The renal length was measured from longitudinal frozen images through the midkidneys showing the largest dimensions.[1, 2] Emamian and group also measured thickness (AP) and width (TRV) from the transverse section through a section near the hilum.[1] Body height was measured and recorded in both studies. Table 1 lists the results by decade and side from both studies.

Source ▪

Emamian's subjects were 665 healthy adult volunteers (307 men, 358 women), who were part of a larger study undergoing a general health survey. There were no morphologic abnormalities of the kidneys at ultrasound.[1] Miletic and group studied 175 subjects (104 men, 71 women) without renal impairment.[2] Emamiam's subjects were exactly 30, 40, 50, 60, or 70 years old whereas Miletic's subjects were roughly evenly distributed from 17 to 85 years.

Comments ▪

In both studies the renal size was significantly larger in men than in women and larger for the left compared with the right. Miletic and coworkers found that the renal length showed a significant correlation with body height such that the ratio of kidney length to body height (KBR) was similar between men and women. The KBR of the left kidney was still larger than that of the right.[2] Both groups found a significant decrease in renal size (both absolute and KBR) with aging, especially after 60 years of age. Emamian and coworkers felt this to be due to a decrease in parenchymal volume since the size of the central echogenic area did not change.[1]

REFERENCES

1. Emamian SA, Nielsen MB, Pedersen JF, Ytte L: Kidney dimensions at sonography: Correlation with age, sex, and habitus in 665 adult volunteers [see comments]. AJR Am J Roentgenol 1993; 160:83–86.
2. Miletic D, Fuckar Z, Sustic A, et al: Sonographic measurement of absolute and relative renal length in adults. J Clin Ultrasound 1998; 26:185–189.

▪: DETERMINATION OF RENAL CORTICAL INDEX[1]
▪ ACR Code: 811 (Renal Parenchyma)

Technique ▪

Central ray: Perpendicular to plane of film centered over midabdomen.
Position: Anteroposterior supine.
Target-film distance: Immaterial.

Measurements ▪ (Figure 1)

The upper and lower poles are marked. The lateral and medial borders are marked. The renal calyceal system is outlined, and the superior, inferior, and lateral calyces are marked. The distances between the marked lines are measured in millimeters.

$$\text{Renal cortical index (RCI)} = \frac{C(\text{mm}) \times D(\text{mm})}{A(\text{mm}) \times B(\text{mm})}$$

RCI (mean value of both kidneys of a patient) = 0.35; SD = 0.04.
RCI/D (difference in RCI between the two kidneys of the same patient) = 0.02; SD = 0.02.

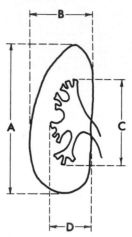

Figure 1 ▪ Measurement of renal cortical index (see text for details). (Adapted from Vuorinen P, et al: Acta Radiol 1962; suppl 211.)

Source ▪

One hundred six normal patients.

REFERENCE

1. Vuorinen P, et al: Acta Radiol 1962; suppl 211.

▪: RELATIONSHIP OF RENAL SURFACE AND PARENCHYMAL AREAS TO RENAL ARTERY SIZE[1]
▪ ACR Code: 811 (Renal Parenchymal); 961 (Renal Artery)

Technique ▪

Central ray: Perpendicular to the plane of the film centered over the interspace between the first and second lumbar vertebral bodies.
Position: Anteroposterior.
Target-film distance: 95 cm.

Measurements ▪ (Figures 1 through 3)

The study was performed using selective renal or abdominal aortography. Serial angiographic films and urographic films were obtained in moderate inspiration. Measurements were made as follows:

1. Renal area is determined with a planimeter from the nephrographic phase.
2. Renal parenchymal area is defined by a line drawn through the calyceal fornices and the intrarenal part of the renal pelvis. The parenchymal area is calculated as the difference between the renal area and the area of the pyelocalyceal system.
3. Renal artery diameter is measured at a distance 1 cm from the origin of the artery. Cross-sectional area of the

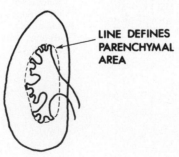

LINE DEFINES
PARENCHYMAL
AREA

Figure 1 ▪ Measurement of renal surface and parenchymal area (see text for details). (From Wojtowicz J: Invest Radiol 1967; 2:231. Used by permission.)

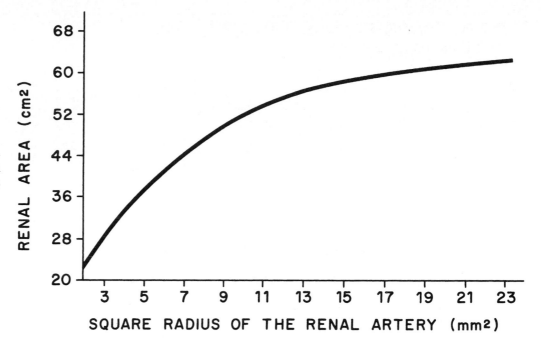

Figure 2 ▪ Renal area versus artery cross-section area. (From Wojtowicz J: Invest Radiol 1967; 2:231. Used by permission.)

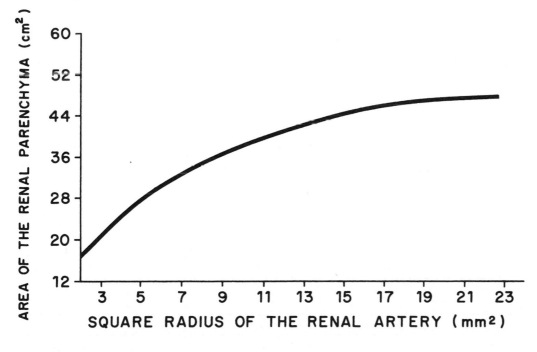

Figure 3 ▪ Renal parenchyma area versus artery cross-section area. (From Wojtowicz J: Invest Radiol 1967; 2:231. Used by permission.)

artery is expressed as the square of the artery radius (the constant π is omitted).

Source ▪

One hundred twenty-four renal angiograms in patients with a single arterial blood supply to each kidney were studied. Some selected cases with pathology were included.

REFERENCE

1. Wojtowicz J: Relationship of the surface parameters of the kidney to the size of the renal artery. Invest Radiol 1967; 2(3):231–242.

▪▐ RENAL PARENCHYMAL THICKNESS AT CT

▪ ACR Code: 811 (Renal Parenchyma)

Table 1 ▪ Renal Parenchymal Thickness in Children

AGE (Yr)	No.	A+B+C+D (mm)		DIAMETER L1 (mm)		(A+B+C+D)/DIAMETER L1	
		Boys	Girls	Boys	Girls	Boys	Girls
0–1	9	130±14	126±12	21±2	21±2	6.19±0.55	6.00±0.50
1–2	7	159±12	142±14	26±2	25±3	6.12±0.51	5.68±0.69
2–3	7	160±18	149±10	27±3	25±2	5.93±0.49	5.96±0.56
3–4	14	165±14	169±15	27±3	26±3	6.11±0.54	6.50±0.49
4–5	10	179±20	157±18	28±4	27±2	6.39±0.66	5.81±0.41
5–6	15	178±19	178±12	29±4	29±3	6.17±0.38	6.17±0.67
6–7	12	193±13	185±14	33±3	29±3	5.88±0.39	6.38±0.56
7–8	9	202±16	186±19	34±3	30±4	5.94±0.50	6.20±0.57
8–9	8	192±17	189±15	34±5	33±4	5.65±0.72	5.73±0.55
9–10	9	207±15	196±18	35±5	33±4	5.91±0.69	5.94±0.61
10–11	12	202±18	208±20	37±4	35±4	5.46±0.63	5.94±0.44
11–12	13	227±18	205±18	37±5	35±5	6.14±0.57	5.86±0.49
12–13	10	218±19	217±20	38±4	36±5	5.74±0.58	6.03±0.61
13–14	12	229±19	223±19	39±5	36±4	5.87±0.68	6.19±0.69
14–15	15	246±22	227±18	40±5	36±5	6.15±0.67	6.31±0.49

a+b+c+d = overall sum of parenchymal thickness measurements at three selected levels through the kidney, given as mean ± standard deviation.
From Prassopoulos P, Cavouras D: Eur Urol 1994; 25:51–54. Used by permission.

Technique ▪

Prassopoulos and Cavouras performed contrast-enhanced CT of the abdomen in children (machine not specified), using 5- to 10-mm slices for younger children and 10-mm slices for older children.[1] Gourtsoyiannis (same institution as reference 1) performed CT of the adult abdomen with an 0450 (Pfizer) machine using 9-mm-slice thickness.[2]

Measurements ▪

On scans through the upper calyx, hilar vessels, and lower calyx, renal parenchymal thickness (PT) was measured in four directions at right angles to each other (a, b, c, and d, in millimeters), using electronic calipers at the CT operator's console. The diameter of the L1 vertebral body (DL1, in millimeters) was also measured, and the summed PT measurements at each level normalized to DL1

([a+b+c+d]/DL1). Figure 1 shows the measurements. Table 1 lists the results in children,[1] and Table 2 lists the results in adults.[2] Figure 2 is a graph of normalized PT versus age, with data from both studies.[1,2]

Source ▪

The study of children included 162 scans (95 boys, 67 girls; age range, 5 months to 14 years).[1] In the adult series there were 360 subjects (180 men, 180 women; age range, 20 to 80 years, 30 women and 30 men in each decade).[2] In both studies, any subject with a history of renal disease, tumor, or abnormal appearance on CT was excluded (preceding numbers are after exclusions).[1,2]

Comments ▪

In childhood, the PT increased with age, though after normalization with DL1 there was no significant change

Table 2 ▪ Renal Parenchymal Thickness in Adults

AGE (Yr)	RIGHT KIDNEY (A+B+C+D)/DIAMETER L1			LEFT KIDNEY (A+B+C+D)/DIAMETER L1			AVERAGE R&L
	Upper Pole	Midpole	Lower Pole	Upper Pole	Midpole	Lower Pole	Sum U+M+L
20–29	2.36±0.28	1.75±0.18	2.12±0.27	2.25±0.26	1.67±0.22	1.94±0.25	5.37
30–39	2.11±0.19	1.58±0.15	1.99±0.32	1.95±0.28	1.51±0.18	1.80±0.22	5.47
40–49	1.86±0.25	1.49±0.15	1.71±0.26	1.76±0.25	1.43±0.22	1.60±0.23	4.92
50–59	1.70±0.21	1.32±0.14	1.56±0.21	1.59±0.21	1.24±0.16	1.44±0.21	4.42
60–69	1.48±0.22	1.17±0.16	1.34±0.20	1.32±0.21	1.07±0.16	1.25±0.20	3.85
70–79	1.22±0.22	1.02±0.17	1.15±0.18	1.14±0.19	0.95±0.16	1.07±0.19	3.25

(a+b+c+d)/Diameter L1 = sum of parenchymal thickness measurements at each level divided by the diameter of the L1 vertebral body listed as mean ± standard deviation. The last column lists summed ratios from all three levels for comparison with data from children.
From Gourtsoyiannis N, Prassopoulos P, Cavouras D, Pantelidis N: AJR Am J Roentgenol 1990; 155(3):541–544. Used by permission.

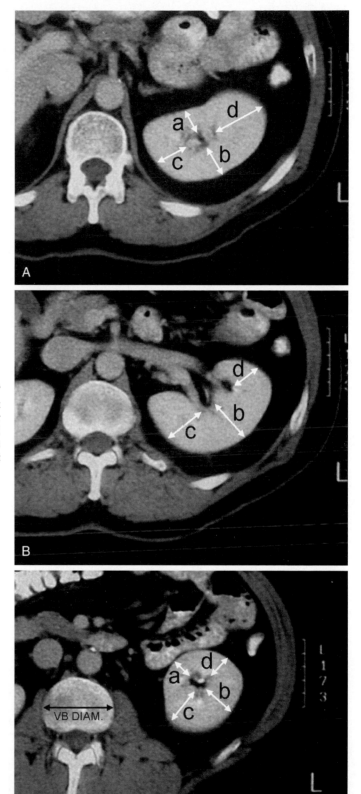

Figure 1 ▪ Measurement of renal parenchymal thickness (PT) on CT scans through *A*, upper calyx; *B*, renal pelvis; and *C*, lower calyx levels. PT was measured at four locations: anterior *(a)*, posterior *(b)*, medial *(c)*, and lateral *(d)*, at right angles to each other and oriented such that a–b paralleled the renal vessels. The width of the L1 vertebral body *(VB DIAM)* was also measured for subsequent normalization.

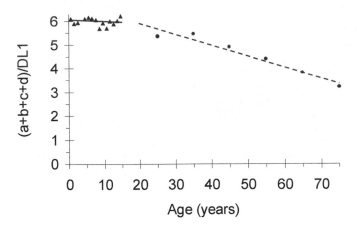

Figure 2 ▪ Renal parenchymal thickness throughout life. Overall sum of measurements at three levels, divided by the diameter of the L1 vertebral body. Data for children[1] are indicated by *triangles* and *solid line* for regression. Data for adults[2] are indicated by *circles* and *dotted line* for regression.

(p > .1). As expected, there was a strong correlation of DL1 with age (r = 0.97, p < .001). There were no significant differences in normalized PT between boys and girls or men and women (p > .1).[1, 2] From 20 to 80 years, there was a significant decrease in normalized PT with age of about 10% per decade such that the PT at age 80 years is 50% to 60% of its thickness at age 20 years.[2]

REFERENCES

1. Prassopoulos P, Cavouras D: Renal parenchymal thickness in children measured by computed tomography. Eur Urol 1994; 25:51–54.
2. Gourtsoyiannis N, Prassopoulos P, Cavouras D, Pantelidis N: The thickness of the renal parenchyma decreases with age: A CT study of 360 patients. AJR Am J Roentgenol 1990; 155(3):541–544.

▪▪ CLASSIFICATION OF CYSTIC RENAL MASSES
▪ ACR Code: 81 (Kidney)

Technique ▪

Computed tomography (CT) is generally held currently to be the most important imaging modality for characterizing renal masses. These are most often discovered as incidental findings at CT or ultrasound performed for other reasons. If the lesion was discovered at ultrasound and is unequivocally a cyst (anechoic, sharp smooth walls, and enhanced through transmission), no specific follow-up is needed. Lesions discovered at routine enhanced abdominal CT often need dedicated CT scanning (see later) and/or ultrasound for further evaluation.[1] Magnetic resonance imaging recently has been recognized as being roughly equal to CT in accuracy and is especially useful in patients with renal insufficiency or contrast allergy.[2]

Ultrasound for characterizing renal lesions should be done with modern equipment and transducers, with frequencies appropriate for the body habitus. Gain settings may be checked by scanning fluid-containing structures (e.g., the bladder) in the same patient to insure that they look anechoic. For the most part, scanning in multiple planes with careful attention to placement of the focal zone(s) suffices to produce gray scale images that allow characterization. Dedicated CT scanning for characterizing renal lesions is best done with a spiral scanner. Scanning of the kidneys is done during a single breathhold, with no more than 5-mm columnation and pitch of no more than 1:1. Typically, this is done both before and after contrast administration (40 gm of iodine, 1.5 to 2.0 ml/sec). Delays of 70 to 100 seconds after the start of injection provide good nephrographic phase (NP) images.[3] Recently, corticomedullary phase scanning has been advocated, which typically is started 30 to 40 seconds after the injection begins. This is followed immediately by a second scan to obtain NP images.[4, 5] Image reconstruction with thin spacing and small field of view is quite helpful.

Measurements ▪

In addition to noting morphologic features, CT density measurements of the mass (unenhanced and after contrast) may be helpful and are incorporated into the Bosniak system of classification (discussed in next paragraph). It should be noted that CT densitometry is somewhat uncertain, with intersubject, intrasubject, interequipment, and intraequipment variability of up to 10 HU or more. Additionally, small lesions (<1.5 cm) may give erroneously high HU measurements owing to adjacent renal parenchyma, though this error is lessened by thin section scanning/reconstruction and careful placement of small regions of interest. With these caveats in mind, the generally accepted cut-off levels are as follows:

For a cyst: <20 to 25 HU,
For fat (as in angiomyolipoma): ≤ − 10,
For "high-density" cysts: 60 to 100 HU,
For abnormal enhancement: >20 to 30 HU above baseline density.[3, 6]

Bosniak has described a system for characterizing renal masses based on imaging characteristics (mostly done with CT) that has been applied widely.[7, 8] The system initially had four classes (I to IV). More recently, he refined the system further and added two subclasses of what were previously called type II lesions.[9–12] Table 1 lists the classification system. We have abbreviated what have been called "hyperdense cysts" as class IIH. Class I and Class II lesions

Table 1 ▪ The Bosniak Classification System for Small (<3.0 cm) Renal Lesions

BOSNIAK CLASS	GENERAL FEATURES	CT SPECIFIC FEATURES	US SPECIFIC FEATURES
I (simple)	Smooth contours No definable wall Clearly defined from normal kidney	<20 HU Homogeneous contents Nonenhancing	Anechoic Sharp back wall Enhanced through transmission
II (minimally complicated, no follow-up)	Small amount of delicate calcification in the wall or in a septum One or two thin septa (≤1.0 mm)	Nonenhancing	
IIH (hyperdense on CT)		Hyperdense (60–100 HU); must also be: nonenhancing, ≤ 3.0 cm, homogeneous, sharply marginated, ≥ 1/4 exophytic	Only 50% will exhibit classic cystic characteristics
IIF (minimally complicated, follow-up)	Slightly thick or irregular calcification in the wall or in a septum >2 septa (not multiloculated though) Septa thicker than 1.0 mm (not irregular)	Hyperdense lesions that do not fulfill all of the above criteria	
III (moderately complicated, indeterminate)	Thick or irregular calcification Thick or irregular septa Uniform wall thickening Irregular outer margins Multiloculation	Enhancing septa Small, nonenhancing areas of nodularity	
IV (cystic neoplasms)	Irregular wall thickening Prominent nodularity Solid areas	Inhomogeneous Enhancement of the wall or areas of nodularity	

We have separated hyperdense cysts and called them IIF.[1, 3, 7-11]

do not need specific follow-up. Class IIF lesions can be followed to see whether they grow, develop enhancement, or acquire additional complicating features. Bosniak recommends 6-month, 1-year, and 2-year follow-up with CT.[12] Cyst puncture, aspiration, and contrast opacification sometimes may be helpful in class IIF (including problematic high-density cysts). Class III and Class IV lesions typically are removed surgically (sometimes with partial nephrectomy), as there is a substantial (III) and high (IV) risk of renal cell carcinoma, respectively, in these lesions.[7]

Comments ▪

Classification of lesions smaller than 1.5 cm can be problematic, even with high-resolution dedicated CT. Lesions less than 20 to 25 HU on unenhanced scans are not studied further and are assumed to be benign cysts. If the lesion measures greater than 25 HU, follow-up may be guided by patient age, clinical condition, and symptomatology. Bosniak's rationale is that even if there is a tiny neoplasm in a patient who is elderly and who has metastatic cancer, heart disease, or other severe illness, such a lesion would be unlikely to decrease ultimate survival. In a younger, healthy patient with such a lesion, dedicated contrast-enhanced CT scanning and ultrasound should be done. If enhancement occurs, or there are other suspicious features, follow-up (as with type IIF larger lesions) may be done.[10]

Note that some angiomyolipomas (AML) might fall into class IV, but the presence of intratumoral fat places them in a distinct group. Although AML are neoplasms, they do not metastasize and often do not require surgery. These tumors are usually followed, and it is helpful to know the expected growth rate. Lamaitre and colleagues studied 55 patients with AML, of which 43 were isolated, 6 were multiple without tuberous sclerosis (TS), and 6 were multiple in patients with TS. The growth rates (transverse area) were 5%, 22%, and 18% per year, respectively.[13]

REFERENCE

1. Gervais DA, Papanicolaou N, Lee MJ: Genitourinary imaging. In Weisslender R, Rieumont MJ, Wittenberg J (eds): Primer of Diagnostic Radiology, 2nd ed. Mosby, St. Louis, 1997, pp 261–263.
2. Rofsky NM, Weinreb JC, Bosniak MA, et al: Renal lesion characterization with gadolinium-enhanced MR imaging: Efficacy and safety in patients with renal insufficiency. Radiology 1991; 180:85–89.
3. Curry NS: Small renal masses (lesions smaller than 3 cm): Imaging, evaluation and management. AJR Am J Roentgenol 1995; 164(2):355–362.
4. Cohan RH, Sherman LS, Korobkin M, et al: Renal masses: Assessment of corticomedullary-phase and nephrographic-phase CT scans. Radiology 1995; 196:445–451.
5. Birnbaum BA, Jacobs JE, Ramchandani P: Multiphasic renal CT: Comparison of renal mass enhancement during the corticomedullary and nephrographic phases. Radiology 1996; 200:753–758.
6. Bosniak MA, Megibow AJ, Hulnick DH, et al: CT diagnosis of renal angiomyolipoma: The importance of detecting small amounts of fat. AJR Am J Roentgenol 1988; 151:497–501.
7. Bosniak MA: The current radiological approach to renal cysts. Radiology 1986; 158:1–10.
8. Bosniak MA: The small (<3.0 cm) renal parenchymal tumor: Detection, diagnosis, and controversies. Radiology 1991; 179:307–317.
9. Bosniak MA: Difficulties in classifying cystic lesions of the kidney. Urol Radiol 1991; 13:91–93.
10. Bosniak MA: Problems in the radiologic diagnosis of renal parenchymal tumors. Urol Clin North Am 1993; 20:217–230.
11. Bosniak MA, Rofsky NM: Problems in the detection and characterization of small renal masses. Radiology 1996; 198:638–641.
12. Bosniak MA: The use of the Bosniak classification system for renal cysts and cystic tumors. Urol 1997; 157:1852–1853.
13. Lemaitre L, Robert Y, Dubrulle F, et al: Renal angiomyolipoma: Growth followed up with CT and/or US. Radiology 1995; 197:598–602.

⁛ ULTRASOUND EVALUATION OF RENAL TRANSPLANTS
▪ ACR Code: 81 (Kidney)

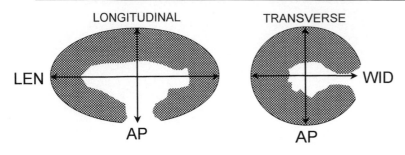

VOLUME (cc) = *0.49 x LEN x WID x AP (cm)

VOLUME% (compared to immediate post op)

ADULTS: 105-130% early, 90-120% late
late<90% (consider chronic rejection, vascular disease)

CHILDREN: 51-220% at 1-3 years.
(normal range too wide to be helpful)

Figure 1 ▪ Measurement of renal transplant volume. Length *(LEN)* is measured from a longitudinal scan through the midkidney, and width *(WID)* is obtained from a transverse section through the hilum. The anteroposterior *(AP)* dimension may be measured from either plane, though oblique transverse scanning can cause error. Calculation of volume can be done using either pi/6 (prolate ellipse) or 0.49 (derived empirically by Hricak and Liets) for the constant.[2] Expected changes in volume are shown.

Technique ▪

Most renal transplants are placed in the pelvis, lying in the iliac fossa. Transducers of 3.5 to 7.0 MHz in sector, linear, or curved-array configuration are used, depending on patient habitus, position of the graft, and desired level of detail. Curved-array transducers with small radius may be the best choice for measuring the length of the graft, and sometimes a stand-off pad can be helpful in this regard. Doppler ultrasound can be very useful, including duplex, color, and power modes, both for detecting vascular problems and screening for rejection.

Measurements ▪

Jurriaans and Dubbins have written an excellent review of the ultrasound examination in normal renal transplants.[1]

There is a great deal of literature about the subject, especially concerning Doppler analysis of transplant vasculature. Here we will briefly outline the most commonly cited measurements of transplant morphology and vascular physiology.

The size of transplants (Figure 1) is typically measured in two planes, and volumes may be calculated and followed for change.[2–4] The relative size of cortex and medullary pyramids (Figure 2) has been evaluated, and thinning of the cortex and swelling of the pyramids may be helpful in diagnosing rejection.[5–9] Duplex Doppler analysis (aided by color Doppler capability) has been studied extensively (Figures 3 and 4). Initially, Doppler indices were found to be diagnostic of rejection by virtue of increased resistance due to perivascular inflammation.[10–12] More recent studies have

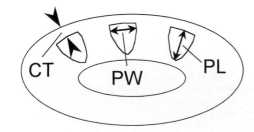

$$MPI = \frac{\frac{1}{2}PL \times PW}{CT}$$

MEAN=5.3-7.0
SD UP TO 2.0
ABNORMAL>8-9

$$CMR = \frac{CT}{PL}$$

MEAN=0.97-1.02
SD UP TO 0.18

CORTICAL
THICKNESS (CT)

MEAN=9.3-9.7 mm
SD UP TO 1.5 mm

Figure 2 ▪ Measurements of renal transplant cortex and pyramid sizes from longitudinal ultrasound. Measurement of cortical thickness *(CT)* may be aided by noting bright arcuate arteries at the corticomedullary junction. Pyramid width *(PW)* and length *(PL)* are measured as shown. The medullary pyramid index *(MPI)* and corticomedullary ratio *(CMR)* are calculated as shown. Normal mean values and SD, as well as cut-off values for MPI, are given.

Figure 3 ▪ Measurement of arterial parameters. Duplex Doppler signals may be obtained from the main *(M)* renal artery and subsequent branches: lobar *(L)*, interlobar *(I)*, arcuate *(AR)*, interlobular *(IL)*. Most studies of intrarenal resistance use measurements from smaller branches *(I-IL)*. Angle correction is not needed for calculating indices but is important in measuring peak systolic velocity *(S)* at or near the arterial anastomosis *(AN)* to detect stenosis. End-diastolic velocity *(D)* is also needed for calculating indices and is given a negative sign if below the Doppler baseline (reversed diastolic flow).

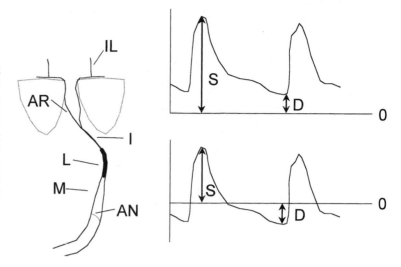

$$RI = \frac{S-D}{S}$$

MEAN=0.64 - 0.73
SD UP TO 0.1
ABNORMAL>0.75-0.9

$$PI = \frac{S-D}{MEAN}$$

MEAN=0.78-1.26
SD UP TO 0.5
ABNORMAL>1.5-1.8

$$SDR = \frac{S}{D}$$

MEAN=2.6-3.6
SD UP TO 0.4
ABNORMAL>4

S (MAX, AT PEDICLE)

100+/-20 cm./sec.
ABNORMAL>190

Figure 4 ▪ Calculation of arterial indices from renal transplant duplex Doppler signals. Resistive index *(RI)* is the most commonly used, followed by pulsatility index *(PI)*. The latter has the advantage of continuous values even when the end-diastolic velocity is below the baseline. The systolic to diastolic ratio *(SDR)* has a linear relationship to RI and is infrequently cited. Most newer machines allow automatic calculation of these indices. Abnormal RI, PI, and SDR indicate rejection. Elevated S at or near the arterial anastomosis denotes stenosis of more than 50%.

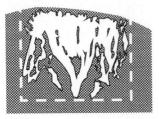

TYPE I

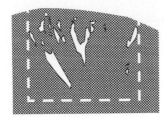

TYPE II

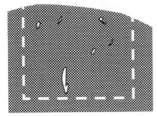

TYPE III

Figure 5 • Power Doppler evaluation of renal transplant parenchymal vessels. The normal scan (type I) appearance depends on machine settings, including frequency, gain, and filter. Typically, there is generous flow *(white)* in small ramifying vessels almost touching the cortex. Rejection leads to geographic areas of decreased or absent flow, tending toward near-absence of small vessel flow in severe cases (types II and III). Grading systems vary from 2 to 5 steps.

found greater overlap between normal and abnormal populations in these indices, rendering them less useful.[9, 13–15] Others have emphasized the intrinsic variability of these measurements and the possibility of abnormal values being caused by factors other than rejection.[16–18] Stenosis at or near the arterial anastomosis can cause increased peak velocity in the main transplant artery.[19] Power Doppler sonography (Figure 5) can show even slow flow in quite small vessels. Since renal transplants are typically close to the transducer, fine vascular detail can be depicted, allowing detection of rejection as regions of little or no parenchymal flow.[20–23]

Morphologic analysis is still very important in the ultrasound evaluation of renal transplants. Features that may explain graft problems should be sought, including hydronephrosis, fluid collections and/or free fluid, pseudoaneurysm, arteriovenous fistula, and vascular thrombosis, among others. Hoddick and colleagues had some success in diagnosing rejection with subjective morphologic analysis, including anteroposterior dimension greater than width (AP > WID) on transverse images, increased size and conspicuousness of the pyramids, decreased renal sinus fat, and thickening of the wall of the collecting system. The accuracy of positive prediction ranged between 83% and 90%, and the accuracy of negative prediction ranged between 17% and 30%.[6]

REFERENCES

1. Jurriaans E, Dubbins PA: Renal transplantation: The normal morphological and Doppler ultrasound examination. J Clin Ultrasound 1992; 20:495–506.
2. Hricak H, Lieto RP: Sonographic determination of renal volume. Radiology 1983; 148:311–312.
3. Asby M, Metreweli C, Matthews C, et al: Changes in transplanted kidney volume measured by ultrasound. Br J Radiol 1983; 148:311–312.
4. Babcock DS, Slovis TL, Han BK, et al: Renal transplants in children: Long-term follow-up using sonography. Radiology 1985; 156:165–167.
5. Hricak H, Toledo-Pereyra LH, Eyler WR, et al: Evaluation of acute post-transplant renal failure by ultrasound. Radiology 1979; 133:443–447.
6. Hoddick W, Filly RA, Backman U, et al: Renal allograft rejection: US evaluation. Radiology 1986; 161:469–473.
7. Fried AM, Woodring JH, Loh FK, et al: The medullary pyramid index: An objective assessment of prominence in renal transplant rejection. Radiology 1983; 149:787–791.
8. Raj D, Hoisala R, Somiah S, et al: Quantitation of change in the medullary compartment in renal allograft by ultrasound. J Clin Ultrasound 1997; 25:265–269.
9. Kelcz F, Pozniak MA, Pirsch JD, Oberly TD: Pyramidal appearance and resistive index: Insensitive and nonspecific sonographic indicators of renal transplant rejection. AJR Am J Roentgenol 1990; 155:531–535.
10. Rigsby CM, Taylor KJW, Weltin G, et al: Renal allografts in acute rejection: Evaluation using duplex sonography. Radiology 1986; 158:375–378.
11. Rigsby CM, Burns PN, Weltin GC, et al: Doppler signal quantitation in renal allografts: Comparison in normal and rejecting transplants. Radiology 1987; 162:39–42.
12. Rifkin MD, Needleman L, Pasto ME, et al: Evaluation of renal transplant rejection by duplex Doppler examination: Value of the resistive index. AJR Am J Roentgenol 1987; 148:759–762.
13. Allen KS, Jorkasky DK, Arger PH, et al: Renal allografts: Prospective analysis of Doppler sonography. Radiology 1988; 169:371–376.
14. Genkins SM, Sanfilippo FP, Carroll BA: Duplex Doppler sonography of renal transplants: Lack of sensitivity and specificity in establishing pathologic diagnosis. AJR Am J Roentgenol 1989; 152:535–539.
15. Perrella R, Duerinckx AJ, Tessler FN, et al: Evaluation of renal transplant dysfunction by duplex Doppler sonography: A prospective study and review of the literature. Am J Kidney Dis 1990; XV:544–550.
16. Pozniak MA, Kelcz F, Stratta RJ, et al: Extraneous factors affecting resistive index. Invest Radiol 1988; 23(12):899–904.
17. Mostbeck GH, Gossinger HD, Mallek R, et al: Effect of heart rate on Doppler measurements of resistive index in renal arteries: Radiology 1990; 175:511–513.
18. Don S, Kopecky KK, Filo R, et al: Duplex Doppler US of renal allografts: Causes of elevated resistive index. Radiology 1989; 171:709–712.
19. Grenier N, Douws C, Morel D, et al: Detection of vascular complications in renal allografts with color Doppler flow imaging. Radiology 1991; 178:217–223.
20. Trillaud H, Merville P, Le Linh PT, et al: Color Doppler sonography in early renal transplantation follow-up: Resistive index measurements versus power Doppler sonography. AJR Am J Roentgenol 1998; 171:1611–1615.
21. Martinoli C, Crespi G, Bertolotto M, et al: Interlobular vasculature in renal transplants: A power Doppler US study with MR correlation. Radiology 1996; 200:111–117.
22. Turetschek K, Nasel C, Wunderbaldinger P, et al: Power Doppler versus color Doppler imaging in renal allograft evaluation. J Ultrasound Med 1996; 15:517–522.
23. Hilborn MD, Bude RD, Murphy KJ, et al: Renal transplant evaluation with power Doppler sonography. Br J Radiol 1997; 70:39–42.

▪ URETERAL DIAMETER IN INFANTS AND CHILDREN AT IVP
▪ ACR Code: 82 (Ureter)

Technique ▪

Intravenous urography was done after injection of Isopaque 260 (n = 156) or 350 (n = 38) (Nyegaard, Oslo), with doses of 4 ml/kg in infants, 30 ml in children weighing 10 to 20 kg, and 40 ml in children weighing more than 20 kg. Supine films were done at 2 to 3 minutes, 10 minutes, and 15 to 20 minutes, and in the prone position at 15 to 20 minutes. Film-focus distance was 100 cm, and the tabletop-film distance was 10 cm.[1]

Measurements ▪

Each adequately visualized ureter was measured at its widest point with a 7× magnifying, graded lens. Care was taken not to measure at the juxtapelvic, cone-shaped portion of the ureter. Correction for magnification was not done. The cephalocaudal distance between the upper end-plate of L1 and the lower end-plate of L3 (L1–L3) was also measured. Figure 1 shows these measurements. A regression equation for ureteral diameter and standard deviations versus age was calculated:

Ureteral diameter = $0.187 \times$ Age (years) + 3.89.

Standard deviation =
$$0.00098 \times \text{Age (years)}^2 + 0.083 \times \text{Age (years)} + 0.60.$$

Similarly, regression between ureteral diameter (mean and standard deviation) and L1–L3 distance yielded:

Ureteral diameter = $0.040 \times$ L1–L3 (mm) + 2.26.

Standard deviation =
$$0.000125 \times \text{L1–L3 (mm)}^2 + 0.00373 \times \text{L1–L3} + 0.56.$$

Figure 2 depicts mean measured ureteral diameter by age up through 12 years, as well as regression lines (mean ± 2 SD) through 16 years. Figure 3 shows regression lines (mean ± 2 SD) of ureteral diameter versus L1–L3 distance.[1]

Source ▪

Subjects were 194 children (100 boys, 94 girls; age range, newborn to 16 years) examined for pain, transient hematuria, enuresis, hypospadias, or screening. Patients with abnormal urograms, history of reflux, or abnormalities of the

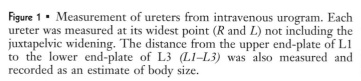

Figure 1 ▪ Measurement of ureters from intravenous urogram. Each ureter was measured at its widest point (*R* and *L*) not including the juxtapelvic widening. The distance from the upper end-plate of L1 to the lower end-plate of L3 *(L1–L3)* was also measured and recorded as an estimate of body size.

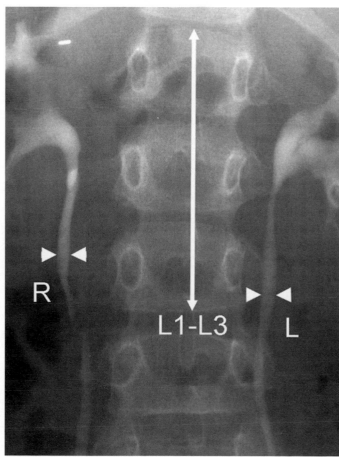

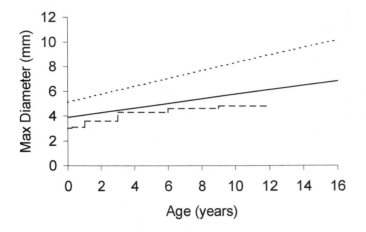

Figure 2 ▪ Ureteral diameter in infants and children versus age. The regression (*solid line*), +2 standard deviation regression (*dotted line*), and measured mean values (*dashed line*) are shown. (From Hellstrom M, Hjelmas K, Jacobson B, et al: Acta Radiol 1985; 26:433–439. Used by permission.)

Figure 3 ▪ Ureteral diameter in infants and children versus L1–L3 distance. The regression (*solid*) and +2 standard deviation regression (*dotted*) lines are shown. (From Hellstrom M, Hjelmas K, Jacobson B, et al: Acta Radiol 1985; 26:433–439. Used by permission.)

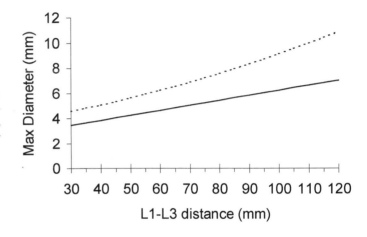

lumbar spine were excluded. Urogram films were initially evaluated for visualization of the ureters, and 330 were filled through more than 50% of their length and subsequently measured.[1]

Comments ▪

There was no difference between the ureteral diameters of boys and girls (p = .45). There was no significant difference in ureteral diameter between the two strengths of contrast or with bladder fullness. The right ureter was wider than the left by an average of 0.6 mm (p < .001). The widest portion of the ureter was most often in the middle third just above the crossing of the iliac vessels (77%).[1]

REFERENCE

1. Hellstrom M, Hjelmas K, Jacobson B, et al: Normal ureteral diameter in infancy and childhood. Acta Radiol 1985; 26:433–439.

▪: GRADING OF VESICOURETERAL REFLUX
▪ ACR Code: 82 (Ureter)

Technique ▪

A standardized method of performing voiding cystourethrography (VCU) has been described, as used in the International Reflux Study in Children.[1, 2] The child should void prior to catheterization. A small catheter (infant feeding of 6–8 French) is inserted into the bladder and residual volume recorded. The bladder is filled with body-temperature 15%–30% concentration contrast by drip infusion, with the bottle no more than 70 cm above the bladder. Infusion is terminated when the child wishes to void or when dripping stops and the volume is recorded. Radio-graphs in the frontal (AP) projection are made to include bladder, ureters, and kidneys at partial filling, with the bladder full, at the height of voiding, and immediately after voiding. If possible, the radiographs are made with fluoroscopic control, with films exposed while reflux is maximal. During the first examination, the urethra should be visualized during voiding, including a lateral view in boys. For follow-up examinations, the amount instilled into the bladder should be at least as much as on the initial examination. Instilled volume may be compared with norms of bladder capacity for age.[3, 4]

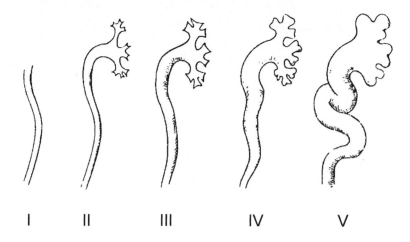

| I | II | III | IV | V |

Figure 1 ▪ Grading of vesicoureteral reflux at voiding cystourethrography. Descriptions of each grade are in Table 1. (From Levitt SB, Obling H, et al: Pediatrics 1981; 67:392–400. Used by permission.)

Table 1 ▪ Grading of Vesicoureteral Reflux

GRADE	INTERNATIONAL SYSTEM[1, 2]	HEIKEL AND PARKKULAINEN[5]	DWOSKIN AND PERLMUTTER[6]
I	Ureter only	Slight reflux confined to the lower part of the ureter, which is of normal width	Lower ureteral filling
II	Ureter, pelvis, and calyces. No dilatation, normal calyceal fornices	Reflux up into the renal pelvis, but the ureter and pelvis are of normal size	Ureteral and pelvicalyceal filling without other changes
III	Mild or moderate dilatation and/or tortuosity of ureter, and mild or moderate dilatation of renal pelvis, but no or slight blunting of the fornices	Shows reflux into a slightly dilated ureter and pelvis	Ureteral and pelvicalyceal filling with mild calyceal blunting but without clubbing and without dilatation of the pelvis or tortuosity of the ureter
IV	Moderate dilatation and/or tortuosity of ureter and moderate dilatation of renal pelvis and calyces. Complete obliteration of sharp angles of fornices but maintenance of papillary impressions in majority of calyces	Reflux into a moderately dilated ureter and pelvis	Ureteral and pelvicalyceal filling, calyceal clubbing, and minor to moderate pelvic dilatation, with slight tortuosity of the ureter
V	Gross dilatation and tortuosity of ureter. Gross dilatation of renal pelvis and calyces. Papillary impressions are no longer visible in the majority of calyces	Massive reflux into a grossly dilated ureter and pelvis	Massive hydronephrosis and hydroureter

The international system (column 1) is a combination of two previous systems (columns 2 and 3). In the system by Dwoskin and Perlmutter, the grades are I, IIA, IIB, III, and IV.

From Lebowitz RL, Olbing H, Parkkulainen KU, et al: Pediatr Radiol 1985; 15:105–109. Used by permission.

Measurements ▪

The new international classification is a combination of one previous classification that emphasized ureteral and pelvic filling and dilation[5] and another that included observations about the calyces.[6] Figure 1 shows the grades of reflux visually, and Table 1 lists the international classification as well as the two that were combined to formulate it.

REFERENCES

1. Lebowitz RL, Olbing H, Parkkulainen KV, et al: International system of radiographic grading of vesicoureteric reflux. Pediatr Radiol 1985; 15:105–109.

2. Levitt SB, Obling H, et al: Medical versus surgical treatment of primary vesicoureteral reflux: Report of the International Reflux Study Committee. Pediatrics 1981; 67:392–400.

3. Koff SA: Estimating bladder capacity in children. Urology 1983; 21:248.

4. Berger RM, Maizels M, Moran GC, et al: Bladder capacity (ounces) equals age (years) plus 2 predicts normal bladder capacity and aids in diagnosis of abnormal voiding patterns. J Urol 1983; 129:347–349.

5. Heikel PE, Parkkulainen KV: Vesicoureteric reflux in children: A classification and results of conservative treatment. Ann Radiol 1966; 9:37–40.

6. Dwoskin JY, Perlmutter AD: Vesicoureteral reflux in children: A computerized review. J Urol 1973; 109:888–890.

▪: MEASUREMENT OF BLADDER VOLUMES BY ULTRASONOGRAPHY FOR DETERMINING RESIDUAL URINE[1]
▪ ACR Code: 83 (Bladder)

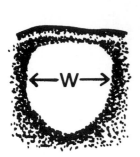
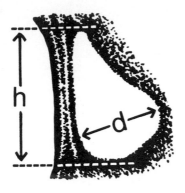

Figure 1 ▪ Width *(w)* is obtained from the transverse scan exhibiting the greatest transverse diameter. A midline longitudinal scan yields both height *(h)* and depth *(d)*; the latter is taken as the longest chord in the anteroposterior plane. The calculated volume *(V_c)* is the product of the three dimensions: $V_c = w \times h \times d$. (From McLean GK, Edell SL: Radiology 1978; 128:181–182. Used by permission.)

Figure 2 ▪ Longitudinal midline scan of bladders filled to total volumes of 300 ml. An acceptable scan clearly shows all bladder boundaries. *a* = anterior abdominal wall; *b* = saline-filled bladder; *f* = Foley balloon. (From McLean GK, Edell SL: Radiology 1978; 128:181–182. Used by permission.)

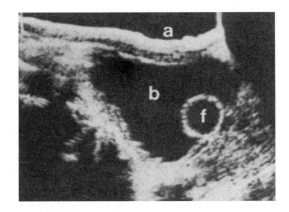

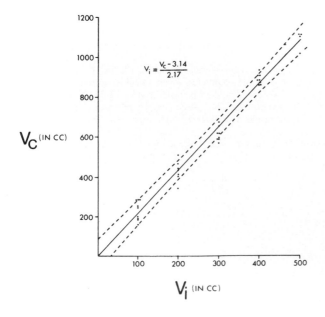

Figure 3 ▪ Computed volumes *(V_c)* are plotted against the volumes of instilled saline *(V_i)*. The calculated linear regression yields the relationship $V_i = (V_c - 3.14) \div 2.17$, with a correlation coefficient of 0.987. *Dashed lines* show the 95% confidence limits. (From McLean GK, Edell SL: Radiology 1978; 128:181–182. Used by permission.)

Technique ▪

1. A Picker 80-L unit with a 2.25-MHz focused transducer was used.
2. Determinations of bladder volumes were made following measured instillation of saline.
3. Bladders were scanned longitudinally and transversely.

Measurements ▪ (Figures 1 and 2)

Computed volumes are plotted against the volumes of instilled saline (Figure 3).

It has been shown that the bladder of a healthy child retains no more than a few millimeters of urine after voiding. Residual urine after normal voiding is abnormal.[2]

Source ▪

Data are based on a total of 48 scans obtained from 14 patients.

REFERENCES

1. Mclean GK, Edell SL: Determination of bladder volumes by gray scale ultrasonography. Radiology 1978; 128(1):181–182.
2. Harrison NW, Parks C, Sherwood T: Ultrasound assessment of residual urine in children. Br J Urol 1975; 47(7):805–814.

▪: ACCURACY OF BLADDER VOLUME DETERMINATION AT ULTRASOUND
▪ ACR Code: 83 (Bladder)

Technique ▪

Transabdominal scanning of the bladder was done with an 860c unit (ATL, Bothel, WA), with a 3-MHz mechanical sector transducer in transverse and longitudinal planes.[1]

Measurements ▪

Scanning of the bladder was done and images were recorded for subsequent measurement prior to micturition. The voided volume (VVoid) was recorded. This procedure was repeated ten times for each subject for a total of 100 volume determinations. One volume per subject was imaged twice to allow assessment of repeatability of imaging.[1] Five different methods of calculating ultrasound volume (UV) were used on each of the 100 sets of images, and these are detailed in Figure 1. For each of 500 pairs of volumes, the ratio of UV/VVoid was determined and recorded. Table 1 lists the results in terms of accuracy (mean of UV/VVoid) and repeatability ([SD of UV/Vvoid]/[mean of UV/Vvoid]) for each method. Numbers closer to 1.0 represent higher accuracy, and lower numbers mean greater repeatability.[1]

Source ▪

Subjects included 10 healthy male volunteers.[1]

Comments ▪

After further analysis of five components of measurement variability, Griffiths and colleagues found the most accurate and repeatable estimate of bladder volume to be the average V2 and V3. Since this method consistently underestimated VVoid by 15%, they suggest multiplying resulting volumes by 1.15.[1] A portable device (BVI 2000/BVI 2500, Diagnostic Ultrasound, Redmond, WA) designed to assess nursing home patients for residual urine volumes has been

Figure 1 ▪ Methods of estimating bladder volume with ultrasound. Five equations (V1–V5) are shown, and they use distances measured from longitudinal and transverse images through the largest portion of the bladder in each plane. The areas (*AT* and *AL*) were determined by tracing the perimeter of the bladder. Most newer units provide a function to calculate area from a closed perimeter. Linear measures from longitudinal images were height (*H*) and depth (*DL*). From transverse images, the width (*W*) and depth (*DT*) were measured.

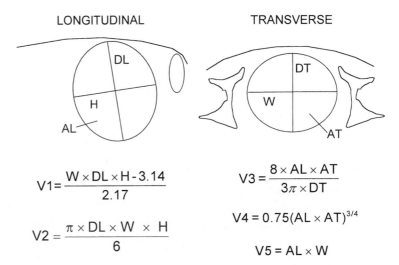

LONGITUDINAL TRANSVERSE

$$V1 = \frac{W \times DL \times H - 3.14}{2.17}$$

$$V2 = \frac{\pi \times DL \times W \times H}{6}$$

$$V3 = \frac{8 \times AL \times AT}{3\pi \times DT}$$

$$V4 = 0.75(AL \times AT)^{3/4}$$

$$V5 = AL \times W$$

Table 1 • Performance of Six Methods of Bladder Volume Determination

| METHOD | U/S VOLUME/VOIDED VOLUME | | | |
| | All Data (n = 100) | | Volume >150 ml (n = 81) | |
	Accuracy (mean)	Repeatability (SD/mean)	Accuracy (mean)	Repeatability (SD/mean)
V1	0.71	0.156	0.73	0.103
V2	0.82	0.151	0.84	0.102
V3	0.89	0.144	0.90	0.103
V4	0.91	0.164	0.93	0.146
V5	1.17	0.131	1.19	0.096
(V2 + V3)/2	0.85	0.134	0.87	0.090

Methods (V1–V5) listed in Figure 1. U/S = ultrasound; SD = standard deviation.

From Griffiths CJ, Murray A, Ramsden PD: J Urol 1986; 136:808–812. Used by permission.

developed. It uses the algorithm recommended above (V2 + V3/2) and has been found to be both precise and accurate when compared with concurrent catheter volumes.[2, 3] It should be noted that many studies have used method V2 (prolate ellipse), and this probably also represents the most common method used in routine practice settings. From the data presented here, a correction factor of 1.17 might be applied to this somewhat simpler method, yielding bladder volume (milliliters) = .613 × W × DL × H (each in centimeters).

REFERENCES

1. Griffiths CJ, Murray A, Ramsden PD: Accuracy and repeatability of bladder volume measurement using ultrasonic imaging. J Urol 1986; 136:808–812.
2. Coombes GM, Millard RJ: The accuracy of portable ultrasound scanning in the measurement of residual urine volume. J Urol 1994; 152(6 Pt 1):2083–2085.
3. Ouslander JG, Simmons S, Tuico E, et al: Use of a portable ultrasound device to measure post-void residual volume among incontinent nursing home residents. J Am Geriatr Soc 1994; 42(11):1189–1192.

⁚ BLADDER CAPACITY IN CHILDREN
- ACR Code: 83 (Bladder)

Technique •

Starfield measured voided urine volumes during diuresis.[1] Koff performed cystometric analysis with subjects under anesthesia, with bladder capacity determined by plateau in the pressure/volume curve.[2] Berger and colleagues measured instilled volume at capacity during cystoscopy or direct nuclear cystography.[3] Treves and colleagues also performed direct nuclear cystography.[4] The end-point of bladder filling was determined by decrease/cessation of flow, spontaneous voiding, or indications by the patient of maximal filling.[3, 4]

Measurements •

In each study the volume voided or instilled was recorded in milliliters. Koff, Berger and colleagues, and Treves and group devised linear relationships between patient age and bladder capacity.[2–4] Treves and group also developed a nonlinear correlation between age and bladder capacity.[4] Figure

(1) oz. = 28 × ml.

(2) Berger / Koff (oz.) = age(years) + 2

(3) Berger / Koff (ml.) = (age(years) + 2) × 28

(4) Berger (ml.) = (32 × age(years) + 73)

(5) Treves linear (ml.) = 22 × age(years) + 136

(6) Treves nonlinear (ml.) = 54 × (10 × age + 1)$^{0.40}$

Figure 1 • Equations for determining bladder capacity in children (1). Conversion of fluid ounces to milliliters is helpful in using the simple Berger/Koff relationship (2). (3) This equation can be directly expressed in terms of milliliters. Linear equations developed by (4) Berger and (5) Treves, as well as a nonlinear relationship from Treves (6), are shown.

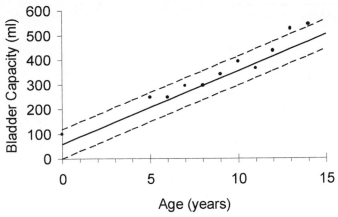

Figure 2 ▪ Bladder capacities *(circles)* in children determined by voided volumes by Starfield, and predicted capacity *(solid line)* by the Berger/Koff relationship (equations 2 and 3 in Figure 1). Plus and minus 2 ounces (56 ml, dashed lines) are also shown. (From Berger RM, Maizels M, Moran GC, et al: J Urol 1983; 129:347349. Used by permission.)

1 lists these equations. Figure 2 shows Starfield's data and the simple equation (number 2 in Figure 1) that both Koff and Berger described (bladder capacity in ounces = age [years] + 2).[1-3] Figure 3 shows the 50th, 10th, and 90th percentiles of the nonlinear model devised by Treves and group, as well as the capacities observed by Berger and Treves.[3, 4] Table 1 lists the mean or 50th percentile predicted bladder capacities from all models.[2-4]

Source ▪

Starfield studied 203 normal, nonenuretic children.[1] Koff's subjects were 35 nonenuretic, uninfected children.[2] Berger and colleagues evaluated 123 children with normal voiding

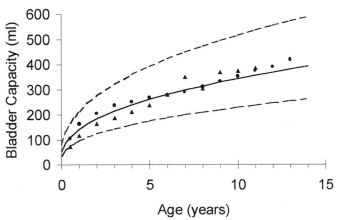

Figure 3 ▪ Observed bladder capacities by Berger *(triangles)* and Treves *(circles)*, as well as 50th *(solid)*, 10th *(dashed)*, and 90th *(dashed)* percentiles from Treves' nonlinear model (equation 6 in Figure 1).

Table 1 ▪ Predicted Bladder Capacity in Children by Four Methods

AGE (Yr)	BERGER/KOFF (3)	BERGER (4)	TREVES LINEAR (5)	TREVES NONLINEAR (6)
Neonate	56	73	136	54
0.25	63	81	142	90
0.5	70	89	147	111
0.75	77	97	153	128
1.0	84	105	158	142
1.5	98	121	169	165
2	112	137	180	184
3	140	169	202	215
4	168	201	224	240
5	196	233	246	262
6	224	265	268	282
7	252	297	290	299
8	280	329	312	315
9	308	361	334	331
10	336	393	356	345
11	364	425	378	358
12	392	457	400	370
13	420	489	422	382
14	448	521	444	394

The numbers in parentheses in column heads refer to the equations in Figure 1. From Treves ST, Zurakowski D, Bauer SB, et al: Radiology 1996; 198:269–272. Used by permission.

patterns.[3] Treves and colleagues reviewed 5165 nuclear cystograms (4018 girls, 1147 boys).[4]

Comments ▪

Following cystography, the total instilled volume of contrast may be compared with these norms to determine the percent predicted. Treves and group found that the nonlinear model performed better than the linear estimate of bladder capacity versus age (r squared = 0.489 and 0.591, respectively), especially above the age of 10 years. They also found that girls had slightly higher bladder capacities than boys.[4] To calculate capacities for girls and boys, 56 and 53 may be substituted for the multiplier (54 for all children) in equation 6 from Figure 1. Bladder capacity was strongly correlated with height and weight, but these factors did not add to the predictive value of age alone as determined by multiple linear regression.[4] The Berger/Koff relationship is the easiest to remember and serves as a fairly accurate "rule of thumb" for children up to 10 years old.[2, 3]

REFERENCES

1. Starfield B: Functional bladder capacity in enuretic and non-enuretic children. J Pediatr 1967; 70:777–781.
2. Koff SA: Estimating bladder capacity in children. Urology 1983; 21:248.
3. Berger RM, Maizels M, Moran GC, et al: Bladder capacity (ounces) equals age (years) plus 2 predicts normal bladder capacity and aids in diagnosis of abnormal voiding patterns. J Urol 1983; 129:347–349.
4. Treves ST, Zurakowski D, Bauer SB, et al: Functional bladder capacity measured during radionuclide cystography in children. Radiology 1996; 198:269–272.

⁚ BLADDER WALL THICKNESS ON ULTRASOUND
▪ ACR Code: 83 (Bladder)

Table 1 ▪ Bladder Wall Thickness by Age and Bladder Volume

AGE	PERCENT OF PREDICTED BLADDER CAPACITY			
	<10%	10–25%	26–90%	>90%
<1 mon	2.62 ± 0.51 (8)	2.10 ± 0.31 (10)	1.92 ± 0.51 (12)	1.67 ± 0.57 (3)
1 mon–1 yr	2.61 ± 0.62 (14)	1.93 ± 0.27 (14)	1.65 ± 0.47 (27)	2 (2)
1–6 yr	2.76 ± 0.73 (29)	2.06 ± 0.35 (39)	1.87 ± 0.37 (57)	1.44 ± 0.52 (9)
6–12 yr	2.82 ± 0.46 (36)	2.17 ± 0.32 (43)	1.97 ± 0.42 (49)	1.43 ± 0.53 (7)
>12 yr	2.83 ± 0.51 (18)	2.18 ± 0.32 (14)	1.89 ± 0.39 (22)	1.64 ± 0.74 (7)
All	2.76 ± 0.59 (105)	2.10 ± 0.33 (120)	1.87 ± 0.42 (167)	1.55 ± 0.66 (28)
All (5th–95th %tile)	(1.54–3.87)	(1.46–2.73)	(1.05–2.52)	(0.29–2.78)

All measurements in millimeters (mean ± standard deviation). Numbers in each group are given in parentheses. The 5th and 95th percentiles (%tile) are given for all patients in the bottom row.

From Jequier S, Rousseau O: AJR Am J Roentgenol 1987; 149:563–566. Used by permission.

Technique ▪

Transabdominal ultrasound of the bladder was done with two machines, ATL (Bothel, WA) or Diasonics (Sunnyvale, CA) using 5- to 7.5-MHz transducers.[1]

Measurements ▪

The bladder wall was measured on transverse and longitudinal images, usually in the area of the bladder floor posterior to the trigone (Figure 1). Care was taken not to include adjacent structures in the measurement. Three axis measurements of the entire bladder were done and bladder volume calculated by summing the measurements and dividing by 8 to obtain the average radius, which was then cubed and multiplied by $4/3 \times \pi$. Calculated volumes were compared with normal bladder capacity for age according to Koff.[2] Bladder volumes (expressed as percentage of age-appropriate capacity) were divided into four ranges. Table 1 lists bladder wall thickness by age and bladder fullness.

Source ▪

Subjects included 410 infants and children (age range, 1 day to 19 years) and 10 adults (age range, 19 to 42 years). There were a total of 218 males and 202 females. Patients having urinary tract symptoms or morphologic abnormalities at ultrasound were excluded.[1]

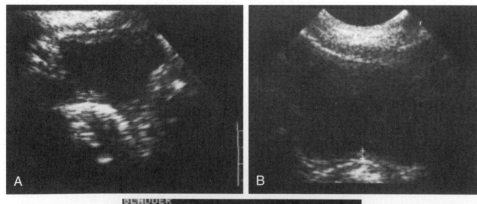

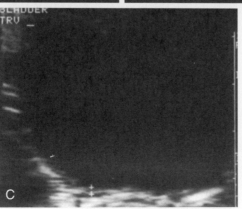

Figure 1 ▪ Measurement of bladder wall thickness. *A*, Empty bladder in a 1 month old boy with a 3.0-mm thick wall. *B*, Partly full bladder in a 7 year old boy; the wall thickness is 2.9 mm. *C*, Full bladder in a 9 year old boy, with a 1.4-mm wall. (From Jequier S, Rousseau O: AJR Am J Roentgenol 1987; 149:563–566. Used by permission.)

Comments ▪

There was a highly significant decrease in wall thickness with greater bladder filling (p < .0001). Boys had minimally thicker walls than girls (2.19 mm versus 2.08 mm, p = .07), and there was a slight increase in thickness with age (p < .04).[1]

Manieri and colleagues measured bladder wall thickness with transabdominal ultrasound in 174 patients (mostly men) and correlated it with uroflowmetry and pressure-flow studies to diagnose bladder outlet obstruction. Of the patients with bladder walls greater than 5 mm, 88% were obstructed, whereas 37% of those whose walls were 5 mm or less were obstructed. Ultrasound wall thickness outperformed flowmetry but was considered not to replace invasive urodynamics.[3] Abu-Yousef and colleagues performed transabdominal bladder ultrasound on 120 patients (mostly men) while studying bladder tumors and found the normal wall to measure 3 to 6 mm.[4]

REFERENCES

1. Jequier S, Rousseau O: Sonographic measurements of the normal bladder wall in children. AJR Am J Roentgenol 1987; 149:563–566.
2. Koff SA: Estimating bladder capacity in children. Urology 1983; 21:248.
3. Manieri C, Carter SS, Romano G, et al: The diagnosis of bladder outlet obstruction in men by ultrasound measurement of bladder wall thickness. J Urol 1998; 159:761–765.
4. Abu-Yousef MM, Narayana AS, Franken EA, Brown RC: Urinary bladder tumors studied by cystosonography. Part I: Detection. Radiology 1984; 153:223–226.

▪▪ MEASUREMENT OF THE URETHROVESICAL ANGLES IN STRESS INCONTINENCE[1]

▪ ACR Code: 833 (Vesicourethral Junction)

Technique ▪

Central ray: At level of greater trochanter perpendicular to plane of film.
Position: Lateral erect straining.
Target-film distance: Immaterial.

Measurements ▪ (Figure 1)

Angles are determined by chain cystourethrography with the patient in the erect position during straining. The angle between the posterior aspect of the urethra and the base of the bladder (posterior urethrovesical angle) normally measures 90° to 100°. Loss of this angle alone indicates Type I stress incontinence. The angle of inclination of the urethra is found by extending a line through the direction of the upper urethra to join a line in the vertical axis of the patient. The normal angle is 10° to 30°, and an angle above 45° is definitely abnormal. Loss of this angle, plus loss of the posterior urethral angle, constitutes Type II stress incontinence.

Source ▪

The data on the posterior urethrovesical angle are based on a study of more than 500 roentgen examinations of the bladder and urethra of 132 nonpregnant women.[2] The data on the angle of inclination of the urethra are based on a study of 350 patients examined by cystourethrography.[3]

Green[1] notes that angle measurements do not apply if a cystocele is present. The chain cystourethrogram is usually abnormal in stress incontinence. However, an abnormal cystourethrogram does not necessarily indicate stress incontinence.

REFERENCES

1. Green TH Jr: Am J Obstet Gynecol 1962; 83:632.
2. Jeffcoate TNA, Roberts H: J Obstet Gynaecol Br Emp 1952; 59:685.
3. Bailey KV: J Obstet Gynaecol Br Emp 1956; 63:663.

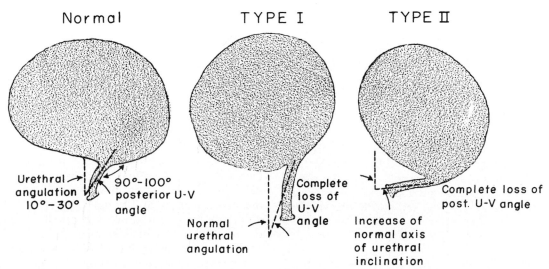

Figure 1 ▪ Measurement of urethrovesical angles from lateral chain cystourethrograms (see text for details). (Adapted from Green TH, Jr: Am J Obstet Gynecol 1962; 83:632.)

▪: THE SACROCOCCYGEAL–INFERIOR PUBIC POINT (SCIPP) LINE AND THE LATERAL CYSTOURETHROGRAM[1]
▪ ACR Code: 833 (Vesicourethral Junction)

Technique ▪

Central ray: At level of greater trochanter perpendicular to plane of film.
Positions: Lateral recumbent, lateral erect straining, lateral erect voiding.
Target-film distance: 36 inches.

Measurements ▪ (Figure 1)

The bladder is filled with opaque medium until the patient experiences discomfort. A small chain of metal beads is used to demonstrate the urethrovesical angle. A line *(SCIPP)* is drawn from the sacrococcygeal joint *(SC)* to the inferior point of the pubic bone *(IPP)*. *BN* is the bladder neck, and the flat base of the bladder is the base plate.

Average measurements (centimeters) in the lateral recumbent position are shown in Table 1.

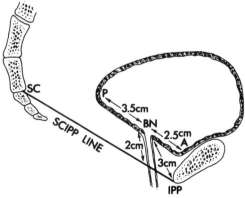

Figure 1 ▪ Composite drawing of lateral recumbent film showing average normal adult female measurements (see text for details). (From Noll LE, Hutch JA: Obstet Gynecol 1969; 33:680. Used by permission.)

In the standing position, the bladder neck drops 1 cm from the recumbent position.

Table 1 ▪ Average Measurements (cm) in the Lateral Recumbent Position

	AVERAGE (cm)
Base plate: Range 5–7 cm	6.0
Base plate: Anterior to bladder neck	2.5
Base plate: Posterior to bladder neck	3.5
Bladder neck above SCIPP line	2.0
Bladder neck to IPP	3.0

From Noll LE, Hutch JA: Obstet Gynecol 1969; 33:680. Used by permission.

In the standing position with straining, the bladder neck drops an additional 1 or 2 cm compared with the recumbent position.

In the standing position with voiding, the bladder neck drops an additional 0.5 to 2.5 cm compared with the recumbent position.

In patients with stress incontinence, the recumbent film showed a rounded base plate for about one half the patients. The bladder neck averaged 1 cm above the SCIPP line. The drop in the bladder neck upon standing, straining, and voiding was greater in distance than for the normal group.

Source ▪

Ninety-five adult women, of whom 20 were urologically normal.

Note: A data sheet has been designed by Noll and Hutch that enables the radiologist to record readily all pertinent cystourethrogram information.

REFERENCE

1. Noll LE, Hutch JA: The SCIPP line — an aid in interpreting the voiding lateral cystourethrogram. Obstet Gynecol 1969; 33(5):680–689.

▪: BLADDER NECK POSITION WITH ULTRASOUND
▪ ACR Code: 833 (Vesicourethral Junction)

Technique ▪

Transperoneal ultrasound was done with a 3.5-MHz curved-array transducer and a 650 scanner (Aloka, Tokyo, Japan), with the bladder comfortably full (about 150 to 250 ml). Sagittal scanning was done to localize the pubic symphysis (PS), vesicourethral junction (VUJ), and proximal urethra. This was done at rest and during the Valsalva maneuver.[1]

Measurements ▪

Measurements of the VUJ position were made with respect to the lower margin of the PS and a horizontal baseline intersecting it and being 120 degrees with respect to the axis of the PS. The baseline corresponded to the reference line between PS and S5 used for lateral chain cystography. Linear measurements included the vertical distance between the baseline and UVJ at rest and during Valsalva/straining (R, S) and the corresponding distance between the lower margin of PS and UVJ (Drest, Dstrain). The difference between R and S was calculated and was termed the descent of the bladder neck (DBN = R − S). The angle between Drest and Dstrain was also measured and was termed rotational angle (RA).[1] These measurements are depicted in Figures 1 and 2. Table 1 lists the results.

Figure 1 ▪ Measurements of the urethrovesical junction *(UVJ)* from sagittal transperoneal ultrasound. A baseline *(dotted line)* was drawn at an angle of 120 degrees to the axis of the pubic symphysis *(solid line)*, intersecting its lower margin *(asterisk)*. The vertical distance *(arrows)* between the baseline and UVJ was measured at rest *(R)* and during Valsalva/straining *(S)*. The descent of the bladder neck was calculated as the difference between R and S (DBN = R − S).

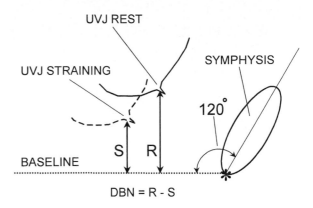

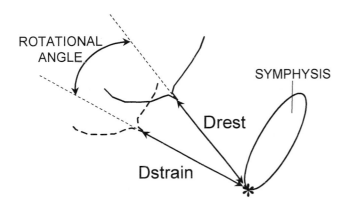

Figure 2 ▪ Measurements of the urethrovesical junction (UVJ) from sagittal transperoneal ultrasound. The distance between the lower margin of the pubic symphysis *(asterisk)* and the UVJ was measured at rest and during Valsalva/straining *(Drest, Dstrain)*. The angle between Drest and Dstrain was measured and termed the rotational angle.

Table 1 ▪ Relationship of the Urethrovesical Junction to the Pubic Symphysis

	CONTINENT		STRESS INCONTINENCE
	Nulliparous	Vag Deliv	
Age range (yr)	Not given	23–49	24–46
Parity	0	1–4	1–4
Number	25	40	37
Drest (mm)	29.3 ± 3.3	29.5 ± 3.6	26.8 ± 4.0
Dstrain (mm)	23.0 ± 3.8	22.4 ± 3.9	19.4 ± 3.5
RA (degrees)	17.6 ± 14.9	22.7 ± 13.6	42.9 ± 19.7
R (mm)	21.3 ± 5.4	22.3 ± 4.6	18.2 ± 5.6
S (mm)	12.3 ± 8.5	11.4 ± 6.0	0.6 ± 6.8
DBN (mm)	9.0 ± 6.9	11.2 ± 5.4	17.6 ± 7.3

All measurements given as mean ± standard deviation. Measurement abbreviations as in text and Figures 1 and 2. Vag Deliv = vaginal delivery.
From Chen GD, Su TH, Lin LY: J Clin Ultrasound 1997; 25:189–194. Used by permission.

Source ▪

Subjects included 37 women with proven genuine stress incontinence (GSI). The control group consisted of 65 continent women (25 nulliparous and 40 with at least one vaginal delivery).[1] Age ranges and parity are listed in Table 1.

Comments ▪

Receiver operating curve (ROC) analysis showed that DBN >13 mm or RA >28 degrees performed equally well in detecting GSI; sensitivity, 73%, specificity, 77%, positive predictive value, 64%, and negative predictive value, 83%. The combination of DBN >13 mm and RA >28 degrees performed as follows: sensitivity, 62%, specificity, 83%, positive predictive value, 68%, and negative predictive value, 79%.[1]

REFERENCE

1. Chen GD, Su TH, Lin LY: Applicability of perineal sonography in anatomical evaluation of bladder neck in women with and without genuine stress incontinence. J Clin Ultrasound 1997; 25:189–194.

▪: MEASUREMENT OF THE URETHRA IN CHILDREN[1]
- ACR Code: 84 (Male Urethra); 85 (Female Urethra)

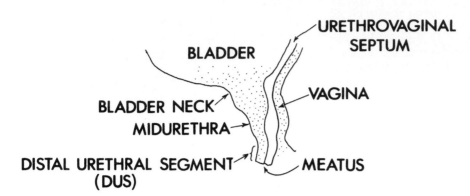

Figure 1 ▪ Measurement of the urethra in girls. (Adapted from Shopfner CE: Radiology 1967; 88:222.)

Table 1 ▪ Urethrogram Measurements (Percentage of Patients)*

DIAMETERS (mm)	GIRLS			BOYS	
	Meatus (%)	DUS (%)	Midurethra (%)	Membranous Urethra (%)	Posterior Urethra (%)
2	4	4		4	
3	16	16		8	
4	20	20	1	16	1
5	31	28	3	26	5
6	25	21	9	24	8
7	4	9	11	16	18
8		2	25	4	24
9			12	2	11
10			4		13
11			5		3
12			17		4
13			4		4
14			1.5		1
15			2		2
16			2		1
17			0.05		1
18			1		1
19			1		1
20			0.05		1
21			0.05		1

*Measurements made during full voiding stream. DUS = distal urethral segment.

From Shopfner CE: Radiology 1967; 88:222. Used by permission.

Technique ▪

Central ray: Television fluoroscopy and spot roentgenograms made during the voiding cycle.
Position: Oblique and lateral views obtained during voiding cystourethrography.
Target-film distance: Variable; Shopfner used a 15% correction for magnification.

Measurements ▪ (Figure 1 and Table 1)

For girls, the meatus was indicated by barium coating of the mucosa or by identification of the urethrovaginal septum. Diameters of meatus, distal urethral segment, and midurethra were measured on films taken during full voiding.

For boys, the urethra was measured at the midpart of the membranous and the posterior urethra.

Source ▪

Fifty-three girls and 67 boys with no urinary tract abnormality. Ages ranged from less than 1 year to 16 years.

REFERENCE

1. Shopfner CE: Roentgen evaluation of distal urethral obstruction. Radiology 1967; 88(2): 222–231.

▪: URETHRAL MEASUREMENTS WITH ULTRASOUND IN CONTINENT WOMEN
▪ ACR Code: 851 (Female Urethra)

Technique ▪

Transvaginal ultrasound was done with an SSA-260A machine (Toshiba, Tokyo, Japan), using a 5.0-MHz vaginal transducer. The patients were supine, and the bladder was comfortably full. The probe was placed adjacent to the introitus just under the external urethral orifice, and scanning was done in the sagittal plane. Scanning was done at rest and during Valsalva maneuver.[1] The vaginal probe is useful because of its configuration, wide field of view, and good near-field image quality. Wise and colleagues have shown that a fully inserted vaginal probe causes significant elevation of the bladder neck and restriction of its descent during straining, and these findings emphasize the importance of not actually inserting the probe into the vagina.[2]

Measurements ▪

On frozen sagittal images centered on the urethra and bladder neck, the urethral inclination (UI), posterior urethrovesical angle (PUVA), urethral thickness (UT), and urethral length (UL) were measured, as shown in Figures 1 and 2. The UI and PUVA were measured at rest and during the Valsalva maneuver. The rotational angle (RA) was defined as the difference in urethral inclination between rest and Valsalva.[1] Table 1 lists the results.

Source ▪

Three groups of women were studied: (1) 103 controls (age range, 17 to 80 years, mean gravidity, 3.7, mean parity, 2.4)

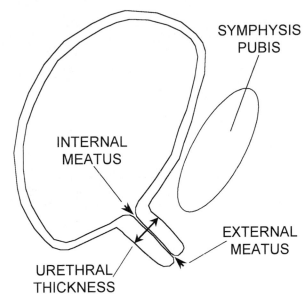

Figure 2 ▪ Measurement of urethral dimensions from sagittal transperoneal ultrasound. Urethral thickness was measured 1 cm distal to the internal urethral meatus (*line with arrowheads*). The urethral length was measured between the internal and external urethral meatus (*arrowheads*).

of whom 10 were postmenopausal (for at least 1 year); (2) 46 pregnant women (age range, 23 to 39 years, mean gravidity, 1.6, mean parity, 0.6, numbers equally distributed between the trimesters); and (3) 15 patients (age range, 34 to 66 years, mean gravidity, 5.4, mean parity, 3.8) with at least third-degree genitourinary prolapse. None of the 154 women had urinary incontinence.[1]

Comments ▪

In general, age, parity, and menopause did not affect the measured parameters in normal women other than a decrease in UT after menopause (p = .026). Pregnant women and those with prolapse had significantly lower urethral position (larger UI, p < .001). Significant hypermotility of the urethra was found only in those with prolapse (larger RA, p < .001). Pregnant women had decreased UL (p = 0.02). The changes noted during pregnancy could help explain the increased incidence of stress incontinence in pregnancy, which usually resolves after delivery.[1]

An increase in the PUVA at rest and hypermotility of the bladder neck during straining are common findings in urethrocystography of incontinent women (none in this study). Though incontinence is not common in prolapse (10% to 30%), measuring urethral mobility may be useful in planning appropriate corrective surgery for prolapse.[1, 3, 4]

Wise performed lateral chain cystourethrography with and without a vaginal U/S probe within the vagina and found that the probe significantly elevates the bladder neck and restricts bladder neck descent.[2] This finding empha-

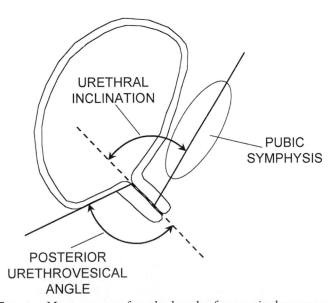

Figure 1 ▪ Measurement of urethral angles from sagittal transperoneal ultrasound. The posterior urethrovesical angle was measured between a line tangential to the base of the bladder from the internal urethral meatus and the midline of the urethral lumen. The urethral inclination was measured between a line through the long axis of the pubic symphysis and the midline of the urethral lumen.

Table 1 ▪ Urethral Angles and Dimensions at Transperoneal Ultrasound

Parameter	Premenopause	Postmenopause	Pregnant	Prolapse
Number	93	10	46	15
Urethral thickness (mm)	16.6±2.6	14.7±2.0	16.4±2.5	14.8±1.3
	(11.0–23.7)	(11.3–17.1)	(13.7–22.8)	(11.3–23.7)
Urethral length (mm)	32.9±4.5	31.4±3.9	30.7±3.9	31.1±3.5
	(26.2–44.2)	(28.0–41.5)	(24.8–37.7)	(27.4–36.5)
Urethral inclination (deg)				
Rest	47±13	48±12	65±14	60±16
	(13–85)	(30–65)	(38–80)	(41–91)
Valsalva	67±19	56±17	83±28	110±19
	(20–133)	(46–64)	(50–123)	(85–131)
Change Valsalva/rest	19±18	21±22	19±19	46±17
(rotational angle)	(−17–80)	(−11–34)	(−8–56)	(27–70)
PUVA (deg)				
Rest	118±20	118±18	119±14	128±27
	(73–175)	(95–159)	(94–150)	(100–174)
Valsalva	135±29	123±28	124±11	121±32
	(80–225)	(85–171)	(103–142)	(87–144)

Measurements are given as mean ± standard deviation and range. PUVA = posterior urethrovesical angle.
From Yang J: J Clin Ultrasound 1996; 24:249–255. Used by permission.

sizes the importance of keeping the transducer at the introitus and not within the vagina.

References

1. Yang J: Factors affecting urethrocystographic parameters in urinary continent women. J Clin Ultrasound 1996; 24:249–255.

2. Wise BG, Burton G, Cutner A, et al: Effect of vaginal ultrasound probe on lower urinary tract function. Br J Urol 1992; 70:12–16.

3. Walters MD, Jackson GM: Urethral mobility and its relationship to stress incontinence in women. J Reprod Med 1990; 35:777–784.

4. Bergman A, Ballard CA, Plat LD: Ultrasonic evaluation of urethrovesical junction in women with stress urinary incontinence. J Clin Ultrasound 1989; 16:295–300.

▪: MEASUREMENT OF THE ADULT MALE URETHRA[1]
▪ ACR Code: 84 (Male Urethra)

Technique ▪

Central ray: Voiding cystourethrography using television fluoroscopy and spot roentgenograms made during the voiding cycle.
Position: Anteroposterior and both obliques. Views obtained during voiding.
Target-film distance: All measurements given are corrected for geometric enlargement.

Measurements ▪ (Figures 1, 2, and 3)

1. The narrowest point between the bladder base and the upper limit of the verumontanum (supracollicular urethra [SCU]).

2. The widest diameter of the prostatic urethra (PRU).
3. The narrowest point between the verumontanum and the cone of the bulbous urethra (membranous urethra [MU]).
4. The widest diameter of the bulbous urethra (BU).
5. The diameter of the penoscrotal junction (PSJ).
6. The narrowest caliber of the penile urethra (PEU).

The measurements were performed with a ruler marked in millimeters. The results were noted as integer numbers. There were three measurements for each segment in Group I and two measurements in Group II. The calibers were corrected for the estimated geometric enlargement

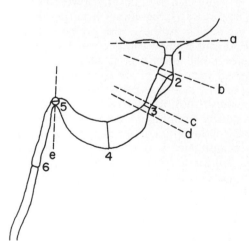

Figure 1 ▪ The anatomic landmarks on the micturition cystourethrogram: *a* = bladder base; *b* = upper limit of verumontanum; *c* = the cone of the prostatic urethra; *d* = the junction between the membranous and bulbous parts; *e* = the penoscrotal junction. The sites where the calibers were measured are indicated by *double lines*: *1* = SCU; *2* = PRU; *3* = MU; *4* = BU; *5* = PSJ; *6* = PEU (see Measurements). (From Manoliu RA: Eur J Radiol 1982; 2:209. Used by permission.)

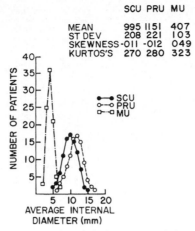

Figure 2 ▪ The average internal diameters of the supracollicular, prostatic, and membranous urethra. (From Manoliu RA: Eur J Radiol 1982; 2:209. Used by permission.)

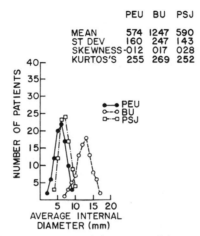

Figure 3 ▪ The average internal diameters of the penoscrotal junction, bulbous, and penile urethra. (From Manoliu RA: Eur J Radiol 1982; 2:209. Used by permission.)

($\times$ 1.3 for the obliques and $\times$ 1.2 for the anteroposterior projections). For each segment an arithmetic mean was computed. This mean was rounded to the nearest millimeter.

Source ▪

Data are based on a study of 92 adult males ranging in age from 18 to 71 years, with a mean age of 43.3 years.

REFERENCE

1. Manolin RA: Urethral calibre measurements on micturition cystourethrograms in adult males. Part 1: normal urethra. Eur J Radiol 1982; 2(3):209–213.

▪▪ TRANSRECTAL ULTRASOUND MEASUREMENT OF PROSTATE VOLUME
▪ ACR Code: 844 (Prostate)

Technique ▪

Terris and Stamey used a model 1846 ultrasound machine (Bruel & Kjaer) equipped with 7.0-MHz transrectal transverse and longitudinal transducers, as well as a ratcheted stepping device that allows recording transverse images at calibrated 2.0-mm intervals from base to apex of the gland.

A constant volume of 30 ml was instilled into the water path balloon attached to the transducers and all measurements were made before any biopsies were performed.[1]

Measurements ▪

From the transverse sections, the largest transverse width (W) and anteroposterior height (H) were measured. With

TRANSVERSE   LONGITUDINAL

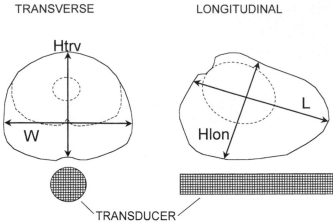

LARGE MEDIAN LOBE

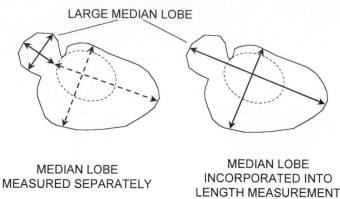

MEDIAN LOBE   MEDIAN LOBE
MEASURED SEPARATELY   INCORPORATED INTO
                              LENGTH MEASUREMENT

Figure 1 ▪ Linear measurements of the prostate for volume determination. The width *(W)* and height *(Htrv)* were measured at their maxima from transverse images. Alternatively, the height *(Hlon)* may be measured from longitudinal images, as described by Littrup.[2] The length *(L)* was measured from an image through the midline from base to apex.

Figure 2 ▪ Incorporating an enlarged median lobe into prostate volume measurements. For planimetry, the beginning of the sweep is extended cephalad to include the median lobe. With linear methods, one may either include the median lobe in the length measurement *(shown on the right)* or make separate measurements *(shown on the left)* and calculate another volume to be added to that of the body of the gland. Terris did not specifically mention this problem.

the transverse transducer mounted in the stepping device, serial transverse sections at 2.0-mm intervals were obtained and the perimeter of the gland traced, yielding an area. This was done from base to apex. During examination with the longitudinal transducer, the greatest cephalocaudal length (L) of the gland was measured from the midline image.[1] Figure 1 shows the linear measurements with two alternatives for gland height measurement.[1, 2] Figure 2 illustrates the problem of an enlarged median lobe (not specifically mentioned by Terris and Stamey).[3] Figure 3 depicts the serial area measurements. The volume was calculated by summation of areas and multiplying by section thickness (planimetry), the popular prolate ellipse formula, seven combinations of linear measurements cubed (sphere), and six products of two linear measurements with one squared (spheroid). Each of the 15 methods of calculating prostate volume was done for each patient.[1] Seven of the best-performing calculation methods are shown in Figure 4.

Since the specific gravity of the prostate has been shown to be 1.050 gm/ml, no correction from volume to weight

was done.[4] The calculated prostate volumes were then compared with the weight of glands removed surgically.[1] Table 1 lists the results from the seven methods that performed best (correlation coefficient > 0.87).

Source ▪

Terris and Stamey evaluated 150 men (age range, 31 to 79 years, mean age, 65.2 years) prior to radical prostatectomy for adenocarcinoma (n = 123) or radical cystoprostatectomy for transitional cell carcinoma of the bladder (n = 27).[1]

Comments ▪

Accurate determination of prostate volume by transrectal scanning is important in classifying the risk of prostate cancer in combination with prostate-specific antigen (PSA) determinations, in cases of prostate cancer being treated with external beam radiation to shrink the tumor/gland prior to interstitial seed placement, and to follow response

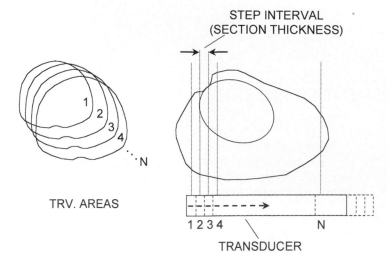

Figure 3 ▪ Measurement of prostate volume by planimetry. Serial transverse sections are made through the gland, using a stepping device to hold the transducer. In addition to allowing calibrated withdrawal, the device holds the transducer in constant orientation. The perimeter of the gland is traced on each image. The resulting areas *(1, 2, 3, 4, . . ., N)* are summed and multiplied by the section thickness to obtain volume.

Table 1 ▪ Performance of Various Methods of Prostate Volume Determination

METHOD	CORRELATION COEFFICIENT	AVERAGE ERROR (grams, mean ± SD)			
		All Volumes	<40 ml	40–80 ml	>80 ml
Spheroid-1	0.94	8.8±7.1	6.6±4.8	9.8±6.4	16.2±9.2
Planimetry	0.93	9.4±7.5	8.6±7.0	10.9±8.1	17.6±9.8
Sphere-1	0.91	10.8±8.2	7.4±4.8	13.0±7.0	24.4±13.6
Sphere-2	0.90	11.7±8.1	8.7±4.7	13.5±7.4	23.9±14.1
Prolate ellipse	0.90	12.1±8.8	8.4±5.0	14.5±7.2	26.4±13.8
Sphere-3	0.88	17.6±12.6	16.4±11.9	18.2±13.0	15.9±9.1
Spheroid-2	0.88	18.9±10.3	14.6±5.5	21.8±8.6	34.7±19.1

Terminology for methods as in Figure 4. The average errors are grouped by excised gland weight and given for all patients (all volumes) as well. SD = standard deviation. From Terris MK, Stamey TA: J Urol 1991; 145:984–987. Used by permission.

to drug treatment of benign hypertrophy. The planimetric method has been well validated[5–7] as the most accurate and precise, and a more rapid computerized method has been described.[6] The methods using linear measurements are attractive because they do not require special equipment, are more rapid, and may be done with the patient in the decubitus position.[7–9]

Terris and Stamey found the spheroid method using W as the major axis and H as the minor axis (spheroid-1 in Figure 4) to be slightly superior overall to planimetry and the spherical method using cubed W (sphere-3 in Figure 4) to be superior at higher prostate volumes. The prolate ellipse method is familiar because it has been used successfully both in uroradiology and other areas, and Terris and Stamey showed that it gave acceptable results.[1] These results have been replicated by others, with the prolate ellipse method performing nearly as well as planimetry and ellipsoid and spherical models in some.[3, 7–9] Littrup and colleagues evaluated area spheroid methods available in the built-in software on some machines and believed that they offered no advantages over the prolate ellipse method.[7]

Bazinet and colleagues caution that linear methods may be subject to as much as 25% variation of consecutive measurements in the same subject.[10]

The normal prostate gland measures 2.5 to 3.0 cm in W as well as H, 2.0 to 2.5 cm in L, and about 20 ml at transrectal scanning.[11] One grading system for hypertrophy has four steps: I <30 gm, II 30 to 50 gm, III 50 to 85 gm, and IV > 85 gm.[12]

REFERENCES

1. Terris MK, Stamey TA: Determination of prostate volume by transrectal ultrasound. J Urol 1991; 145:984–987.
2. Littrup PJ: Reply to comments in Radiology 1992; 183:625–626. Radiology 1992; 183:626–627.
3. Tewari A, Indudhara R, Shinohara K, et al: Comparison of transrectal ultrasound prostatic volume estimation with magnetic resonance imaging volume estimation and surgical specimen weight in patients with benign prostatic hyperplasia. J Clin Ultrasound 1996; 24:169–174.
4. Watanabe H, Igari D, Tanahashi Y, et al: Measurements of size and weight of prostate by means of transrectal ultrasonography. Tohoku J Exp Med 1974; 114:277–285.
5. Hastak SM, Gammelgaard J, Holm HH: Transrectal ultrasonic volume determination of the prostate—A preoperative and postoperative study. J Urol 1982; 127:1115–1118.
6. Sehgal CM, Broderick GA, Whittington R, et al: Three-dimensional US and volumetric assessment of the prostate. Radiology 1994; 192:274–278.
7. Littrup PJ, Williams CR, Egglin TK, Kane RA: Determination of prostate volume with transrectal US for cancer screening. Part II. Accuracy of in vitro and in vivo techniques [see comments]. Radiology 1991; 179(1):49–53.
8. Aus G, Bergdahl S, Hugosson J, Norlen L: Volume determinations of the whole prostate and of adenomas by transrectal ultrasound in patients with clinically benign prostatic hyperplasia: Correlation of resected weight, blood loss and duration of operation. Br J Urol 1994; 73:659–663.
9. Wolff JM, Boeckmann W, Mattelaer P, et al: Determination of prostate gland volume by transrectal ultrasound: Correlation with radical prostatectomy specimens. Eur Urol 1995; 28:10–12.
10. Bazinet M, Karakiewicz PI, Aprikian AG, et al: Reassessment of nonplanimetric transrectal ultrasound prostate volume estimates. Urology 1996; 47:857–862.
11. Kastlunger W, Bartsch G, Jenewein K: Benign prostatic hyperplasia revealed by transrectal ultrasonography. In Resnick MI (ed): Prostatic Ultrasonography. BC Decker Inc, Philadelphia, 1990, vol 1, pp 49–54.
12. Aguirre CR, Tallada MB, Mayayo TD, et al: Evaluation comparative du volume prostatique par l'echographic transabdominale, le profil uretral et la radiologie. J Urol 1980; 86:675–679.

$$\text{PLANIMETRY} = \sum_{N}^{1} (\text{TRV AREA} \times \text{SECTION THICKNESS})$$

$$\text{PROLATE ELLIPSE} = \frac{\pi}{6} \times W \times H \times L$$

$$\text{SPHEROID - 1} = \frac{\pi}{6} \times W^2 \times H$$

$$\text{SPHEROID - 2} = \frac{\pi}{6} \times H^2 \times W$$

$$\text{SPHERE - 1} = \frac{\pi}{6} \times ((W + H + L) / 3)^3$$

$$\text{SPHERE - 2} = \frac{\pi}{6} \times ((W + H) / 2)^3$$

$$\text{SPHERE - 3} = \frac{\pi}{6} \times W^3$$

Figure 4 ▪ Formulas for various methods of prostate volume determination by transrectal ultrasound as evaluated by Terris. Abbreviations for linear measurements are as in Figure 1. *Trv Area* = transverse area.

▪: SIZE OF THE SEMINAL VESICLES IN NORMAL SUBJECTS AND IN PROSTATE CANCER STAGING

▪ ACR Code: 845 (Seminal Vesicle)

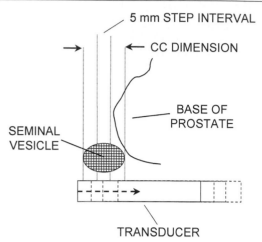

Figure 1 ▪ Measurement of prostate volume was done by summing transverse areas obtained at 5-mm intervals as shown. The cephalocaudal *(CC)* dimension was determined by noting transducer position at the top and bottom of the gland.[1]

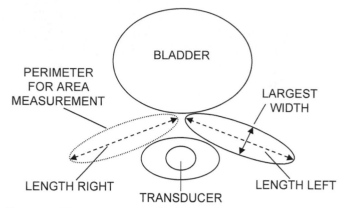

Figure 2 ▪ Measurements made from axial sections through the seminal vesicles included transverse lengths, largest width, and areas by perimeter tracing as shown.[1]

Technique ▪

Terasaki and colleagues used a USI-51 chair-type transrectal ultrasound machine (Aloka, Tokyo), which allowed transverse radial scanning at calibrated 5.0-mm intervals.[1] Cummings and colleagues used a Combison 310A transrectal ultrasound unit (Kretz), with a 7.5-MHz biplanar probe, and patients were scanned in decubitus position.[2]

Measurements ▪

Terasaki and colleagues measured anteroposterior width, transverse length, and the area of each gland on serial sections. The cephalocaudal dimension was determined by noting the transducer position at the top and bottom of the gland. The volume (of both sides) was obtained by summing the areas and dividing by 2 to correct for the 5.0-mm section interval. Figures 1 and 2 show these measurements. Table 1 lists results by age from the 3rd through 9th decades.[1] Cummings and colleagues measured each seminal vesicle in three axes and multiplied the dimensions

to obtain volumes on each side. No correction factor was employed in this calculation, as the gland shape was assumed to be rectangular. Table 2 lists the largest single volume and summed bilateral volumes by stage of prostate cancer as determined by pathologic examination of radical prostatectomy specimens. Table 3 gives test performances of single largest volume, bilateral volume, and side-to-side asymmetry in predicting stage C prostate cancer with extraprostatic tumor extension.[2]

Source ▪

Terasaki and group studied 76 men ranging in age from 20 to 89 years, with 10 to 12 subjects per decade. The men had presented with complaints unrelated to the seminal vesicles, prostate, or urethra, and no abnormalities of those structures were subsequently found.[1] Cummings and group evaluated 47 men with prostate carcinoma prior to lymphadectomy and modified radical prostatectomy. All had negative nodes (inclusion criteria for the study). Prostatectomy specimens were step-sectioned for evidence of capsular invasion or seminal vesicle involvement.[2]

Table 1 ▪ Prostate Dimensions, Areas, and Volume in Men Aged 20 to 89 Years, by Decade

AGE RANGE (Yr)	BILATERAL VOLUME (ml)	BILATERAL AREA (sq cm)	SUM OF LENGTHS (cm)	LARGEST WIDTH (cm)	CEPHALOCAUDAL DIMENSION (cm)
20–29	9.3 ± 3.9	4.8 ± 1.2	6.1 ± 0.8	1.1 ± 0.2	2.3 ± 0.5
30–39	9.7 ± 1.3	5.8 ± 1.0	6.5 ± 0.6	1.3 ± 0.2	2.3 ± 0.3
40–49	10.1 ± 2.6	5.5 ± 1.1	6.7 ± 0.6	1.1 ± 0.2	2.4 ± 0.3
50–59	9.3 ± 2.4	6.3 ± 2.0	6.8 ± 0.8	1.1 ± 0.4	1.9 ± 0.4
60–69	7.5 ± 1.7	4.6 ± 1.1	6.0 ± 0.7	0.9 ± 0.1	2.1 ± 0.4
70–79	6.1 ± 1.4	4.5 ± 0.9	6.1 ± 0.6	1.0 t 0.2	2.0 ± 0.3
80–89	5.1 ± 1.1	3.2 ± 0.5	5.8 ± 0.7	0.8 ± 0.1	2.2 ± 0.3

All measurements given as mean ± standard deviation.
From Terasaki T, Watanabe H, Kamoi K, Naya Y: J Urol 1993; 150:914–916. Used by permission.

Table 2 ▪ Volumes of Seminal Vesicles in Various Stages of Prostate Cancer

STAGE	NO.	BILATERAL VOLUME (ml)		LARGEST SINGLE VOLUME (ml)	
		Mean ± SD	Range	Mean ± SD	Range
B1	12	7.6 ± 4.6	1.6–15.8	4.2 ± 2.5	0.8–9.2
B2	19	8.8 ± 5.8	1.6–22.5	5.0 ± 2.9	1.4–11.3
All B	31	8.4 ± 5.3	1.6–22	4.7 ± 2.7	0.8–11.3
All C	16	20.7 ± 31.9	1.5–13	11.7 ± 16.9	2.5–70.0
C with seminal vesicle invasion	6	18.1 ± 13.8	5.1–39.4	10.9 ± 8.7	2.5–26.3

From Cummings JM, Boullier JA, Sankari BR, Parra RO: Urology 1994; 44:206–210. Used by permission.

Table 3 ▪ Performance of Transrectal Ultrasound Volume Estimation of Seminal Vesicles in Predicting Stage C Prostate Cancer

CRITERIA	BILATERAL VOLUME > 15 cc	ASYMMETRY OF VOLUME (Larger/Smaller > 1.5)	LARGEST VOLUME > 10 ml OR ASYMMETRY	BILATERAL VOLUME > 15 ml OR ASYMMETRY
Sensitivity (%)	38	38	63	69
Specificity (%)	84	90	87	77
PPV (%)	54	55	61	58
NPV (%)	72	73	81	82

PPV = positive predictive value, NPV = negative predictive value.
From Cummings JM, Boullier JA, Sankari BR, Parra RO: Urology 1994; 44:206–210. Used by permission.

Comments ▪

In Cummings' patients with stage C prostate cancer, there was no significant difference in seminal vesicle volume between those with and without direct seminal vesicle invasion, though the volumes were significantly higher than with stage B disease. Using combined criteria of absolute volumes and asymmetry is useful in staging prostate cancer, as shown in Table 3. For example, if the total seminal vesicle volume is less than 15 ml and the seminal vesicles are symmetric (larger/smaller < 1.5), the patient has only an 18% chance of capsular penetration. This method compares favorably with a 66% detection rate of sonography for advanced disease reported in a multi-institutional study.[3]

REFERENCES

1. Terasaki T, Watanabe H, Kamoi K, Naya Y: Seminal vesicle parameters at 10-year intervals measured by transrectal ultrasonography. J Urol 1993; 150:914–916.
2. Cummings JM, Boullier JA, Sankari BR, Parra RO: Seminal vesicle volume as a sonographic predictor of prostate cancer stage. Urology 1994; 44:206–210.
3. Rifkin MD, Zerhouni EA, Gatsonis CA: Comparison of magnetic resonance imaging and ultrasonography in staging early prostate cancer. Results of a multi-institutional cooperative study. N Engl J Med 1990; 323:621–626.

▪: DOPPLER ULTRASOUND EVALUATION FOR IMPOTENCE
▪ ACR Code: 847 (External Genitalia)

Technique ▪

Ultrasound of the penis is done with 7.5- to 10-MHz linear transducers and modern equipment capable of color Doppler, duplex Doppler, and high-quality gray scale imaging. The patient is placed supine and the flaccid penis may be supported by a rolled towel placed between the legs. Copious amounts of coupling gel help minimize transducer pressure. After initial survey scanning to locate any morphologic abnormalities (such as Peyronie plaques), the vascular system is examined near the base of the penis for most of the remaining procedure. Baseline measurements of diameter and flow parameters in the deep arteries are done in the longitudinal plane, and transverse scanning may be helpful to locate anatomy. The dorsal arteries and vein are sometimes evaluated also. Figure 1 depicts the relevant anatomy in diagrammatic cross-section.

The second phase of the examination is done after injection of a vasoactive agent with a small-bore needle or butterfly device. Papaverine is often used, and reported doses vary from 15 to 60 mg. Injection may be made into one or both (split-dose) corpora cavernosa, and a tourniquet or rubber band is often placed at the base of the penis at the time of injection. Scanning is then resumed and carried out at 3- to 5-minute intervals up to 30 to 40 minutes (depending on response). During this time the most important structures to evaluate are the deep arteries of the penis, though some workers also interrogate the dorsal arteries and vein.

Measurements ▪

The temporal pattern of the penile vascular response to injected vasodilators may be divided into five phases,[10, 11]

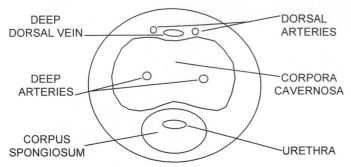

Figure 1 ▪ Cross-section of the penis with relevant anatomy indicated.

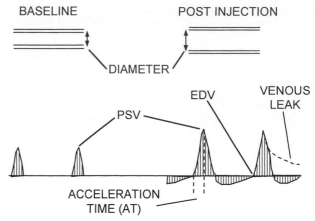

Figure 3 ▪ Measurements of the deep arteries include diameter, peak systolic velocity *(PSV)*, end-diastolic velocity *(EDV)*, and acceleration time *(AT)*. The time-averaged velocity may also be measured over one or more cardiac cycles and used to calculate volume flow. With venous leakage, there will be persistent antegrade diastolic flow *(dotted line)*, resulting in a positive value for EDV.

and Figure 2 shows these as described by Lue.[1] Full response usually occurs within 5 minutes but may be delayed up to 30 minutes.[13] The diameters (D) of the deep arteries are measured, usually in longitudinal plane, and right/left may be averaged or the largest one recorded. The percent change in diameter from baseline (Dbase) to maximal diameter (Dmax) is calculated by $(Dmax - Dbase)/Dbase \times 100$.

Several parameters may be measured from angle-corrected (45 to 65 degrees) duplex Doppler tracings of the deep arteries, including peak systolic velocity (PSV), end-diastolic velocity (EDV), acceleration time (AT), and time-averaged velocity (TAV). The volume flow may be calculated by multiplying TAV by area ($pi/4 \times D$ squared) and the acceleration by dividing $PSV - EDV$ by AT. Figure 3 shows these measurements. Lopez and colleagues have developed a penile blood flow index (PBFI), which is the sum of the percent diameter increase and the PSV from both right and left deep arteries.[12] Some or all of these parameters may be measured/calculated from the dorsal artery as well, though these are rather less commonly cited. The dorsal vein flow is typically slow and is variably seen with color Doppler at baseline and during early response. There should be no flow at full erectile response; persistent flow indicates venous leakage but is not always seen in this condition since there other pathways for venous return.

Typical values for the aforementioned parameters are listed in Table 1 for baseline and at maximal (full) response, and published criteria for abnormal are also included. The arterial diameters typically reach maximum values prior to full response (latent phase).[4] For diagnostic purposes, the maximum value of each arterial parameter after injection is used and applied to the criteria. The only exception is AT,

for which the minimum time is used.[19] Abnormal values of all arterial criteria except EDV indicate arterial insufficiency. Increased EDV and persistent dorsal vein flow suggest venous leak. Some care must be taken in interpreting the EDV, since during the latent and tumescent phases there is continuous diastolic flow that reverses as penile pressure rises toward the time of full response.[13]

The most frequently cited criteria for normal response involve the deep arteries and include PSV >25 to 35 cm/sec, EDV <5 cm/sec, and diameter increase >60% to 70%. Maximum diameter,[6] acceleration time,[19] acceleration,[18] side-to-side difference in PSV,[9] volume flow rate,[15, 16] and persistent dorsal vein flow[9, 13] are more recently described and/or less commonly used. For arterial insufficiency, the index (PBFI) described by Lopez is attractive because it avoids the problem of deciding on which of the paired deep arteries to use and combines change in size with velocity into one number.[12]

Source ▪

The subject of ultrasound evaluation of the penile vasculature for impotence has been well reviewed[1-4] and extensively studied.[5-19] The techniques, normative values, and

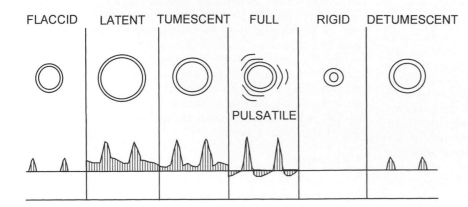

Figure 2 ▪ Phases of response of deep penile arteries to vasodilator injection. The arteries reach maximal diameter in the latent phase and are visibly pulsatile at full response. Typical Doppler waveforms in the deep arteries are depicted at the bottom. (From Lue TF: WB Saunders, Philadelphia, 1998, vol 2, pp 1181–1214. Used by permission.)

Table 1 ▪ Normative Values and Criteria for Abnormal for Various Measured and Calculated Parameters from Penile Ultrasound

PARAMETER	UNITS	BASELINE	POSTINJECTION	ABNORMAL CRITERIA (Postinjection)
Deep artery				
Diameter	mm	0.3–0.6	0.7–1.0	<0.7
Diameter increase	%	—	60–100	<60–70*
Peak systolic velocity	cm/sec	8–30	30–50	<25*
				25–35 borderline
End-diastolic velocity	cm/sec	—	0–10	>5*
Systolic acceleration time	msec	—	60–120	>110
Systolic acceleration	cm/sec²	—	300–750	<400
Side-to-side difference in PSV	cm/sec	—	0–7	>10
Volume flow rate	ml/min	3–5	10–15	<10
Penile blood flow index (sum of R & L diameter increase and PSV)	—	—	200–500	<285
Dorsal artery				
Peak systolic velocity	cm/sec	10–30	25–75	No definite criteria
Volume flow rate	ml/min	5–10	15–30	No definite criteria
Dorsal vein flow	—	Variable	None	Persistent flow

*Most commonly used parameters/criteria.
PSV = peak systolic velocity.

diagnostic criteria contained herein are based on these works. This area is still being actively investigated, and some controversy remains concerning the optimal measurements and normative criteria.

REFERENCES

1. Lue TF: Physiology of penile erection and pathophysiology of impotence. In Walsh PC, Retik AB, Stamey TA, Vaughan ED (eds): Campbell's Urology. WB Saunders, Philadelphia, 1998, vol 2, pp 1181–1214.
2. Krysiewicz S, Mellinger BC: The role of imaging in the diagnostic evaluation of impotence. AJR Am J Roentgenol 1989; 153:1133–1139.
3. Rosen MP, Schwartz AN, Levine FJ, Greenfield AJ: Radiologic assessment of impotence: Angiography, sonography, cavernosography, and scintigraphy. AJR Am J Roentgenol 1991; 157:923–931.
4. Connolly J, Borirakchanyavat S, Lue TF: Ultrasound evaluation of the penis for assessment of impotence. J Clin Ultrasound 1996; 24:481–486.
5. Lue TF, Hricak H, Marich KW, Tanagho EA: Vasculogenic impotence evaluated by high-resolution ultrasonography and pulsed Doppler spectrum analysis. Radiology 1985; 155:777–781.
6. Lue TF, Tanagho EA: Physiology of erection and pharmacological management of impotence. J Urol 1987; 137:829–836.
7. Shabsigh R, Fishman IJ, Quesada ET, et al: Evaluation of vasculogenic erectile impotence using penile duplex ultrasonography. J Urol 1989; 142:1469–1474.
8. Quam JP, King BF, James EM, et al: Duplex and color Doppler sonographic evaluation of vasculogenic impotence. AJR Am J Roentgenol 1989; 153:1141–1147.
9. Benson CB, Vickers MA: Sexual impotence caused by vascular disease: Diagnosis with duplex sonography. AJR Am J Roentgenol 1989; 153:1149–1153.
10. Schwartz AN, Wang KY, Mack LA, et al: Evaluation of normal erectile function with color flow Doppler sonography. AJR Am J Roentgenol 1989; 153:1155–1160.
11. Schwartz AN, Lowe M, Berger RE, et al: Assessment of normal and abnormal erectile function: Color Doppler flow sonography versus conventional techniques. Radiology 1991; 180:105–109.
12. Lopez JA, Espeland MA, Jarow JP: Interpretation and quantification of penile blood flow studies using duplex ultrasonography. J Urol 1991; 146:1271–1275.
13. Fitzgerald SW, Erickson SJ, Foley WD, et al: Color Doppler sonography in the evaluation of erectile dysfunction: Patterns of temporal response to papaverine. AJR Am J Roentgenol 1991; 157:331–336.
14. Chiang PH, Chiang CP, Wu CC, et al: Colour duplex sonography in the assessment of impotence. Br J Urol 1991; 68:181–186.
15. Meuleman EJH, Bemelmans BLH, van Asten WNJC, et al: Assessment of penile blood flow by duplex ultrasonography in 44 men with normal erectile potency in different phases of erection. J Urol 1992; 147:51–56.
16. Lee B, Suresh CS, Randrup ER, et al: Standardization of penile blood flow parameters in normal men using intracavernous prostaglandins E1 and visual sexual stimulation. J Urol 1993; 149:49–52.
17. Benson CB, Aruny JE, Vickers MA: Correlation of duplex sonography with arteriography in patients with erectile dysfunction. AJR Am J Roentgenol 1993; 160:71–73.
18. Valji K, Bookstein JJ: Diagnosis of arteriogenic impotence: Efficacy of duplex sonography as a screening tool. AJR Am J Roentgenol 1993; 160:65–69.
19. Oates CP, Pickard RS, Powell PH, et al: The use of duplex ultrasound in the assessment of arterial supply to the penis in vasculogenic impotence. J Urol 1995; 153:354–357.

⁛ DETERMINATION OF OVARIAN VOLUME BY ULTRASOUND[1]
▪ ACR Code: 852 (Ovary)

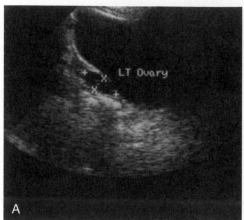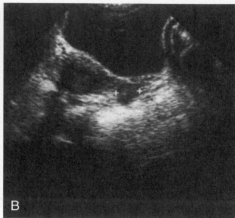

Figure 1 ▪ *A*, Longitudinal scan shows typical length and AP thickness measurements. *B*, Transverse scan demonstrates measurements of ovarian width. (From Munn CS, et al: Radiology 1986; 159:731–732. Used by permission.)

Technique ▪

Ultrasound examination performed with a real-time Diasonics DRF 400 scanner, using a 3.5-MHz oscillating transducer.

Measurements ▪ (Figure 1)

The greatest length, transverse dimension (width), and AP thickness were determined. Volumes were calculated using the formula for the volume of an ellipsoid:

$$\text{Volume} = 0.523 \times \text{length} \times \text{width} \times \text{thickness}$$

The derived data show that the normal volume ranged as high as 13.84 cm³, with an average of 6.48 cm³.

Source ▪

Data are based on ultrasonographic study of 15 women aged 18 to 47 years.

REFERENCE

1. Munn CS, Kiser L, Wetzner SM, Baer J: Ovary volume in young and premenopausal adults: US determination. Radiology 1986; 159:731–732.

⁛ OVARIAN VOLUMES THROUGHOUT LIFE
▪ ACR Code: 852 (Ovary)

Technique ▪

Cohen and colleagues performed transvesical ultrasound of the uterus with different machines, using real-time transducers from 3.0 to 7.0 MHz. Higher-frequency transducers were used for younger patients.[1, 2] Tepper and colleagues did transvaginal scanning of the uterus with an SSD-680 machine (Aloka Ltd, Tokyo, Japan) and a 5-MHz probe.[3]

Measurements ▪

In all three studies, ovarian volume was determined by three axis measurements: anteroposterior (AP), transverse (TRV), and cephalocaudal length (LEN) multiplied together and the product multiplied by 0.523, assuming the shape to be a prolate ellipse.[1–3] The percentage of adequate visualization of both ovaries for measurement was noted. Table 1 lists ovarian volumes and percentage visualization by age, menstrual status, and menstrual cycle phase from Cohen and group.[1, 2] Table 2 lists ovarian volumes versus years after menopause from Tepper and group.[3]

Source ▪

Cohen and colleagues studied 762 girls and women examined for various reasons. Any ovary containing a cyst or cysts of 2.0 cm or more was excluded from the analysis of normal ovaries, leaving a total of 998 ovaries.[1] They also evaluated 77 infant girls (mostly scanned for urinary tract infection), with a total of 98 ovaries included in the analysis.[2] Age ranges and numbers in each age group are included in Table 1. Tepper and colleagues studied 311 menopausal women (age range, 48 to 78 years, mean age, 50 years). Any ovary containing a cyst of 2.0 cm or more was excluded. Otherwise, the largest ovary was measured and included in the analysis.[3]

Comments ▪

Tepper et al noted that in 97% of postmenopausal patients scanned transvaginally, both ovaries were seen,[3] whereas Cohen et al found a decreasing percentage with age on

Table 1 ▪ Ovarian Volumes Throughout Life

SUBJECT GROUPS	BOTH OVARIES SEEN (%)	NO. OF OVARIES	VOLUME (cc) MEAN ± SD	VOLUME (cc) 95% CI
Age				
NB–3 mon	29	34	1.06 ± 0.96	0.03–3.56
4–12 mon	62	34	1.05 ± 0.67	0.18–2.71
13–24 mon	45	30	0.67 ± 0.35	0.15–1.68
0–9 yr	75	19	1.7 ± 1.4	0.2–4.9
10–19 yr	94	83	7.8 ± 4.4	1.7–18.5
20–29 yr	73	308	10.2 ± 6.2	2.6–23.1
30–39 yr	77	358	9.5 ± 5.4	2.6–20.7
40–49 yr	61	206	9.0 ± 5.8	2.1–20.9
50–59 yr	51	57	6.2 ± 5.7	1.6–14.2
>60 yr	26	44	6.0 ± 3.8	1.0–15.0
Menstrual Status				
Premenarchal	—	32	3.0 ± 2.3	0.2–9.1
Menstruating	—	866	9.8 ± 5.8	2.5–21.9
Postmenopausal	—	100	5.8 ± 3.6	1.2–14.1
Cycle phase (days)	—			
Follicular (1–10)	—	81	9.7 ± 6.1	2.4–21.0
Preovulatory (11–16)	—	55	10.2 ± 7.1	2.7–23.3
Luteal (17–35)	—	129	9.4 ± 5.6	1.9–23.2

SD = standard deviation, CI = confidence intervals.
From Cohen HL, Tice HM, Mandel FS: Radiology 1990; 177:189–192. Used by permission.

Table 2 ▪ Ovarian Volumes in Menopausal Women

YEARS SINCE MENOPAUSE	AGE RANGE (Yr)	NO.	VOLUME (cc) MEAN ± SD
Perimenopausal	48–54	33	8.6 ± 2.3
1–2	49–57	56	6.2 ± 2.7
3–4	53–58	30	5.2 ± 1.6
5–6	54–59	36	4.0 ± 1.8
7–8	55–60	36	3.1 ± 1.3
9–10	58–63	31	2.8 ± 2.1
11–12	60–74	28	2.4 ± 1.3
13–14	64–68	27	2.2 ± 1.3
≥15	60–78	34	2.2 ± 1.4

From Tepper R, Zalel Y, Markov S, et al: Acta Obstet Gynecol 1995; 74:208–211. Used by permission.

transabdominal scanning.[1] Tepper and associates found no significant difference in ovarian volume from side to side.[3]

REFERENCES

1. Cohen HL, Tice HM, Mandel FS: Ovarian volumes measured by US: Bigger than we think. Radiology 1990; 177:189–192.
2. Cohen HL, Shapiro MA, Mandel FS, Shapiro ML: Normal ovaries in neonates and infants: A sonographic study of 77 patients 1 day to 24 months old. AJR Am J Roentgenol 1993; 160:583–586.
3. Tepper R, Zalel Y, Markov S, et al: Ovarian volume in postmenopausal women—suggestions for an ovarian size nomogram for menopausal age. Acta Obstet Gynecol 1995; 74:208–211.

▪▪ UTERINE AND OVARIAN VOLUMES IN INFANCY AND CHILDHOOD
▪ ACR Code: 852 (Ovary); 854 (Uterus)

Technique ▪

Real-time transabdominal ultrasound of the pelvis was done with a 128 machine (Acuson, Mountain View, CA) and 3.5- to 5.0-MHz transducers. The patients were supine, with a comfortably full bladder.[1]

Measurements ▪

The maximal transverse (TRV), anteroposterior (AP), and cephalocaudal (LEN) dimensions of the uterus and each ovary were measured. The volume of each structure was

Table 1 ▪ Uterine and Ovarian Volumes in Girls by Age and Pubertal Stage

AGE	NO. OF UTERI	UTERINE VOLUME (cc)	NO. OF OVARIES	OVARIAN VOLUME (cc)
0–1 mon	15	3.4 ± 1.2	6	0.5 ± 0.4
3 mon	7	0.9 ± 0.2	4	0.4 ± 0.1
1 yr	19	1.0 ± 0.2	6	0.5 ± 0.2
3 yr	26	1.0 ± 0.3	17	0.7 ± 0.4
5 yr	26	1.0 ± 0.3	13	0.7 ± 0.5
7 yr	28	0.9 ± 0.3	15	0.8 ± 0.6
9 yr	18	1.3 ± 0.4	12	0.6 ± 0.4
11 yr	16	1.9 ± 0.9	10	1.3 ± 1.0
13 yr	8	11.0 ± 10.5	8	3.7 ± 2.1
15 yr	15	21.2 ± 13.5	9	6.7 ± 4.8
Pubertal stage				
B 1	130	1.0 ± 0.3	69	0.7 ± 0.4
B 2	10	2.3 ± 0.6	9	1.6 ± 0.9
B 3	11	10.3 ± 6.1	8	3.5 ± 1.8
B 4–5	12	24.6 ± 14.4	8	7.4 ± 4.8

Measurements are given as mean ± standard deviation.
From Haber HP, Mayer EI: Pediatr Radiol 1994; 24(1):11–13. Used by permission.

calculated by 0.5233 × TRV × AP × LEN (prolate ellipse). The ovarian volumes were the average of right and left, and any ovary containing a cyst larger than 2.0 cm was excluded from the analysis.[1] Table 1 lists the results by age and developmental stage.[1]

Source ▪

Subjects included 178 normal girls (age range, 1 day to 14 and 11/12 years) examined for non-endocrinologic acute symptoms. Age, weight, height, and pubertal development[2] were noted and recorded. All the subjects had appropriate pubertal development for age.[1]

REFERENCES

1. Haber HP, Mayer EI: Ultrasound evaluation of uterine and ovarian size from birth to puberty [see comments]. Pediatr Radiol 1994; 24(1):11–13.
2. Tanner JM, Whitehouse RH: Clinical longitudinal standards for height, weight, height velocity, weight velocity, and stages of puberty. Arch Dis Child 1976; 51:170–179.

▪: SCORING SYSTEM FOR OVARIAN MASSES USING ULTRASOUND
▪ ACR Code: 852 (Ovary)

Technique ▪

Transvaginal ultrasound was done with various machines and transducer types to evaluate ovarian masses.[1–10]

Measurements ▪

Sassone and colleagues developed a scoring system that has possible integer values of 4 to 15, which combines commonly described morphologic characteristics of ovarian masses.[1] The characteristics are shown in Figures 1 through 4, and the overall system is detailed in Table 1. In addition to applying the scoring system to their patients,[1] Sassone and colleagues applied the same system to masses, as reported in seven additional papers.[2–8] Subsequently Timor-Tritsch[9] and Schneider[10] and their associates used the same scoring system to evaluate two additional groups of ovarian masses. Table 2 lists the performance of the scoring system as reported, with a cut-off for abnormal of 9 or more, and Table 3 lists likelihood ratios (LR) calculated from the reported data.[1–10]

Source ▪

The studies described here for the most part included women ranging in age from young adulthood through the 8th decade.[1–10] The number of patients and ovaries examined, as well as the prevalence of malignancy among them, are detailed in Table 2.

Comments ▪

A combination of gray scale morphology and Doppler characteristics is superior to one or the other alone in characterizing ovarian masses. This has been validated numerous times.[9–14] Other gray scale scoring systems may work equally as well as the one described here, and we have described Sassone's because it seems to be one of the most widely used.[1]

Note that the size of the ovary or the mass is not included in this scoring system, which relies instead on morphology alone. With regard to screening asymptomatic women, ovarian volumes have been used, with 8 ml and 18

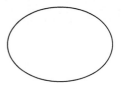

SMOOTH
SCORE=1

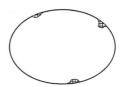

IRREGULARITIES
< 3 mm
SCORE=2

Figure 1 ▪ Depiction of ovarian tumor scores relating to inner wall structure.[1]

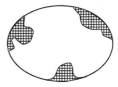

PAPILLARITIES
> 3 mm
SCORE=3

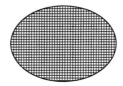

MOSTLY SOLID
SCORE=4

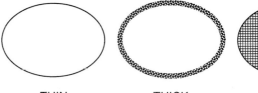

THIN
< 3 mm
SCORE=1

THICK
> 3 mm
SCORE=2

MOSTLY
SOLID
SCORE=3

Figure 2 ▪ Depiction of ovarian tumor scores relating to wall thickness.[1]

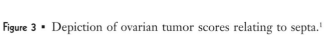

Figure 3 ▪ Depiction of ovarian tumor scores relating to septa.[1]

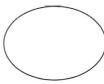

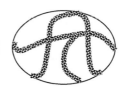

NO SEPTA
SCORE=1

THIN SEPTA
< 3 mm
SCORE=2

THICK SEPTA
> 3 mm
SCORE=3

SONOLUCENT
SCORE=1

LOW ECHOGENICITY
SCORE=2

Figure 4 ▪ Depiction of ovarian tumor scores relating to echogenicity.[1]

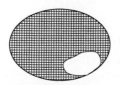

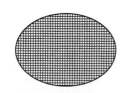

LOW ECHOGENICITY
& ECHOGENIC CORE
SCORE=3

MIXED
ECHOGENICITY
SCORE=4

HIGH
ECHOGENICITY
SCORE=5

Table 1 ▪ Scoring System to Quantify Gray Scale Ultrasound Findings of Ovarian Tumors

SCORE VALUE	INNER WALL STRUCTURE	WALL THICKNESS	SEPTA	ECHOGENICITY
1	Smooth	Thin < 3 mm	None	Sonolucent
2	Irregularities < 3 mm	Thick > 3 mm	Thin < 3 mm	Low echogenicity
3	Papillarities > 3 mm	Mostly solid	Thick > 3 mm	Low echogenicity with echogenic core
4	Mostly solid	—	—	Mixed echogenicity
5	—	—	—	High echogenicity
Maximum possible score	4	3	3	5

Scores may range from 4 to 15; tumors with scores of 9 or more are suspicious for malignancy.
From Sassone AM, Timor-Tritsch IE, Artner A, et al: Obstet Gynecol 1991; 78:70–76. Used by permission.

Table 2 ▪ Performance of Gray Scale Ultrasound Scoring System for Predicting Malignancy in Ovarian Tumors

REFERENCE	NO.	PREVALENCE OF MALIGNANCY (%)	PPV (%)	NPV (%)	SENSITIVITY (%)	SPECIFICITY (%)
Sassone	143	10	37	100	100	83
Kobayashi	406	15	31	93	72	73
Meire	51	35	83	91	83	91
Pussell	25	48	83	91	83	84
Herrmann	241	21	75	95	82	93
Finkler	102	36	88	81	62	95
Benacerraf	100	30	72	91	80	87
Granberg	180	22	74	95	82	92
Timor-Tritsch*	94	17	60	99	94	87
Schneider*	55	29	58	93	88	74

All results as reported by Sassone et al,[1] except Timor-Tritsch et al[9] and Schneider et al,[10] which are marked with an asterisk. PPV = positive predictive value; NPV = negative predictive value. A positive test was a score of 9 or higher.
From Sassone AM, Timor-Tritsch IE, Artner A, et al: Obstet Gynecol 1991; 78:70–76. Used by permission.

Table 3 ▪ Likelihood Ratios for Ultrasound Tumor Score in Predicting Malignancy in Ovarian Masses

REFERENCE	SENSITIVITY (%)	SPECIFICITY (%)	LR POSITIVE SCORE ≥ 9	LR NEGATIVE SCORE < 9
Sassone	100	83	5.88	0.00
Kobayashi	72	73	2.67	0.38
Meire	83	91	9.22	0.19
Pussell	83	84	5.19	0.20
Herrmann	82	93	11.71	0.19
Finkler	62	95	12.40	0.40
Benacerraf	80	87	6.15	0.23
Granberg	82	92	10.25	0.20
Timor-Tritsch*	94	87	7.23	0.07
Schneider*	88	74	3.38	0.16
Averages	82.6	85.9	7.41	0.20

Likelihood ratios (LR) have been calculated from reported sensitivity and specificity. Averages are simple means of the reported/calculated values.[1–10]

ml cited as the upper limits of normal for postmenopausal and premenopausal women, respectively.[15, 16] Herrmann and colleagues used 10 cm (greatest diameter) for simple cystic adnexal masses as the cut-off for suspicious lesions.[5]

REFERENCES

1. Sassone AM, Timor-Tritsch IE, Artner A, et al: Transvaginal sonographic characterization of ovarian disease: Evaluation of a new scoring system to predict ovarian malignancy. Obstet Gynecol 1991; 78:70–76.
2. Kobayashi M: Use of diagnostic ultrasound in trophoblastic neoplasms and ovarian tumors. Cancer 1976; 38:441–452.
3. Meire HB, Farrant P, Guha T: Distinction of benign from malignant ovarian cysts by ultrasound. Br J Obstet Gynaecol 1978; 85:893–899.
4. Pussell SJ, Cosgrove DO, Hinton J, et al: Carcinoma of the ovary: Correlation of ultrasound with second look laparotomy. Br J Obstet Gynaecol 1980; 87:1140–1144.
5. Herrmann IJ, Locher GW, Goldhirsh A: Sonographic patterns of ovarian tumors: Prediction of malignancy. Obstet Gynecol 1987; 69:777–781.
6. Finkler NJ, Benacerraf BR, Lavin PT, et al: Comparison of CA 125, clinical impression, and ultrasound in the postoperative evaluation of ovarian masses. Obstet Gynecol 1988; 72:659–664.
7. Benacerraf BR, Finkler NJ, Wojciechowski C, Knapp RC: Sonographic accuracy in the diagnosis of ovarian masses. J Reprod Med 1990; 35:491–495.
8. Granberg S, Norstrom A, Wikland M: Tumors in the lower pelvis as imaged by vaginal sonography. Gynecol Oncol 1990; 37:224–229.
9. Timor-Tritsch IE, Lerner J, Monteagudo A, et al: Transvaginal sonographic characterization of ovarian masses using color-flow directed Doppler measurements. Ultrasound Obstet Gynecol 1992; 2(Suppl):171–176.
10. Schneider VL, Schneider A, Reed KL, Hatch KD: Comparison of Doppler with two-dimensional sonography and CA 125 for prediction of malignancy of pelvic masses. Obstet Gynecol 1993; 81:983–988.
11. Kurjak A, Predanic M: New scoring system for prediction of ovarian malignancy based on transvaginal color Doppler sonography. J Ultrasound Med 1992; 11(12):631–638.
12. Jain K: Prospective evaluation of adnexal masses with endovaginal gray-scale and duplex and color Doppler US: Correlation with pathologic findings. Radiology 1994; 191:63–67.
13. Predanic M, Vlahos N, Pennisi JA, et al: Color and pulsed Doppler sonography, gray-scale imaging, and serum CA 125 in the assessment of adnexal disease. Obstet Gynecol 1996; 88:283–288.
14. Buy JN, Ghossain MA, Hugol D, et al: Characterization of adnexal masses: Combination of color Doppler and conventional sonography compared with spectral Doppler analysis alone and conventional sonography alone. AJR Am J Roentgenol 1996; 166:385–393.
15. van Nagell JR, Defriest PD, Puls PD, et al: Ovarian cancer screening in asymptomatic postmenopausal women by transvaginal sonography. Cancer 1991; 68:458–462.
16. Taylor KJ, Schwartz PE: Screening for early ovarian cancer [review]. Radiology 1994; 192(1):1–10.

▪: DOPPLER MEASUREMENTS OF OVARIAN TUMORS
▪ ACR Code: 852 (Ovary)

Technique ▪

Transvaginal ultrasound was done with an Ultramark 9 machine (Advanced Technology Laboratories, Bothell, WA) and a 5.0-MHz vaginal probe. Color Doppler and duplex Doppler examination was carried out, with special attention to vascularity associated with the ovarian mass in question. During the examination, the probe was tilted until the maximum blood flow velocity and quality of signal were obtained at each site chosen for measurement of vessels associated within and adjacent to the tumor. The wall filter was set at 100 Hz to eliminate low-frequency signals. When the patient was menstruating, the examination was done in the first half of the cycle.[1]

Measurements ▪

Duplex measurements were done at each location within the tumor or its capsule, where significant color Doppler flow was visible. These included peak systolic velocity (PSV), end-diastolic velocity (EDV), and mean flow velocity (MFV). Calculated parameters included resistive index (RI), pulsatility index (PI), and PSV/EDV. The highest PSV, EDV, MFV, and PSV/EDV were recorded for each tumor. The lowest RI and PI were recorded. Vascularity was present in 98% of tumors (both benign and malignant). Table 1 lists the results.

Source ▪

Over 3 years, 120 women (age range, 14 to 83 years) with adnexal tumors found at physical examination or conventional ultrasound examination were examined. Histopathology following laparotomy was used as the gold standard for diagnosis. Of these patients, 80 had benign tumors of various types, and 40 had malignant masses. The malignant tumors were mostly cystadenocarcinomas (n = 32), followed in frequency by metastases (n = 4).[1]

Table 1 ▪ Performance of Doppler Ultrasound Parameters in Differentiating Benign from Malignant Adnexal Masses

PARAMETER	BENIGN (n = 80) (Mean ± SD)	MALIGNANT (n = 40) (Mean ± SD)	CUT-OFF FOR MALIGNANT	SENSITIVITY (%)	SPECIFICITY (%)
RI	0.56±0.14	0.33±0.13	≤ 0.40	82	97
PI	1.0±0.6	0.4±0.3	< 0.50	74	99
PSV (cm/sec)	12.4±7.6	12.4±5.1	≥ 18 cm/sec	13	86
EDV (cm/sec)	4.2±2.7	6.4±3.0	≥ 5 cm/sec	64	86
PSV/EDV	5.3±2.7	2.8±1.2	< 3	36	42
MFV (cm/sec)	6.2±2.8	8.4±3.7	≥ 6 cm/sec	74	62

Parameter abbreviations are standard and are given in the text.
From Takac I: J Ultrasound Med 1998; 17:637–642. Used by permission.

Comments ▪

The subject of Doppler ultrasound for characterizing ad-nexal/ovarian masses has been extensively studied. There are scores of papers in the medical literature, with a comprehensive review by Taylor and Schwartz.[2] We chose Takac's study since it was recent and gave measurements for all previously reported duplex Doppler parameters.[1] Most studies that include premenopausal patients stress the importance of scanning during the first portion of the cycle (often within 1 week of the menses). This is important to avoid confusion caused by robust neovascularity that may display rather brisk, low-resistance flow associated with functional ovarian cysts (especially the dominant follicle) during the later portions of the cycle. As Takac described, most workers have recorded the lowest RI, the lowest PI, and the highest PSV (when evaluated) found in each tumor under study.

Of the available Doppler parameters, RI seems to be most commonly used, and cut-offs for malignancy of less than 0.40 to 0.46 have been cited most often.[2] Tepper and colleagues found that when the RI cut-off was increased from 0.40 to 0.53, the malignancy detection rate went from 68% to 100%, with a concomitant increase in false-positives of from 4% to 26%.[3] The PI has been evaluated almost as extensively as the RI. Cited cut-off values for malignancy range between 0.50 and 1.25, with less than 1.0 being most commonly cited.[2] The PSV is more controversial, with one researcher finding lower values in malignant masses than in benign ones.[4] Others have cited cut-off values for PSV of more than 15 to 16 cm/sec for malignancy.[5, 6] The other parameters (EDV, PSV/EDV, and MFV) studied by Takac have not received much attention elsewhere.[1]

Several workers have noted that benign tumors and normal ovaries often (60% to 89%) have a diastolic notch in the Doppler waveform, whereas malignancies do not display this feature.[7–9] Figure 1 shows typical benign and malignant arterial Doppler waveforms. The diagnostic potential of diastolic notching has been questioned, with one study finding it in only 13% of benign masses and in one malignancy.[10] In addition to measured duplex Doppler

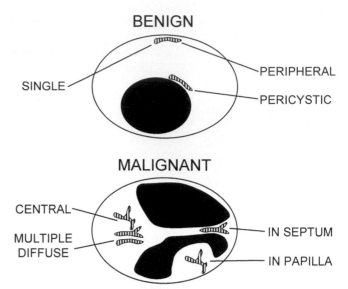

Figure 2 ▪ Depiction of described morphologies of color Doppler flow from within benign *(top)* and malignant *(bottom)* adnexal masses.[11, 12]

parameters, the distribution of intratumoral flow at color Doppler examination can add useful information. Kurjak and associates developed a scoring system to describe these findings.[11, 12] In general, peripheral and pericystic location of a single vessel was associated with benign lesions, whereas multiple vessels located within septa, papillary projections, and in the center of the tumor were malignant. Figure 2 shows the salient features of this type of analysis in benign and malignant masses.

Finally, note that there is a substantial body of evidence to support the idea that Doppler flow has limited or no value at all in differentiating benign from malignant adnexal masses.[13–17] These results emphasize the value of gray scale tumor morphology, the importance of which is almost universally agreed upon. Therefore, during any examination of a pelvic mass, echoarchitecture should be carefully assessed—scoring systems (separate section) are available to help with this. A complex, solid-appearing tumor with no color flow must be considered suspicious for malignancy even if no Doppler flow is measurable.

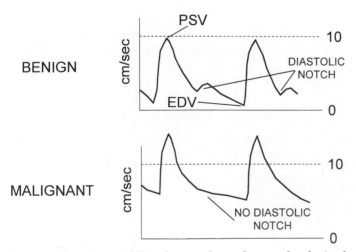

Figure 1 ▪ Typical arterial Doppler waveforms that may be obtained from benign *(top)* and malignant *(bottom)* adnexal masses.[7–9]

REFERENCES

1. Takac I: Receiver operating characteristic curves of transvaginal Doppler blood flow measurements in benign and malignant adnexal tumors. J Ultrasound Med 1998; 17:637–642.
2. Taylor KJ, Schwartz PE: Screening for early ovarian cancer [review]. Radiology 1994; 192(1):1–10.
3. Tepper R, Lerner-Geva L, Altaras MM, et al: Transvaginal color flow imaging in the diagnosis of ovarian tumors. J Ultrasound Med 1995; 14:731–734.
4. Predanic M, Vlahos N, Pennisi JA, et al: Color and pulsed Doppler sonography, gray-scale imaging, and serum CA 125 in the assessment of adnexal disease. Obstet Gynecol 1996; 88:283–288.
5. Hata K, Hata T, Kitao M: Intratumoral peak systolic velocity as a new possible predictor for detection of adnexal malignancy. Am J Obstet Gynecol 1995; 172:1496–1500.
6. Buy JN, Ghossain MA, Hugol D, et al: Characterization of adnexal masses: Combination of color Doppler and conventional sonography compared with spectral Doppler analysis alone and conventional sonography alone. AJR Am J Roentgenol 1996; 166:385–393.
7. Fleischer AC, Rodgers WH, Rao BK, et al: Assessment of ovarian

tumor vascularity with transvaginal color Doppler sonography [see comments]. J Ultrasound Med 1991; 10:563–568.

8. Fleischer AC, Rodgers WH, Kepple DM, et al: Color Doppler sonography of ovarian masses: A multiparameter analysis. J Ultrasound Med 1993; 12:41–48.

9. Maly Z, Riss P, Deutinger J: Localization of blood vessels and qualitative assessment of blood flow in ovarian tumors. Obstet Gynecol 1995; 85:33–36.

10. Angeid-Backman E, Coleman BG, Arger PH, et al: Comparison of resistive index versus pulsatility index in assessing the benign etiology of adnexal masses. Clin Imaging 1998; 22:284–291.

11. Kurjak A, Predanic M, Kupesic-Urek S, et al: Transvaginal color and pulsed Doppler assessment of adnexal tumor vascularity. Gynecol Oncol 1993; 50:3–9.

12. Kurjak A, Predanic M: New scoring system for prediction of ovarian malignancy based on transvaginal color Doppler sonography. J Ultrasound Med 1992; 11(12):631–638.

13. Brown DL, Frates MC, Laing FC, et al: Ovarian masses: Can benign and malignant lesions be differentiated with color and pulsed Doppler US? Radiology 1994; 190:333–336.

14. Valentin L, Sladkevicius P, Marsal K: Limited contribution of Doppler velocimetry to the differential diagnosis of extrauterine pelvic tumors. Obstet Gynecol 1994; 83:425–433.

15. Levine D, Feldstein VA, Babcook CJ, Filly RA: Sonography of ovarian masses: Poor sensitivity of resistive index for identifying malignant lesions. AJR Am J Roentgenol 1994; 162:1355–1359.

16. Antonic J, Rakar S: Colour and pulsed Doppler US and tumour marker CA 125 in differentiation between benign and malignant ovarian masses. Anticancer Res 1995; 15:1527–1532.

17. Stein SM, Laifer-Narin S, Johnson MB, et al: Differentiation of benign and malignant adnexal masses: Relative value of gray-scale, color Doppler, and spectral Doppler sonography. AJR Am J Roentgenol 1995; 164:381–386.

▪: SIZE AND WEIGHT OF THE ADULT UTERUS
- ACR Code: 854 (Uterus)

Technique ▪

Langlois obtained data from pathologic reports of hysterectomy specimens.[1] Platt and colleagues performed transvesical ultrasound of the uterus on several machines with 3.5- to 5.0-MHz transducers prior to hysterectomy within 3 months of surgery.[2]

Measurements ▪

Langlois recorded measurements of the specimens of the anteroposterior (AP) and transverse (TRV) dimensions, cephalocaudal length (LEN), and weight. The volume product (AP × TRV × LEN) was calculated as well.[1] Platt and colleagues measured AP and TRV dimensions from transverse images through the midbody and LEN from a longitudinal scan through the miduterus, including the cervix.[2] Table 1 lists the linear dimensions, volume (product multiplied by $\pi/6$), and weights of the uterus by age, parity, and menopausal status from both studies.[1, 2] Table 2 lists uterine weights by parity and menopausal status from Platt and group.[2]

Table 1 ▪ Size, Volume, and Weight of the Adult Uterus

PARAMETER	NO.	AP (cm)	TRV (cm)	LON (cm)	VOLUME (cc)	WEIGHT (gm)
Age						
10–19	3	2.8±0.7	5.0±0.5	8.0±0.0	59.0±14.9	56.0±13.9
20–29	68	4.1±0.8	5.5±0.8	9.2±1.6	113.1±48.8	107.0±34.5
30–39	223	4.1±1.5	5.7±1.5	9.4±1.5	121.9±61.8	114.9±36.1
40–49	114	4.2±1.1	5.9±1.1	9.5±1.1	130.7±65.4	118.1±44.7
50–59	38	3.2±1.2	5.0±1.2	8.1±1.8	78.6±52.6	84.3±41.9
60+	15	2.8±0.8	4.5±0.8	8.0±1.9	55.9±28.6	56.1±20.3
Gravidity						
0	22	2.8±0.9	4.7±0.5	7.6±1.4	55.8±34.1	61.1±21.6
1	23	3.3±1.0	4.8±1.0	8.1±1.4	74.5±48.7	82.7±40.0
2–3	138	3.9±1.2	5.5±1.2	9.0±1.2	107.5±59.0	100.9±36.2
4–5	123	4.2±1.1	5.8±1.1	9.4±1.1	127.4±64.5	114.7±39.3
6+	155	4.2±1.2	5.9±1.2	9.6±1.2	131.4±58.0	124.5±38.3
Parity						
0	30	2.9±1.1	4.7±0.5	7.7±1.1	58.5±31.5	63.2±21.4
1	26	3.5±1.0	5.0±1.0	8.6±1.5	85.1±49.7	90.4±39.8
2–3	173	3.9±1.3	5.6±1.3	9.2±1.3	113.6±63.4	104.1±36.0
4–5	115	4.2±1.1	5.8±1.1	9.4±1.1	129.2±61.8	118.5±42.2
6+	117	4.2±1.1	5.9±1.1	9.7±1.1	131.0±56.1	125.7±36.9
Premenopause (nulliparous)*	9	3.3±0.8	4.6±0.6	7.1±0.8	56.4	60±20
Premenopause (parous)*	52	4.3±0.6	5.8±0.8	8.9±1.0	124.3	116.7±33
Postmenopause*	76	3.2±0.7	4.9±0.8	7.9±1.2	64.9	58±26

All measurements are given as mean ± standard deviation.
From Platt and colleagues[2]; other parameters are from Langlois.[1]

Table 2 ▪ Weights of the Adult Uterus by Menopausal
Status and Parity

GROUP	NO.	WEIGHT
Premenopausal (by parity)		
0	9	60 ± 20
1	9	109 ± 26
2	18	108 ± 28
3	12	121 ± 35
>4	13	130 ± 35
TOTAL	61	109 ± 37
Postmenopausal (by years postmenopause)		
0–5	15	84 ± 22
5–10	18	58 ± 21
10–20	19	56 ± 27
>20	24	43 ± 18
TOTAL	76	58 ± 26
Postmenopausal (by parity)		
0	8	40 ± 21
1	7	53 ± 28
2	28	56 ± 26
3	14	58 ± 25
>4	19	70 ± 26
TOTAL	76	58 ± 26

Measurements in grams (mean ± standard deviation).
From Platt JF, Bree RL, Davidson D: J Clin Ultrasound 1990; 18:15–19. Used
by permission.

Source ▪

Langlois evaluated a total of 468 pathologic reports from specimens with no leiomyomata larger than 1.0 cm, adenomyosis, or endometrial hyperplasia.[1] Platt's subjects had no leiomyomata larger than 1.0 cm nor any other significant abnormalities.[2] Age ranges and numbers of patients are listed in Table 1.

Comments ▪

Platt and colleagues found that the actual volume differed from the calculated volume (AP × TRV × LEN × 0.5233) by an average of 1.6%. The standard deviation of the differences was 13% (random error). The uterine density was determined to be 1.03 gm/cc, which was not significantly different from 1.0 so that volume and weight were interchangeable.[2] Wiener and Newcombe performed a study similar to Platt's and compared uterine volume calculated from linear ultrasound measurements (0.5236 × TRV × AP × LON) with that obtained by water displacement. The overall average error was 2.0%. However, at smaller uterine volumes (<140 cc) the error was rather larger, ranging from −33.6% to 37.6%.[3]

REFERENCES

1. Langlois PL: The size of the normal uterus. J Reprod Med 1970; 4:221–226.
2. Platt JF, Bree RL, Davidson D: Ultrasound of the normal non-gravid uterus: Correlation with gross and histopathology. J Clin Ultrasound 1990; 18:15–19.
3. Wiener JJ, Newcombe RG: Measurements of uterine volume: A comparison between measurements by ultrasonography and by water displacement. J Clin Ultrasound 1992; 20:457–460.

▪▪ MEASUREMENT OF PELVIC ORGANS IN PREMENARCHAL GIRLS BY ULTRASOUND[1]

▪ ACR Code: 852 (Ovary); 854 (Uterus)

Technique ▪

1. Studies were performed with a 3-MHz mechanical sector scanner (SRT L/S GE), with electronic calipers calibrated to a velocity of 1540 m/sec.
2. The examinations were performed with the bladder distended.
3. Serial longitudinal and transverse scans were obtained in the supine position.

Measurements ▪

When the largest available uterine section was displayed in the longitudinal axis, the image was frozen and the total uterine length (TUL) and AP diameters of the corpus (COAP) and the cervix (CEAP) were measured on the screen. The transducer was then rotated through 90° and scanning was performed in the transverse axis of the uterus to measure the widest transverse diameter of the corpus.

Serial longitudinal scans of the pelvis with the uterus as a landmark were made by tilting the transducer and scanning through the bladder from the contralateral side. The ovaries appeared as oval structures, more transonic than surrounding tissues, about halfway from the uterus to the iliopsoas muscle. The ovarian vessels were useful as additional landmarks.

Table 1 ▪ Uterine Diameters and Volume*

AGE (Yr)	NO. OF PATIENTS	UTERINE DIAMETERS (mm)				UTERINE VOLUME (cm³)	
		TUL	COAP	CEAP	COAP/CEAP	By Chronologic Age	By Bone Age
		Mean ± SD	Mean ± SD	Mean ± SD	Mean ± SD	Mean ± SD	Mean ± SD
2	7	33.1 ± 4.4	7.0 ± 3.4	8.3 ± 2.0	0.84 ± 0.29	1.98 ± 1.58	1.76 ± 0.72
3	8	32.4 ± 4.3	6.4 ± 1.3	7.6 ± 2.2	0.89 ± 0.29	1.63 ± 0.81	1.80 ± 0.74
4	15	32.9 ± 3.3	7.6 ± 1.8	8.6 ± 1.8	0.90 ± 0.22	2.10 ± 0.57	1.97 ± 0.74
5	7	33.1 ± 5.5	8.0 ± 2.8	8.4 ± 1.6	0.95 ± 0.28	2.36 ± 1.39	2.19 ± 1.16
6	9	33.2 ± 4.1	6.7 ± 2.9	7.5 ± 1.8	0.86 ± 0.18	1.80 ± 1.57	1.65 ± 0.93
7	9	32.3 ± 3.9	8.0 ± 2.2	7.7 ± 2.5	1.08 ± 0.26	2.32 ± 1.07	2.81 ± 1.44
8	11	35.8 ± 7.3	9.0 ± 2.8	8.4 ± 1.7	1.05 ± 0.20	3.12 ± 1.52	2.70 ± 1.43
9	11	37.1 ± 4.4	9.7 ± 3.0	8.8 ± 2.0	1.10 ± 0.24	3.70 ± 1.62	2.69 ± 1.83
10	13	40.3 ± 6.4	12.8 ± 5.3	10.7 ± 2.6	1.17 ± 0.31	6.54 ± 3.78	4.66 ± 3.03
11	13	42.2 ± 5.1	12.8 ± 3.1	10.7 ± 2.6	1.22 ± 0.26	6.66 ± 2.87	6.24 ± 3.07
12	6	54.3 ± 8.4	17.3 ± 5.3	14.3 ± 5.2	1.23 ± 0.16	16.18 ± 9.15	8.88 ± 3.65
13	5	53.8 ± 11.4	15.8 ± 4.5	15.0 ± 2.4	1.03 ± 0.15	13.18 ± 5.64	15.55 + 5.98

*As determined by ultrasonography in 114 girls from ages 2 to 13 years. TUL = total uterine length; COAP = AP diameter of the corpus; CEAP = AP diameter of the cervix.

From Orsini LF: Radiology 1984; 153:113–116. Used by permission.

Table 2 ▪ Ovarian Volume*

AGE (Yr)	NO. OF PATIENTS	OVARIAN VOLUME (cm³)	
		By Chronologic Age	By Bone Age
		Mean ± SD	Mean ± SD
2	5	0.75 ± 0.41	0.78 ± 0.38
3	6	0.66 ± 0.17	0.64 ± 0.18
4	14	0.82 ± 0.36	1.00 ± 0.45
5	4	0.86 ± 0.02	0.95 ± 0.52
6	9	1.19 ± 0.36	1.05 ± 0.65
7	8	1.26 ± 0.59	1.23 ± 0.47
8	10	1.05 ± 0.50	1.29 ± 0.33
9	11	1.98 ± 0.76	1.35 ± 0.71
10	12	2.22 ± 0.69	1.47 ± 0.56
11	12	2.52 ± 1.30	2.45 ± 0.86
12	6	3.80 ± 1.40	3.10 + 1.29
13	4	4.18 ± 2.30	4.38 ± 2.74

*As determined by ultrasonography in 101 girls from ages 2 to 13 years.
From Orsini LF: Radiology 1984; 153:113–116. Used by permission.

Ovarian length and longitudinal inclination were evaluated on the scan displaying the largest section of the ovary. Transverse and AP diameters were measured from a transverse scan perpendicular to the longitudinal inclination.

Uterine and ovarian volumes (UV, OV) were determined by the formula for a prolate ellipsoid (volume = 0.5233 × D1 × D2 × D3; where D1, D2, D3 are the three maximal longitudinal, AP, and transverse diameters).

Uterine diameters and volumes are given in Table 1.
Ovarian volumes are shown in Table 2.

Source ▪

Data are based on study of 114 normal premenarchal girls ranging in age from 2 to 13 years.

REFERENCE

1. Orsini LF: Pelvic organs in premenarcheal girls: Real time ultrasonography. Radiology 1984; 159:731–732.

∵ VOLUME OF THE GRAVID UTERUS
- ACR Code: 854 (Uterus)

Technique •

Ultrasound of the gravid uterus was done with 3.5-MHz contact B or real-time linear array techniques.[1]

Measurements •

The maximal transverse (TRV), anteroposterior (AP), and cephalocaudal (LEN) dimensions of the uterus (including myometrium) were measured. Volume was calculated by $0.52 \times TRV \times AP \times LEN$ (prolate ellipse) and correlated with gestational age determined by dates and/or ultrasound measurements.[1] Table 1 lists the volumes for each week of gestation from 5 to 20.

Source •

A total of 126 pregnant women with gestational ages of from 5 to 20 weeks were included in the analysis. The gestational age from ultrasound measurements was within 1 week of that predicted by dates.[1]

Comments •

It is useful to be able to express uterine volume in nonpregnant women in terms of weeks of gestation since this is a standard nomenclature for expressing uterine enlargement. In cases of diffuse uterine enlargement by myomata, the volume/gestational age nomogram may be used. When there are discrete exophytic or pedunculated myomas, it is more accurate to report their locations and measurements separately, along with the uterine measurements/volume.[1]

Table 1 • Total Uterine Corpus Volume in Normal Pregnancy

WEEKS' GESTATION	NO.	UTERINE VOLUME (cc)
5	7	79 ± 16
6	16	109 ± 21
7	13	161 ± 17
8	27	190 ± 17
9	7	249 ± 26
10	6	296 ± 12
11	8	339 ± 25
12	15	383 ± 29
13	5	454 ± 15
14	4	494 ± 31
15	4	574 ± 47
16	13	684 ± 123
17	37	795 ± 81
18	12	924 ± 112
19	7	1056 ± 59
20	5	1243 ± 124

Measurements are given as mean ± standard deviation.
From Goldstein SR, Horii SC, Snyder JR, et al: Obstet Gynecol 1988; 72:86–90. Used by permission.

REFERENCE

1. Goldstein SR, Horii SC, Snyder JR, et al:. Estimation of nongravid uterine volume based on a nomogram of gravid uterine volume: Its value in gynaecologic uterine abnormalities. Obstet Gynecol 1988; 72:86–90.

∵ ENDOMETRIAL THICKNESS IN POSTMENOPAUSAL WOMEN
- ACR Code: 854 (Endometrium)

Technique •

Transvaginal ultrasound was performed using a variety of machines, with 5.0- to 7.5-MHz vaginal probes.[1–3]

Measurements •

From sagittal images through the body and fundus of the uterus, the thickest portion of the endometrium (ET) was measured between the boundaries separating the hyperechoic endometrium from the adjacent layer of myometrium. The double thickness was measured in each study, mostly in the fundus and occasionally in the body.[1–3] Lin and Levine and their colleagues excluded any fluid from the measurements by subtracting the thickness of any fluid (at the site of measurement) from the double layer endometrial thickness.[1, 2] Karlsson and colleagues did not exclude fluid from the ET measurement.[3] Figure 1 shows the measurement. Table 1 lists the results grouped by hormone replacement regimen in asymptomatic women[1, 2] and by biopsy results in those with bleeding.[3] Figure 2 is a receiver operating characteristic curve showing the performance of ET to identify abnormal endometrium (any diagnosis on biopsy other than normal or hormonal effect).[3] Figure 3 is a flow chart proposed by Levine and colleagues for management of women with various ET measurements, symptoms, and hormone regimens.[2]

Source •

Lin's and Levine's subjects included 112 and 121 unselected, self-referred, asymptomatic women who were all over the age of 50 years and were at least 1 year postmenopausal by clinical and historic criteria.[1, 2] Karlsson and colleagues evaluated 1168 women (age range, 41 to 91 years, mean age, 64 years) scanned within 3 days of endometrial curettage who were at least 1 year postmenopausal and presented with vaginal bleeding. The study included 351 women who were receiving hormone replacement (165, estriol, 186, sequential estrogen-progesterone).[3]

Comments •

There have been numerous studies of ET to discriminate causes of postmenopausal bleeding. Various cut-off levels have been advocated, ranging from 4 to 7 mm.[4–10] Studies

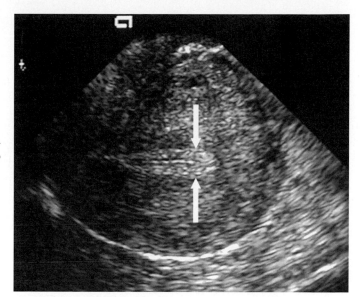

Figure 1 · Measurement of endometrial thickness. The double thickness of the endometrium (*arrows*) was measured from junction to junction at the widest portion.

Table 1 · Endometrial Thickness in Postmenopausal Women

| REFERENCE (GROUP) | NO. | ENDOMETRIAL THICKNESS (mm) | |
		Mean ± SD	Range
Lin (asymptomatic—hormone regimen)[1]			
None	58	5.2 ± 4.5	0–25
Unopposed estrogen	10	6.8 ± 5.3	0–14
Continuous estrogen & progesterone	9	5.3 + 1.7	2–7
Sequential estrogen & progesterone	35	6.6 ± 3.9	0–17
Levine (asymptomatic—hormone regimen)[2]			
None	61	5.0 ± 2.9	1–18
Unopposed estrogen	7	6.6 ± 4.0	1–13
Continuous estrogen & progesterone	15	6.2 ± 2.4	1–13
Sequential estrogen & progesterone	40	8.3 ± 3.9	1–18
Karlsson (bleeding–biopsy results)[3]			
Atrophy	667	3.9 ± 2.5	1–22
Hormonal effect	77	7.8 ± 4.0	2–28
Endometrial polyp	140	12.9 ± 8.1	2–53
Endometrial cancer	114	21.1 ± 11.8	5–68
Hyperplasia	112	12.0 ± 6.0	2–72
Other	19	15.1 ± 7.9	7–35

A measurement of 0 indicates that the endometrium was not visible.

Figure 2 · Receiver operating characteristics of endometrial thickness in postmenopausal women with vaginal bleeding. Disease positive is any diagnosis other than normal or hormonal effect on subsequent biopsy. Cut-off values are indicated (*triangles*) around the inflection point of the curve. (From Karlsson B, Granberg S, Wikland M, et al: Am J Obstet Gynecol 1995; 172(5):1488–1494. Used by permission.)

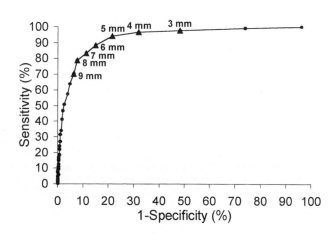

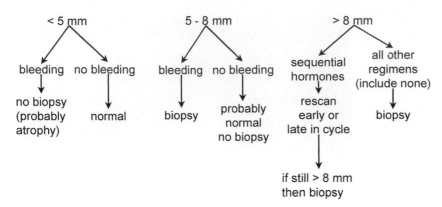

Figure 3 ▪ Algorithm for endometrial thickness management. (From Levine D, Gosink BB, Johnson LA: Radiology 1995; 197:603–608. Used by permission.)

of ET in asymptomatic women have produced recommendations for cut-off levels of from 8 to 10 mm.[11–13] The algorithm presented in Figure 3 represents only one set of cut-off numbers, and the reader may choose to modify them. However, it provides a clear outline for how to proceed.

Delisle and colleagues evaluated intra- and interobserver reproducibility and found coefficients of agreement of 94% to 97% and 94%, respectively. They advocate that ET measurements of 4 or 5 mm be managed with attention to the amount of bleeding and associated risk factors.[14] The endometrium of women undergoing tamoxifen therapy for breast cancer is significantly thicker than that of controls. Lahti and colleagues found mean ET in tamoxifen-treated women and controls of 10.4 mm versus 4.2 mm.[15] Hann and colleagues found that 47% of tamoxifen-treated women had endometrial thickness of 8 mm or more, of whom four had polyps, three hyperplasia, one papillary syncytial metaplasia, and two endometrial cancer.[16] This is a difficult problem as there are conflicting reports concerning the increased risk of endometrial cancer in this population,[17, 18] in addition to a probably increased risk associated with breast cancer alone in older women.[19] Andolf and colleagues have shown an association between body habitus and ET in asymptomatic postmenopausal women, with thicker measurements (>4 mm) being associated with greater body mass index.[20] Tsuda and colleagues compared ET in postmenopausal Japanese and white women of similar ages and found that the cut-off for Japanese women (and perhaps for other Asian populations) should be >3 mm.[21]

REFERENCES

1. Lin MC, Gosink BB, Wolf SI, et al: Endometrial thickness after menopause: Effect of hormone replacement [see comments]. Radiology 1991; 180(2):427–432.
2. Levine D, Gosink BB, Johnson LA: Change in endometrial thickness in postmenopausal women undergoing hormone replacement therapy. Radiology 1995; 197:603–608.
3. Karlsson B, Granberg S, Wikland M, et al: Transvaginal ultrasonography of the endometrium in women with postmenopausal bleeding—a Nordic multicenter study [see comments]. Am J Obstet Gynecol 1995; 172(5):1488–1494.
4. Goldstein SR, Nachtigal M, Snyder JR, et al: Endometrial assessment by vaginal ultrasonography before endometrial sampling in patients with postmenopausal bleeding. Am J Obstet Gynecol 1990; 163:119–123.
5. Granberg S, Wikland M, Karlsson B, et al: Endometrial thickness as measured by endovaginal ultrasonography for identifying endometrial abnormality. Am J Obstet Gynecol 1991; 164:47–52.
6. Dorum A, Kristensen GB, Langebrekke A, et al: Evaluation of endometrial thickness measured by endovaginal ultrasound in women with postmenopausal bleeding. Acta Obstet Gynecol 1993; 72:116–119.
7. Karlsson B, Granberg S, Wikland M, et al: Endovaginal scanning of the endometrium compared to cytology and histology in women with postmenopausal bleeding. Gynecol Oncol 1993; 50:173–178.
8. Tongsong T, Pongnarisorn C, Mahanuphap P: Use of vaginosonographic measurements of endometrial thickness in the identification of abnormal endometrium in peri- and postmenopausal bleeding. J Clin Ultrasound 1994; 22:479–482.
9. Emanuel MH, Verdel MJ, Wamsteker K, Lammes FB: A prospective comparison of transvaginal ultrasonography and diagnostic hysteroscopy in the evaluation of patients with abnormal uterine bleeding: clinical implications [see comments]. Am J Obstet Gynecol 1995; 172(2 Pt 1):547–552.
10. Van den Bosch T, Vandendael A, Van Schoubroeck D, et al: Combining vaginal ultrasonography and office endometrial sampling in the diagnosis of endometrial disease in postmenopausal women [see comments]. Obstet Gynecol 1995; 85(3):349–352.
11. Aleem F, Predaniac M, Calame R, et al: Transvaginal color and pulsed Doppler sonography of the endometrium: A possible role in reducing the number of dilation and curettage procedures. J Ultrasound Med 1995; 14:139–145.
12. Malpani A, Singer J, Wolverson MK, Merenda G: Endometrial hyperplasia: Value of endometrial thickness in ultrasonographic diagnosis and clinical significance. J Clin Ultrasound 1990; 18:173–177.
13. Shipley CF 3rd, Simmons CL, Nelson GH: Comparison of transvaginal sonography with endometrial biopsy in asymptomatic postmenopausal women. J Ultrasound Med 1994; 13(2):99–104.
14. Delisle MF, Villeneuve M, Boulvain M: Measurement of endometrial thickness with transvaginal ultrasonography: Is it reproducible? J Ultrasound Med 1998; 17:481–484.
15. Lahti E, Blanco G, Kauppila A, et al: Endometrial changes in postmenopausal breast cancer patients receiving tamoxifen. Obstet Gynecol 1993; 81:660–664.
16. Hann LE, Giess CS, Bach AM, et al: Endometrial thickness in tamoxifen-treated patients: Correlation with clinical and pathological findings. AJR Am J Roentgenol 1997; 168:657–661.
17. Breast Cancer Trials Committee, Scottish Cancer Trials Office: Adjuvant tamoxifen in the management of operable breast cancer: The Scottish trial. Lancet 1987; 2:171–175.
18. Fornander T, Rutqvist LE, Cedermark B, et al: Adjuvant tamoxifen in early breast cancer: Occurrence of new primary cancers. Lancet 1989; 1:117–119.
19. Adami HO, Krusemo UB, Bergkvist L, et al: On the age-dependent association between cancer of the breast and of the endometrium: A nationwide cohort study. Br J Cancer 1987; 55:77–80.
20. Andolf E, Dahlander K, Aspenberg P: Ultrasonic thickness of the endometrium correlated to body weight in asymptomatic postmenopausal women. Obstet Gynecol 1993; 82(6):936–940.
21. Tsuda H, Kawabata M, Kawabata K, et al: Differences between occidental and oriental postmenopausal women in cutoff level of endometrial thickness for endometrial cancer screening by vaginal scan. Am J Obstet Gynecol 1995; 172:1495–1495.

⁚ NEONATAL ADRENAL GLAND SIZE ON ULTRASOUND
▪ ACR Code: 86 (Adrenal)

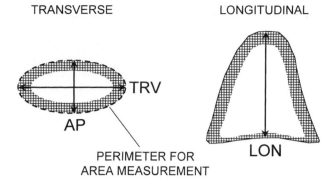

Figure 1 ▪ Measurement of the neonatal adrenal gland with ultrasound. From longitudinal images the anteroposterior *(AP)* and transverse *(TRV)* dimensions, as well as the perimeter *(dotted line)*, were determined. Area was calculated from the traced perimeter. From longitudinal images, the cephalocaudal length (LON) was measured from apex to midbase.

Technique ▪

Real-time ultrasound of the renal/adrenal fossae was done with a 128 machine (Acuson, Mountain View, CA) and a 5.0-MHz sector transducer. The right adrenal was visualized with the baby prone and the left side with the baby in the right-side-down decubitus position.[1]

Measurements ▪

From transverse images through the gland, anteroposterior (AP) and transverse (TRV) dimensions, as well as area by tracing the circumference, were measured. From the longitudinal image through each gland, the cephalocaudal length (LEN) was measured from the apex to the midpoint of the base of the gland.[1] Figure 1 shows the measurements. Table 1 lists the results, including change (decrease) over time expressed as percentage size at the time in question compared with the size at birth.[1]

Source ▪

Subjects included 12 healthy term infants (mean ± SD birth weight, 3260 ± 400 gm) who were each serially scanned six times from day 1 through days 42 to 45 after birth.[1]

Comments ▪

At birth the adrenal represents 0.2% to 0.3% of total body weight, compared with 0.001% in adults.[2] Scott's longitudinal data show a continuous decrease in linear dimensions and transverse area during the first 6 weeks of life, accounting for about half of the total decrease in bulk between birth and adulthood. The right gland was easier to see in general, but there were no significant side-to-side differences in measurements.[1]

Kangarloo and colleagues performed a cross-sectional study of normal term and premature neonates, as well as healthy infants up to 6 months of age, in which the length of the right adrenal was measured using ultrasound. They found a continuous decrease in size during the first 6 months (20 mm at birth to 9 mm at 6 months) in the healthy babies.[3] In healthy neonates, there were positive linear relationships between body weight and gland length (20 mm for 2500 gm to 30 mm for 5000 gm, r = 0.74, p <.001) and between body length and gland length (21 mm for 48 cm to 30 mm for 57 cm, r = 0.55, p <.01). In the premature neonates there was a linear relationship between gestational age and gland size (10 mm for 24 weeks to 28 mm for 32 weeks, r = 0.93, p <.001, no significant change from 32 weeks to term). The change in appearance of the

Table 1 ▪ Neonatal Adrenal Gland Measurements from Birth Through 42 Days

DAY	TRANSVERSE	ANTEROPOSTERIOR	CIRCUMFERENCE	AREA (cm²)	LENGTH
1	17.9±2.7	9.6±2.1	44.5±5.3	1.35±0.3	17.3±1.8
3	14.8±3.3	7.5±2.2	36.7±8.4	0.95±0.5	12.8±3.2
%day 3/1	(84.0±19.9)	(78.6±16.9)	(82.4±16.3)	(68.3±24.5)	(73.9±18.7)
5	13.7±2.1	6.9±1.6	33.4±5.1	0.75±0.2	11.4±2.7
%day 5/1	(77.5±11.3)	(74.6±21.6)	(75.3±9.1)	(56.3±16.9)	(66.1±16.9)
11	11.8±2.5	5.9±1.4	28.6±6.1	0.57±0.3	8.9±2.0
%day 11/1	(67.4±17.2)	(62.0±20.6)	(65.2±19.4)	(44.5±29.2)	(51.9±12.6)
21	10.8±1.9	5.6±0.5	25.3±3.9	0.45±0.1	8.2±1.2
%day 21/1	(61.5±13.4)	(61.1±16.3)	(57.8±11.3)	(35.7±13.7)	(47.9±80)
42	9.5±1.5	5.7±1.0	23.8±2.8	0.4±0.1	7.7±0.9
%day 42/1	(53.9±11.6)	(61.3±14.8)	(54.4±10.4)	(32.5±11.5)	(45.0±6.4)

Measurements in millimeters (except Area, which is in square centimeters), given as mean ± standard deviation. The change in size expressed as mean ± standard deviation percentage compared with day 1 is given in parentheses for each time interval.

From Scott EM, Thomas A, McGarrigle HHG, Lachelin GCL: J Ultrasound Med 1990; 9:279–283. Used by permission.

Table 2 • Changes in Ultrasound Appearances of the Adrenal During the First Year of Life

AGE	SHAPE AND SIZE	ECHOGENICITY
Neonate	Cortex large, with convex borders; medulla small	Cortex hypoechoic; medulla hyperechoic
1.5–2 mon	Cortex smaller, with convex borders; medulla proportionately larger and more uniform	Cortex hypoechoic; medulla hyperechoic
5–6 mon	Gland smaller, with straight borders	Gland hyperechoic (difficult to differentiate cortex and medulla)
1 yr and older	Borders straight or concave, similar to adult gland	Gland hypoechoic

From Kangarloo H, Diament MJ, Gold RH, et al: J Clin Ultrasound 1986; 14:43–47. Used by permission.

gland during the first year was described and is reproduced in Table 2.[3]

REFERENCES

1. Scott EM, Thomas A, McGarrigle HHG, Lachelin GCL: Serial adrenal ultrasonography in normal neonates. J Ultrasound Med 1990; 9:279–283.

2. Bech K, Tygstrup I, Nerup J: The involution of the fetal adrenal cortex. Acta Pathol Microbiol Scand 1969; 76:391–400.

3. Kangarloo H, Diament MJ, Gold RH, et al: Sonography of adrenal glands in neonates and children: Changes in appearance with age. J Clin Ultrasound 1986; 14:43–47.

∷ MEASUREMENT OF NORMAL SIZE AND SHAPE OF ADRENAL GLANDS BY CT[1]

- ACR Code: 86 (Adrenal)

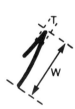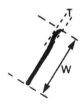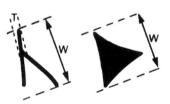

Figure 1 • Method of measuring with *(W)* and thickness *(T)* of adrenal glands. (From Montagne JP, et al: AJR Am J Roentgenol 1978; 130:963. Used by permission.)

Technique •

1. EMI 5000 scanner with 160 × 160 matrix or GE 8800 CT/T scanner with 320 × 320 matrix.
2. Slice thickness 1 cm. Use of intravenous contrast not noted.

Measurements • (Figures 1 and 2; Tables 1, 2, and 3)

The right adrenal is located just posterior to the inferior vena cava as it enters the liver. The left adrenal is somewhat more anterior than the right, lateral to the left crus of the diaphragm, posterior to the tail of the pancreas.

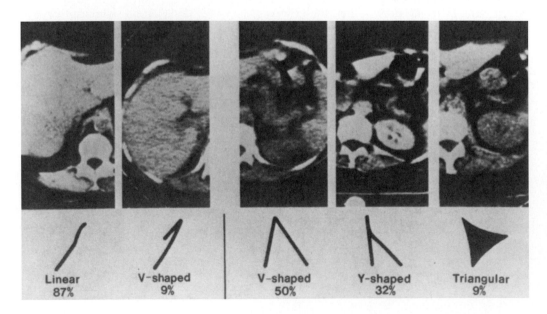

Linear
87%

V-shaped
9%

V-shaped
50%

Y-shaped
32%

Triangular
9%

Figure 2 • Most frequent shapes of normal adrenal glands. (From Montagne JP, et al: AJR Am J Roentgenol 1978; 130:963. Used by permission.)

Table 1 • Length of Adrenal Glands

NO. SECTIONS*	RIGHT		LEFT	
	No.	%	No.	%
1	3	6	—	—
2	20	43	16	34
3	23	49	29	62
4	1	2	2	4

*Nonoverlapping adjacent slices either 10 or 13 mm thick.
From Montagne JP, et al: AJR Am J Roentgenol 1978; 130:963. Used by permission.

Table 3 • Thickness of Adrenal Glands

CM	RIGHT		LEFT	
	No.	%	No.	%
<1.0	35	72	10	23
1.0	12	26	33	77
1.5	1	2	—	—

*Measurements not made in 4 left and 1 right triangular-shaped glands.
From Montagne JP, et al: AJR Am J Roentgenol 1978; 130:963. Used by permission.

The shape of the right adrenal is usually linear, and the left is usually V- or Y-shaped (Figure 2).

The length of each adrenal gland was estimated by counting the number of transverse cross-sections on which each was visualized (Table 1). The width of each gland was

Table 2 • Width of Adrenal Glands

CM	RIGHT		LEFT	
	No.	%	No.	%
1.0	2	4	1	2
1.5	3	6	4	9
2.0	21	45	25	53
2.5	15	32	16	34
3.0	6	13	1	2

From Montagne JP, et al: AJR Am J Roentgenol 1978;130:963. Used by permission.

determined on the section in which the adrenal appeared largest during the examination (Figure 1). The thickness of the adrenal gland was defined as its dimension perpendicular to the long axis of the gland or one of its limbs. The greatest thickness at any site was the measurement recorded. In the linear glands this tended to occur at the anterior portion, whereas in the V- and Y-shaped glands the site was usually at the junction of the limbs.

Source •

Sixty random patients were reviewed who had complete studies of the adrenal region and who had no clinical evidence of adrenal disease. Thirty-three men and 27 women ranged in age from 27 to 80 years (mean, 56 years).

REFERENCE

1. Montagne JP, Kressel HY, Korobkin M, Moss AA: Computed tomography of the normal adrenal glands. AJR Am J Roentgenol 1978; 130(5):963–966.

▪: SIZE OF THE ADRENAL GLAND AT CT
▪ ACR Code: 86 (Adrenal)

Technique •

CT scanning of the abdomen on a 9800 scanner (General Electric Corp., Milwaukee, WI) using 10-mm contiguous slices.[1, 2]

Measurements •

The adrenal gland was measured at the operator's console with electronic calipers. The maximal width of the body of the gland was measured just above the junction of the limbs

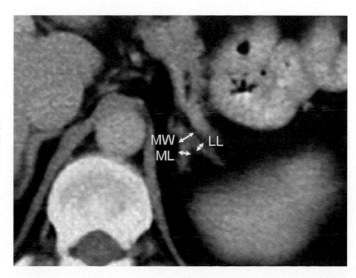

Figure 1 • Measurements of the adrenal gland from CT scans. Measurements of the maximal width of the body (MW), of the medial limb (ML), and of the lateral limb (LL) were made from the slice showing the measured portion to best advantage. On this scan through the left adrenal, the body and both limbs are visible on one slice.

Table 1 ▪ Adrenal Gland Size on CT in Normal Subjects, Patients with Solid Tumors, and Those with Lymphoma

	RIGHT ADRENAL GLAND			LEFT ADRENAL GLAND		
	Maximum Width	Medial Limb	Lateral Limb	Maximum Width	Medial Limb	Lateral Limb
Normal	6.1 ± 2.0 (3.0–12.3)	2.8 ± 0.8 (1.4–4.9)	2.8 ± 0.6 (1.4–4.9)	7.9 ± 2.1 (4.1–12.3)	3.3 ± 0.9 (1.7–5.1)	3.0 ± 1.0 (1.3–5.2)
Lymphoma	7.4 ± 2.4 (3.1–16.0)	3.8 ± 1.3 (2.2–8.3)	3.7 ± 1.0 (1.8–5.9)	9.6 ± 2.7 (3.8–16.2)	4.1 ± 1.2 (2.2–8.2)	3.7 ± 1.3 (1.5–6.5)
Tumor	8.1 ± 1.9 (3.8–12.6)	3.9 ± 1.1 (1.5–8.2)	3.8 ± 1.2 (1.4–8.5)	10.1 ± 2.6 (5.5–22.4)	4.7 ± 1.5 (1.6–9.3)	4.3 ± 1.5 (1.6–12.1)
P Values						
Normal vs. lymphoma	0.0102	0.002	0.0001	0.0064	0.0081	0.0059
Normal vs. tumor	0.0001	0.0001	0.0001	0.0001	0.0001	0.0001

Measurements are in millimeters, given as mean ± standard deviation as well as range (parentheses). P values are listed in the last two rows for comparisons between normal subjects and each malignancy group.

From Vincent JM, Morrison ID, Armstrong P, Reznek RH: Clin Radiol 1994; 49:456–460. Used by permission.

perpendicular to the long axis. The maximal width of each limb was also measured perpendicular to each long axis.[1, 2] Figure 1 shows the measurements on the left. Table 1 lists the results for normal subjects, patients with lymphoma, and those with solid tumors.

Source ▪

Subjects were 55 controls with no known disease that would affect the size of the adrenals,[1] 144 patients with nonendocrine malignant solid tumors, and 47 patients with lymphoma.[2] None of the patients with malignancy had undergone radiation or chemotherapy or had discrete adrenal masses either by history or on the scans from which measurements were made, which were all done for initial staging or recurrent disease.[2]

Comments ▪

The mean widths of the adrenal glands of those with lymphoma and solid tumors were significantly larger than those of normal controls (p values in Table 1). This was felt to be due to hyperplasia, perhaps from release of bioactive ACTH from lymphocytes in response to tumor antigens.[2]

REFERENCES

1. Vincent JM, Morrison ID, Armstrong P, Reznek RH: The size of normal adrenal glands on computed tomography [published erratum appears in Clin Radiol 1995; 50(3):202]. Clin Radiol 1994; 49:453–455.
2. Vincent JM, Morrison ID, Armstrong P, Reznek RH: Computed tomography of diffuse, non-metastatic enlargement of the adrenal glands in patients with malignant disease. Clin Radiol 1994; 49:456–460.

▪: CT ATTENUATION OF ADRENAL MASSES
▪ ACR Code: 86 (Adrenal)

Technique ▪

Boland and colleagues[1] analyzed ten studies[2–11] concerning CT attenuation values of adrenal masses to distinguish benign adenomas from other (malignant) etiologies. Individual attenuation values of all masses from unenhanced CT were abstracted from the paper (n = 9) or obtained from the authors (n = 1). Individual study technical details are listed in Table 1.

Measurements ▪

Regions of interest (ROI) were drawn over the lesion in question (described as encompassing at least half of its area in most papers) and the CT density in Hounsfield units (HU) recorded. Table 1 lists the numbers of lesions, threshold value used, and test performance for detecting malignancy from each study[2–11] as presented in the meta-analysis.[1] Boland and colleagues used receiver operating characteristic analysis techniques[12, 13] to calculate test performance of CT density in predicting benign etiology of the lesions.[1] Table 2 details the results of this analysis,

using varying threshold values in terms of sensitivity and specificity. Included in Table 2 are the likelihood ratios (calculated by us for lesion density above or below threshold) for benignity as described by Black and Armstrong.[14] These may be useful in combination with the prior odds of a benign lesion based on history of a primary tumor and size of the lesion in question.

Source ▪

From the ten studies analyzed, a total of 495 adrenal lesions were reported, of which 272 (55%) were benign and 223 (45%) were malignant.

Comments ▪

Adrenal cortex neoplasms and many benign adrenal neoplasms (adenomas and myelolipomas, for example) contain fat, and they may be distinguished from malignant lesions because they will have lower attenuation values at unenhanced CT.[15]

Table 1 • Details of CT Studies of Adrenal Mass Density

STUDY (Reference)	CT MANUFACTURER	CT TECHNIQUE	SLICE THICKNESS (mm)	ADENOMAS/ NONADENOMAS	THRESHOLD (HU)	SENSITIVITY (%)	SPECIFICITY (%)
Paivansalo[2]	Siemens	C	4	20/35	—	—	—
Miyake[3]	GE	C	5,10	22/8	—	—	—
Lee[4]	GE	C	10	38/28	0	47	100
van Erkel[5]	Philips	C	5,10	24/17	16.5	95	100
Miyake[6]	GE	C	5,10	14/19	15	64	100
McNicholas[7]	GE	C	5	18/19	12	94	100
Korobkin[8]	GE	C	5,10	41/20	18	85	100
Outwater[9]	GE	Hel,C	1,5,10	27/17	18	70	100
Szolar[10]	Siemens	Hel	5	41/37	11	61	100
Boland[11]	GE	Hel,C	5	23/23	13	100	100

HU = Hounsfield units, GE = General Electric, Hel = helical, C = conventional.
From Boland GW, Lee MJ, Gazelle G, et al: AJR Am J Roentgenol 1998; 171:201–204. Used by permission.

Table 2 • Test Performance of CT Density to Predict Benign Etiology of Adrenal Masses

THRESHOLD VALUE (HU)	SENSITIVITY (%)	SPECIFICITY (%)	LR FOR BENIGN (Lesion < Threshold)	LR FOR BENIGN (Lesion > Threshold)
0	41	100	infinity	0.59
2	47	100	infinity	0.53
3	51	99	51.0	0.49
4	55	99	55.0	0.45
8	65	98.5	43.3	0.36
10	71	98	35.5	0.30
12	73	97	24.3	0.28
14	80	94.5	14.5	0.21
16	84	92	10.5	0.17
18	86	88	7.2	0.16
20	88	84	5.5	0.14

HU = Hounsfield units, LR = likelihood ratio.
From Boland GW, Lee MJ, Gazelle G, et al: AJR Am J Roentgenol 1998; 171:201–204. Used by permission.

REFERENCES

1. Boland GW, Lee MJ, Gazelle G, et al: Characterization of adrenal masses using unenhanced CT: An analysis of the CT literature. AJR Am J Roentgenol 1998; 171:201–204.
2. Paivansalo M, Lahde S, Merikanto J, Kallionen M: Computed tomography in primary and secondary adrenal tumors. Acta Radiol 1988; 29:519–522.
3. Miyake H, Meada H, Tashiro M, et al: CT of adrenal tumors: Frequency and clinical significance of low-attenuation lesions. AJR Am J Roentgenol 1989; 152:1005–1007.
4. Lee MJ, Hahn PF, Papanicolaou N, et al: Benign and malignant adrenal masses: CT distinction with attenuation coefficients, size, and observer analysis. Radiology 1991; 179:415–418.
5. van Erkel AR, van Gils APG, Lequin M, et al: CT and MR distinction of adenomas and nonadenomas of the adrenal gland. J Comput Assist Tomogr 1994; 18:432–438.
6. Miyake H, Takaki H, Matsumoto S, et al: Adrenal nonhyperfunctioning and nonadenoma: CT attenuation value as a discriminative index. Abdom Imaging 1995; 20:559–562.
7. McNicholas MMJ, Lee MJ, Mayo-Smith WW, et al: An imaging algorithm for the differential diagnosis of adrenal adenomas and metastases. AJR Am J Roentgenol 1995; 165:1453–1459.
8. Korobkin M, Brodeur FJ, Yutzy GG, et al: Differentiation of adrenal adenomas from nonadenomas using CT attenuation values. AJR Am J Roentgenol 1996; 166(3):531–536.
9. Outwater EK, Siegelman ES, Abbott BH, Birnbaum BA: Adrenal masses: Correlation between CT attenuation value and chemical shift ratio at MR imaging with in-phase and opposed-phase sequences. Radiology 1996; 200:749–752.
10. Szolar DH, Kammerhuber F: Quantitative CT evaluation of adrenal gland masses: A step forward in the differentiation between adenomas and nonadenomas? Radiology 1997; 20:517–521.
11. Boland GW, Hahn PF, Pena C, Mueller PR: Adrenal masses: Characterization with delayed contrast-enhanced CT. Radiology 1997; 202:693–696.
12. Metz CE: ROC methodology in radiologic imaging. Invest Radiol 1986; 21:720–733.
13. Metz CE: Some practical issues of experimental design and data analysis in radiologic ROC studies. Invest Radiol 1989; 24:234–245.
14. Black WC, Armstrong P: Communicating the significance of radiologic test results: The likelihood ratio. AJR Am J Roentgenol 1986; 147:1313–1318.
15. Korobkin M, Giordano TJ, Brodeur GJ, et al: Adrenal adenomas: Relationship between histologic lipid and CT and MR findings. Radiology 1996; 200:743–747.

CHAPTER 13

Biometry and Pelvimetry in Pregnancy

▪: MEASUREMENTS OF THE CERVIX IN PREGNANCY

▪ ACR Code: 854 (Cervix During Pregnancy)

Technique ▪

Transvaginal scanning of the cervix in pregnant women was done with a variety of machines and 5- to 7.5-MHz vaginal probes.[1-3] Patients were in lithotomy position after voiding. The probe was gently placed in the introitus and not advanced if bulging membranes were seen. Otherwise, the probe was gently advanced until the cervix could be seen in sagittal/longitudinal section for its entire length. To avoid distortion by the probe, some advocate withdrawing until the image blurs and reapplying just enough pressure to restore clarity.[4, 5] Andersen also performed transabdominal scanning (3.5-MHz transducer) with a comfortably full bladder for measurements of the cervix.[3]

Measurements ▪

From images through the long axis of the cervix, including the internal os, external os, and canal, the length was measured from internal to external os.[1-3] The width was measured midway between the internal and external os.[1] Figure 1 shows the measurements. Figure 2 graphically depicts cervical length as reported by Smith and Kushnir

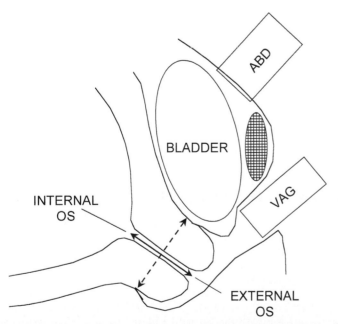

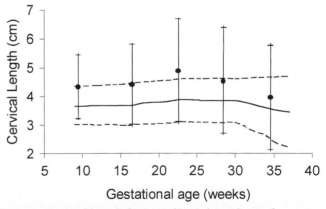

Figure 1 ▪ Measurements of the cervix in pregnancy. Positions of transvaginal *(VAG)* and transabdominal *(ABD)* probes are shown. The length *(solid line with arrows)* is measured between the internal os and external os on images through the long axis of the cervix. The width *(dotted line with arrows)* is measured from the same image at the midpoint.

Figure 2 ▪ Cervical length from weeks 10 through 37 of pregnancy. 10th *(lower dashed)*, 50th *(solid)*, and 90th *(upper dashed)* percentiles are from Smith and associates.[1] Data from Kushnir et al *(circles with error bars)* are also shown.[2] (From Smith CV, Anderson JC, Matamoros A, Rayburn WF: J Ultrasound Med 1992; 11(9):465–467. Used by permission.)

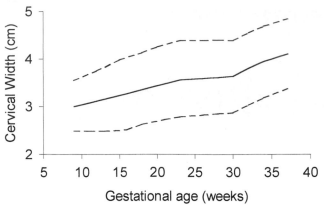

Figure 3 ▪ Cervical width from 10 to 37 weeks of pregnancy. 10th (*lower dashed*), 50th (*solid*), and 90th (*upper dashed*) percentiles are shown. (From Smith CV, Anderson JC, Matamoros A, Rayburn WF: J Ultrasound Med 1992; 11(9):465–467. Used by permission.)

and their associates.[1, 2] Figure 3 is a graph of cervical width from Smith and colleagues.[1] Table 1 lists cervical length by gestational age and parity for transabdominal and transvaginal scanning, as reported by Andersen.[3]

Source ▪

Smith's subjects were 109 normal, well-dated singleton pregnancies in which the women delivered at or near term and were scanned from 9 to 37 weeks.[1] Kushnir evaluated 166 women with normal singleton pregnancies, of whom 50 were primagravida and 116 were multigravid. Scans were done between 8 and 37 weeks.[2] Andersen studied 186 singleton pregnancies, of which 81 were in nulliparous women and 105 women had prior birth. Transabdominal and transvaginal determination of cervical length was done from 6 weeks to term. Eight women had findings of cervical incompetence requiring cerclage, and these were excluded from further analysis.[3]

Comments ▪

Kushnir and colleagues found no significant difference in cervical length based on gravidity, whereas Andersen found

Table 1 ▪ Cervical Length in Pregnancy by Transvaginal and Transabdominal Scanning[3]

PARITY	GEST. AGE (wk)	NO.	LENGTH (cm) (Mean ± SD)	LENGTH (cm) (Range)
			Transabdominal Scanning	
Multiparous	6–28	78	4.72 ± 1.38	2.5–8.4
Nulliparous	6–28	57	4.16 ± 1.48	1.8–9.2
Both	6–13	32	5.32 ± 1.69	2.9–9.2
	14–27	67	4.37 ± 1.38	2.1–8.4
	28–40	36	3.95 ± 0.98	1.8–6.3
			Transvaginal Scanning	
Multiparous	6–28	98	3.96 ± 1.21	1.2–7.2
Nulliparous	6–28	79	3.58 ± 0.97	1.3–6.2
Both	6–13	38	3.98 ± 0.85	2.3–5.9
	14–27	77	4.16 ± 1.02	2.7–7.2
	28–40	62	3.23 ± 1.16	1.2–6.1

that multiparous women had a mean cervical length of 4.0 mm (average 10% difference) greater than nulliparous women.[2, 3] Andersen did not think that this small difference requires separate norms for these two groups.[3] Cervical length determined by transvaginal scanning was significantly less than that measured with transabdominal scanning, with an average difference of 5.2 mm and p < .001.[3] Andersen noted cervical funneling (protrusion of membranes into the internal os) in 22 of 178 patients (12%) who did not require cerclage, and 3 of 8 (38%) who received cerclage.[3]

REFERENCES

1. Smith CV, Anderson JC, Matamoros A, Rayburn WF: Transvaginal sonography of cervical width and length during pregnancy. J Ultrasound Med 1992; 11(9):465–467.
2. Kushnir O, Vigil DA, Izquierdo L, et al: Vaginal ultrasonographic assessment of cervical length changes during normal pregnancy. Am J Obstet Gynecol 1990; 162:991–993.
3. Andersen HF: Transvaginal and transabdominal ultrasonography of the uterine cervix during pregnancy. J Clin Ultrasound 1991; 19:77–83.
4. Berghella V, Kuhlman K, Weiner S, et al: Cervical funneling: Sonographic criteria predictive of preterm delivery. Ultrasound Obstet Gynecol 1997; 10:161–166.
5. Iams JD, Goldenberg RL, Mercer BM: The preterm prediction study: Recurrence risk of spontaneous preterm birth. Am J Obstet Gynecol 1998; 178:1035–1040.

▪ PERFORMANCE OF CERVICAL MEASUREMENTS TO PREDICT PRETERM DELIVERY
▪ ACR Code: 854 (Cervix During Pregnancy)

Technique ▪

Transvaginal ultrasound in the lithotomy position with an empty bladder was performed to evaluate the gravid cervix as described in a previous section of this book.[1, 2] Berghella and colleagues performed either translabial (3.5-MHz transducer) or transvaginal scans.[3] No attempts were made to perform transfundal pressure or any other provocative maneuvers.[1–3]

Measurements ▪

The length of the cervix (CX-length) was measured from frozen longitudinal/sagittal images through its midportion.[1–3] This was called functional cervical length by Berghella and colleagues.[3] Funneling was considered to be present by Iams et al if membranes bulged into the internal os by 3 mm or more, as measured along the lateral border of the funnel.[1] Berghella and group measured the amount of

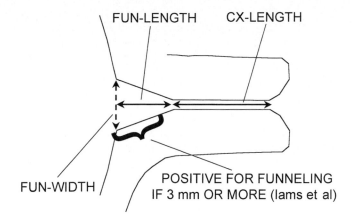

Figure 1 ▪ Measurements of the cervix were done from a frozen longitudinal image through the midportion. The length of the closed portion (*CX-length*) was measured in all three studies.[1–3] The width (*FUN-width*) and length (*FUN-length*) of bulging membranes (called funneling) was measured in one, and in another funneling was considered to be present when the lateral border was 3 mm or more.

funneling along the projected axis of the cervical canal (FUN-length) and the width of the funnel (FUN-width) at the fetal end, and calculated the percentage of funneling: FUN-% = (FUN-length/CX-length + FUN-length) × 100.[3] Figure 1 shows these measurements. Table 1 lists performance of these parameters in predicting premature delivery. Table 2 lists probability of and likelihood ratios for preterm delivery at different cervical length ranges and cut-off values, respectively.[1, 2]

Source ▪

The paper by Iams and colleagues describes a multi-institutional study including 2915 pregnant women examined at

Table 2 ▪ Probabilities and Likelihood Ratios of Cervical Lengths in Predicting Preterm Delivery[1, 2]

CERVICAL LENGTH RANGE (cm)	PROBABILITY (Delivery <35 Wk)
<1.5	0.34
1.5–2.3	0.20
2.4–2.7	0.08
2.8–3.0	0.05
3.1–4.0	0.03
>4.0	0.02

CERVICAL LENGTH CUT-OFF (cm)	LIKELIHOOD RATIO (Delivery <37 Wk)
2.0	3.23
2.5	2.48
3.0	1.75
3.5	1.07
4.0	1.04
4.5	1.01
5.0	1.00
5.5	1.00

24 weeks, of whom 2531 had a second evaluation at 28 weeks. The frequency of preterm delivery (prior to 35 weeks) was 4.3% among the subjects examined at 24 weeks and 3.3% among those examined again at 28 weeks.[1] Tongsong and colleagues evaluated 730 women with well-dated singleton pregnancies at 28 to 30 weeks. Of these, 12.5% delivered before 37 weeks.[2] Berghella's subjects were retrospectively selected from ultrasounds (23 translabial, 20 transvaginal) of pregnant women showing cervical funneling. The scans were done between 16 and 28 weeks. Preterm delivery (prior to 37 weeks) occurred in 42% of these women.[3]

Table 1 ▪ Performance of Cervical Measurements for Predicting Preterm Delivery

REFERENCE/ PARAMETER	CUT-OFF VALUE	SENSITIVITY (%)	SPECIFICITY (%)	PPV (%)	NPV (%)
Iams		Scanned at 24/28 Wk, Delivery <35 Wk			
CX-Length	≤2.0 cm	23/31	97/95	26/17	97/98
	≤2.5 cm	37/49	92/87	18/11	97/98
	≤3.0 cm	54/70	76/69	9.3/7.0	97/99
Funneling	present	25/33	95/92	17/12	97/98
Tongsong		Scanned at 28–30 Wk, Delivery <37 Wk			
CX-Length	≤2.0 cm	3.3	100	—	—
	≤2.5 cm	5.5	98	—	—
	≤3.0 cm	31	88	—	—
	≤3.5 cm	66	62	—	—
	≤4.0 cm	81	24	—	—
	≤4.5 cm	95	9.2	—	—
	≤5.0 cm	100	2.5	—	—
	≤5.5 cm	100	0.6	—	—
Berghella		Scanned at 16–28 Wk, Delivery <37 Wk			
CX-Length	≤1.5 cm	50	88	75	71
	≤2.0 cm	78	56	56	78
FUN-Length	≥25 mm	56	96	91	75
	≥16 mm	67	76	67	76
FUN-Width	≥16 mm	33	88	67	65
	≥14 mm	72	76	68	79
FUN-%	≥55	56	88	77	73
	≥40	78	76	70	83

PPV = positive predictive value, NPV = negative predictive value. Other abbreviations in text and Figure 1.[1–3]

REFERENCES

1. Iams JD, Goldenberg RL, Meis PJ, et al: The length of the cervix and the risk of spontaneous premature delivery. N Engl J Med 1996; 334:567–572.

2. Tongsong T, Kamprapanth P, Srisomboon J, et al: Single transvaginal sonographic measurement of cervical length early in the third trimester as a predictor of preterm delivery. Obstet Gynecol 1995; 86:184–187.
3. Berghella V, Kuhlman K, Weiner S, et al: Cervical funneling: Sonographic criteria predictive of preterm delivery. Ultrasound Obstet Gynecol 1997; 10:161–166.

▪▪ AMNIOTIC FLUID VOLUME IN THE FIRST TRIMESTER
▪ ACR Code: 856 (Amniotic Fluid)

Technique ▪

Transvaginal ultrasound of the gravid uterus was done with 650 (Aloka, Tokyo, Japan) or ESI-1000 (Elscint, Haifa, Israel) machines and 5- to 6.5-MHz vaginal probes.[1]

Measurements ▪

The anteroposterior (AP), transverse (TRV), and longitudinal (LON) dimensions of the gestational sac were measured. The volume was calculated by the prolate ellipse formula ($\frac{4}{3}\pi \times$ (AP/2 $\times$ TRV/2 $\times$ LON/2). No attempt was made to subtract the volume of the embryo/fetus from the volumes thus obtained.[1] Table 1 lists volumes (as mean $\pm$ 95% confidence interval) and range versus gestational age (GA) and embryonic/fetal crown-rump length (CRL).

Source ▪

Study subjects included 95 pregnant women (all singleton) referred for routine examination to confirm GA. In all subjects, the ultrasound GA was within 4 days of GA by last menstrual period (LMP). There was no history of vaginal bleeding, subsequent abortion, morphologically abnormal ultrasound, or other complicating feature.[1]

REFERENCES

1. Weissman A, Itskovitz-Eldor J, Jakobi P: Sonographic measurement of amniotic fluid volume in the first trimester of pregnancy. J Ultrasound Med 1996; 15:771–774.

Table 1 ▪ Amniotic Fluid Volume by Ultrasound in Normal Singleton Pregnancies

WEEKS	NO.	MEAN ± 95% CI	Range
		F Volume (ml)	
7	8	1.5 ± 0.7	0.8–3.4
8	18	3.9 ± 0.9	0.9–11.2
9	19	12.5 ± 3.0	5.2–28.6
10	15	24.2 ± 5.8	9.3–37.8
11	13	48 ± 6.8	23.8–86
12	12	58 ± 8.8	27.4–80
13	10	100 ± 13.5	67–158
		CRL (mm)	
10–19	18	2.5 ± 0.8	0.9–7
20–29	21	9.2 ± 2.3	3.2–18
30–39	14	27.7 ± 5.5	15–51
40–49	17	54 ± 9.7	33–99
50–59	12	59 ± 11.4	27–82
60–69	8	90 ± 22.2	56–134
70–79	5	101 ± 45.3	67–158

CI = confidence interval, AF = amniotic fluid, CRL = crown-rump length. From Weissman A, Itskovitz-Eldor J, Jakobi P: J Ultrasound Med 1996; 15:771–774. Used by permission.

▪▪ AMNIOTIC FLUID INDEX IN NORMAL SINGLETON AND TWIN PREGNANCIES
▪ ACR Code: 856 (Amniotic Fluid)

Technique ▪

Ultrasound of the gravid uterus was performed with real-time 3.5 to 5.0-MHz linear transducers.[1,2]

Measurements ▪

The amniotic fluid index (AFI) for singletons was measured by Moore and Cayle as shown in Figure 1.[1] Chau and colleagues measured aggregate AFI for the entire gravid uterus in their study of twins.[2] Table 1 lists the 5th, 50th, and 95th percentiles of AFI from 16 weeks through term as reported by Moore and Cayle in singletons and calculated from Chau's polynomial regression equation for twins.[1,2] Figures 2 and 3 are graphic depictions of these same data. Figure 4 is a graph of weekly percentage change in AFI for singleton pregnancies.[1]

Source ▪

Moore and Cayle studied 791 normal singleton term pregnancies that were dated by last menstrual period (LMP) and ultrasound crown-rump length (CRL) in the first trimester or by ultrasound in the second trimester.[1] Chau and colleagues evaluated 91 normal diamniotic twin pregnancies delivered from 37 to 40 weeks, having birth weight discrepancies ranging from 0 to 19% and average birth weights of 2723 gm. There were 42 dichorionic and 49 monochorionic pregnancies. Each patient had follow-up

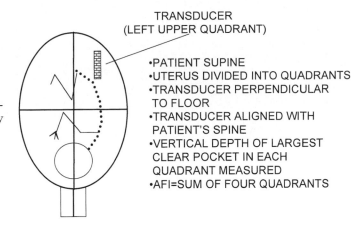

TRANSDUCER
(LEFT UPPER QUADRANT)

•PATIENT SUPINE
•UTERUS DIVIDED INTO QUADRANTS
•TRANSDUCER PERPENDICULAR
 TO FLOOR
•TRANSDUCER ALIGNED WITH
 PATIENT'S SPINE
•VERTICAL DEPTH OF LARGEST
 CLEAR POCKET IN EACH
 QUADRANT MEASURED
•AFI=SUM OF FOUR QUADRANTS

Figure 1 ▪ Measurement of amniotic fluid index *(AFI)*. The transducer is shown in the left upper quadrant and would be similarly positioned (over the largest pocket) in the other three quadrants.

Table 1 ▪ Amniotic Fluid Index (AFI) in Normal Singleton and Twin Pregnancies

WEEKS	AFI (cm) SINGLETONS			AFI (cm) TWINS		
	5th	50th	95th	5th	50th	95th
16	7.9	12.1	18.5	7.7	12.1	19.0
17	8.3	12.7	19.4	8.0	12.5	19.6
18	8.7	13.3	20.2	8.2	12.9	20.2
19	9.0	13.7	20.7	8.4	13.2	20.7
20	9.3	14.1	21.2	8.6	13.6	21.3
21	9.5	14.3	21.4	8.8	13.9	21.8
22	9.7	14.5	21.6	9.0	14.2	22.3
23	9.8	14.6	21.8	9.2	14.4	22.7
24	9.8	14.7	21.9	9.3	14.7	23.0
25	9.7	14.7	22.1	9.5	14.9	23.3
26	9.7	14.7	22.3	9.6	15.0	23.6
27	9.5	14.6	22.6	9.6	15.1	23.7
28	9.4	14.6	22.8	9.6	15.1	23.8
29	9.2	14.5	23.1	9.6	15.1	23.7
30	9.0	14.5	23.4	9.6	15.0	23.6
31	8.8	14.4	23.8	9.5	14.8	23.3
32	8.6	14.4	24.2	9.3	14.6	22.9
33	8.3	14.3	24.5	9.1	14.3	22.4
34	8.1	14.2	24.8	8.9	13.9	21.8
35	7.9	14.0	24.9	8.6	13.5	21.1
36	7.7	13.8	24.9	8.2	12.9	20.3
37	7.5	13.5	24.4	7.9	12.3	19.4
38	7.3	13.2	23.9	7.4	11.7	18.4
39	7.2	12.7	22.6	7.0	11.0	17.3
40	7.1	12.3	21.4	6.5	10.3	16.1
41	7.0	11.6	19.4	6.0	9.5	14.9
42	6.9	11.0	17.5	5.5	8.7	13.7

Data are as observed for singletons and were calculated from the given polynomial regression equation for twins.

From Moore TR, Cayle JE: Am J Obstet Gynecol 1990; 162:1168–1173. Used by permission.

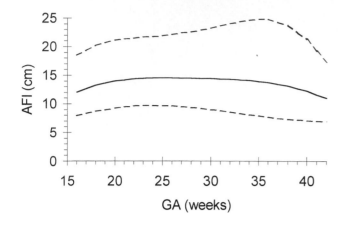

Figure 2 ▪ Amniotic fluid index *(AFI)* in normal singleton pregnancies. 50th (solid), 5th *(lower dashed)*, and 95th *(upper dashed)* percentiles are shown. *GA* = gestational age. (From Moore TR, Cayle JE: Am J Obstet Gynecol 1990; 162:1168–1173. Used by permission.)

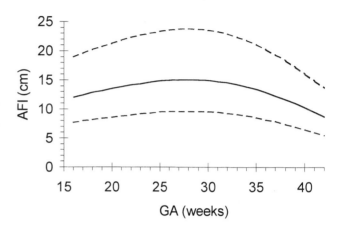

Figure 3 ▪ Amniotic fluid index *(AFI)* in normal twin pregnancies. 50th (solid), 5th *(lower dashed)*, and 95th *(upper dashed)* percentiles are shown. *GA* = gestational age. (From Chau AC, Kjos SL, Kovacs BW: Am J Obstet Gynecol 1996; 174(3):1003–1007. Used by permission.)

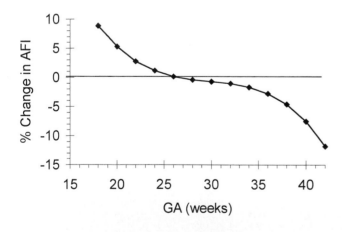

Figure 4 ▪ Weekly percentage change in amniotic fluid index *(AFI)* in normal singleton pregnancies. *GA* = gestational age. (From Moore TR, Cayle JE: Am J Obstet Gynecol 1990; 162:1168–1173. Used by permission.)

scans every 4 to 6 weeks, and a total of 376 scans were available for analysis.[2]

Comments ▪

Moore and Cayle evaluated intra- and interobserver variability and found them to average 0.5 cm (3.1%) and 0.97 cm (6.7%), respectively. Chau and colleagues found a mean intraobserver error of 0.37 cm (2.9%).[1, 2] There was no significant difference in AFI values between normal dichorionic and monochorionic twins.[2]

References

1. Moore TR, Cayle JE: The amniotic fluid index in normal pregnancy. Am J Obstet Gynecol 1990; 162:1168–1173.
2. Chau AC, Kjos SL, Kovacs BW: Ultrasonographic measurement of amniotic fluid volume in normal diamniotic twin pregnancies. Am J Obstet Gynecol 1996; 174(3):1003–1007.

⦂ PERFORMANCE OF ULTRASOUND ESTIMATES OF AMNIOTIC FLUID VOLUME

■ ACR Code: 856 (Amniotic Fluid)

Table 1 ■ Methods of Amniotic Fluid Volume Determination or Estimation with Normal Values

METHOD	ABREVIATION	DESCRIPTION	REFERENCE: NORMAL VALUES
Dye dilution	DDil	Hippurate injected into amnion, sample withdrawn and volume calculated based on concentration in sample	Magann: 500–1500 ml Croom: from Brace[3]
Amniotic fluid index	AFI	Sum of AP measurement of largest pocket in each quadrant	Magann: 5–18 cm Croom: 5–20 cm
Largest vertical pocket	LVP	AP measurement of the largest pocket in any quadrant	Magann: 2–8 cm Croom: 2–8 cm
Two-diameter pocket	TDP	AP × TRV measurements of largest pocket in any quadrant	Magann: 15–50 sq cm

Technique ■

Magann and colleagues performed obstetric ultrasound with an Ultramark 4 machine (ATL, Bothell, WA), and Croom and colleagues used a 128 machine (Acuson, Mountain View, CA).[1, 2] Croom et al used a 3.5-MHz linear array transducer for amniotic fluid measurements; the transducer type was not specified by Magann et al. Both teams performed amniocentesis at the time of the scan, during which amniotic fluid (AF) volume was determined by the dye dilution (DDil) technique using (para)aminohippurate.[1, 2]

Measurements ■

Table 1 lists the three measurements performed to assess AF volume by ultrasound, including the abbreviations, method, and normal ranges as defined by each group of workers.[1, 2] The normal range of AF volume for diagnosing oligo- or polyhydramnios used by Croom and colleagues was taken from a meta-analysis of AF volumes throughout pregnancy by Brace and Wolf.[3] Figure 1 is a scatterplot of AF volume by DDil versus amniotic fluid index (AFI) and largest vertical pocket (LVP) from Croom's data.[2] Table 2 lists the performance of AFI, LVP, and Magann's two-diameter pocket (TDP) method in diagnosing oligo- and polyhydramnios, using DDil as the gold standard.[1, 2]

Source ■

Magann and colleagues studied 40 pregnant women undergoing 3rd trimester amniocentesis for fetal lung maturity determination (gestational age, 28 to 37 weeks). There were 15 with oligohydramnios (DDil <500 cc), 9 with polyhydramnios (DDil >1500 cc), and 19 with normal AF volumes.[1] Croom's subjects included 50 pregnant women undergoing 3rd trimester amniocentesis for fetal lung maturity determination (mean gestational age, 38.6 ± 1.2 weeks). None had polyhydramnios, two had oligohydramnios, and the rest had normal AF volumes by Brace's nomogram.[2, 3]

Comments ■

We have calculated regression equations for amniotic fluid volume versus AFI and LVP from Croom's scatterplot data as follows:

$$\text{AF volume } (cc) = 38.538 + 117.456 \times \text{AFI (cm)}, (r = 0.752).$$
$$\text{AF volume } (cc) = 84.070 + 158.499 \times \text{LVP (cm)}, (r = 0.597).$$

The linear regression r values given by Croom and associates were 0.773 and 0.599, respectively, though they did not list the coefficients or constants.

Both groups concluded that AFI was superior to LVP for estimating AF volume, in terms of correlation with DDil volume as well as sensitivity and specificity for detecting oligo- and polyhydramnios. Magann and colleagues

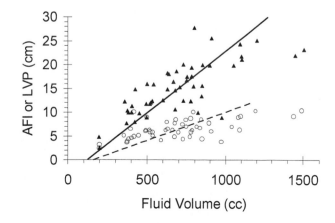

Figure 1 ■ Amniotic fluid volume by dilution at amniocentesis versus amniotic fluid index *(AFI, triangles)* and largest vertical pocket *(LVP, circles)* measurements at ultrasound. Linear regression lines are shown for AFI *(solid)* and LVP *(dashed)* (From Croom CS, Banias BB, Ramos-Santos E, et al: Am J Obstet Gynecol 1992; 167:995–999. Used by permission.)

Table 2 ▪ Performance of Ultrasound Estimates of Amniotic Fluid Volume

REFERENCE/CONDITION (Criteria)	MEASUREMENT (Criteria)	SENSITIVITY %	SPECIFICITY %
Magann			
Oligohydramnios (DDil < 500 ml)	Amniotic fluid index (<5 cm)	6.7	100
	Largest vertical pocket (<2 cm)	0.0	100
	Two-diameter pocket (<15 sq cm)	60.0	84
Polyhydramnios (DDil > 1500 ml)	Amniotic fluid index (>20 cm)	83.3	85.3
	Largest vertical pocket (>8 cm)	50	97
	Two-diameter pocket (>50 sq cm)	50	97
Croom			
Oligohydramnios (from Brace)	Amniotic fluid index (<5 cm)	100	100
	Largest vertical pocket (<2 cm)	0	100
Polyhydramnios (from Brace)	Amniotic fluid index (>18 cm)	—	76
	Largest vertical pocket (>8 cm)	—	84

DDil = dye dilution.

believed that the TDP method was superior to AFI in detecting oligohydramnios.[2]

REFERENCES

1. Magann EF, Nolan TE, Hess LW, et al: Measurement of amniotic fluid volume: Accuracy of ultrasonography techniques [see comments]. Am J Obstet Gynecol 1992; 167:1533–1537.

2. Croom CS, Banias BB, Ramos-Santos E, et al: Do semiquantitative amniotic fluid indexes reflect actual volume? Am J Obstet Gynecol 1992; 167:995–999.

3. Brace RA, Wolf EJ: Normal amniotic fluid volume changes throughout pregnancy. Am J Obstet Gynecol 1989; 161:382–388.

▪: RELATIONSHIP BETWEEN SAC SIZE, CROWN-RUMP LENGTH, AND PREGNANCY OUTCOME
▪ ACR Code: 856 (Early Pregnancy)

Technique ▪

Transvaginal ultrasound of the gravid uterus was done with a variety of machines and 3.5- to 5.0-MHz transducers.[1–3]

Measurements ▪

The mean gestational sac diameter (MSD) was measured with electronic calipers by averaging three orthogonal measurements made from frozen images.[1, 2] The embryonic/fetal crown-rump length (CRL) was measured from frozen images through the long axis.[1, 3] Tables 1 and 2 list normal MSD and CRL percentiles versus menstrual age (MA) in days as given by Dickey and colleagues.[2, 3] Figure 1 is a graph of MSD − CRL versus MA from Rowling and colleagues.[1] Dickey and colleagues correlated numbers of patients having spontaneous abortions with initial MSD and CRL, and these data are presented in Tables 3 and 4.[2, 3]

Source ▪

Rowling and associates collected MSD and CRL measurements from 595 pregnancies with normal outcomes to determine normative values of MSD − CRL. Records from 17 additional patients with MSD − CRL < 5 mm were also reviewed.[1] Dickey and associates prospectively evaluated 700[2] and 837[3] well-dated singleton pregnancies to determine the relationship of initial MSD (measured before 45 menstrual days) and CRL (measured after 42 menstrual days) to outcome. A subset of 74 patients (224 scans) who delivered after 34 weeks, whose exact postovula-

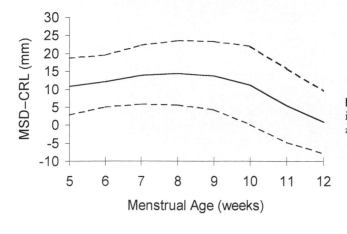

Figure 1 ▪ Mean sac diameter (MSD) minus crown to rump length (CRL) in normal pregnancy. (From Rowling SE, Coleman BG, Langer JE, et al: Radiology 1997; 203:211–217. Used by permission.)

Table 1 ▪ Centile Growth Curves for Mean Sac Diameter Versus
Menstrual Age

MA (Days)	MEAN SAC DIAMETER (mm) PERCENTILES				
	10th	25th	50th	75th	90th
30	0.6	0.8	1.2	1.9	2.6
31	0.9	1.2	1.6	2.5	3.4
32	1.2	1.5	2.1	3.2	4.2
33	1.5	2.0	2.6	3.9	5.0
34	1.9	2.4	3.3	4.7	6.0
35	2.4	3.0	3.9	5.6	7.0
36	2.9	3.6	4.7	6.5	8.1
37	3.4	4.2	5.5	7.5	9.2
38	4.0	4.9	6.3	8.5	10.4
39	4.6	5.7	7.2	9.6	11.6
40	5.3	6.5	8.1	10.7	12.8
41	6.0	7.3	9.1	11.8	14.0
42	6.8	8.1	10.1	13.0	15.3
43	7.6	9.0	11.1	14.2	16.6
44	8.4	10.0	12.2	15.4	17.9
45	9.2	10.9	13.3	16.6	19.2
46	10.1	11.9	14.4	17.9	20.5
47	10.9	12.9	15.5	19.1	21.8
48	11.8	13.9	16.6	20.4	23.1
49	12.8	14.9	17.8	21.6	24.4
50	13.7	15.9	19.0	22.9	25.7
51	14.6	17.0	20.1	24.2	27.0
52	15.6	18.0	21.3	25.4	28.3
53	16.6	19.1	22.5	26.7	29.6
54	17.5	20.1	23.6	27.9	30.8
55	18.5	21.2	24.8	29.2	32.1
56	19.5	22.2	26.0	30.4	33.3
57	20.5	23.3	27.1	31.6	34.6
58	21.4	24.4	28.3	32.8	35.8
59	22.4	25.4	29.4	34.0	37.0
60	23.4	26.5	30.6	35.2	38.1
61	24.4	27.6	31.7	36.4	39.4
62	25.3	28.6	32.9	37.6	40.5
63	26.3	29.6	34.0	38.7	41.7

MA = menstrual age.
From Dickey RP, Gasser R, Olar TT, et al: Hum Reprod 1994; 9(3):559–565.
Used by permission.

Table 2 ▪ Centile Growth Curves for Crown-Rump Length Versus Menstrual Age

MA (Days)	CROWN-RUMP LENGTH (mm) PERCENTILES				
	10th	25th	50th	75th	90th
40	0.7	1.0	1.4	2.0	2.2
41	0.9	1.2	1.7	2.4	2.7
42	1.1	1.5	2.1	2.8	3.2
43	1.4	1.8	2.5	3.4	3.7
44	1.7	2.2	3.0	3.9	4.3
45	2.0	2.6	3.5	4.5	5.0
46	2.4	3.1	4.0	5.2	5.7
47	2.5	3.6	4.6	5.9	6.5
48	3.3	4.1	5.3	6.8	7.3
49	3.8	4.7	5.7	7.5	8.2
50	4.3	5.4	6.1	8.3	9.1
51	4.9	6.0	7.5	9.1	10.1
52	5.6	6.8	8.3	10.1	11.0
53	6.2	7.5	9.1	11.1	12.1
54	7.0	8.3	10.0	12.1	13.2
55	7.8	9.2	11.0	13.1	14.3
56	8.6	10.1	11.9	14.2	15.4
57	9.4	11.0	13.0	15.3	16.6
58	10.3	12.0	14.0	16.4	17.5
59	11.2	13.0	15.1	17.6	19.0
60	12.2	14.1	16.2	18.7	20.3
61	13.2	15.1	17.3	19.9	21.6
62	14.3	16.2	18.3	21.2	22.9
63	15.4	17.3	19.7	22.4	24.2
64	16.5	18.5	20.9	23.7	25.5
65	17.6	19.7	22.1	25.0	26.9
66	18.8	21.0	23.4	26.3	28.3
67	20.0	22.2	24.6	27.6	29.7
68	21.3	23.5	25.9	28.9	31.1
69	22.5	24.5	27.2	30.2	32.5
70	23.8	26.1	28.6	31.6	33.9
71	25.1	27.4	29.9	33.0	35.4
72	26.5	28.8	31.2	34.3	36.8
73	27.9	30.2	32.6	35.7	38.3
74	29.2	31.6	34.0	37.1	39.8
75	30.6	33.0	35.4	38.5	41.2
76	32.1	34.4	36.8	39.9	42.7
77	33.5	35.9	38.2	41.3	44.2

MA = menstrual age.
From Dickey RP, Gasser RF, Olar TT, et al: Hum Reprod 1994; 9:366–373. Used by permission.

Table 3 ▪ Spontaneous Abortion Rates Versus Mean Sac Diameters Determined Before 45 Menstrual Days

AGE GROUP MSD CENTILE	NUMBER IN CENTILE	SPONT. AB NO.	SPONT. AB %	95% CI OF PERCENT
Maternal age < 35 years				
≤10th	88	24	27.3	18.0–36.6
<50th	230	41	17.8	12.9–22.7
≥75th	308	15	4.9	2.5–7.3
≥90th	79	2	2.5	0.0–5.9
Maternal age > 35 years				
≤10th	29	15	51.7	33.5–69.9
<50th	77	32	41.6	31.6–52.6
≥75th	85	11	12.9	5.8–20.0
≥90th	26	5	19.2	15.3–23.1
All maternal ages				
≤10th	117	39	33.3	24.8–41.8
<50th	307	73	23.8	19.0–28.6
≥75th	393	26	6.7	4.2–9.2
≥90th	105	7	6.7	1.9–11.5

MSD = mean sac diameter, Spont. AB = spontaneous abortion, CI = confidence interval.

From Dickey RP, Gasser R, Olar TT, et al: Hum Reprod 1994; 9(3):559–565. Used by permission.

Table 4 ▪ Spontaneous Abortion Rates Versus Crown-Rump Lengths Determined After 42 Menstrual Days

AGE GROUP CRL CENTILE	NUMBER IN CENTILE	SPONT. AB NO.	SPONT. AB %	95% CI OF PERCENT
Maternal age < 35 years				
≤10th	131	26	19.8	13.0–26.6
<50th	292	41	14.0	10.0–18.0
≥75th	281	7	2.5	0.7–10.6
≥90th	113	4	6.2	1.8–10.6
Maternal age > 35 years				
≤10th	33	20	60.6	43.9–77.3
<50th	78	31	39.7	28.8–50.5
≥75th	82	5	6.1	0.9–11.3
≥90th	35	1	2.8	0.0–8.3
All maternal ages				
≤10th	164	46	28.0	21.1–34.8
<50th	370	72	19.4	15.4–23.4
≥75th	363	12	3.3	1.5–5.1
≥90th	148	5	3.4	0.5–5.8

CRL = crown-rump length, Spont. AB = spontaneous abortion, CI = confidence interval.

From Dickey RP, Gasser RF, Olar TT, et al: Hum Reprod 1994; 9:366–373. Used by permission.

tion ages were known because of in vitro fertilization (IVF) or gamete intrafallopian transfer (GIFT), was used to establish norms for MSD.[2] A subset of 74 patients (201 scans) who delivered after 28 weeks, with exact postovulation ages from IVF or GIFT, was used to establish norms for CRL.[3]

Comments ▪

Dickey's normative and predictive data on MSD and CRL are very useful when the gestational/menstrual age is known.[2, 3] Otherwise, the MSD − CRL can be used, and several workers have cited a cut-off of 5.0 mm for this value. Rowling and group found a survival rate of at least 35% in 17 cases in which the MSD − CRL was less than 5 mm.[1] This finding is contrasted with Bromley's report that 94% of such cases resulted in spontaneous abortion.[4] In an earlier study, Dickey and group found fetal death rates of 80% when MSD − CRL was < 5 mm, 26.5% when it was 5.0 to 7.9 mm, and 10.6% when it was 8 mm or more.[5] Dickey has concluded that it is the small sac size that is significant relative to outcome when considering the MSD-CRL relationship. MSD − CRL does not work well after 9 to 10 weeks, as it decreases (Figure 1) when the

CRL growth accelerates relative to MSD (perhaps related to increased placental flow).[6] Therefore, though a small sac is certainly associated with an increased rate of subsequent spontaneous abortion, follow-up scanning is useful in questionable cases.

REFERENCES

1. Rowling SE, Coleman BG, Langer JE, et al: First-trimester US parameters of failed pregnancy. Radiology 1997; 203:211–217.
2. Dickey RP, Gasser R, Olar TT, et al: Relationship of initial chorionic sac diameter to abortion and abortus karyotype based on new growth curves for the 16th to 49th post-ovulation day. Hum Reprod 1994; 9(3):559–565.
3. Dickey RP, Gasser RF, Olar TT, et al: The relationship of initial crown-rump length to pregnancy outcome and abortus karyotype based on new growth curves for the 2–31 mm embryo. Hum Reprod 1994; 9:366–373.
4. Bromley B, Harlow BL, Laboda LA, Benacerraf BR: Small sac size in the first trimester: A predictor of poor fetal outcome. Radiology 1991; 178:375–377.
5. Dickey RP, Olar TT, Taylor SN, et al: Relationship of small gestational sac–crown-rump length differences to abortion and abortus karyotypes. Obstet Gynecol 1992; 79(4):554–557.
6. Dickey RP: Personal communication, 1999.

▪▪ YOLK SAC SIZE IN NORMAL PREGNANCY
▪ ACR Code: 856 (Early Pregnancy)

Technique ▪

Transvaginal ultrasound of the gravid uterus with ESI 1000 or 2000 (Elscint, Haifa, Israel) or Sonoline 2 (Siemens, Erlangen, Germany) scanners and 6.5- to 7.5-MHz probes.[1]

Measurements ▪

From frozen images, the yolk sac diameter (YSD) was measured with electronic calipers. Likewise, the gestational

sac was measured in three planes, and these measurements were summed and divided by 3 to obtain the mean sac diameter (MSD). The crown-rump length (CRL) was measured from an image through the embryo in the sagittal plane.[1] Figure 1 shows these measurements. Table 1 lists YSD versus menstrual age (MA), Table 2 lists YSD versus CRL, and Table 3 lists YSD versus MSD (all in the normal group). Table 4 gives regression equations for normal YSD versus MA, CRL, and MSD.

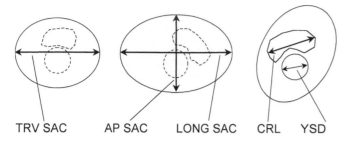

TRV SAC   LONG SAC   LONG EM/FET

TRV SAC   AP SAC   LONG SAC   CRL   YSD

Figure 1 ▪ Measurements from transvaginal ultrasound of the gravid uterus. Gestational sac diameters were measured from transverse *(TRV SAC)* and longitudinal *(LONG SAC)* images. From images through the long axis of the embryo/fetus *(LONG EM/FET)*, the crown-rump length *(CRL)* was measured. The yolk sac diameter *(YSD)* was measured as shown (though it can be measured in other planes as it is almost spherical).

Source ▪

The total study population numbered 486, including 327 women with normal singleton pregnancies of which 281 progressed into the late 3rd trimester and 46 had elective termination before 20 weeks. There were also 159 patients who had abnormal pregnancy outcomes (first-trimester demise or demonstrable fetal abnormality).[1]

Comments ▪

The relationship of YSD and MSD showed the best promise in predicting abnormal pregnancy outcome. Based on the MSD table, YSD >2 standard deviations (SD) above the mean was 16% sensitive and 97% specific, YSD <2 SD below the mean was 16% sensitive and 95% specific, and YSD >2 SD above or <2 SD below the mean had sensitivity of 27% and specificity of 93% in predicting abnormal outcome.[1] The previously described finding that an absent yolk sac with MSD >8 mm is always abnormal

Table 1 ▪ Normal Values for Yolk Sac Diameter Versus Menstrual Age

| MA (days) | YS DIAMETER (mm) | |
	Mean	95% CI
31	0.4	0–2.0
32	0.7	0–2.2
33	1.0	0–2.5
34	1.2	0–2.7
35	1.4	0–2.9
36	1.6	0.1–3.1
37	1.7	0.2–3.2
38	1.9	0.4–3.4
39	2.0	0.5–3.6
40	2.2	0.7–3.7
41	2.3	0.8–3.8
42	2.4	0.9–3.9
43	2.5	1.0–4.0
44	2.6	1.1–4.1
45	2.7	1.2–4.2
46	2.7	1.2–4.2
47	2.8	1.3–4.3
48	2.8	1.3–4.3
49	2.9	1.4–4.4
50	2.9	1.4–4.4
51	3.0	1.5–4.5
52	3.0	1.5–4.5
53	3.0	1.5–4.5
54	3.1	1.6–4.6
55	3.1	1.6–4.6
56	3.1	1.6–4.6
57	3.2	1.7–4.7
58	3.2	1.7–4.7
59	3.2	1.7–4.7
60	3.3	1.8–4.8
61	3.3	1.8–4.8
62	3.4	1.8–4.9
63	3.4	1.9–4.9
64	3.5	1.9–5.0
65	3.5	2.0–5.0
66	3.6	2.1–5.1
67	3.7	2.1–5.2
68	3.8	2.2–5.3

MA = menstrual age; YS = yolk sac; CI = confidence interval.
From Lindsay DJ, Lovett IS, Lyons EA, et al: Radiology 1992; 183(1):115–118. Used by permission.

Table 2 ▪ Normal Values for Yolk Sac Diameter Versus Crown-Rump Length

| CRL (mm) | YS DIAMETER (mm) | |
	Mean	95% CI
0	2.1	0.0–3.8
1	2.2	0.6–3.9
2	2.3	0.6–3.9
3	2.4	0.7–4.0
4	2.4	0.8–4.1
5	2.5	0.9–4.2
6	2.6	0.9–4.2
7	2.7	1.0–4.3
8	2.7	1.1–4.4
9	2.8	1.2–4.5
10	2.9	1.2–4.5
11	3.0	1.3–4.6
12	3.0	1.4–4.7
13	3.1	1.5–4.8
14	3.2	1.5–4.8
15	3.3	1.6–4.9
16	3.3	1.7–5.0
17	3.4	1.8–5.1
18	3.5	1.8–5.1
19	3.6	1.9–5.2
20	3.6	2.0–5.3
21	3.7	2.0–5.4
22	3.8	2.1–5.4
23	3.9	2.2–5.5
24	3.9	2.3–5.6
25	4.0	2.3–5.7

CRL = crown-rump length, YS = yolk sac, CI = confidence interval.
From Lindsay DJ, Lovett IS, Lyons EA, et al: Radiology 1992; 183(1):115–118. Used by permission.

Table 3 ▪ Normal Values for Yolk Sac Diameter Versus Mean Sac Diameter

MSD (mm)	YS DIAMETER (mm)	
	Mean	95% CI
2	0.4	0–1.8
3	0.6	0–2.1
4	0.9	0–2.4
5	1.2	0–2.7
6	1.5	0–2.9
7	1.7	0.3–3.2
8	1.9	0.5–3.4
9	2.1	0.7–3.6
10	2.3	0.8–3.7
11	2.4	1.0–3.9
12	2.6	1.1–4.0
13	2.7	1.2–4.1
14	2.8	1.3–4.2
15	2.8	1.4–4.3
16	2.9	1.5–4.3
17	3.0	1.5–4.4
18	3.0	1.6–4.4
19	3.0	1.6–4.5
20	3.1	1.6–4.5
21	3.1	1.6–4.5
22	3.1	1.6–4.5
23	3.1	1.6–4.5
24	3.1	1.6–4.5
25	3.1	1.6–4.5
26	3.1	1.6–4.5
27	3.1	1.6–4.5
28	3.1	1.6–4.5
29	3.1	1.6–4.5
30	3.1	1.7–4.6
31	3.1	1.7–4.6
32	3.1	1.7–4.6
33	3.2	1.7–4.6
34	3.2	1.8–4.7
35	3.3	1.8–4.7
36	3.3	1.9–4.8
37	3.4	1.9–4.9
38	3.5	2.0–5.0
39	3.6	2.1–5.1
40	3.7	2.2–5.2
41	3.9	2.3–5.4
42	4.1	2.5–5.6
43	4.2	2.6–5.8
44	4.4	2.7–6.0
45	4.5	2.8–6.1

MSD = mean sac diameter, YS = yolk sac, CI = confidence interval.
From Lindsay DJ, Lovett IS, Lyons EA, et al: Radiology 1992; 183(1):115–118. Used by permission.

Table 4 ▪ Regression Equations for Yolk Sac Diameter

PARAMETERS	EQUATION	r VALUE
YSD vs. MA	$-21.1 + 1.256 (MA) - 0.02 (MA)^2 + 0.0001 (MA)^3$	0.387
YSD vs. CRL	$2.127 + 0.075 (CRL)$	0.253
YSD vs. MSD	$-0.47 + 0.418 (MSD) - 0.016 (MSD)^2 + 0.0002 (MSD)^3$	0.435

YSD = yolk sac diameter, MA = menstrual age, CRL = crown-rump length, MSD = mean sac diameter.[1]

was confirmed.[2] Also, a YSD of >5.6 mm in a pregnancy of less than 10 weeks (menstrual age) and visualization of an embryo without demonstration of the yolk sac were always abnormal.[1]

Note: Others have determined that the yolk sac may be invisible at MSD up to 18 mm[3] and 19 mm[4] in pregnancies that progress normally. Rowling and colleagues found 30 cases of normal pregnancy in which the yolk sac was not seen when the MSD was 8 to 19 mm; they believed that an MSD of 20 mm was a better discriminatory value.[4]

REFERENCES

1. Lindsay DJ, Lovett IS, Lyons EA, et al: Yolk sac diameter and shape at endovaginal US: Predictors of pregnancy outcome in the first trimester. Radiology 1992; 183(1):115–118.
2. Levi CS, Lyons EA, Lindsay DJ: Early diagnosis of nonviable pregnancy with endovaginal US. Radiology 1988; 167:383–385.
3. Kurtz AB, Needleman L, Pennell RG, et al: Can detection of the yolk sac in the first trimester be used to predict the outcome of pregnancy? AJR Am J Roentgenol 1992; 158:843–847.
4. Rowling SE, Coleman BG, Langer JE, et al: First-trimester US parameters of failed pregnancy. Radiology 1997; 203:211–217.

": HEART RATE IN EARLY PREGNANCY
■ ACR Code: 856 (Early Pregnancy)

Technique ■

Vaginal sonography of the gravid uterus was done with a 128 10XP machine (Acuson, Mountain View, CA) and a 5.0-MHz probe. Gray scale imaging was used for measurements and to visualize cardiac activity. M-mode scanning over the site was then done to determine heart rate in beats per minute (bpm).[1, 2]

Measurements ■

The presence or absence of visible and/or M-mode cardiac activity was noted. If seen, heart rate (HR) was calculated from frozen M-mode tracings by means of electronic calipers and software built into the machine.[1, 2] The mean gestational sac diameter (MSD) and embryonic/fetal crown-rump length (CRL) were measured from frozen images with electronic calipers.[2] Table 1 lists the results, including number with positive cardiac activity/number scanned, measured heart rates, CRL, and MSD.[1, 2]

Source ■

A total of 426 1st-trimester examinations was done between 24 and 56 menstrual days. All pregnancies resulted from assisted reproductive procedures, and the menstrual age (MA) was calculated by normalizing day 14 as the day of ovulation. Pregnancies were included only if follow-up beyond the first trimester revealed normal gestations.[1] A second series included 235 well-dated singleton pregnancies evaluated with ultrasound (n = 361) during the 1st trimester. All these pregnancies had successful outcomes.[2]

Table 1 ■ Heart Rate, Crown-Rump Length, and Mean Sac Diameter in Early Pregnancy

MA (days)	NUMBER CA/NE (%)	MSD (mm) (Mean ± SD)	CRL (mm) (Mean ± SD)	HEART RATE (Mean ± SD)	HEART RATE (Range)
<34	0/65 (0)	—	—	—	—
34	2/13 (15)	8 ± 0.1	1.6 ± 0.2	94 ± 5	89–99
35	8/28 (29)	10 ± 4	1.9 ± 0.4	93 ± 15	79–126
36	16/19 (82)	8 ± 2	2.1 ± 0.7	99 ± 8	77–113
37	9/9 (100)	9 ± 2	2.2 ± 0.8	97 ± 9	86–110
38	10	11 ± 3	2.6 ± 0.8	98 ± 6	85–108
39	9	12 ± 2	2.6 ± 0.5	104 ± 9	90–120
40	14	13 ± 4	3.2 ± 0.6	107 ± 7	97–118
41	23	14 ± 8	3.4 ± 1.2	109 ± 13	83–135
42	30	13 ± 4	4.0 ± 1.2	111 ± 11	90–131
43	23	12 ± 4	3.9 ± 1.2	118 ± 12	89–143
44	24	15 ± 3	5.0 ± 1.7	121 ± 8	108–135
45	29	16 ± 4	5.5 ± 2.0	123 ± 9	108–151
46	24	16 ± 5	6.2 ± 2.1	130 ± 8	111–147
47	18	17 ± 5	6.4 ± 2.0	128 ± 15	104–164
48	23	18 ± 4	8.2 ± 1.8	134 ± 8	118–148
49	17	20 ± 6	9.1 ± 1.4	148 ± 16	123–185
50	10	22 ± 5	9.5 ± 1.3	145 ± 20	118–182
51	13	20 ± 7	9.6 ± 1.9	144 ± 12	126–164
52	17	21 ± 5	9.9 ± 1.9	152 ± 13	118–169
53	11	24 ± 5	12.8 ± 3.8	154 ± 14	126–175
54	8	23 ± 3	14.7 ± 2.7	158 ± 12	132–175
55	8	29 ± 3	15.3 ± 2.0	163 ± 10	147–181
56	15	27 ± 7	14.0 ± 2.0	166 ± 13	139–181

MA = menstrual age, MSD = mean sac diameter, CRL = crown-rump length, SD = standard deviation, CA/NE (%) = number with cardiac activity/number examined (percent). After 36 days, cardiac activity was always seen.

From Coulam CB, Britten S, Soenksen DM: Hum Reprod 1996; 11(8):1771–1774. Used by permission.

Comments ▪

Measurable cardiac activity was always present after 36 menstrual days. The fetal HR increased linearly with MA, MSD, and CRL as follows:

$$HR \text{ (bpm)} = 3.591 \times MA \text{ (days)} + 36.25 \text{ (r} = 0.857)[1]$$

$$HR \text{ (bpm)} = 2.6 \times MSD \text{ (mm)} + 82 \text{ (r} = 0.73)[2]$$

$$HR \text{ (bpm)} = 4.6 \times CRL \text{ (mm)} + 96 \text{ (r} = 0.85)[2]$$

To be normal, gestations with MSD of 20 mm and 30 mm should contain embryos with a CRL of at least 2 mm and 5 mm, having an HR of at least 75 bpm and 100 bpm, respectively. Embryos with a CRL of 2 mm, 5 mm, 10 mm, and 15 mm should display an HR of at least 75 bpm, 100 bpm, 120 bpm, and 130 bpm, respectively.[2] If gestational age is known, the HR norms on Table 1 may be used directly. If accurate dating is not available, the MSD/CRL columns in Table 1 can be used to find the expected HR and to estimate menstrual age.

Stefos and colleagues studied 2164 singleton pregnancies and found an HR (mean ± SD) of 111 ± 14 from 42 to 45 days, 125 ± 15 from 46 to 49 days, 145 ± 14 from 50 to 52 days, and 157 ± 13 from 53 to 56 days. Embryos with heart rates below 85 bpm measured during 6 to 8 weeks did not survive.[3] Merchiers and colleagues studied 170 pregnancies and found that the combination of HR <100 bpm and declining HR between weeks 5 and 10 had a sensitivity of 98%, specificity of 83%, positive predictive value (PPV) of 77%, and negative predictive value (NPV) of 99% for subsequent embryonic death.[4] A single determination of HR at 7 weeks being <100 bpm was 88% sensitive and 88% specific for prediction of embryonic loss. Likewise, HR <80 bpm at 7 weeks had sensitivity of 71% and specificity of 98%.[4]

REFERENCES

1. Britton S, Soenksen DM, Bustillo M, Coulam CB: Very early (24–56 days from the LMP) embryonic heart rate in normal pregnancies. Hum Reprod 1994; 9:2424–2426.
2. Coulam CB, Britten S, Soenksen DM: Early (34–56 days from last menstrual period) ultrasonographic measurements in normal pregnancies. Hum Reprod 1996; 11(8):1771–1774.
3. Stefos TI, Lolis DE, Sotiriadis AJ, Ziakas GV: Embryonic heart rate in early pregnancy. J Clin Ultrasound 1998; 26:33–36.
4. Merchiers EH, Dhont M, DeSutter PA, et al: Predictive value of early embryonic cardiac activity for pregnancy outcome. Am J Obstet Gynecol 1991; 165:11–14.

▪▪ GESTATIONAL AGE DETERMINATION BY SAC SIZE AT TRANSVAGINAL SONOGRAPHY
▪ ACR Code: 856 (Biometry)

Technique ▪

Transvaginal ultrasound of the gravid uterus was done with an SSD-650 unit (Aloka) and a 5-MHz vaginal probe.[1]

Measurements ▪

Three orthogonal measurements of the gestational sac (in millimeters) were made from frozen images with electronic calipers and averaged to form the mean sac diameter (MSD) (Figure 1). The gestational age (GA) was determined by counting from the first day of the last menstrual period (LMP) and by comparison of serial beta-human chorionic gonadotropin (βhCG) determination with a locally developed normal curve. The difference between these two methods of GA determination was 0.44 ± 0.43 days (mean ± SD). Regression analysis of GA versus MSD was done and yielded the following relationships:

$$GA \text{ by LMP (days)} = 0.821 \text{ (MSD)} + 35.081.$$

$$GA \text{ by serial } \beta hCG = 0.882 \text{ (MSD)} + 33.117.$$

Figure 1 ▪ Measurement of gestational sac diameter from transvaginal ultrasound. Anteroposterior *(AP)* and longitudinal *(LON)* dimensions of the sac are determined from a longitudinal image through the uterus. The transverse *(TRV)* dimension of the sac is measured from a transverse image through the uterus. Mean sac diameter *(MSD)* is the average of these three measurements, as shown.

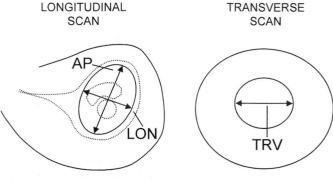

$$MSD = \frac{LON + AP + TRV}{3}$$

Table 1 ▪ Mean Gestational Sac Diameter and Corresponding
Estimate of Gestational Age

MSD (mm)	WEEKS	DAYS	95% PI
2	5.0	34.9	31.6–38.2
3	5.1	35.8	32.5–39.1
4	5.2	36.6	33.3–39.9
5	5.4	37.5	34.2–40.8
6	5.5	38.4	35.1–41.7
7	5.6	39.3	36.0–42.6
8	5.7	40.2	36.9–43.5
9	5.9	41.1	37.8–44.3
10	6.0	41.9	38.7–45.2
11	6.1	42.8	39.5–46.1
12	6.2	43.7	40.4–47.0
13	6.4	44.6	41.3–47.9
14	6.5	45.5	42.2–48.7
15	6.6	46.3	43.1–49.6
16	6.7	47.2	44.0–50.5
17	6.9	48.1	44.8–51.4
18	7.0	49.0	45.7–52.3
19	7.1	49.9	46.6–53.2
20	7.3	50.8	47.5–54.0
21	7.4	51.6	48.3–54.9
22	7.5	52.5	49.2–55.8
23	7.6	53.4	50.1–56.7
24	7.8	54.3	51.0–57.6
25	7.9	55.2	51.9–58.5
26	8.0	56.0	52.7–59.4
27	8.1	56.9	53.6–60.3
28	8.3	57.8	54.5–61.1
29	8.4	58.7	55.4–62.0
30	8.5	59.6	56.2–62.9

MSD = mean sac diameter; 95% PI = 95 percent prediction interval (days).
From Daya S, Woods S, Ward S, et al: J Can Med Assoc 1991; 144:441–446.
Used by permission.

Table 1 lists GA predictions based on the second formula. The variability between GA predicted by MSD from Table 1 and actual GA was 1 day (mean = 0.2 ± 0.6 days).[1]

Source ▪

Subjects were 20 women with normal singleton pregnancies that progressed beyond 20 weeks. Transvaginal ultrasound was done every 1 to 2 weeks through 8 weeks, and serial βhCG determination was done every 2 to 7 days through 60 days.[1]

Reference

1. Daya S, Woods S, Ward S, et al: Early pregnancy assessment with transvaginal ultrasound scanning. J Can Med Assoc 1991; 144:441–446.

▪: CROWN-RUMP LENGTH FOR DETERMINATION OF GESTATIONAL AGE
▪ ACR Code: 856 (Biometry)

Technique ▪

Ultrasound of the gravid uterus was done using a variety of machines and vaginal probes. For the most part, transvaginal scanning was done during the first trimester and transabdominal thereafter.[1–3]

Measurements ▪

The crown-rump length (CRL) of the embryo/fetus was measured from frozen images through its long axis. The measurement was made from the cephalic to the caudal ends of the embryonic pole or from the vertex to the distal sacrum/buttocks in fetuses.[1–3] Data analysis included linear regression,[1] polynomial regression,[2] and logarithmic regression.[3] Table 1 lists the regression equations reported from each study. Figure 1 shows plots of predicted gestational age (GA) calculated from each equation for CRL from 0 to 12 cm.[1–3] Note how the linear and quadratic prediction lines bend away from the logarithmic quaternary prediction near the stated upper limits for CRL of each model (2.5 cm for linear and 8.0 cm for quadratic). Table 2 lists the predicted GA (in menstrual days) for each model as reported.[1–3]

A note about terminology: Goldstein and coworker and Daya used the term *gestational age* whereas Hadlock used the term *menstrual age*. Though the term gestational age is

Table 1 ▪ Equations for Gestational Age Prediction Using Crown-Rump Length

STUDY	USEFUL CRL RANGE (mm)	EQUATION UNITS	EQUATION	CORRELATION (95% CI)
Goldstein	1–25	GA = days CRL = mm	GA = 42 + CRL	r = 0.87 ±3 days
Daya	2–80	GA = days CRL = mm	GA = 40.447 + 1.125 (CRL) − 0.0058 (CRL)^2	r = 0.99 ±5 days
Hadlock	20–120	MA = weeks CRL = cm	ln(MA) = 1.684969 + 0.315646 (CRL) − 0.049306 (CRL)^2 　　+ 0.004057 (CRL)^3 − 0.000120456 (CRL)^4	r = 0.99 ±8%
Proposed linear	25–120	GA = days CRL = mm	GA = 51 + 0.6 (CRL)	0.99 —

GA = gestational age, CRL = crown-rump length, MA = menstrual age, ln = logarithm (natural), CI = confidence interval.[1-3]

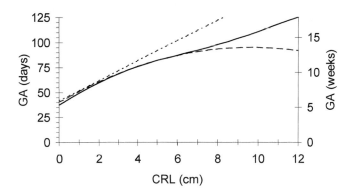

Figure 1 ▪ Predicted gestational age *(GA)* by crown-rump length *(CRL)*, using Goldstein's linear *(dotted)*, Daya's quadratic *(dashed)*, and Hadlock's logarithmic quaternary *(solid)* equations.

Table 2 ▪ Predicted Gestational Age by Crown-Rump Length

CRL	DAYS	CRL	DAYS	CRL	DAYS	CRL	DAYS
1	-/-/43	31	70/70/-	61	88/87/-	91	105/-/-
2	40/43/44	32	71/71/-	62	88/88/-	92	106/-/-
3	41/44/45	33	71/71/-	63	89/88/-	93	106/-/-
4	43/45/46	34	72/72/-	64	90/89/-	94	107/-/-
5	43/46/47	35	73/73/-	65	90/89/-	95	107/-/-
6	45/47/48	36	74/73/-	66	90/89/-	96	108/-/-
7	46/48/49	37	74/74/-	67	91/90/-	97	109/-/-
8	47/49/50	38	75/75/-	68	92/90/-	98	109/-/-
9	48/50/51	39	76/75/-	69	92/90/-	99	110/-/-
10	50/51/52	40	76/76/-	70	92/91/-	100	111/-/-
11	50/52/53	41	77/77/-	71	93/91/-	101	112/-/-
12	52/53/54	42	78/77/-	72	94/91/-	102	113/-/-
13	53/54/55	43	78/78/-	73	94/92/-	103	113/-/-
14	54/55/56	44	78/79/-	74	95/92/-	104	114/-/-
15	55/56/57	45	79/79/-	75	95/92/-	105	115/-/-
16	56/57/58	46	80/80/-	76	96/92/-	106	116/-/-
17	57/58/59	47	81/80/-	77	97/93/-	107	116/-/-
18	58/59/60	48	81/81/-	78	97/93/-	108	117/-/-
19	59/60/61	49	82/82/-	79	97/93/-	109	118/-/-
20	60/61/62	50	82/82/-	80	98/93/-	110	118/-/-
21	61/62/63	51	83/83/-	81	99/-/-	111	119/-/-
22	62/62/64	52	83/83/-	82	99/-/-	112	120/-/-
23	63/63/65	53	84/84/-	83	99/-/-	113	120/-/-
24	64/64/66	54	84/84/-	84	100/-/-	114	121/-/-
25	64/65/67	55	85/85/-	85	101/-/-	115	122/-/-
26	66/66/-	56	85/85/-	86	102/-/-	116	123/-/-
27	67/67/-	57	86/86/-	87	102/-/-	117	123/-/-
28	67/67/-	58	86/86/-	88	103/-/-	118	124/-/-
29	68/68/-	59	87/87/-	89	104/-/-	119	125/-/-
30	69/69/-	60	88/87/-	90	104/-/-	120	125/-/-

Days = Hadlock / Daya / Goldstein; CRL = crown-rump length in millimeters.

sometimes used to denote time since conception, in this setting it was used synonymously with menstrual age and we have used the abbreviation GA.

Source ■

Goldstein and Wolfson studied 143 pregnant women having normal, well-dated by last menstrual period (LMP), singleton pregnancies during the first trimester.[1] Daya's subjects included 94 infertile women who had successful in vitro fertilization (singleton) and ultrasounds in the first trimester. Dates were established by setting the day of oocyte retrieval as day 14 so as to correspond with menstrual age.[2] Hadlock and colleagues evaluated obstetric ultrasounds of normal singleton pregnancies done from 5 to 20 weeks. The women all had regular menses, knew the day of their LMP, and had not taken birth control pills for 3 months prior.[3]

Comments ■

The simplest linear prediction: GA (days) = CRL (mm) + 42, can be remembered as a "rule of thumb," though it is accurate only through a CRL of 25 mm.[1] Daya found no significant improvement in predictive power for cubic or quaternary models over a quadratic function through a CRL of 8.0 cm, whereas Hadlock's logarithmic quaternary model remained accurate through 12.0 cm.[2,3] Hadlock and colleagues found CRL to be equivalent in accuracy with biparietal diameter from 14 to 18 weeks using their model.[3] We noted that Hadlock's GA versus CRL data seemed roughly linear above 25 mm and calculated a linear equation for this interval (bottom row in Table 1). Figure 2

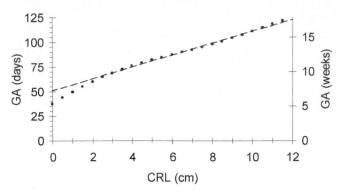

Figure 2 ■ Proposed linear prediction (*dashed line*) for gestational age (*GA*) by crown-rump length (*CRL*), compared with Hadlock's log quaternary prediction equation (*circles*).

compares this linear model with Hadlock's logarithmic quaternary equation and shows it to be quite closely superimposed. A second linear equation above 2.5 cm would be useful as it is rather easier to compute, though we do not know of any studies to support its use.

References

1. Goldstein SR, Wolfson R: Endovaginal ultrasonographic measurement of early embryonic size as a means of assessing gestational age. J Ultrasound Med 1994; 13(1):27–31.
2. Daya S: Accuracy of gestational age estimation by means of fetal crown-rump length measurement. Am J Obstet Gynecol 1993; 168:903–908.
3. Hadlock FP, Shah YP, Kanon DJ, Lindsey JV: Fetal crown-rump length: Reevaluation of the relation to menstrual age (5–18 weeks) with high resolution real-time ultrasound. Radiology 1992; 182:501–505.

⠶ STANDARD FETAL BIOMETRY
■ ACR Code: 856 (Fetal Biometry)

Technique ■

Ultrasound of the gravid uterus was done transabdominally with 3.5-MHz real-time linear transducers.[1–4]

Measurements ■

The biparietal diameter (BPD) and head circumference (HC) were measured from hard copy images with calipers and a hand-held map measurer, respectively.[1,2] The abdominal circumference (AC) was measured from hard copy images with a hand-held map measurer.[3] The femur length (FL) was measured from frozen images using electronic calipers.[4] Figure 1 illustrates the measurements. Mean values of each measurement and the standard deviations (SD) were calculated for each menstrual week. Mathematical modeling with linear, linear-quadratic, and linear-cubic models was done for menstrual age (MA) versus measured parameters. The optimal model was chosen based on coefficient of determination (r squared), the variances of the estimates of regression coefficients, and the distribution of residuals.[1–4] The experimental data were grouped by menstrual weeks (five groups for BPD, HC, and AC and two groups for FL) for purposes of calculating variability

(SD of MA about the regression line) associated with the model as pregnancy progressed.[1–4]

Tables 1 through 4 list the predicted menstrual age for each measured parameter. Table 5 lists the best-fit regression equations. Table 6 lists the estimated variability of prediction at various MA ranges.[1–4]

Source ■

Hadlock and colleagues studied well-dated normal singleton pregnancies, including 533 from 12 to 40 weeks for BPD, 400 from 15 to 41 weeks for HC, 400 from 15 to 41 weeks for AC, and 338 from 12 to 40 weeks for FL.[1–4]

Comments ■

Though there have certainly been many studies published since the ones contained herein, they continue to be very commonly quoted and widely used. In another section we detail an additional study by Hadlock and colleagues concerning estimation of fetal age from multiple biometric parameters obtained at ultrasound. If perimeter tracing or other method of circumference measurement is not available, the HC may be estimated by π/2 × (OFD + BPD). Likewise, the abdominal circumference may be estimated

Text continued on page 546

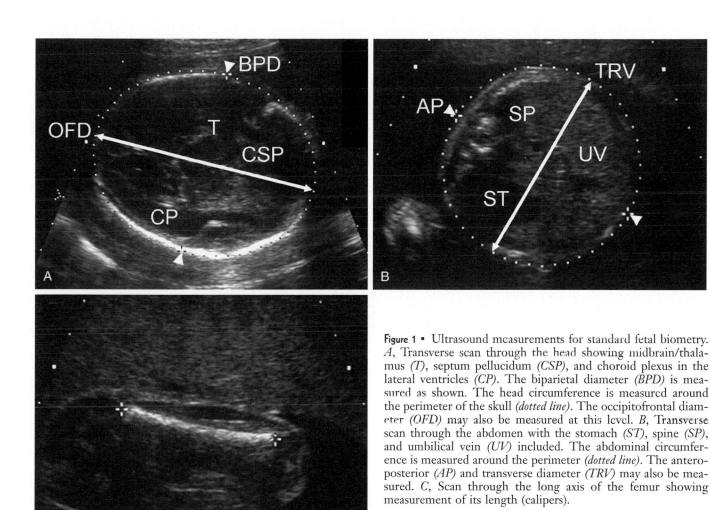

Figure 1 ▪ Ultrasound measurements for standard fetal biometry. *A,* Transverse scan through the head showing midbrain/thalamus *(T),* septum pellucidum *(CSP),* and choroid plexus in the lateral ventricles *(CP).* The biparietal diameter *(BPD)* is measured as shown. The head circumference is measured around the perimeter of the skull *(dotted line).* The occipitofrontal diameter *(OFD)* may also be measured at this level. *B,* Transverse scan through the abdomen with the stomach *(ST),* spine *(SP),* and umbilical vein *(UV)* included. The abdominal circumference is measured around the perimeter *(dotted line).* The anteroposterior *(AP)* and transverse diameter *(TRV)* may also be measured. *C,* Scan through the long axis of the femur showing measurement of its length (calipers).

Table 1 ▪ Predicted Menstrual Ages for Biparietal Diameter from 2.0 to 10.0 Cm

BPD (cm)	MA (wk)	BPD (cm)	MA (wk)
2.0	12.2	6.1	25.0
2.1	12.5	6.2	25.3
2.2	12.8	6.3	25.7
2.3	13.1	6.4	26.1
2.4	13.3	6.5	26.4
2.5	13.6	6.6	26.8
2.6	13.9	6.7	27.2
2.7	14.2	6.8	27.6
2.8	14.5	6.9	28.0
2.9	14.7	7.0	28.3
3.0	15.0	7.1	28.7
3.1	15.3	7.2	29.1
3.2	15.6	7.3	29.5
3.3	15.9	7.4	29.9
3.4	16.2	7.5	30.4
3.5	16.5	7.6	30.8
3.6	16.8	7.7	31.2
3.7	17.1	7.8	31.6
3.8	17.4	7.9	32.0
3.9	17.7	8.0	32.5
4.0	18.0	8.1	32.9
4.1	18.3	8.2	33.3
4.2	18.6	8.3	33.8
4.3	18.9	8.4	34.2
4.4	19.2	8.5	34.7
4.5	19.5	8.6	35.1
4.6	19.9	8.7	35.6
4.7	20.2	8.8	36.1
4.8	20.5	8.9	36.5
4.9	20.8	9.0	37.0
5.0	21.2	9.1	37.5
5.1	21.5	9.2	38.0
5.2	21.8	9.3	38.5
5.3	22.2	9.4	38.9
5.4	22.5	9.5	39.4
5.5	22.8	9.6	39.9
5.6	23.2	9.7	40.5
5.7	23.5	9.8	41.0
5.8	23.9	9.9	41.5
5.9	24.2	10.0	42.0
6.0	24.6		

BPD = biparietal diameter, MA = menstrual age.
From Hadlock FP, Deter RL, Harrist RB, et al: J Ultrasound Med 1982; 1:97–104. Used by permission.

Table 2 ▪ Predicted Menstrual Ages for Head Circumference from 8.0 to 36.0 Cm

HC (cm)	MA (wk)	HC (cm)	MA (wk)
8.0	13.4	22.5	24.4
8.5	13.7	23.0	24.9
9.0	14.0	23.5	25.4
9.5	14.3	24.0	25.9
10.0	14.6	24.5	26.4
10.5	15.0	25.0	26.9
11.0	15.3	25.5	27.5
11.5	15.6	26.0	28.0
12.0	15.9	26.5	28.1
12.5	16.3	27.0	29.2
13.0	16.6	27.5	29.8
13.5	17.0	28.0	30.3
14.0	17.3	28.5	31.0
14.5	17.7	29.0	31.6
15.0	18.1	29.5	32.2
15.5	18.4	30.0	32.8
16.0	18.8	30.5	33.5
16.5	19.2	31.0	34.2
17.0	19.6	31.5	34.9
17.5	20.0	32.0	35.5
18.0	20.4	32.5	36.3
18.5	20.8	33.0	37.0
19.0	21.2	33.5	37.7
19.5	21.6	34.0	38.5
20.0	22.1	34.5	39.2
20.5	22.5	35.0	40.0
21.0	23.0	35.5	40.8
21.5	23.4	36.0	41.6
22.0	23.9		

HC = head circumference, MA = menstrual age.
From Hadlock FP, Deter RL, Harrist RB, Park SK: AJR Am J Roentgenol 1982; 138:649–653. Used by permission.

Table 3 ▪ Predicted Menstrual Ages for Abdominal Circumference
from 10.0 to 36.5 Cm

AC (cm)	MA (wk)	AC (cm)	MA (wk)
10.0	15.6	23.5	27.7
10.5	16.1	24.0	28.2
11.0	16.5	24.5	28.7
11.5	16.9	25.0	29.2
12.0	17.3	25.5	29.7
12.5	17.8	26.0	30.1
13.0	18.2	26.5	30.6
13.5	18.6	27.0	31.1
14.0	19.1	27.5	31.6
14.5	19.5	28.0	32.1
15.0	20.0	28.5	32.6
15.5	20.4	29.0	33.1
16.0	20.8	29.5	33.6
16.5	21.3	30.0	34.1
17.0	21.7	30.5	34.6
17.5	22.2	31.0	35.1
18.0	22.6	31.5	35.6
18.5	23.1	32.0	36.1
19.0	23.6	32.5	36.6
19.5	24.0	33.0	37.1
20.0	24.5	33.5	37.6
20.5	24.9	34.0	38.1
21.0	25.4	34.5	38.7
21.5	25.9	35.0	39.2
22.0	26.3	35.5	39.7
22.5	26.8	36.0	40.2
23.0	27.3	36.5	40.8

AC = abdominal circumference, MA = menstrual age.
From Hadlock FP, Deter RL, Harrist RB, Park SK: AJR Am J Roentgenol 1982;
139:367–370. Used by permission.

Table 4 ▪ **Predicted Menstrual Ages for Femur Length from 10.0 to 79.0 mm**

FL (mm)	MA (wk)	FL (mm)	MA (wk)
10	12.8	45	24.5
11	13.1	46	24.9
12	13.4	47	25.3
13	13.6	48	25.7
14	13.9	49	26.1
15	14.2	50	26.5
16	14.5	51	27.0
17	14.8	52	27.4
18	15.1	53	27.8
19	15.4	54	28.2
20	15.7	55	28.7
21	16.0	56	29.1
22	16.3	57	29.6
23	16.6	58	30.0
24	16.9	59	30.5
25	17.2	60	30.9
26	17.6	61	31.4
27	17.9	62	31.9
28	18.2	63	32.3
29	18.6	64	32.8
30	18.9	65	33.3
31	19.2	66	33.8
32	19.6	67	34.2
33	19.9	68	34.7
34	20.3	69	35.2
35	20.7	70	35.7
36	21.0	71	36.2
37	21.4	72	36.7
38	21.8	73	37.2
39	22.1	74	37.7
40	22.5	75	38.3
41	22.9	76	38.8
42	23.3	77	39.3
43	23.7	78	39.8
44	24.1	79	40.4

FL = femur length, MA = menstrual age.
From Hadlock FP, Deter RL, Harrist RB, Park SK: AJR Am J Roentgenol 1982; 138:875–878. Used by permission.

Table 5 ▪ Best-Fit Regression Equations for Estimating Menstrual Age from Biometric Parameters

PARAMETER	REGRESSION EQUATION FOR MENSTRUAL AGE	r SQUARED
BPD	MA = 6.8954 + 2.6345 (BPD) + 0.008771 (BPD)^3	.987
HC	MA = 8.8 + 0.55 (HC) + 0.00028 (HC)^3	.979
AC	MA = 7.6070 + 0.7645 (AC) + 0.00393 (AC)^2	.978
FL	MA = 10.38 + 0.2256 (FL) + 0.001948 (FL)^2	.973

MA = menstrual age; parameter abbreviations in text.[1-4]

Table 6 ▪ Variability of Menstrual Age Determination from Fetal Biometry

AGE RANGE (wk)	BPD (±2 SD wk)	HC (±2 SD wk)	AC (±2 SD wk)	FL (±2 SD wk)
12–18	0.8	1.3	1.9	1.3
18–24	1.4	1.6	2.0	1.3
24–30	1.3	2.3	2.2	3.1
30–36	2.0	2.7	3.0	3.1
36–40	3.6	3.4	2.5	3.1

SD = standard deviation; parameter abbreviations in text.[1-4]

by $\pi/2 \times$ (AP + TRV). These linear diameter measurements are also shown in Figure 1.

REFERENCES

1. Hadlock FP, Deter RL, Harrist RB, et al: Fetal biparietal diameter: A critical reevaluation of the relation to menstrual age by means of realtime ultrasound. J Ultrasound Med 1982; 1:97–104.

2. Hadlock FP, Deter RL, Harrist RB, Park SK: Fetal head circumference: Relation to menstrual age. AJR Am J Roentgenol 1982; 138:649–653.

3. Hadlock FP, Deter RL, Harrist RB, Park SK: Fetal abdominal circumference as a predictor of menstrual age. AJR Am J Roentgenol 1982; 139:367–370.

4. Hadlock FP, Deter RL, Harrist RB, Park SK: Fetal femur length as a predictor of menstrual age: Sonographically measured. AJR Am J Roentgenol 1982; 138:875–878.

▪▪ FETAL AGE ESTIMATION WITH MULTIPLE ULTRASOUND PARAMETERS

▪ ACR Code: 856 (Fetal Biometry)

Technique ▪

Ultrasound of the gravid uterus was done transabdominally with 3.5-MHz real-time linear transducers.[1]

Measurements ▪

Biparietal diameter (BPD) and femur length (FL) measurements were made with electronic calipers from appropriate images. Head circumference (HC) and abdominal circumference (AC) were measured either from hard copy images by tracing the perimeter of the skull or abdomen or by means of two axis measurements summed and multiplied by $\pi/2$.[1] Mathematical models for predicting menstrual age from various combinations of these parameters, including linear, quadratic, and cubic terms, were developed by stepwise regression. The efficacy of each equation in estimating menstrual age was assessed by comparing the standard deviation (SD) and r squared. The 361 known menstrual age data points were divided into 6-week intervals, and they assess changes in model output variability with increasing gestational age. Table 1 lists the various regression models developed in the analysis, along with SD, r squared, and error terms. Table 2 lists the prediction variability for each equation at 6-week intervals.[1]

Source ▪

Subjects consisted of 361 middle-class white women with normal singleton pregnancies, a history of regular menses, and unequivocal knowledge of the beginning day of the last menstrual period (LMP). Scans were done from 14 to 42 menstrual weeks.[1]

Comments ▪

The investigators found that combinations of parameters performed better than individual parameter estimates (the best candidates in Table 1 are marked with asterisks) in estimating gestational age. They developed regressions for each parameter as the dependent variable based on known menstrual age (Table 3) and have combined the output of these into a single chart (Table 4). To use this table, simply find the entry matching the measured parameter and record the menstrual age for that row. The menstrual age may be estimated by the simple average of these. Indeed, the researchers found that this method was just as accurate (p <.05) as any of the multiple parameter equations in Table 1.

REFERENCE

1. Hadlock FP, Deter LR, Harrist RB, Park SK: Estimating fetal age: Computer-assisted analysis of multiple fetal growth parameters. Radiology 1984; 152:497–501.

Table 1 ▪ Regression Equations for Predicting Menstrual Age

PARAMETERS USED	REGRESSION EQUATION FOR MENSTRUAL AGE	SD (wk)	MAX ERR (wk)	r SQUARED
BPD	$09.54 + 1.482 \, (BPD) + 0.1676 \, (BPD)^2$	1.36	5.1	.967
HC	$08.96 + 0.540 \, (HC) + 0.0003 \, (HC)^3$	1.23	4.1	.973
AC	$08.14 + 0.753 \, (AC) + 0.0036 \, (AC)^2$	1.31	4.6	.969
FL	$10.35 + 2.460 \, (FL) + 0.170 \, (FL)^2$	1.28	4.9	.971
BPD, AC	$09.57 + 0.524 \, (AC) + 0.1220 \, (BPD)^2$	1.18	3.8	.975
BPD, HC	$10.32 + 0.009 \, (HC)^2 + 1.3200 \, (BPD) + 0.00012 \, (HC)^3$	1.21	3.5	.974
BPD, FL	$10.50 + 0.197 \, (BPD) \, (FL) + 0.9500 \, (FL) + 0.7300 \, (BPD)$	1.10	3.6	.978
HC, AC	$10.31 + 0.012 \, (HC)^2 + 0.3850 \, (AC)$	1.15	4.3	.976
HC, FL*	$11.19 + 0.070 \, (HC) \, (FL) + 0.2630 \, (HC)$	1.04	3.3	.980
AC, FL	$10.47 + 0.442 \, (AC) + 0.3140 \, (FL)^2 - 00121 \, (FL)^3$	1.11	3.8	.978
BPD, AC, FL*	$10.61 + 0.175 \, (BPD) \, (FL) + 0.2970 \, (AC) + 0.7100 \, (FL)$	1.06	3.4	.980
BPD, HC, FL*	$11.38 + 0.070 \, (HC) \, (FL) + 0.9800 \, (BPD)$	1.04	3.2	.981
HC, AC, FL*	$10.33 + 0.031 \, (HC) \, (FL) + 0.3610 \, (HC) + 0.0298 \, (AC) \, (FL)$	1.03	3.4	.981
HC, AC, BPD	$10.58 + 0.005 \, (HC)^2 + 0.3635 \, (AC) + 0.02864 \, (BPD) \, (AC)$	1.14	4.0	.977
BPD, HC, AC, FL*	$10.85 + 0.060 \, (HC) \, (FL) + 0.6700 \, (BPD) + 0.1680 \, (AC)$	1.02	3.2	.981

*Equations that provided the best estimates. SD = standard deviation, Max Err = maximum error; parameter abbreviations given in the text.
From Hadlock FP, Deter LR, Harrist RB, Park SK: Radiology 1984; 152:497–501. Used by permission.

Table 2 ▪ Subgroup Variability in Predicting Menstrual Age, Using Equations in Table 1

PARAMETERS USED	SUBGROUP VARIABILITY (±2 SD)				
	12–18 wk (n = 43)	18–24 wk (n = 69)	24–30 wk (n = 76)	30–36 wk (n = 95)	36–40 wk (n = 78)
BPD	1.19	1.73	2.18	3.08	3.20
HC	1.19	1.48	2.06	2.98	2.70
AC	1.66	2.06	2.18	2.96	3.04
FL	1.38	1.80	2.08	2.96	3.12
BPD, AC	1.26	1.68	1.92	2.60	2.88
BPD, HC	1.08	1.49	1.99	2.86	2.64
BPD, FL	1.12	1.46	1.84	2.60	2.62
HC, AC	1.20	1.52	1.98	2.68	2.52
HC, FL*	1.08	1.34	1.86	2.52	2.28
AC, FL	1.32	1.64	1.88	2.66	2.60
BPD, AC, FL*	1.20	1.52	1.82	2.50	2.52
BPD, HC, FL*	1.04	1.35	1.81	2.52	2.34
HC, AC, FL*	1.14	1.46	1.86	2.52	2.34
HC, AC, BPD	1.21	1.58	1.94	2.60	2.52
BPD, HC, AC, FL*	1.08	1.40	1.80	2.44	2.30

*Equations that provided the best estimates. SD = standard deviation; parameter abbreviations given in text.
From Hadlock FP, Deter LR, Harrist RB, Park SK: Radiology 1984; 152:497–501. Used by permission.

Table 3 ▪ Equations Used to Produce Table 4

PARAMETER	REGRESSION EQUATION FOR PARAMETER	r SQUARED	SD
Biparietal diameter (BPD)	$-3.08 + 0.41 \, (MA) - 0.000061 \, MA^3$	.976	3.0 mm
Head circumference (HC)	$-11.48 + 1.56 \, (MA) - 0.0002548 \, MA^3$	.981	1.0 cm
Abdomen circumference (AC)	$-13.3 + 1.61 \, (MA) - 0.00998 \, MA^2$	.972	1.34 cm
Femur length (FL)	$-3.91 + 0.427 \, (MA) - 0.0034 \, MA^2$	.975	3.0 mm

MA = known menstrual age (by LMP), SD = standard deviation; parameter abbreviations given in text.
From Hadlock FP, Deter LR, Harrist RB, Park SK: Radiology 1984; 152:497–501. Used by permission.

Table 4 ▪ **Predicted Fetal Measurements at Specific Menstrual Ages**

MA	BPD	HC	AC	FL	MA	BPD	HC	AC	FL
12.0	1.7	6.8	4.6	0.7	26.0	6.5	24.6	21.9	4.9
12.5	1.9	7.5	5.3	0.9	26.5	6.7	25.1	22.4	5.0
13.0	2.1	8.2	6.0	1.1	27.0	6.8	25.6	23.0	5.1
13.5	2.3	8.9	6.7	1.2	27.5	6.9	26.1	23.5	5.2
14.0	2.5	9.7	7.3	1.4	28.0	7.1	26.6	24.0	5.4
14.5	2.7	10.4	8.0	1.6	28.5	7.2	27.1	24.6	5.5
15.0	2.9	11.0	8.6	1.7	29.0	7.3	27.5	25.1	5.6
15.5	3.1	11.7	9.3	1.9	29.5	7.5	28.0	25.6	5.7
16.0	3.2	12.4	9.9	2.0	30.0	7.6	28.4	26.1	5.8
16.5	3.4	13.1	10.6	2.2	30.5	7.7	28.8	26.6	5.9
17.0	3.6	13.8	11.2	2.4	31.0	7.8	29.3	27.1	6.0
17.5	3.8	14.4	11.9	2.5	31.5	7.9	29.7	27.6	6.1
18.0	3.9	15.1	12.5	2.7	32.0	8.1	30.1	28.1	6.2
18.5	4.1	15.8	13.1	2.8	32.5	8.2	30.4	28.6	6.3
19.0	4.3	16.4	13.7	3.0	33.0	8.3	30.8	29.1	6.4
19.5	4.5	17.0	14.4	3.1	33.5	8.4	31.2	29.5	6.5
20.0	4.6	17.7	15.0	3.3	34.0	8.5	31.5	30.0	6.6
20.5	4.8	18.3	15.6	3.4	34.5	8.6	31.8	30.5	6.7
21.0	5.0	18.9	16.2	3.5	35.0	8.7	32.2	30.9	6.8
21.5	5.1	19.5	16.8	3.7	35.5	8.8	32.5	31.4	6.9
22.0	5.3	20.1	17.4	3.8	36.0	8.9	32.8	31.8	7.0
22.5	5.5	20.7	17.9	4.0	36.5	8.9	33.0	32.3	7.1
23.0	5.6	21.3	18.5	4.1	37.0	9.0	33.3	32.7	7.2
23.5	5.8	21.9	19.1	4.2	37.5	9.1	33.5	33.2	7.3
24.0	5.9	22.4	19.7	4.4	38.0	9.2	33.8	33.6	7.4
24.5	6.1	23.0	20.2	4.5	38.5	9.2	34.0	34.0	7.4
25.0	6.2	23.5	20.8	4.6	39.0	9.3	34.2	34.4	7.5
25.5	6.4	24.1	21.3	4.7	39.5	9.4	34.4	34.8	7.6
					40.0	9.4	34.6	35.3	7.7

All measurements in cm, MA = menstrual age (in weeks); parameter abbreviations given in text.

From Hadlock FP, Deter LR, Harrist RB, Park SK: Radiology 1984; 152:497–501. Used by permission.

▪: FETAL BIOMETRY EQUATIONS
▪ ACR Code: 856 (Fetal Biometry)

Table 1 ▪ Equations for Calculating Biometric Parameters Based on Study of 663 Fetuses

MEASUREMENT	MEAN (50th Percentile)	STANDARD DEVIATION
Biparietal diameter (outer-inner) (BPD)	$-28.36 + 3.967w - 0.0005543w^3$	$+1.225 + 0.06883w$
Occipitofrontal diameter (OFD)	$-41.58 + 5.550w - 0.0009141w^3$	$+4.795 - 0.2283w + 0.007089w^2$
Cephalic index [BPD/OFD]	$+0.8927 - 0.008276w + 0.0001533w^2$	$+0.03673$
Head circumference (plotted)	$-109.9 + 15.29w - 0.002378w^3$	$+3.644 + 0.2311w$
Head circumference [π(BPD + OFD)/2]	$-109.7 + 15.16w - 0.002388w^3$	$+3.913 + 0.2329w$
Abdominal circumference (plotted)	$-87.05 + 12.28w - 0.0008088w^3$	$+0.4930 + 0.4576w$
Abdominal circumference [π(AP + TRV)/2]	$-85.84 + 11.92w - 0.0007902w^3$	$-3.080 + 0.6018w$
Femur length	$-32.43 + 3.416w - 0.0004791w^3$	$+1.060 + 0.05833w$

w = Gestational age in weeks, AP = anteroposterior (diameter), TRV = transverse (diameter); parameters defined in text.[2-4]

Technique ▪

Standard obstetric ultrasound was done with an EUB-340 scanner (Hitachi Medical Corp., Tokyo, Japan).[1-4]

Measurements ▪

The biparietal diameter (BPD) was measured from outer-inner tables of the skull as well as from outer-outer tables. The occipital frontal diameter (OFD) was measured from the leading edge of the frontal bone to the outer border of the occiput. The head circumference was measured by tracing the perimeter and calculated by using BPD and OFD (formula in Table 1). The cephalic index (BPD/OFD) was calculated also. The outer-inner BPD was used for both these calculations. The abdominal circumference was measured by tracing the perimeter and also calculated from anteroposterior (AP) and transverse (TRV) diameters as shown in Table 1. The femur length was measured between diaphyses disregarding curvature.

The mean of each measurement versus gestational age (GA) was modeled by fitting polynomial regression equations (quadratic, cubic, or linear cubic) to the data. Variability was also modeled by use of polynomial regression on standard deviation (SD) of observed measurements as a function of GA. Goodness of fit for each proposed model was evaluated by a multistep procedure, which, in addition to calculating correlation of model output with observed values, takes into account variability of data by the method of standard deviation scores. The models were also checked visually by plotting observed data and superimposing predicted mean and percentile curves (see later). The simplest accurate models for predicting mean and SD by GA were chosen.[1] Table 1 lists these equations.

Source ▪

The fetuses of 663 pregnant (singleton) women whose ultrasound and menstrual dates agreed within 10 days were included in the study. A set of measurements was included from each fetus at one point between 12 and 42 weeks, and the numbers of measurement sets for each week ranged from 10 to 27. Maternal ethnicity was European or Afro-Caribbean (study done at a London teaching hospital). There was no maternal disease or medication likely to affect fetal growth, and there were no detected fetal malformations or abnormal karyotypes.[1]

Comments ▪

To use the equations listed in Table 1, calculate the predicted means by gestational age (12 to 42 weeks) from the equations in the second column. The percentiles may be calculated using the equations in the third column to calculate SD for GA (12 to 42 weeks) and then determining mean ± Z SD, where Z = -1.88, -1.28, 0, 1.28, and 1.88 for 3rd, 10th, 50th, 90th, and 97th centiles, respectively.[2]

REFERENCES

1. Altman DG, Chitty LS: Charts of fetal size. 1. Methodology. Br J Obstet Gynaecol 1994; 101:29–34.
2. Chitty LS, Altman DB, Henderson A, et al: Charts of fetal size. 2. Head measurements. Br J Obstet Gynaecol 1994; 101:35–43.
3. Chitty LS, Altman DG, Henderson A, et al: Charts of fetal size. 3. Abdominal measurements. Br J Obstet Gynaecol 1994; 101:125–131.
4. Chitty LS, Altman DG, Henderson A, et al: Charts of fetal size. 4. Femur length. Br J Obstet Gynaecol 1994; 101:132–135.

▪: NEW FETAL BIOMETRY CHART
▪ ACR Code: 856 (Fetal Biometry)

Technique ▪

Ultrasound of the gravid uterus was done with several machines and different transducers. All machines were regularly calibrated (3-month intervals) using an American Institute of Ultrasound in Medicine (AIUM) test object.[1]

Measurements ▪

Up to 10 measurements were made from frozen images with built-in software at each visit. Thoracic circumference (TC) was measured from an axial image, with the true cross-section of the spine and plane of maximal tricuspid

Table 1 ▪ Fetal Biometry Chart for a North American White Population

WEEKS	BPD	HC	AC	TC	FL
12	17 / 20 / 24	64 / 76 / 87	48 / 59 / 68	47 / 53 / 60	5 / 7 / 10
13	21 / 24 / 27	76 / 89 / 99	59 / 70 / 80	56 / 63 / 71	8 / 11 / 14
14	24 / 27 / 31	90 / 101 / 112	71 / 81 / 92	65 / 73 / 82	11 / 14 / 17
15	28 / 31 / 34	103 / 114 / 124	82 / 93 / 104	75 / 83 / 93	14 / 17 / 20
16	31 / 34 / 37	116 / 127 / 137	94 / 105 / 117	84 / 93 / 104	17 / 20 / 23
17	34 / 38 / 41	128 / 139 / 150	106 / 117 / 129	92 / 103 / 115	21 / 23 / 26
18	37 / 41 / 44	140 / 151 / 163	117 / 129 / 142	101 / 112 / 126	23 / 26 / 29
19	40 / 44 / 47	152 / 163 / 175	128 / 141 / 155	109 / 122 / 136	26 / 29 / 32
20	43 / 47 / 51	163 / 175 / 188	140 / 153 / 168	117 / 132 / 146	29 / 32 / 35
21	46 / 50 / 54	174 / 188 / 201	151 / 165 / 181	126 / 141 / 156	32 / 35 / 38
22	49 / 53 / 58	186 / 200 / 214	162 / 177 / 193	135 / 151 / 166	34 / 37 / 41
23	52 / 57 / 61	197 / 212 / 227	172 / 188 / 205	143 / 161 / 176	37 / 40 / 44
24	55 / 60 / 65	208 / 224 / 240	183 / 200 / 217	152 / 170 / 185	40 / 43 / 47
25	58 / 63 / 68	220 / 236 / 252	193 / 211 / 229	160 / 180 / 194	42 / 45 / 49
26	61 / 66 / 71	231 / 247 / 264	203 / 222 / 240	169 / 188 / 203	45 / 48 / 52
27	64 / 69 / 74	242 / 258 / 275	214 / 234 / 252	176 / 196 / 212	47 / 51 / 55
28	67 / 72 / 77	252 / 268 / 286	224 / 245 / 263	184 / 204 / 220	49 / 53 / 57
29	70 / 75 / 79	262 / 277 / 296	235 / 255 / 274	190 / 211 / 229	51 / 55 / 59
30	73 / 77 / 82	271 / 286 / 305	246 / 266 / 285	197 / 217 / 237	53 / 57 / 61
31	75 / 80 / 84	279 / 295 / 314	257 / 277 / 296	203 / 224 / 245	55 / 59 / 63
32	78 / 82 / 86	286 / 303 / 321	267 / 287 / 307	209 / 231 / 254	56 / 61 / 65
33	79 / 84 / 89	293 / 310 / 328	276 / 297 / 317	216 / 238 / 262	58 / 63 / 67
34	81 / 86 / 91	299 / 317 / 334	285 / 306 / 327	221 / 244 / 269	60 / 65 / 69
35	83 / 87 / 93	304 / 322 / 340	294 / 315 / 336	227 / 250 / 276	62 / 67 / 71
36	84 / 89 / 94	309 / 327 / 345	301 / 324 / 345	231 / 256 / 282	63 / 69 / 72
37	85 / 90 / 96	313 / 332 / 350	308 / 332 / 354	236 / 260 / 288	65 / 70 / 74
38	87 / 92 / 97	317 / 335 / 354	314 / 340 / 361	240 / 264 / 294	66 / 72 / 75
39	88 / 93 / 98	320 / 339 / 359	319 / 349 / 370	244 / 268 / 299	67 / 73 / 77
40	88 / 94 / 99	323 / 342 / 364	324 / 358 / 378	248 / 271 / 304	68 / 74 / 78
41	89 / 95 / 100	326 / 345 / 370	329 / 367 / 387	252 / 274 / 310	69 / 75 / 79
42	90 / 96 / 100	329 / 348 / 375	333 / 377 / 397	256 / 277 / 315	71 / 77 / 80

Weeks = menstrual age, BPD = biparietal diameter, HC = head circumference, AC = abdominal circumference, TC = thoracic circumference, FL = femur length. All measurements are in millimeters, and 10th / 50th / 90th percentiles are given.

From Lessoway VA: Personal communication, 1999. Used by permission.

and mitral valve motion for orientation.[2] Biparietal diameter (BPD), head circumference (HC), abdominal circumference (AC), and femur length (FL) were measured with standard criteria for image orientation. Circumferences (HC, TC, and AC) were measured by means of perimeter tracing and linear measurements. BPD and FL measurements were made with electronic calipers. Each measurement was repeated four times and averaged.

The cross-sectional measurements of each parameter were related to menstrual age (MA) in days, and a 7-day sliding window was created about each day to read the data. From observations within each window, 7 percentiles were calculated using Tukey's method.[3] The estimates were smoothed with the cubic spline method, with tensions varying from 5 to 8.[4] Table 1 gives 10th, 50th, and 90th percentile parameter estimates for each menstrual week from 12 to 42.[5]

Source ▪

After excluding multiple gestations, intrapartum obstetric complications, prematurity, and fetal abnormalities in utero or at birth, 790 normal singleton pregnancies were available for evaluation. All the women had regular normal menstrual cycles and knew the date of the beginning of their last menstrual period (LMP). They all had ultrasound prior to 14 weeks and the MA from crown-rump length agreed

with LMP to within 1 week; these dates were used in the analysis. Subjects were all North American whites (British Columbia).[1, 5]

Comments ▪

The cited paper[1] contains tabulated biometry data by menstrual day from 12 to 42 weeks, for a total of 10 measurements, and numerous graphs of these measurements. Table 1 may be used to asses fetal size when dates are known by using the percentile entries for MA. When dates are uncertain, the 50th percentile values may be used in estimating gestational age. The researchers caution against using their cross-sectional data to track fetal growth.[1] This may be done using longitudinal fetal growth charts contained in a separate section of this book.

REFERENCES

1. Lessoway VA, Schulzer M, Wittmenn BK, et al: Ultrasound fetal biometry charts for a North American Caucasian population. J Clin Ultrasound 1998; 26:433–453.
2. Nimrod C, Davies D, Iwanicki S, et al: Ultrasound prediction of pulmonary hypoplasia. Obstet Gynecol 1986; 68:495.
3. Hoaglin DC, Mostell F, Tukey JW: Understanding Robust and Exploratory Data Analysis. John Wiley & Sons, New York, 1983, pp 33–55.
4. CSSMH: Cubic spline software routine. IMSL Inc, Houston, 1989.
5. Lessoway VA: Personal communication, 1999.

▪: MEASUREMENT OF TWIN AND SINGLETON FETAL GROWTH PATTERNS BY ULTRASOUND[1]

▪ ACR Code: 856 (Fetal Biometry)

Table 1 ▪ Mean Twin and Singleton Biparietal Diameter (BPD) for 27th to 37th Week of Gestation

GESTATIONAL AGE (wk)	NO.	MEAN TWIN BPD (cm)	SD (cm)	SINGLETON BPD (cm)	p VALUE*
27	20	6.9	.4	6.9	.999
28	20	7.4	.4	7.2	.057
29	22	7.4	.4	7.4	.919
30	26	7.4	.5	7.6	.028
31	18	7.8	.5	7.9	.466
32	20	7.9	.4	8.1	.028
33	24	8.1	.4	8.3	.047
34	16	8.2	.3	8.5	.002
35	18	8.4	.4	8.7	.006
36	14	8.5	.3	8.9	.005
37	6	8.5	.3	9.1	.003

*Student's t-test.
From Grumbach K, et al: Radiology 1986; 158:237–241. Used by permission.

Table 2 ▪ Mean Twin and Singleton Fetal Femur Length (FFL) for 27th to 37th Week of Gestation

GESTATIONAL AGE (wk)	NO.	MEAN TWIN FFL (cm)	SD (cm)	MEAN SINGLETON FFL (cm)	p VALUE*
27	10	5.1	.3	5.1	.99
28	8	5.7	.2	5.4	.60
29	4	5.2	.3	5.6	.60
30	16	5.9	.4	5.8	.12
31	8	5.9	.6	6.0	.44
32	10	6.3	.5	6.3	.99
33	10	6.4	.5	6.5	.68
34	10	6.6	.3	6.7	.62
35	8	6.9	.3	6.9	.22
36	8	6.9	.3	7.1	.24
37	4	7.2	.3	7.3	.62

*Student's t-test.
From Grumbach K, et al: Radiology 1986; 158:237–241. Used by permission.

Table 3 ▪ Mean Twin and Singleton Abdominal Circumference (AC) for 27th to 37th Week of Gestation

GESTATIONAL AGE (wk)	NO.	MEAN TWIN AC (cm)	SD (cm)	MEAN SINGLETON AC (cm)	p VALUE*
27	12	23.6	1.7	22.7	.07
28	19	23.9	2.7	23.8	.68
29	12	24.9	2.5	24.9	.56
30	18	25.3	1.9	26.0	.11
31	12	26.9	1.9	27.1	.68
32	18	27.2	1.8	28.2	.035
33	14	27.1	2.1	29.3	.002
34	14	28.9	1.9	30.4	.012
35	14	29.6	1.7	31.5	.001
36	10	29.8	1.6	32.6	.001
37	8	29.2	2.6	33.7	.009

*Student's t-test.
From Grumbach K, et al: Radiology 1986; 158:237–241. Used by permission.

Table 4 ▪ Predicted Biparietal Diameters (BPD) of Twin Fetuses Between 20 and 37 Weeks of Gestation

WK OF GESTATION	MEAN BPD (cm)	10th PERCENTILE (cm)	90th PERCENTILE (cm)
20	5.1	4.9	5.3
21	5.1	4.9	5.7
22	5.4	5.0	6.5
23	5.7	4.5	5.9
24	6.0	5.3	7.4
25	6.3	5.5	7.5
26	6.6	5.9	7.8
27	6.8	6.5	7.5
28	7.1	6.9	8.2
29	7.3	6.8	7.9
30	7.5	6.8	8.1
31	7.7	6.9	8.6
32	7.9	7.3	8.4
33	8.0	7.4	8.6
34	8.2	7.9	8.5
35	8.3	7.9	8.9
36	8.5	8.0	9.0
37	8.6	8.2	8.8

From Grumbach K, et al: Radiology 1986; 158:237–241. Used by permission.

Table 5 ▪ Predicted Abdominal Circumferences (AC) of Twin Fetuses Between 20 and 37 Weeks of Gestation

WK OF GESTATION	MEAN AC (cm)	10th PERCENTILE (cm)	90th PERCENTILE (cm)
20	16.8	14.9	17.1
21	17.5	15.7	19.0
22	18.6	15.8	20.9
23	19.4	16.3	19.6
24	20.2	16.7	23.9
25	21.1	18.8	23.9
26	21.9	18.9	26.2
27	22.7	21.5	25.9
28	23.6	19.9	27.7
29	24.4	21.6	27.4
30	25.2	22.4	26.6
31	26.0	24.5	28.9
32	26.7	24.7	29.6
33	27.4	23.2	29.0
34	28.3	25.9	30.3
35	29.1	26.9	31.1
36	29.8	27.5	31.5
37	30.5	23.9	32.1

From Grumbach K, et al: Radiology 1986; 158:237–241. Used by permission.

Technique ▪

1. Examinations were performed using a 3.5-MHz focused transducer on mechanical sector scanners.
2. Examinations were performed at 4- to 6-week intervals once twin gestation had been established.

Measurements ▪

A complete fetal anatomic survey was carried out for each twin and included biparietal diameter (BPD), fetal femur length (FFL), and abdominal circumference (AC).

The data for these measurements are given in Tables 1 through 5.

Source ▪

Data are based on a study of 103 twin gestations.

REFERENCE

1. Grumbach K, Coleman BG, Arger PH, et al: Twin and singleton growth patterns compared using US. Radiology 1986; 158:237–241.

▪: GROWTH RATES OF NORMAL FETUSES FROM 17 TO 36 WEEKS
▪ ACR Code: 856 (Fetal Biometry)

Technique ▪

Standard obstetric ultrasound was done with multiple machines and transducers.[1]

Measurements ▪

All measurements were made from frozen images with electronic calipers. The biparietal diameter (BPD) was obtained from an axial image centered on the thalami or midbrain by measuring from the outer table of the closer temporoparietal bone to the inner table of the farther one. The abdominal diameter (AD) was measured from axial images through the abdomen with the left portal vein centrally located. Two orthogonal (anteroposterior and transverse) outer edge to outer edge measurements were averaged, and the abdominal circumference was calculated by multiplying the AD by π. The femur length (FL) was measured along the long axis of the ossified shaft.[1] Cubic regression growth curves were calculated for each parameter, and quadratic growth rate (millimeter/week) equations were calculated as their derivatives. For each growth parameter, standard deviations (SD) were derived from the variance associated with the fitted growth curve regression.[1] Tables 1 through 4 list the 10th, 50th, and 90th percentiles of growth rate for each of four intervals (4, 6, 8, and 10 or more weeks). Table 5 lists the quadratic growth rate equations and the associated SD.[1]

Source ▪

Subjects included 510 pregnant (singleton only) women followed for prenatal care in the authors'[1] clinic. Eighty percent were African-American, 15% were white, and 5% were of Hispanic or Asian background. Initial dating was done from measurements made during the first ultrasound, as accurate menstrual dates generally were not available. Reference was made to the appropriate table for crown-rump length or BPD.[2,3] Estimated gestational age (GA) at the time of delivery ranged from 37 to 42 weeks, and the birth weight ranged from 2340 to 4050 gm (mean ± SD = 3262 ± 310 gm). A total of 1450 sonograms were made on the 510 patients during their pregnancies (range, 2 to 6, mean, 2.8 examinations per patient).[1]

Comments ▪

To use these tables, consider the following example: A patient had a first-trimester scan giving GA as 10 weeks and a second scan 10 weeks later (GA, 20 weeks), at which time the BPD measured 50 mm. A third scan was performed 10 weeks later (GA, 30 weeks) and the BPD was 80 mm. To calculate growth rate, simply subtract the two measurements (80 − 50 = 30 mm) and divide by the interval to get a rate (30 mm/10 wk = 3 mm/wk). The mean gestational age (MGA) is calculated by averaging the

	Table 1 ▪ Growth of Singleton Fetuses at Intervals of 4 Weeks											
	BPD (mm/wk)			AVERAGE AD (mm/wk)			AC (mm/wk)			FL (mm/wk)		
WEEKS	10th	50th	90th	10th	50th	90th	10th	50th	90th	10th	50th	90th
17	2.5	3.5	4.4	2.3	3.7	5.1	7.2	11.5	15.9	2.1	3.1	4.2
18	2.5	3.4	4.4	2.3	3.7	5.0	7.1	11.5	15.8	2.0	3.0	4.1
19	2.4	3.4	4.4	2.2	3.6	5.0	7.0	11.4	15.7	1.9	2.9	4.0
20	2.4	3.3	4.3	2.2	3.6	5.0	6.9	11.3	15.6	1.8	2.8	3.9
21	2.3	3.3	4.3	2.2	3.5	4.9	6.8	11.1	15.5	1.7	2.7	3.8
22	2.3	3.2	4.2	2.1	3.5	4.9	6.6	11.0	15.4	1.6	2.6	3.7
23	2.2	3.2	4.1	2.1	3.5	4.9	6.5	10.9	15.3	1.5	2.6	3.6
24	2.1	3.1	4.0	2.0	3.4	4.8	6.4	10.7	15.1	1.4	2.5	3.5
25	2.0	3.0	3.9	2.0	3.4	4.8	6.2	10.6	14.9	1.4	2.4	3.4
26	1.9	2.9	3.8	1.9	3.3	4.7	6.0	10.4	14.8	1.3	2.3	3.3
27	1.8	2.8	3.7	1.9	3.3	4.6	5.8	10.2	14.6	1.2	2.2	3.3
28	1.7	2.6	3.6	1.8	3.2	4.6	5.7	10.0	14.4	1.1	2.2	3.2
29	1.5	2.5	3.5	1.7	3.1	4.5	5.5	9.8	14.2	1.1	2.1	3.1
30	1.4	2.4	3.4	1.7	3.1	4.5	5.2	9.6	14.0	1.0	2.0	3.1
31	1.3	2.2	3.2	1.6	3.0	4.4	5.0	9.4	13.8	0.9	2.0	3.0
32	1.1	2.1	3.1	1.5	2.9	4.3	4.8	9.2	13.5	0.9	1.9	3.0
33	0.9	1.9	2.9	1.4	2.8	4.2	4.5	8.9	13.3	0.8	1.9	2.9
34	0.8	1.7	2.7	1.4	2.8	4.2	4.3	8.7	13.0	0.8	1.8	2.9
35	0.6	1.6	2.5	1.3	2.7	4.1	4.0	8.4	12.8	0.7	1.8	2.8
36	0.4	1.4	2.3	1.2	2.6	4.0	3.7	8.1	12.5	0.7	1.7	2.8

10th, 50th, 90th = percentiles. Measurement abbreviations are standard (in text).
From Nazarian LN, Halpern EJ, Kurtz AB, et al: J Ultrasound Med 1995; 14(11):829–836. Used by permission.

Table 2 ▪ Growth of Singleton Fetuses at Intervals of 6 Weeks

WEEKS	BPD (mm/wk)			AVERAGE AD (mm/wk)			AC (mm/wk)			FL (mm/wk)		
	10th	50th	90th	10th	50th	90th	10th	50th	90th	10th	50th	90th
17	2.8	3.5	4.1	2.7	3.7	4.6	8.6	11.5	14.5	2.4	3.1	3.8
18	2.8	3.4	4.1	2.7	3.7	4.6	8.5	11.5	14.4	2.3	3.0	3.7
19	2.7	3.4	4.0	2.7	3.6	4.6	8.4	11.4	14.3	2.2	2.9	3.6
20	2.7	3.3	4.0	2.7	3.6	4.5	8.3	11.3	14.2	2.1	2.8	3.5
21	2.6	3.3	3.9	2.6	3.5	4.5	8.2	11.1	14.1	2.0	2.7	3.4
22	2.6	3.2	3.9	2.6	3.5	4.4	8.1	11.0	14.0	1.9	2.6	3.3
23	2.5	3.2	3.8	2.5	3.5	4.4	7.9	10.9	13.8	1.9	2.6	3.2
24	2.4	3.1	3.7	2.5	3.4	4.4	7.8	10.7	13.7	1.8	2.5	3.2
25	2.3	3.0	3.6	2.4	3.4	4.3	7.6	10.6	13.5	1.7	2.4	3.1
26	2.2	2.9	3.5	2.4	3.3	4.2	7.5	10.4	13.3	1.6	2.3	3.0
27	2.1	2.8	3.4	2.3	3.3	4.2	7.3	10.2	13.2	1.5	2.2	2.9
28	2.0	2.6	3.3	2.3	3.2	4.1	7.1	10.0	13.0	1.5	2.2	2.9
29	1.9	2.5	3.2	2.2	3.1	4.1	6.9	9.8	12.8	1.4	2.1	2.8
30	1.7	2.4	3.0	2.1	3.1	4.0	6.7	9.6	12.6	1.3	2.0	2.7
31	1.6	2.2	2.9	2.1	3.0	3.9	6.5	9.4	12.3	1.3	2.0	2.7
32	1.4	2.1	2.7	2.0	2.9	3.9	6.2	9.2	12.1	1.2	1.9	2.6
33	1.3	1.9	2.6	1.9	2.8	3.8	6.0	8.9	11.9	1.2	1.9	2.6
34	1.1	1.7	2.4	1.8	2.8	3.7	5.7	8.7	11.6	1.1	1.8	2.5
35	0.9	1.6	2.2	1.7	2.7	3.6	5.5	8.4	11.3	1.1	1.8	2.5
36	0.7	1.4	2.0	1.7	2.6	3.5	5.2	8.1	11.1	1.0	1.7	2.4

10th, 50th, 90th = percentiles. Measurement abbreviations are standard (in text).
From Nazarian LN, Halpern EJ, Kurtz AB, et al: J Ultrasound Med 1995; 14(11):829–836. Used by permission.

Table 3 ▪ Growth of Singleton Fetuses at Intervals of 8 Weeks

WEEKS	BPD (mm/wk)			AVERAGE AD (mm/wk)			AC (mm/wk)			FL (mm/wk)		
	10th	50th	90th	10th	50th	90th	10th	50th	90th	10th	50th	90th
17	3.0	3.5	4.0	3.0	3.7	4.4	9.3	11.5	13.7	2.6	3.1	3.7
18	2.9	3.4	3.9	2.9	3.7	4.4	9.2	11.5	13.7	2.5	3.0	3.7
19	2.9	3.4	3.9	2.9	3.6	4.3	9.1	11.4	13.6	2.4	2.9	3.4
20	2.9	3.3	3.8	2.9	3.6	4.3	9.0	11.3	13.5	2.3	2.8	3.3
21	2.8	3.3	3.8	2.8	3.5	4.3	8.9	11.1	13.4	2.2	2.7	3.3
22	2.7	3.2	3.7	2.8	3.5	4.2	8.8	11.0	13.2	2.1	2.6	3.2
23	2.7	3.2	3.6	2.8	3.5	4.2	8.7	10.9	13.1	2.0	2.6	3.1
24	2.6	3.1	3.6	2.7	3.4	4.1	8.5	10.7	12.9	1.9	2.5	3.0
25	2.5	3.0	3.5	2.7	3.4	4.1	8.3	10.6	12.8	1.9	2.4	2.9
26	2.4	2.9	3.4	2.6	3.3	4.0	8.2	10.4	12.6	1.8	2.3	2.8
27	2.3	2.8	3.3	2.5	3.3	4.0	8.0	10.2	12.4	1.7	2.2	2.8
28	2.2	2.6	3.1	2.5	3.2	3.9	7.8	10.0	12.2	1.6	2.2	2.7
29	2.0	2.5	3.0	2.4	3.1	3.8	7.6	9.8	12.0	1.6	2.1	2.6
30	1.9	2.4	2.9	2.4	3.1	3.8	7.4	9.6	11.8	1.5	2.0	2.6
31	1.7	2.2	2.7	2.3	3.0	3.7	7.2	9.4	11.6	1.5	2.0	2.5
32	1.6	2.1	2.6	2.2	2.9	3.6	6.9	9.2	11.4	1.4	1.9	2.4
33	1.4	1.9	2.4	2.1	2.8	3.5	6.7	8.9	11.1	1.3	1.9	2.4
34	1.3	1.7	2.2	2.1	2.8	3.5	6.4	8.7	10.9	1.3	1.8	2.3
35	1.1	1.6	2.1	2.0	2.7	3.4	6.2	8.4	10.6	1.3	1.8	2.3
36	0.9	1.4	1.9	1.9	2.6	3.3	5.9	8.1	10.3	1.2	1.7	2.3

10th, 50th, 90th = percentiles. Measurement abbreviations are standard (in text).
From Nazarian LN, Halpern EJ, Kurtz AB, et al: J Ultrasound Med 1995; 14(11):829–836. Used by permission.

Table 4 ▪ Growth of Singleton Fetuses at Intervals of 10 or More Weeks

WEEKS	BPD (mm/wk)			AVERAGE AD (mm/wk)			AC (mm/wk)			FL (mm/wk)		
	10th	50th	90th	10th	50th	90th	10th	50th	90th	10th	50th	90th
17	3.1	3.5	3.9	3.1	3.7	4.2	9.7	11.6	13.3	2.7	3.1	3.6
18	3.0	3.4	3.8	3.1	3.7	4.2	9.7	11.5	13.3	2.6	3.0	3.5
19	3.0	3.4	3.8	3.0	3.6	4.2	9.6	11.4	13.2	2.5	2.9	3.3
20	3.0	3.3	3.7	3.0	3.6	4.2	9.5	11.3	13.1	2.4	2.8	3.2
21	2.9	3.3	3.7	3.0	3.5	4.1	9.3	11.1	13.0	2.3	2.7	3.2
22	2.8	3.2	3.6	2.9	3.5	4.1	9.2	11.0	12.8	2.2	2.6	3.1
23	2.8	3.2	3.6	2.9	3.5	4.0	9.1	10.9	12.7	2.1	2.6	3.0
24	2.7	3.1	3.5	2.8	3.4	4.0	8.9	10.7	12.5	2.0	2.5	2.9
25	2.6	3.0	3.4	2.8	3.4	3.9	8.8	10.6	12.4	2.0	2.4	2.8
26	2.5	2.9	3.3	2.7	3.3	3.9	8.6	10.4	12.2	1.9	2.3	2.7
27	2.4	2.8	3.2	2.7	3.3	3.8	8.4	10.2	12.0	1.8	2.2	2.7
28	2.3	2.6	3.0	2.6	3.2	3.8	8.2	10.0	11.8	1.7	2.2	2.6
29	2.1	2.5	2.9	2.6	3.1	3.7	8.0	9.8	11.6	1.7	2.1	2.5
30	2.0	2.4	2.8	2.5	3.1	3.6	7.8	9.6	11.4	1.6	2.0	2.5
31	1.8	2.2	2.6	2.4	3.0	3.6	7.6	9.4	11.2	1.6	2.0	2.4
32	1.7	2.1	2.5	2.3	2.9	3.5	7.4	9.2	11.0	1.5	1.9	2.3
33	1.5	1.9	2.3	2.3	2.8	3.4	7.1	8.9	10.7	1.4	1.9	2.3
34	1.4	1.7	2.1	2.2	2.8	3.3	6.9	8.7	10.5	1.4	1.8	2.2
35	1.2	1.6	2.0	2.1	2.7	3.2	6.6	8.4	10.2	1.4	1.8	2.2
36	1.0	1.4	1.8	2.0	2.6	3.2	6.3	8.1	9.9	1.3	1.7	2.2

10th, 50th, 90th = percentiles. Measurement abbreviations are standard (in text).
From Nazarian LN, Halpern EJ, Kurtz AB, et al: J Ultrasound Med 1995; 14(11):829–836. Used by permission.

Table 5 ▪ Quadratic Growth Rate Equations from 17 to 36 Weeks in Singleton Pregnancies

MEASUREMENT	GROWTH RATE EQUATION	SD
BPD	$2.59 + 0.127 (MGA) - 0.000447 (MGA)^2$	0.306
Average AD	$3.61 + 0.0325 (MGA) - 0.0017 (MGA)^2$	0.444
AC	$11.3 + 0.102 (MGA) - 0.00534 (MGA)^2$	1.39
FL	$5.49 + 0.17 (MGA) - 0.00181 (MGA)^2$	0.327

MGA = mean gestational age, SD = standard deviation (see text for derivation). Measurement abbreviations are standard (in text).[1]

GA from the two scans in question ([20 + 30]/2 = 25 weeks). The appropriate chart in this case is found in Table 4 (10 or more weeks' follow-up interval), and the BPD column at 25 weeks is consulted to find the expected growth rate percentiles, which show that the growth is at the 50th percentile in this case.[1]

REFERENCES

1. Nazarian LN, Halpern EJ, Kurtz AB, et al: Normal interval fetal growth rates based on obstetrical ultrasonographic measurements. J Ultrasound Med 1995; 14(11):829–836.
2. Robinson HP, Fleming JE: A critical evaluation of sonar "crown-rump length" measurements. Br J Obstet Gynaecol 1975; 82(9):702–710.
3. Kurtz AB, Wapner RJ, Kurtz RJ, et al: Analysis of biparietal diameter as an accurate indicator of gestational age. J Clin Ultrasound 1980; 8(4):319–326.

": NORMAL FETAL BODY RATIOS
- ACR Code: 856 (Fetal Biometry)

Technique •

Standard transabdominal ultrasound studies of the gravid uterus with a variety of transducers and machines.[1-7]

Measurements •

Hadlock and colleagues combined the results of six studies into a single table concerning fetal biometric ratios.[1] The measurements contained in these ratios include biparietal diameter (BPD), occipitofrontal diameter (OFD), head circumference (HC), abdominal circumference (AC), and femur length (FL). These were all measured in standard fashion.[1-7] Table 1 lists four reported ratios of these measurements from 14 weeks to term.

Source •

Six studies of well-dated singleton fetuses, whose sample size ranged from 156 to 1770 gm, are abstracted in Table 1.[2-7]

Comments •

The cephalic index (CI) is useful in determining whether dolichocephaly (CI < 75.9) or brachycephaly (CI > 81) is present, which can adversely affect the accuracy of gestational age calculations based on BPD.[2, 4] Down syndrome may be suspected if the BPD/FL is greater than 1.5 SD above the mean.[3] Short femurs, as reflected in the FL/BPD and FL/HC ratio, may be seen in dwarfism.[5, 6] The FL/AC ratio is relatively independent of gestational age and may be useful to detect intrauterine growth retardation (abnormally high) or macrosomia (abnormally low).[7]

Table 1 • Normal Fetal Body Ratios from 14 to 40 Weeks				
MENSTRUAL WEEKS	BPD/OFD	FL/BPD × 100	FL/HC × 100	FL/AC × 100
	SD = 3.7[2]	SD = 4.0[3]	SD = 1.0[3]	SD = 1.3[3]
14	81.5	58.0	15.0	19.0
15	81.0	59.0	15.7	19.3
16	80.5	61.0	16.4	19.8
17	80.1	63.0	16.9	20.3
18	79.7	65.0	17.5	20.8
19	79.4	67.0	18.1	21.0
20	79.1	69.0	18.4	21.3
21	78.8	70.0	18.6	21.5
	SD = 4.4[4]	SD = 5.0[5]	SD = 1.1[6]	SD = 1.3[7]
22	78.3	77.4	18.6	21.6
23	78.3	77.6	18.8	21.7
24	78.3	77.8	19.0	21.7
25	78.3	78.0	19.2	21.8
26	78.3	78.2	19.4	21.8
27	78.3	78.4	19.6	21.9
28	78.3	78.6	19.8	21.9
29	78.3	78.8	20.0	21.9
30	78.3	79.0	20.3	22.0
31	78.3	79.2	20.5	22.0
32	78.3	79.4	20.7	22.1
33	78.3	79.6	20.9	22.1
34	78.3	79.8	21.1	22.2
35	78.3	80.0	21.4	22.2
36	78.3	80.2	21.6	22.2
37	78.3	80.4	21.8	22.3
38	78.3	80.6	22.0	22.3
39	78.3	80.8	22.2	22.3
40	78.3	81.0	22.4	22.4

SD = standard deviation; other abbreviations as in the text.
From Hadlock FP: WB Saunders, Philadelphia, 1994, vol 1, pp 86–101. Used by permission.

REFERENCES

1. Hadlock FP: Ultrasound determination of menstrual age. In Callen PW (ed): Ultrasonography in Obstetrics and Gynecology. WB Saunders, Philadelphia, 1994, vol 1, pp: 86–101.
2. Gray DL, Songster GS, Parvin CA, Crane JP: Cephalic index: A gestational age-dependent biometric parameter. Obstet Gynecol 1989; 74:600–603.
3. Hadlock FP, Harrist RB, Martinez-Poyer J: Fetal body ratios in second trimester: A useful tool for identifying chromosomal abnormalities. J Ultrasound Med 1992; 11:81–85.
4. Hadlock FP, Deter RL, Carpenter RJ, Park SK: Estimating fetal age: Effect of head shape on BPD. AJR Am J Roentgenol 1981; 137:83–85.
5. Hohler CW, Quetel TA: Comparison of ultrasound femur length and biparietal diameter in late pregnancy. Am J Obstet Gynecol 1981; 141:759–762.
6. Hadlock FP, Harrist RB, Shah Y, Park SK: The femur length/head circumference relation in obstetric sonography. J Ultrasound Med 1984; 3:439–442.
7. Hadlock FP, Deter RL, Harrist RB, et al: A date-independent predictor of intrauterine growth retardation: Femur length/abdominal circumference ratio. AJR Am J Roentgenol 1983; 141:979–984.

": FETAL LIMB BIOMETRY
- ACR Code: 856 (Fetal Biometry)

Technique •

Ultrasound of the gravid uterus with real time scanners.[1, 2] The transducer was specified as being a linear array in the second study.[2]

Measurements •

Each bone was measured from images through its long axis from end to end. The biparietal diameter (BPD) of the skull was also measured in standard fashion.

Table 1 • Length of Fetal Long Bones in Millimeters from 11 to 40 Weeks

WEEKS	HUMERUS PERCENTILE			ULNA PERCENTILE			RADIUS PERCENTILE			FEMUR PERCENTILE			TIBIA PERCENTILE			FIBULA PERCENTILE		
	5th	50th	90th	5th	50th	90th	5th	50th	90th	5th	50th	90th	5th	50th	90th	5th	50th	90th
11	—	6	—	—	5	—	—	5	—	—	6	—	—	4	—	—	2	—
12	3	9	10	—	8	—	—	7	—	—	9	—	—	7	—	—	5	—
13	5	13	20	3	11	18	—	10	—	6	12	19	4	10	17	—	8	—
14	5	16	20	4	13	17	8	13	12	5	15	19	2	13	19	6	11	10
15	11	18	26	10	16	22	12	15	19	11	19	26	5	16	27	10	14	18
16	12	21	25	8	19	24	9	18	21	13	22	24	7	19	25	6	17	22
17	19	24	29	11	21	32	11	20	29	20	25	29	15	22	29	7	19	31
18	18	27	30	13	24	30	14	22	26	19	28	31	14	24	29	10	22	28
19	22	29	36	20	26	32	20	24	29	23	31	38	19	27	35	18	24	30
20	23	32	36	21	29	32	21	27	28	22	33	39	19	29	35	18	27	30
21	28	34	40	25	31	36	25	29	32	27	36	45	24	32	39	24	29	34
22	28	36	40	24	33	37	24	31	34	29	39	44	25	34	39	21	31	37
23	32	38	45	27	35	43	26	32	39	35	41	48	30	36	43	23	33	44
24	31	41	46	29	37	41	27	34	38	34	44	49	28	39	45	26	35	41
25	35	43	51	34	39	44	31	36	40	38	46	54	31	41	50	33	37	42
26	36	45	49	34	41	44	30	37	41	39	49	53	33	43	49	32	39	43
27	42	46	51	37	43	48	33	39	45	45	51	57	39	45	51	35	41	47
28	41	48	52	37	44	48	33	40	45	45	53	57	38	47	52	36	43	47
29	44	50	56	40	46	51	36	42	47	49	56	62	40	49	57	40	45	50
30	44	52	56	38	47	54	34	43	49	49	58	62	41	51	56	38	47	52
31	47	53	59	39	49	59	34	44	53	53	60	67	46	52	58	40	48	57
32	47	55	59	40	50	58	37	45	51	53	62	67	46	54	59	40	50	56
33	50	56	62	43	52	60	41	46	51	56	64	71	49	56	62	43	51	59
34	50	57	62	44	53	59	39	47	53	57	65	70	47	57	64	46	52	56
35	52	58	65	47	54	61	38	48	57	61	67	73	48	59	69	51	54	57
36	53	60	63	47	55	61	41	48	54	61	69	74	49	60	68	51	55	56
37	57	61	64	49	56	62	45	49	53	64	71	77	52	61	71	55	56	58
38	55	61	66	48	57	63	45	49	53	62	72	79	54	62	69	54	57	59
39	56	62	69	49	57	66	46	50	54	64	74	83	58	64	69	55	58	62
40	56	63	69	50	58	65	46	50	54	66	75	81	58	65	69	54	59	62

From Jeanty P. Radiology 1983; 147:601–602. Used by permission.

Table 2 • Polynomial Regression Equations of Limb Lengths in Normal Pregnancies

BONE	REGRESSION EQUATION
Femur	$-36.040470 + 4.1626390\,w - 0.034636367\,w^2$
Tibia	$+3.8822362\,w - 0.03519398\,w^2 - 34.226237$
Fibula	$+3.7979563\,w - 0.035979828\,w^2 - 35.049953$
Humerus	$-33.895341 + 4.1233654\,w - 0.042461521\,w^2$
Ulna	$+3.8984839\,w - 0.040382251\,w^2 - 33.169956$
Radius	$+3.8008120\,w - 0.043570568\,w^2 - 32.018781$

w = weeks.
From Jeanty P, Dramaix-Wilmet M, van Kerkem J, et al: Radiology 1982; 143:751–754. Used by permission.

Source •

The BPD, femur, and humerus were measured in 520 normal pregnancies and the distal long bones measured in 220. Gestational age (GA) ranged from 11 weeks to term.[1,2] Dr. Jeanty subsequently combined the data into a single nomogram, and these are listed in Table 1.[3] Table 2 lists regression equations of limb length versus GA.[2]

REFERENCES

1. Jeanty P, Kirkpatric C, Dramaix-Wilmet M, Struyven J: Ultrasonic evaluation of fetal limb growth. Radiology 1981; 140:165–168.
2. Jeanty P, Dramaix-Wilmet M, van Kerkem J, et al: Ultrasonic evaluation of fetal limb growth. Part II. Radiology 1982; 143:751–754.
3. Jeanty P: Fetal limb biometry [letter]. Radiology 1983; 147:601–602.

⁚ MEASUREMENT OF THE FETAL CEREBELLUM
▪ ACR Code: 856 (Fetal Biometry)

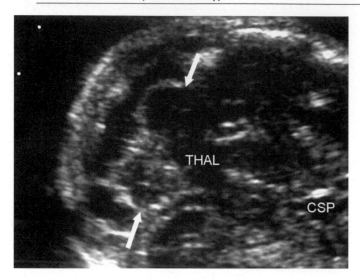

Figure 1 ▪ Measurement of transverse cerebellar diameter from an axial scan through the fetal head angled to include the posterior fossa, the thalamus/midbrain *(THAL)*, and the frontal horns/septum pellucidum *(CSP)*. The cerebellum is measured at its widest point *(arrows)*.

Technique ▪

Transabdominal ultrasound of the gravid uterus was done with a variety of real-time scanners and appropriate transducers.[1–3]

Measurements ▪

The transverse cerebellar diameter (TCD) was measured from an axial section through the fetal head, angled to include the posterior fossa, thalamus/midbrain, and frontal horns/septum pellucidum regions.[1–3] Figure 1 shows the measurement. Table 1 lists cubic regression equations for gestational age (GA), developed by Goldstein and Hill and their colleagues, along with reported variability of GA prediction by Hill and associates.[1, 2] Table 2 lists predicted GA for TCD from 13 to 56 mm, as calculated from Goldstein's equation and reported by Hill and group.[1, 2] In addition to TCD, Meyer and colleagues measured abdominal circumference (AC) in the standard fashion and calculated a ratio (TCD/AC) for each scan.[3] Table 3 lists the 10th, 50th, and 90th percentiles of TCD and TCD/AC by

gestational age, as reported by Goldstein et al and Hill et al.[1, 2]

Source ▪

Goldstein's subjects included 371 women with normal pregnancies at 13 to 40 weeks.[1] Hill and associates studied 675 pregnant women scanned from 14 to 42 weeks.[2] Meyer and associates evaluated 603 normal pregnancies from 14 to 42 weeks.[3] The pregnancies were all considered to be

Table 1 ▪ Regression Equations for Gestational Age Versus Transverse Cerebellar Diameter

Goldstein regression	Weeks = 6.329 + 0.4807 TCD + 0.01484 TCD^2 − 0.0002474 TCD^3	
Hill regression	Weeks = 6.37 + 0.54 TCD + 0.0078 TCD^2 − 0.00013 TCD^3	
Hill variability	Weeks	SD of Regression
	12–17	±0.5
	18–23	±0.9
	24–29	±1.01
	30–35	±1.2
	≥36	±1.6

TCD = transverse cerebellar diameter (in millimeters); SD = standard deviation.[1, 2]

Table 2 ▪ Gestational Age Predicted by Transverse Cerebellar Diameter

TCD (mm)	GA GOLDSTEIN	GA HILL	TCD (mm)	GA GOLDSTEIN	GA HILL
13	14.5	—	35	30.7	29.4
14	15.3	15.2	36	31.3	30.0
15	16.0	15.8	37	31.9	30.6
16	16.8	16.5	38	32.5	31.2
17	17.6	17.2	39	33.0	31.8
18	18.3	17.9	40	33.5	32.3
19	19.1	18.6	41	34.0	32.8
20	19.9	19.3	42	34.4	33.4
21	20.7	20.0	43	34.8	33.9
22	21.5	20.7	44	35.2	34.4
23	22.2	21.4	45	35.5	34.8
24	23.0	22.1	46	35.8	35.3
25	23.8	22.8	47	36.1	35.7
26	24.5	23.5	48	36.3	36.1
27	25.3	24.2	49	36.5	36.5
28	26.0	24.9	50	36.6	36.8
29	26.7	25.5	51	36.7	37.2
30	27.4	26.2	52	36.7	37.5
31	28.1	26.9	53	36.7	—
32	28.8	27.5	54	36.7	38.0
33	29.5	28.1	55	36.6	38.3
34	30.1	28.8	56	36.4	38.5

Hill = as reported, Goldstein = calculated from cubic regression equation. GA = gestational age (in weeks), TCD = transverse cerebellar diameter (in millimeters).[1, 2]

Table 3 ▪ Transverse Cerebellar Diameter and Abdominal Circumference Ratio Versus Gestational Age

GA (wk)	TCD (mm)			TCD/AC		
	10th	50th	90th	10th	50	90th
14	—	—	—	12.50	14.04	14.61
15	10.0	14.0	16.0	12.74	14.04	15.66
16	14.0	16.0	17.0	13.58	14.47	15.42
17	16.0	17.0	18.0	12.93	14.17	15.09
18	17.0	18.0	19.0	13.08	14.52	15.57
19	18.0	19.0	22.0	12.67	13.85	15.55
20	18.0	20.0	22.0	12.42	13.45	14.65
21	19.0	22.0	24.0	11.90	13.38	14.37
22	21.0	23.0	24.0	12.28	13.35	14.11
23	22.0	24.0	26.0	12.43	13.41	15.03
24	22.0	25.0	28.0	12.43	13.16	14.66
25	23.0	28.0	29.0	12.67	13.40	14.15
26	25.0	29.0	32.0	12.50	13.71	14.73
27	26.0	30.0	32.0	12.26	13.54	15.18
28	27.0	31.0	34.0	12.66	13.52	14.98
29	29.0	34.0	38.0	12.18	13.54	14.66
30	31.0	35.0	40.0	12.60	13.77	15.32
31	32.0	38.0	43.0	12.27	13.21	14.66
32	33.0	38.0	42.0	12.88	14.08	15.09
33	32.0	40.0	44.0	12.58	13.91	14.58
34	33.0	40.0	44.0	12.54	14.18	14.76
35	31.0	40.5	47.0	12.50	13.72	14.57
36	36.0	43.0	55.0	11.66	13.62	14.84
37	37.0	45.0	55.0	13.04	14.04	14.88
38	40.0	48.5	55.0	13.35	13.71	14.72
39	52.0	52.0	55.0	11.53	13.40	15.70
40	—	—	—	12.30	13.20	14.66
41	—	—	—	12.30	13.26	13.85
42	—	—	—	12.39	13.77	14.01

10th, 50th, and 90th percentiles are given. GA = gestational age, TCD = transverse cerebellar diameter, TCD/AC = transverse cerebellar diameter divided by abdominal circumference.[1,2]

well dated in that the menstrual history correlated well with ultrasound measurements.[1-3]

Comments ▪

In pregnancies that are suspected to be large for gestational age (LGA) or complicated by intrauterine growth retardation (IUGR), the traditional biometric parameters may be altered by the underlying growth abnormality rendering them inaccurate. The fetal cerebellum is relatively unaffected by these processes and can serve as an alternative means of estimating gestational age.[1-5] The TCD/AC ratio remains quite stable through the second and third trimesters in normal pregnancy, and deviations from the normal range may be indicative of LGA (lower than normal) or IUGR (higher than normal).

REFERENCES

1. Goldstein I, Reece EA, Pilu G, et al: Cerebellar measurements with ultrasonography in the evaluation of fetal growth and development. Am J Obstet Gynecol 1987; 156:1065–1069.
2. Hill LM, Guzick D, Fries J, et al: The transverse cerebellar diameter in estimating gestational age in the large for gestational age fetus. Obstet Gynecol 1990; 75:981–985.
3. Meyer WJ, Gauthier DW, Goldenberg B, et al: The fetal transverse cerebellar diameter/abdominal circumference ratio: A gestational age–independent method of assessing fetal size. J Ultrasound Med 1993; 12(7):379–382.
4. Reece EA, Goldstein I, Pilu G, Hobbins JC: Fetal cerebellar growth unaffected by IUGR: A new parameter for prenatal diagnosis. Am J Obstet Gynecol 1987; 157:632–638.
5. Co E, Raju TN, Aldana O: Cerebellar dimensions in assessment of gestational age in neonates [see comments]. Radiology 1991; 181(2):581–585.

⁚ EQUATIONS FOR ESTIMATING FETAL WEIGHT
▪ ACR Code: 856 (Fetal Weight Determination)

Table 1 ▪ Details of Studies of Estimation of Fetal Weight by Ultrasound

REFERENCE	YEAR	NO.	SCAN-DELIV TIME (days)	BIRTH WEIGHT RANGE (gm)	PARAMETERS USED	% ERROR (mean ± SD)	COMMENTS
Warsof	1977	85	0–2	174–4760	BPD, AC	± 10.6	
Shepard	1982	73	0–2	740–4125	BPD, AC	− 0.4 ± 11.7	In common use
Hadlock	1984	167	0–7	600–4600	HC, AC, FL	0.3 ± 7.6	Still commonly cited
Hadlock	1985	276	0–7	600–4600	AC, FL	0.3 ± 8.0	Used if head cannot be measured
					HC, AC, FL	0.0 ± 7.5	Considered an optimal equation by Hadlock
					BPD, HC, AC, FL	0.1 ± 7.4	
Roberts	1985	50	0–2	480–2380	BPD, HC, AC, FL	0.2 ± 6.6	
Combs	1993	380	0–3	500–4500	HC, AC, FL	2.0 ± 11	Based on volumetric models (head, abdomen)
Scott	1996	167	0–7	410–1385	HC, AC, FL	− 1.7 ± 12	Good for <1 kg

Scan-Deliv = interval between scan and delivery, % Error = described in text, SD = standard deviation, parameter abbreviations given in text.[1–7]

Technique ▪

Transabdominal ultrasound of the gravid uterus was done with a variety of machines and transducers.[1–7]

Measurements ▪

Standard biometric parameters, including biparietal diameter (BPD), head circumference (HC), abdominal circumference (AC), and femur length (FL), were measured.[1–7] Multiple regression analysis was done, typically producing several models for predicting fetal weight. Comparison with birth weight was done to determine accuracy of the formulas. One commonly used statistic is percent error, which is calculated by (predicted weight − actual weight)/ actual weight × 100. This is calculated for each subject and the simple mean, standard deviation, and mean of the absolute value reported. The simple mean (sometimes called signed mean) percent error can be negative if the predictions tend to underestimate actual weight and will be positive in the case of overestimation. However, the simple (signed) mean may be near zero even with larger errors if they cancel each other out. The standard deviation is not subject to this.

Table 1 lists characteristics of the studies included here.

Table 2 lists the equation(s) selected by the researchers as being the optimum in terms of accuracy, precision, and ease of use. Figure 1 was produced by applying each equation listed in Table 2 to a table of normative biometric

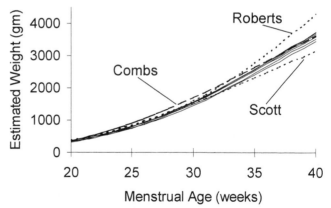

Figure 1 ▪ Outputs of equations listed in Table 2 when each are given inputs (appropriate parameters) from a table of biometric normative data. Dotted and dashed lines indicate output curves that are visually different. The remainder are plotted as solid lines.[1–7]

Table 2 ▪ Equations for Fetal Weight Estimation by Ultrasound

REFERENCE	YEAR	EQUATION FOR FETAL WEIGHT
Warsof	1977	$\log(w) = -1.599 + 0.144\,(BPD) + 0.032\,(AC) - 0.111\,(BPD^2 \times AC)/1000$
Shepard	1982	$\log(w) = -1.7492 + 0.166\,(BPD) + 0.046\,(AC) - 2.646\,(AC \times BPD)/1000$
Hadlock	1984	$\log(w) = 1.5662 - 0.0108\,(HC) + 0.0468\,(AC) + 0.171\,(FL) + 0.00034\,(HC)^2 - 0.003685\,(AC \times FL)$
Hadlock	1985	$\log(w) = 1.304 + 0.05281\,(AC) + 0.1938\,(FL) - 0.004\,(AC \times FL)$
Hadlock	1985	$\log(w) = 1.335 - 0.0034\,(AC \times FL) + 0.0316\,(BPD) + 0.0457\,(AC) + 0.1623\,(FL)$
Hadlock	1985	$\log(w) = 1.326 - 0.00326\,(AC \times FL) + 0.0107\,(HC) + 0.0438\,(AC) + 0.158\,(FL)$
Hadlock	1985	$\log(w) = 1.3596 - 0.00386\,(AC \times FL) + 0.0064\,(HC) + 0.00061\,(BPD \times AC) + 0.0424\,(AC) + 0.174\,(FL)$
Roberts	1985	$\log(w) = 1.6758 + 0.01707\,(AC) + 0.042478\,(BPD) + 0.05216\,(FL) + 0.01604\,(HC)$
Combs	1993	$w = 0.23718\,(AC)^2\,(FL) + 0.03312\,(HC)^3$
Scott	1996	$\ln(w) = 0.66\,\ln(HC) + 1.04\,\ln(AC) + 0.985\,\ln(FL)$

w = weight, log = logarithm (base 10), ln = logarithm (natural); parameter abbreviations given in text.[1–7]

data.[8] This reveals that most equations,[1-4] when given the same inputs, produce similar estimates, with those by Roberts,[5] Combs,[6] and Scott and their associates[7] deviating from the rest. Of course, it is hard to say why this is as each study population was unique. It is interesting to note that the mathematical form of these latter three models is somewhat different from the earlier ones.

Source ▪

Table 1 lists numbers of patients, birth weight range, and time intervals between the scans and delivery for all studies.[1-7] In general, the babies were weighed immediately after birth for comparison with ultrasound estimated weight.

Comments ▪

The equations have been reproduced in Table 2 exactly as reported in the original papers, with one exception. In Robert's equation, the term 0.42478 (BPD) has been changed to 0.042478 (BPD), which was needed to make the equation produce meaningful weight estimates in our testing.[5] This may have been a misprint in the original article. The equations from Warsof and associates[1] and Shepard and associates[2] produce weight estimates in kilograms, whereas the remainder[3-7] yield gram estimates. To change a logarithmic (base 10) equation to produce gram

instead of kilogram estimates, simply add 3.0 as a constant prior to taking the exponent. For Warsof's equation, the first term would change from −1.599 to 1.401 and for Shepard's equation the first term changes from −1.7492 to 1.2508.[1, 2]

References

1. Warsof SL, Gohari P, Berkowitz RL, Hobbins JC: The estimation of fetal weight by computer-assisted analysis. Am J Obstet Gynecol 1977; 128:881–892.
2. Shepard MJ, Richards VA, Berkowitz FL, et al: An evaluation of two equations for predicting fetal weight by ultrasound. Am J Obstet Gynecol 1982; 142:47–54.
3. Hadlock FP, Harrist RB, Carpenter RJ, et al: Sonographic estimation of fetal weight: The value of femur length in addition to head and abdomen measurements. Radiology 1984; 150:535–540.
4. Hadlock FP, Harrist RB, Sharman RS, et al: Estimation of fetal weight with the use of head, body, and femur measurements: A prospective study. Am J Obstet Gynecol 1985; 151:333–337.
5. Roberts AB, Lee AJ, James AG: Ultrasonic estimation of fetal weight: A new predictive model incorporating femur length for the low-birthweight fetus. J Clin Ultrasound 1985; 13:555–559.
6. Combs CA, Jaekle RK, Rosenn B, et al: Sonographic estimation of fetal weight based on a model of fetal volume. Obstet Gynecol 1993; 82(3):365–370.
7. Scott F, Beeby P, Abbott J, et al: New formula for estimating fetal weight below 1000g: Comparison with existing formulas. J Ultrasound Med 1996; 15:669–672.
8. Hadlock FP, Deter LR, Harrist RB, Park SK: Estimating fetal age: Computer-assisted analysis of multiple fetal growth parameters. Radiology 1984; 152:497–501.

▪▪ STANDARDS FOR ULTRASOUND-DETERMINED FETAL WEIGHT
▪ ACR Code: 856 (Fetal Weight Determination)

Technique ▪

Hadlock and Yarkoni and their colleagues performed transabdominal ultrasound of the gravid uterus with real-time equipment and 3.5- to 5.0-MHz transducers.[1, 2]

Measurements ▪

Ultrasound biometric parameters were measured in standard fashion.[1, 2] Hadlock and colleagues applied a formula for estimating fetal weight developed previously in their laboratory to each set of biometric measurements.[3] Yarkoni and colleagues[2] used the formula developed by Shepard and associates[4] to calculate estimated fetal weight from

each ultrasound. Nomograms of fetal weight were produced based on regression of fetal weight on menstrual age, and these are presented in Tables 1 and 2. Figure 1 is a graph of mean/50th percentile fetal weight versus menstrual age for singletons and twins.

Source ▪

Hadlock's subjects were 392 predominantly middle-class white women with well-dated normal singleton pregnancies. Scans were done from 10 weeks through term.[1] Yarkoni and colleagues evaluated 35 healthy women with twin pregnancies and no obstetric complications or fetal abnor-

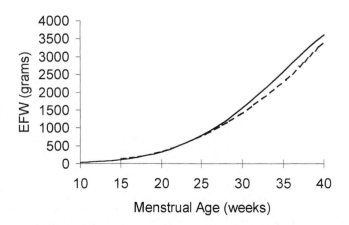

Figure 1 ▪ In utero fetal weight (by ultrasound) for singleton (*solid*) and twin (*dashed*) pregnancies.[1, 2] EFW = estimated fetal weight.

Table 1 ▪ In Utero Fetal Weight Standards for
Normal Singleton Pregnancies

	PERCENTILES OF FETAL WEIGHT (gm)				
WEEKS	3rd	10th	50th	90th	97th
10	26	29	35	41	44
11	34	37	45	53	56
12	43	48	58	68	73
13	55	61	73	85	91
14	70	77	93	109	116
15	88	97	117	137	146
16	110	121	146	171	183
17	136	150	181	212	226
18	167	185	223	261	279
19	205	227	273	319	341
20	248	275	331	387	414
21	299	331	399	467	499
22	359	398	478	559	598
23	426	471	568	665	710
24	503	556	670	784	838
25	589	652	785	918	981
26	685	758	913	1068	1141
27	791	876	1055	1234	1319
28	908	1004	1210	1416	1513
29	1034	1145	1379	1613	1724
30	1169	1294	1559	1824	1649
31	1313	1453	1751	2049	2189
32	1465	1621	1953	2285	2441
33	1622	1794	2162	2530	2703
34	1783	1973	2377	2781	2971
35	1946	2154	2595	3036	3244
36	2110	2335	2813	3291	3516
37	2271	2513	3028	3543	3785
38	2427	2686	3236	3786	4045
39	2576	2851	3435	4019	4294
40	2714	3004	3619	4234	4524

From Hadlock FP, Harrist RB, Martinez-Poyer J: Radiology 1991; 181:129–133. Used by permission.

Table 2 ▪ In Utero Fetal Weight Standards for
Normal Twin Pregnancies

	PERCENTILES OF FETAL WEIGHT (gm)				
WEEKS	5th	25th	50th	75th	95th
16	132	141	154	189	207
17	173	194	215	239	249
18	214	248	276	289	291
19	223	253	300	333	412
20	232	259	324	378	534
21	275	355	432	482	705
22	319	452	540	586	876
23	347	497	598	684	880
24	376	543	656	783	885
25	549	677	793	916	1118
26	722	812	931	1049	1352
27	755	978	1087	1193	1563
28	789	1145	1244	1337	1774
29	900	1266	1395	1509	1883
30	1011	1387	1546	1682	1992
31	1198	1532	1693	1875	2392
32	1385	1677	1840	2068	2793
33	1491	1771	2032	2334	3000
34	1597	1866	2224	2601	3208
35	1703	2093	2427	2716	3336
36	1809	2321	2631	2832	3465
37	2239	2540	2824	3035	3679
38	2669	2760	3017	3239	3894

From Yarkoni S, Reece EA, Holford T, et al: Obstet Gynecol 1987; 69:636–639. Used by permission.

malities. Scans were done every 3 weeks from 15 weeks through delivery.[2]

Comments ▪

These tables may be used in assessment of fetal growth, and Hadlock and colleagues considered that the 3rd and 97th percentiles (for singletons) may be used as limits of normal.[1] The 5th and 95th percentiles should serve the same purpose for twins. Yarkoni and group found that the variability in weights between twin pairs increased with gestational age though the overall mean weights between them was not significantly different.[2] The percentage weight difference between twins (bigger−smaller/bigger × 100) remained fairly constant, with 25th, 50th, 75th, and 95th percentiles of 1.5%, 3.8%, 9.0%, and 27.5%,

respectively.[2] In twins, growth of the biparietal diameter (BPD) and abdominal circumference (AC) remained linear through the 2nd trimester, after which BPD growth slowed somewhat and the AC increase remained constant.[2]

REFERENCES

1. Hadlock FP, Harrist RB, Martinez-Poyer J: In utero analysis of fetal growth: A sonographic weight standard. Radiology 1991; 181:129–133.
2. Yarkoni S, Reece EA, Holford T, et al: Estimated fetal weight in the evaluation of growth in twin gestations: A prospective longitudinal study. Obstet Gynecol 1987; 69:636–639.
3. Hadlock FP, Harrist RB, Sharman RS, et al: Estimation of fetal weight with the use of head, body, and femur measurements: A prospective study. Am J Obstet Gynecol 1985; 151:333–337.
4. Shepard MJ, Richards VA, Berkowitz FL, et al: An evaluation of two equations for predicting fetal weight by ultrasound. Am J Obstet Gynecol 1982; 142:47–54.

▪▪ UMBILICAL ARTERY DOPPLER INDICES
▪ ACR Code: 856 (Umbilical Artery, Vein)

Technique ▪

Erskine and Ritchie performed transabdominal scanning of the gravid uterus with a Mark V scanner (ATL, Bothel, WA). Arduini and Rizzo did transvaginal scanning of the gravid uterus with an Esacord 81 machine (Ansaldo), with a 5.0-MHz vaginal probe.[2] Sonesson and colleagues used a Sonos 100 machine (Hewlett-Packard) to perform transabdominal obstetric scans with 3.5- to 5.0-MHz transducers.[3] All investigators used duplex Doppler to obtain tracings of the umbilical artery. Arduini and Rizzo placed the gate in the midcord, and Sonesson and colleagues made separate measurements at the fetal end and placental end of the cord.[2, 3]

Measurements ▪

Once an optimal tracing was obtained, the peak systolic velocity (PSV), end-diastolic velocity (EDV), and mean velocity were determined. The systolic to diastolic (S:D) ratio, resistive index (RI), and pulsatility index (PI) were calculated as shown in Figure 1. In general, tracings were obtained when there was no significant fetal movement,

breathing, or cardiac rhythm disturbance.[1–3] Figures 2, 3 and 4 are graphs of S:D ratio, RI, and PI from 16 to 40 weeks from Erskine's study.[1] Figure 5 depicts the PI at 7 to 16 weeks from Arduini and Rizzo.[2] Tables 1 and 2 list the three parameters obtained from the fetal and placental ends of the cord, respectively, as reported by Sonesson and colleagues.[3]

Source ▪

Erskine and Ritchie evaluated 15 normal singleton fetuses at 24 and 28 weeks, then at fortnightly intervals until delivery. A subset of eight subjects was also scanned at monthly intervals from 16 to 24 weeks.[1] Arduini's subjects included 202 women with normal singleton pregnancies who were scanned from 7 to 16 weeks.[2] Sonesson and colleagues scanned 269 women with normal singleton pregnancies from 17 weeks to term.[3]

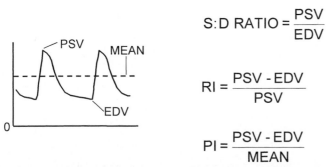

$$\text{S:D RATIO} = \frac{\text{PSV}}{\text{EDV}}$$

$$\text{RI} = \frac{\text{PSV - EDV}}{\text{PSV}}$$

$$\text{PI} = \frac{\text{PSV - EDV}}{\text{MEAN}}$$

Figure 1 ▪ Umbilical artery Doppler waveform characterization. The peak systolic velocity *(PSV)*, end-diastolic velocity *(EDV)*, and mean velocity *(MEAN)* are determined from a frozen tracing of the umbilical artery. Three parameters may be calculated: systolic to diastolic *(S:D)* ratio, resistive index *(RI)*, and pulsatility index *(PI)*, as shown.

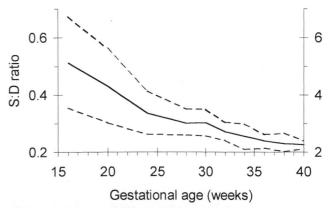

Figure 2 ▪ Systolic to diastolic (S:D) ratio from 16 weeks to term. Mean *(solid line)* and ± 2 SD *(dashed lines)* are shown. The fractional labels on the left Y axis are as given by Erskine. Often, whole numbers are reported (right Y axis). (From Erskine RLA, Ritchie JWK: Br J Obstet Gynaecol 1985; 92:605–610. Used by permission.)

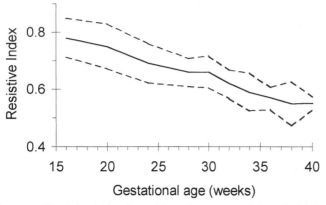

Figure 3 ▪ Resistive index from 16 weeks to term. Mean *(solid line)* ± 2 SD *(dashed lines)* are shown. (From Erskine RLA, Ritchie JWK: Br J Obstet Gynaecol 1985; 92:605–610. Used by permission.)

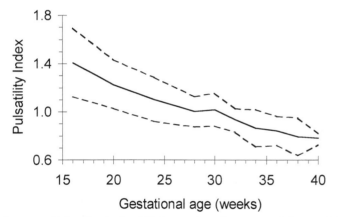

Figure 4 ▪ Pulsatility index (PI) from 16 weeks to term. Mean *(solid line)* ± 2 SD *(dashed lines)* are shown. (From Erskine RLA, Ritchie JWK: Br J Obstet Gynaecol 1985; 92:605–610. Used by permission.)

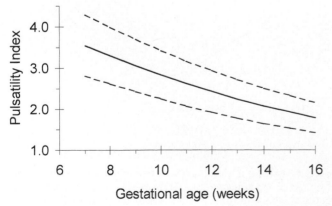

Figure 5 ▪ Pulsatility index (PI) from 7 to 16 weeks. Mean *(solid line)* ± 2 SD *(dashed lines)* are shown. (From Arduini D, Rizzo G: J Clin Ultrasound 1991: 19:335–339. Used by permission.)

Table 1 ▪ Umbilical Artery Measurements from the Fetal End of the Cord

| | 95% CONFIDENCE INTERVAL (3rd–97th %tiles) | | |
WEEKS	S:D Ratio	RI	PI
17	4.27–6.63	0.76–0.84	1.27–1.54
18	4.20–6.97	0.76–0.86	1.29–1.73
19	2.42–9.55	0.58–0.90	0.83–1.90
20	2.94–8.29	0.66–0.87	0.98–1.71
21	3.20–5.49	0.68–0.82	1.10–1.56
22	3.06–5.98	0.67–0.83	1.08–0.67
23	3.55–7.00	0.71–0.85	1.14–1.61
24	3.31–6.66	0.70–0.85	1.05–1.52
25	2.22–5.60	0.55–0.82	0.76–1.51
26	2.90–5.50	0.66–0.82	1.00–1.54
27	2.67–4.67	0.63–0.79	0.86–1.37
28	2.55–4.43	0.61–0.78	0.91–1.42
29	2.27–5.45	0.56–0.82	0.77–1.37
30	2.34–5.85	0.57–0.83	0.81–1.50
31	2.06–4.94	0.52–0.80	0.73–1.35
32	2.24–4.28	0.55–0.77	0.74–1.39
33	2.21–3.31	0.55–0.70	0.77–1.15
34	2.08–3.60	0.52–0.72	0.72–1.15
35	1.95–3.00	0.49–0.67	0.69–1.10
36	2.00–5.15	0.50–0.81	0.69–1.53
37	2.23–4.17	0.55–0.76	0.75–1.23
38	2.09–4.11	0.52–0.76	0.70–1.27
39	2.01–4.49	0.50–0.78	0.67–1.30

S:D = systolic to diastolic ratio, RI = resistive index, PI = pulsatility index, %tile = percentile.
From Sonesson SE, Fouron JC, Drblik SP, et al: J Clin Ultrasound 1993; 21(5):317–324. Used by permission.

Table 2 ▪ Umbilical Artery Measurements from the Umbilical End of the Cord

| | 95% CONFIDENCE INTERVAL (3rd–97th %tiles) | | |
WEEKS	S:D Ratio	RI	PI
17	3.59–4.78	0.72–0.79	1.16–1.52
18	3.39–5.10	0.71–0.80	1.16–1.60
19	1.82–5.85	0.45–0.83	0.82–1.59
20	2.41–5.69	0.59–0.82	0.85–1.60
21	3.00–4.17	0.67–0.76	1.07–1.33
22	2.18–4.28	0.54–0.76	0.85–1.29
23	2.72–3.50	0.63–0.71	0.96–1.21
24	2.52–5.08	0.60–0.80	0.86–1.51
25	2.21–4.11	0.55–0.80	0.73–1.30
26	2.20–3.99	0.54–0.79	0.78–1.45
27	2.33–4.03	0.57–0.75	0.79–1.31
28	1.99–4.29	0.49–0.77	0.68–1.48
29	2.10–3.30	0.52–0.69	0.73–1.09
30	1.99–3.44	0.49–0.71	0.67–1.18
31	2.24–3.65	0.55–0.74	0.76–1.16
32	1.63–4.60	0.39–0.78	0.57–1.39
33	1.83–2.81	0.44–0.54	0.71–0.99
34	1.90–3.36	0.47–0.71	0.63–1.10
35	1.89–4.01	0.47–0.75	0.63–1.30
36	1.94–4.17	0.49–0.88	0.65–1.41
37	1.97–3.66	0.49–0.73	0.65–1.33
38	1.90–3.43	0.47–0.71	0.65–1.10
39	1.74–3.43	0.43–0.72	0.54–1.19

S:D = systolic to diastolic ratio, RI = resistive index, PI = pulsatility index, %tile = percentile.
From Sonesson SE, Fouron JC, Drblik SP, et al: J Clin Ultrasound 1993; 21(5):317–324. Used by permission.

Comments ▪

These measurements are useful in screening for intrauterine growth retardation (IUGR) and in following patients with known IUGR, in combination with ultrasound biometry, to assess interval growth, estimation of fetal weight, amniotic fluid determination, and biophysical profile evaluation, as appropriate. Placental insufficiency is thought to cause increased resistance to umbilical artery inflow, which causes increases in all three parameters. There is considerable debate concerning which of the indices are the most reliable, so we have included normative data for all three. Morphologic analysis of the waveforms may reveal absence of diastolic flow or reversal of diastolic flow described as indicating increasingly severe compromise.[4–6] These waveform morphologies are shown in Figure 6.

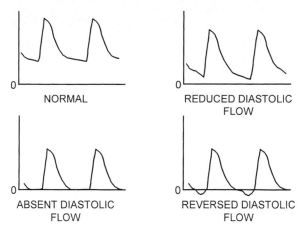

Figure 6 ▪ Umbilical artery morphologies are shown in order of increasing abnormality.

REFERENCES

1. Erskine RLA, Ritchie JWK: Umbilical artery blood flow characteristics in normal and growth retarded fetuses. Br J Obstet Gynaecol 1985; 92:605–610.
2. Arduini D, Rizzo G: Umbilical artery velocity waveforms in early pregnancy: A transvaginal color Doppler study. J Clin Ultrasound 1991: 19:335–339.
3. Sonesson SE, Fouron JC, Drblik SP, et al: Reference values for Doppler velocimetric indices from the fetal and placental ends of the umbilical artery during normal pregnancy. J Clin Ultrasound 1993; 21(5):317–324.

4. Park YW, Cho JS, Kim HS, et al: The clinical implications of early diastolic notch in third trimester Doppler waveform analysis of the uterine artery. J Ultrasound Med 1996; 15(1):47–51.
5. Johnstone FD, Haddad NG, Hoskins P, et al: Umbilical artery Doppler flow velocity waveform: The outcome of pregnancies with absent end diastolic flow. Eur J Obstet Gynecol Reprod Biol 1988; 28:171–178.
6. Brar HS, Platt LD: Reverse end-diastolic flow velocity on umbilical artery velocimetry in high-risk pregnancies: An ominous finding with adverse pregnancy outcome. Am J Obstet Gynecol 1988; 159:559–561.

▪: THE FETAL BIOPHYSICAL PROFILE
▪ ACR Code: 856 (Biophysical Profile)

Technique ▪

The fetal biophysical profile score (BPS) is determined at the time of obstetric ultrasound, usually in conjunction with morphologic evaluation of the pregnancy and measurement of biometric parameters. Table 1 lists the five variables/parameters that make up the score and defines normal/abnormal findings as described by Manning.[1] Although the criteria allow up to 30 minutes of observation, Manning found the mean testing time to be 8 minutes, since the test may be terminated when all criteria for normal have been satisfied.

Measurements ▪

The ultrasound BPS is the sum (X) of individual scores (normal = 2, abnormal = 0) for each of the four ultrasound criteria and is expressed as "X out of 8" or "X/8." When fetal cardiac monitoring is performed to determine whether there is a reactive fetal heart rate (nonstress test = NST), the BPS score is expressed as "X out of 10" or "X/10." Manning has found that when the ultrasound portion is normal (8/8), the NST does not add any prognostically useful information, and this was the case about 95% of the time.[1]

Table 1 ▪ **Fetal Biophysical Profile Scoring System**

VARIABLE	NORMAL FINDING (Score = 2)	ABNORMAL FINDING (Score = 0)
Fetal breathing movements (FBM)	At least 1 episode of FBM of at least 30 sec duration in 30 min observation	Absent FBM or no episode of >30 sec in 30-min observation
Gross body movement	At least 3 discrete body/limb movements in 30 min (episodes of active continuous movement considered as single movement)	2 or fewer episodes of body/limb movements in 30 min
Fetal tone	At least 1 episode of active extension with return to flexion of fetal limb(s) or trunk. Opening and closing of hand considered normal tone	Either slow extension with return to partial flexion or movement of limb in full extension. Absent fetal movement
Reactive fetal heart rate (FHR)	At least 2 episodes of FHR acceleration of >15 beats/min and of at least 15 sec duration, associated with fetal movement in 30 min	<2 episodes of acceleration of FHR or acceleration of <15 beats/min in 30 min
Qualitative amniotic fluid (AF) volume	At least 1 pocket of AF that measures at least 2 cm in 2 perpendicular planes	Either no AF pockets or largest pocket <2 cm in 2 perpendicular planes

From Manning FA: Clin Obstet Gynecol 1995; 38:26–44. Used by permission.

Table 2 ▪ Interpretation of Fetal Biophysical Score and Management Recommendations

TEST SCORE RESULT	INTERPRETATION	PNM WITHIN 1 WEEK WITHOUT INTERVENTION	MANAGEMENT
10/10 8/10 (normal fluid) 8/8 (NST not done)	Risk of fetal asphyxia extremely rare	1/1000	Intervention only for obstetric and maternal factors No indication for intervention for fetal disease
8/10 (abnormal fluid)	Probable chronic fetal compromise	89/1000	Determine that there is functioning renal tissue and intact membranes; if so, deliver for fetal indications
6/10 (normal fluid)	Equivocal test, possible fetal asphyxia	Variable	If the fetus is mature, deliver. In the immature fetus, repeat test within 24 hr. If <6/10, deliver
6/10 (abnormal fluid)	Probable fetal asphyxia	89/1000	Deliver for fetal indications
4/10	High probability of fetal asphyxia	91/1000	Deliver for fetal indications
2/10	Fetal asphyxia almost certain	125/1000	Deliver for fetal indications
0/10	Fetal asphyxia certain	600/1000	Deliver for fetal indications

PNM = perinatal mortality, NST = nonstress test.
From Manning FA: Clin Obstet Gynecol 1995; 38:26–44. Used by permission.

Source ▪

Since the initial prospective study of 216 patients,[2] there are reports of more than 100,000 biophysical profile evaluations in over 55,000 high-risk pregnancies.[3-6] These have informed Manning's comprehensive review of the subject abstracted here.[1]

Comments ▪

Table 2 is a guideline for interpretation of BPS obtained in high-risk pregnancies, with suggested management for various scores as outlined by Manning.[1] In addition to (inverse) correlation of BPS with perinatal mortality, there is also strong correlation between BPS and antepartum umbilical cord pH values.[1] Though these findings and suggestions are based on extensive clinical experience and several large studies, management in these difficult cases must be individualized based on local/regional standards of care, physician experience, and particulars of the case at hand.

REFERENCES

1. Manning FA: Dynamic ultrasound-based assessment: The fetal biophysical profile score. Clin Obstet Gynecol 1995; 38:26–44.
2. Manning FA, Platt LD, Sipos L: Antepartum fetal evaluation: Development of a fetal biophysical profile. Am J Obstet Gynecol 1980; 136:787–795.
3. Manning FA, Baskett TF, Morrison I, Lange I: Fetal biophysical profile scoring: A prospective study in 1,184 high-risk patients. Am J Obstet Gynecol 1981; 140:289–294.
4. Baskett TF, Allen AC, Gray JH, et al: Fetal biophysical profile scoring and prenatal death. Obstet Gynecol 1987; 70:357–370.
5. Platt LD, Eglington GS, Sipos L: Further experience with the fetal biophysical profile score. Obstet Gynecol 1983; 61:480–485.
6. Manning FA, Morrison I, Harman CR, et al: Fetal assessment based on fetal biophysical profile scoring: Experience in 19,221 referred high risk pregnancies. II: An analysis of false negative fetal death. Am J Obstet Gynecol 1987; 157:880–884.

▪: MEASUREMENT OF THE PELVIS—COLCHER-SUSSMAN METHOD[1]
▪ ACR Code: 859 (Pelvimetry)

Technique ▪

Central ray: Lateral: to greater trochanter of femur. Anteroposterior: to superior margin of pubic symphysis.
Positions: Lateral (Figure 1A): true lateral with patient lying on either right or left side; knees and thighs semiflexed. Anteroposterior (Figure 1B): patient supine with knees and thighs semiflexed and separated.
Target-film distance: 36 or 40 inches.

A specially devised ruler* is used to make measurement corrections. When positioned as described, the ruler will have the same distortion as the diameters on the same level. Therefore, the ruler markings on the film become the centimeter scale. Placement of ruler:

1. *Lateral view* (Figure 2A): The ruler is placed at the midsacral spine parallel with the spine and film. The centimeter rule markings are projected on the film for direct mensuration.
2. *Anteroposterior view* (Figure 2B): The ruler is placed at the level of the tuberosities of the ischium by direct manual palpation or by lowering the ruler 10 cm below the superior border of the symphysis pubis.

Description of Intersecting Diameters ▪ (Figure 2C and D)

Inlet:

▪ Anteroposterior diameter (I–G): Extends from the upper inner margin of the symphysis to the interior sur-

---

*This ruler, devised by Colcher and Sussman, may be obtained from the Picker X-ray Corporation.

POSITIONING

A

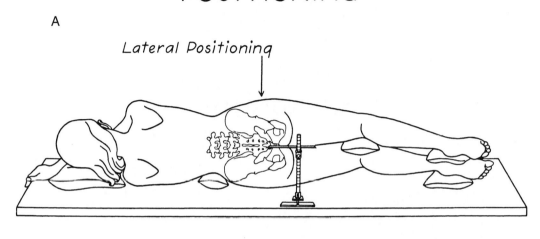

Lateral Positioning

B

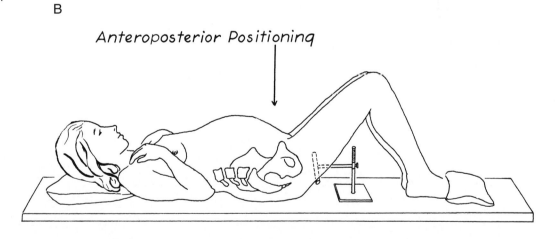

Anteroposterior Positioning

Figure 1 ▪ Technique for radiologic pelvimetry (see text for details). (From Colcher AE, Sussman W: AJR 1944; 51:207. Used by permission.)

Table 1 ▪ Inlet, Midpelvis, and Outlet Diameters

DIAMETERS	REF.	AVERAGE NORMAL	AVERAGE TOTAL	LOW NORMAL
Actual inlet				
Anteroposterior	I to G	12.5	25.5	22.0
Transverse	A to A'	13.0		
Midpelvis				
Anteroposterior	M to P	11.5	22.0	20.0
Transverse (bispinous)	B to B'	10.5		
Outlet				
Anteroposterior (post. sagittal)	S to T	7.5	18.0	16.0
Transverse (bituberal)	C to C'	10.5		

Reference points are found on Figure 2*C* and *D*.

POSITIONING WITH RULER

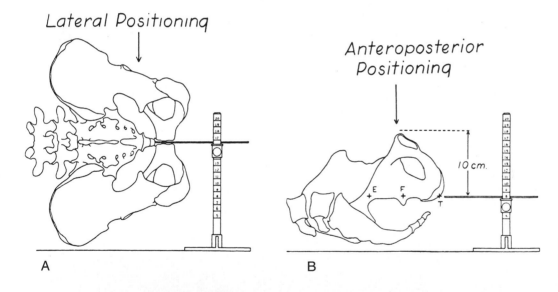

A

B

Figure 2 ▪ Measurements from pelvimetry radiographs (see text for details). (From Colcher AE, Sussman W: AJR 1944; 51:207. Used by permission.)

INTERSECTING DIAMETERS

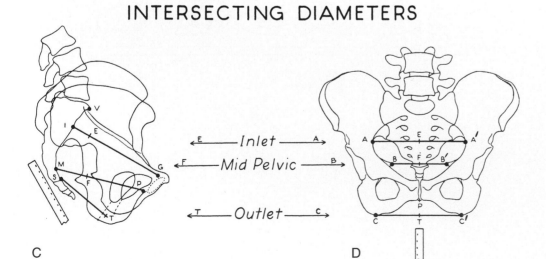

C

D

face of the sacrum following the level of the iliopectineal line, passing through a midpoint between the brim of the pelvis and the apices of the sacrosciatic notches. The apices of the notches must approximate each other.

▪ Transverse diameter *(A–A')*: Widest transverse diameter of the inlet *(E)*.

Midpelvis

▪ Anteroposterior diameter *(P–M)*: Extends from the inner lower border of the pubic symphysis through the point halfway between the contours of the two ischial spines to the anterior margin of the sacrum.

▪ Transverse diameter *(B–B')*: Transverse interspinous diameter *(F)*.

Outlet

▪ Anteroposterior diameter (postsagittal, *S–T*): Extends from the midbituberal point *(T)* to the lower anterior margin of the last sacral segment *(S)*.

Point *T* is found as follows: On the lateral view, straight lines are projected from the lower border of each obturator foramen to the lowest point on the shadow of the ischial tuberosity. These lowest points (the bituberal points) are connected by a straight line. The midbituberal point *T* is halfway between these two points.

▪ Transverse diameter (bituberal) *(C–C')*: On the film, the points *C* and *C'* are obtained by projecting a straight line from the lateral margin of the inlet along the lateral wall of the forepelvis, which appears as a dense white line on the film, to the lower margin of ischial tuberosity.

Measurements ▪

Diameters of inlet, midpelvis, and outlet (see Figure 2C and *D* and Table 1).

Source ▪

The number of patients studied is not stated by Colcher and Sussman. However, the measurements are in good agreement with those obtained in other extensive studies.

REFERENCE

1. Colcher AE, Sussman W: A practical technique for roentgen pelvimetry with a new positioning. AJR Am J Roentgenol 1944; 51:207–214.

▪: TECHNIQUE OF CT PELVIMETRY
▪ ACR Code: 859 (Pelvimetry)

Technique ▪

The technique of computed tomographic (CT) pelvimetry was first proposed by Federle and colleagues to assess pelvic proportions in the third trimester of pregnancy as an alternative to standard pelvimetry.[1] The patient lies supine on the CT couch, centered carefully (with the spine and sacrum parallel to the Z axis and centered over the X axis). The patient's hips may be flexed slightly for comfort, though it is best to have them extended. Lateral (LAT) and anteroposterior (AP) scout views (digital radiographic) are obtained through the pelvis.

Some reported technical factors are 120 to 130 kVp, 30 to 70 mA for the AP scout, and 120 to 130 kVp, 100 to 120 mA for the lateral scout.[2, 3] A single axial slice is done through the ischial spines. Technical factors reported include 80 to 130 kVp, 40 to 50 mA, and collimation up to 10 mm.[2, 3]

To determine the level of the ischial spines, first look at the LAT scout and they will be seen 70% of the time, allowing prescription of the slice level.[3] The initial reports described an unangled slice, and Ferguson and colleagues have proposed angling the gantry, as shown in Figure 1, to decrease radiation to the presenting part of the fetus.[2] The spines can sometimes be seen on the AP scout; if not visualized, the fovea of the femoral heads may be used.

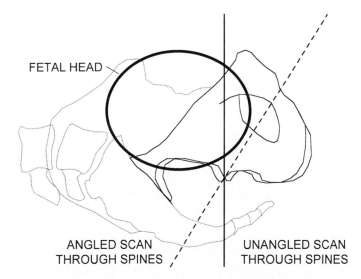

FETAL HEAD

ANGLED SCAN THROUGH SPINES

UNANGLED SCAN THROUGH SPINES

Figure 1 ▪ Prescription of an axial slice through the ischial spines is best done from the lateral scout view when the spines are visible. Angled *(dashed)* and unangled *(solid)* scan planes are shown intersecting at the ischial spines.

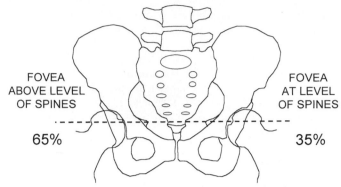

Figure 2 ▪ Relationship of the fovea of the femoral heads to the ischial spines during pelvimetry of pregnant patients. The spines (*dashed line*) typically lie at or just below the level of the inferior margin of the fovea, as shown.

Aronson and Kier found that the ischial spines were at the level of the fovea in 35% of pelvimetry patients, below them in 65% (mean 1.2 cm), and never above.[3] Therefore, if the spines are not included on an axial slice centered on the inferior margins of the fovea, the next attempt should be 1 cm lower. These relationships are shown in Figure 2.

Measurements ▪

Measurements are made from the LAT scout (anteroposterior pelvic inlet and midpelvis), as shown in Figure 3; from the AP scout (transverse pelvic inlet), as shown in Figure 4; and from the axial slice through the ischial spines (transverse midpelvis), as shown in Figure 5. These may be abbreviated as AP-IN, AP-MID, TRV-IN, and TRV-MID, respectively.

Assuming that the patient is correctly centered on the CT couch, the only measurement subject to geometric error is TRV-IN from the AP scout. Smith and McCarthy have proposed a solution to this problem that involves

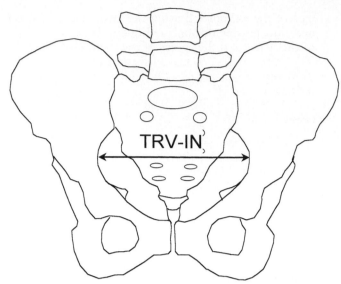

Figure 4 ▪ Measurement from anteroposterior digital radiograph (scout). The transverse pelvic inlet (*TRV-IN*) is measured at its widest point, as shown.

determining the distance (*d*) between the pelvic inlet and the gantry isocenter. Figure 6 depicts the method, and Table 1 lists correction factors for different values of d.[4]

Source ▪ None

Comments ▪

Federle and colleagues cited absorbed radiation doses of 22 mrad for the scout views and 380 mrad for the axial slice, as opposed to 885 mrad for conventional radiography.[1] Wright and colleagues calculated relative doses (conventional view = 1.0) of 0.09 for a single scout view and 0.15 for an axial slice.[5] Ferguson and associates found the dose to the fetal vertex from an unangled axial slice to average 439 mrad and from an angled axial slice— "as far as possible given patient and machine limitations"—to average 36 mrad.[2] The decision of whether or not to routinely perform an axial CT slice to visualize the ischial spines is not a

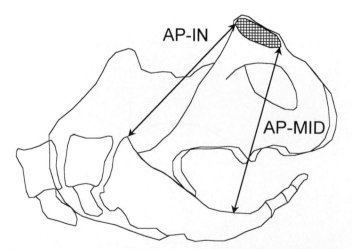

Figure 3 ▪ Measurements from lateral digital radiograph (scout). The anteroposterior pelvic inlet (*AP-IN*) is measured between the upper margin of the symphysis (*shaded*) and the sacral promontory. The anteroposterior midpelvis (*AP-MID*) is measured from the inferior margin of the symphysis through the ischial spines to the anterior margin of the sacrum/coccyx.

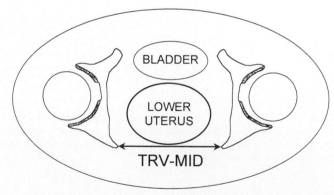

Figure 5 ▪ Measurement from an unangled axial slice through the ischial spines. The transverse midpelvis (*TRV-MID*) is measured between the spines as shown. On angled scans, the symphysis is sometimes included.

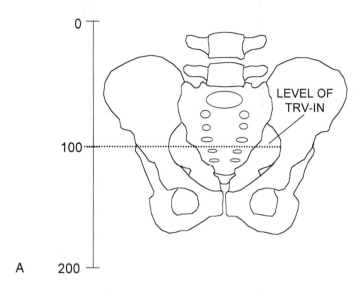

Figure 6 ▪ Method of correcting for geometric error in measurement of transverse pelvic inlet *(TRV-IN). A,* After the measurement of TRV-IN is made from the anteroposterior scout, the table position is determined. *B,* From the lateral scout, at the same table position *(dotted line),* the distance *(d)* between the line for the anteroposterior inlet *(AP-IN)* and the gantry isocenter *(dashed line)* is measured. Table 1 lists correction factors to be applied to *TRV-IN* based on *d.*

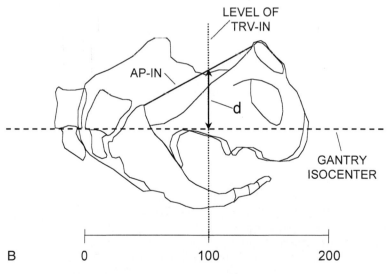

Table 1 ▪ Correction Factors for Transverse Pelvic Inlet Based on Its Relationship to the Gantry Isocenter

DISTANCE d (cm)	CORRECTION FACTOR ABOVE ISOCENTER $(63 - d)/63$	CORRECTION FACTOR BELOW ISOCENTER $(63 + d)/63$
0.5	0.992	1.008
1.0	0.984	1.016
1.5	0.976	1.024
2.0	0.968	1.032
2.5	0.960	1.040
3.0	0.952	1.048
3.5	0.944	1.056
4.0	0.937	1.063
4.5	0.929	1.071
5.0	0.921	1.079
5.5	0.913	1.087
6.0	0.905	1.095
6.5	0.897	1.103
7.0	0.889	1.111
7.5	0.881	1.120
8.0	0.873	1.127
8.5	0.865	1.135
9.0	0.857	1.143
9.5	0.849	1.151
10.0	0.841	1.159

The correction factors assume a target-detector radius of 63 cm (GE 9800 scanner). d = distance between gantry isocenter and pelvic inlet.
From Smith RC, McCarthy S: J Comput Assist Tomogr 1991; 15(5):787–789. Used by permission.

trivial one since it increases the total radiation from the procedures by a factor of 10. Some investigators maintain that the axial image is not needed to measure TRV-MID, since it can be done from the AP scout radiograph (with appropriate magnification correction), and should not be performed.[6, 10]

When compared with true dimensions of dried pelvises, measurements from CT images gave errors of about 1% and from conventional radiographs gave errors of 10%.[6] Comparisons of measurements made from CT and conventional radiographs of the same patients, as well as dried cadaveric pelvises in two small studies, gave absolute differences ranging from 2 to 11 mm.[7, 8] Morris and colleagues compared CT and conventional pelvimetry in 10 nonpregnant females of childbearing age.[9] The mean and ± standard deviations (in millimeters) of the differences were as follows: AP-MID = 0.8 ± 1.9, AP-MID = 1.3 ± 2.6, TRV-IN (measured from the axial CT slice) = 0.2 ± 2.7, TRV-IN (measured from the CT scout) = 0.6 ± 1.6, TRV-MID = −0.3 ± 2.7. In all dimensions except TRV-MID (negative mean difference), CT gave higher measurements.[9]

REFERENCES

1. Federle MP, Cohen HA, Rosenwein MF, et al: Pelvimetry by digital radiography: A low-dose examination. Radiology 1982; 143:733–735.
2. Ferguson JE, DeAngelis GA, Newberry YG, et al: Fetal radiation exposure is minimal after pelvimetry by modified digital radiography. Am J Obstet Gynecol 1996; 175:260–269.
3. Aronson D, Kier R: CT pelvimetry: The foveae are not an accurate landmark for the level of the ischial spines. AJR Am J Roentgenol 1991; 156(3):527–530.
4. Smith RC, McCarthy S: Improving the accuracy of digital CT pelvimetry. J Comput Assist Tomogr 1991; 15(5):787–789.
5. Wright DJ, Godding L, Kirkpatrick C: Technical note: Digital radiographic pelvimetry—a novel, low dose, accurate technique. Br J Radiol 1995; 68(809):528–530.
6. Alberge AY, Castellano S, Kassab M, Escude B: Pelvimetry by digital radiography. Clin Radiol 1985; 36:327–330.
7. Gimovsky ML, Willard K, Neglio M, et al: X-ray pelvimetry in a breech protocol: A comparison of digital radiography and conventional methods. Am J Obstet Gynecol 1985; 153:887–888.
8. Lotz H, Ekelund L, Hietela SO, et al: Low dose pelvimetry with biplane digital radiography. Acta Radiol 1987; 28:577–580.
9. Morris CW, Heggie JCP, Action CM: Computed tomography pelvimetry: Accuracy and radiation dose compared with conventional pelvimetry. Australas Radiol 1993; 37:186–191.
10. Lenke RR, Shuman WP: Computed tomographic pelvimetry. J Reprod Med 1986; 31:958–960.

▪: PELVIMETRY BY MAGNETIC RESONANCE IMAGING[1]
▪ ACR Code: 859 (Pelvimetry)

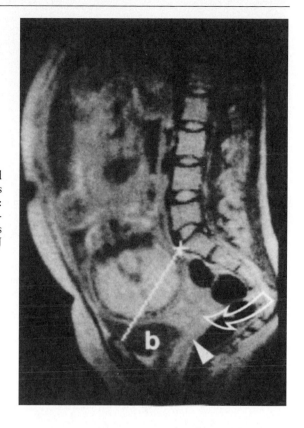

Figure 1 ▪ Sagittal, midline MRI. Fetus in vertex presentation with fetal head imaged coronally, maternal pelvis imaged sagittally. Electronic cursor measures distance between inner cortex of symphysis pubis and sacral promontory (+): AP pelvic inlet diameter. Maternal cervix *(arrow)*, vagina *(arrowhead)*, and urinary bladder *(b)* are well seen. Bony fetal calvaria is of low intensity and is covered by scalp fat of high intensity. (From Stark DD, et al: AJR Am J Roentgenol 1985; 144:947–950. Used by permission.)

Technique ▪

1. MRI is performed with a superconducting magnet at 0.35 T. An elliptical body coil with a 50 × 58 cm aperture is used.
2. Position: Supine. Spin echo technique using 1.0-sec TR for both sagittal and transverse planes.

Measurements ▪

Sagittal images are centered 5 cm below the maternal umbilicus (Figure 1).

A transverse series of 10 multislice images centered 5 cm above the symphysis pubis includes one section through the widest transverse inlet diameter (Figure 2).

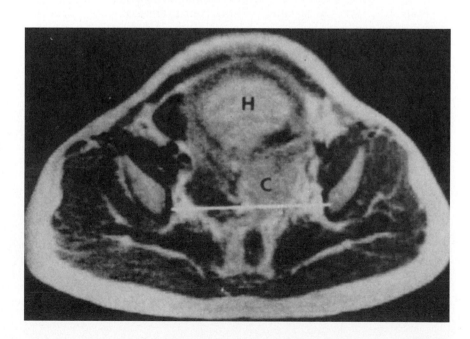

Figure 2 ▪ Transverse MRI at pelvic inlet. Vertex of fetal head *(H)* and part of cervix *(C)* are identified. Transverse inlet diameter is measured at its widest point. (From Stark DD, et al: AJR Am J Roentgenol 1985; 144:947–950. Used by permission.)

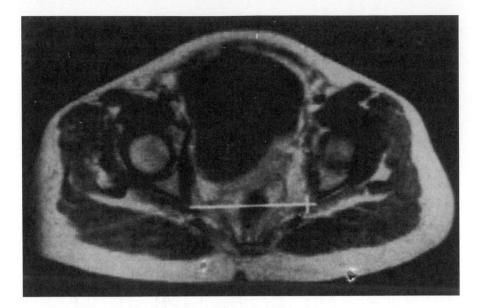

Figure 3 ▪ Transverse MRI at midpelvis. Measurement of transverse (bispinous) midpelvis diameter is shown. (From Stark DD, et al: AJR Am J Roentgenol 1985; 144:947–950. Used by permission.)

Another more caudal section obtained through the ischial spines allows measurement of the transverse midpelvis diameter (Figure 3). See next section for normal pelvic dimensions.

Source ▪

Data are based on MR examination of 10 3rd-trimester women.

REFERENCE

1. Stark DD, McCarthy SM, Filly RA, et al: Pelvimetry by magnetic resonance imaging. AJR Am J Roentgenol 1985; 144:947–950.

": CLINICAL USE OF PELVIMETRY
- ▪ ACR Code: 859 (Pelvimetry)

Technique ▪

Computed tomographic or conventional (x-ray) pelvimetry in pregnant women was performed as outlined in separate sections. It is also very useful to perform concurrent ultrasound with standard biometric measurements, including head circumference (HC) and abdominal circumference (AC), as described separately.

Measurements ▪

Measurements available from MRI, CT, or x-ray pelvimetry include the anteroposterior and transverse dimensions of the pelvic inlet and midpelvis (AP-IN, TRV-IN, AP-MID, and TRV-MID, respectively). The diameters of the pelvic inlet and midpelvis may be summed (SUM-IN and SUM-MID). Colcher and Sussman defined an adequate pelvis by SUM-IN > 22 cm and SUM-MID >20 cm.[1] The areas of the pelvic inlet and midpelvis may be approximated by multiplying the diameters (PROD-IN and PROD-MID). Mengert defined adequate "areas" as PROD-IN > 123 cm and PROD-MID > 106 cm.[2] These numbers represent 85% of the population average.[2] Patients with measurements falling below these normative values were considered to have contracted pelves.

Mengert also cited averages for the linear measurements as follows: AP-IN = 11.6 cm, TRV-IN = 12.5 cm, AP-MID = 12.1 cm, and TRV-IN = 10.3 cm.[2] Normative values of single linear measurements have not been cited much subsequently as most authors favor the sum of product of AP and TRV dimensions. However, a standard obstetrics text gives the following critical values: AP-IN = 10.0 cm, TRV-IN = 12.0 cm, AP-MID = 11.5 cm, and TRV-IN = 9.5 cm.[3]

Morgan and Thurnau have defined the fetal-pelvic index (FPI) that relates pelvimetry and ultrasound fetal measurements (definition in Table 1). They studied the value of FPI >0 in predicting operative (mostly cesarean) delivery in several groups of patients and also reported the performance of the Colcher-Sussman indices in the same papers. Table 1 lists commonly cited measurements/indices and shows the calculation of the FPI. Tables 2 and 3 list Thurnau and Morgan's results.[4–9]

Ferguson's recent study of pelvimetry yielded rather disappointing results, in contrast to those of Thurnau and Morgan, for the utility of the FPI in predicting clinical outcomes in pregnant patients suspected of having fetal-pelvic disproportion. Tables 4 and 5 list the results as well as performance of FPI, the Colcher-Sussman cut-offs, and the Mengert criteria to predict failure of a trial of labor (ending in cesarean delivery), as reported by Ferguson and colleagues.[10]

Table 1 ▪ Measurements and Indices Used in Pelvimetry

PARAMETER	ABBREVIATION	HOW OBTAINED OR CALCULATED	CRITICAL VALUE
Anteroposterior pelvic inlet	AP-IN	Directly measured from pelvimetry	10.0 cm
Transverse pelvic inlet	TRV-IN	Directly measured from pelvimetry	12.0 cm
Anteroposterior midpelvis	AP-MID	Directly measured from pelvimetry	11.5 cm
Transverse midpelvis	TRV-MID	Directly measured from pelvimetry	9.5 cm
Sum of pelvic inlet diameters	SUM-IN	AP-IN + TRV-IN	22 cm
Sum of midpelvis diameters	SUM-MID	AP-MID + TRV-IN	20 cm
Product of pelvic inlet diameters	PROD-IN	AP-IN × TRV-IN	123 cm²
Product of midpelvis diameters	PROD-MID	AP-MID × TRV-MID	106 cm²
Pelvic inlet circumference	CIR-IN	(AP-IN + TRV-IN) × $\pi/2$	—
Midpelvic circumference	CIR-MID	(AP-MID + TRV-MID) × $\pi/2$	—
Fetal head circumference	HC	Directly measured at ultrasound	—
Fetal abdominal circumference	AC	Directly measured at ultrasound	—
Abdominal-pelvic (inlet) difference	APID	AC − CIR-IN	—
Abdominal-pelvic (mid) difference	APMD	AC − CIR-MID	—
Cephalopelvic (inlet) difference	CPID	HC − CIR-IN	—
Cephalopelvic (mid) difference	CPMD	HC − CIR-MID	—
Fetal-pelvic index	FPI	Sum of the two most positive differences	0

Table 2 ▪ Performance of Colcher-Sussman Criteria in Predicting Operative Delivery

REFERENCE	GROUP	OPERATIVE		SPONTANEOUS VAGINAL		PERFORMANCE (%)	
		Cont.	Adeq.	Cont.	Adeq.	Sensitivity	Specificity
4	Original study	5	22	0	48	19	100
5	Fetal macrosomia	0	18	0	16	0	100
6	Labor inductions	1	13	0	35	7	100
7	Labor augmentations	1	23	0	22	4	100
8	Vaginal after cesarean	3	15	0	47	17	100
9	Nulliparous	22	51	3	61	22	98
4–9	Combined	32	142	3	229	18	99

Cont = contracted (SUM-IN < 22 cm or SUM-MID < 20 cm). Adeq = adequate (SUM-IN > 22 cm and SUM-MID > 20 cm).[4–9]

Table 3 ▪ Performance of Fetal Pelvic Index in Predicting Operative Delivery

REFERENCE	GROUP	OPERATIVE		SPONTANEOUS VAGINAL		PERFORMANCE (%)	
		FPI +	FPI −	FPI +	FPI −	Sensitivity	Specificity
4	Original study	27	4	0	44	87	100
5	Fetal macrosomia	17	1	1	15	94	94
6	Labor inductions	12	2	0	35	86	100
7	Labor augmentations	17	7	1	23	71	95
8	Vaginal after cesarean	13	5	0	47	72	100
9	Nulliparous	55	18	2	62	75	97
4–9	Combined	141	37	4	226	79	98

FPI = fetal pelvic index.[4–9]

Table 4 ▪ Measurements Obtained in Vaginal and Cesarean Delivery Patients

PARAMETER	CESAREAN MEAN ± SD	VAGINAL MEAN ± SD	STATISTICAL SIGNIFICANCE
Birth weight (gm)	3792 ± 440	3555 ± 474	p = .02
Ultrasound measurements			
Head circumference (cm)	34.3 ± 2.3	33.6 ± 4.6	NS
Abdominal circumference (cm)	35.2 ± 2.3	34.3 ± 4.9	NS
CT pelvimetry measurements			
Pelvic inlet circumference (cm)	40.8 ± 2.6	39.9 ± 5.9	NS
Midpelvic circumference (cm)	36.4 ± 2.4	36.8 ± 5.4	NS
Fetal-pelvic index	−2.4 ± 5.8	−5.4 ± 5.3	p = .02

CT = computed radiography/tomography, SD = standard deviation, NS = not significant.
From Ferguson JE 2nd, Newberry YG, DeAngelis GA, et al: Am J Obstet Gynecol 1998, 179:1186–1192. Used by permission.

Table 5 ▪ Performance of Pelvimetry in Predicting Cesarean Delivery

PARAMETER	CESAREAN DELIVERY	VAGINAL DELIVERY	SENSITIVITY (%)	SPECIFICITY (%)
Estimated fetal weight (U/S)			17	90
>4100 grams	5	6		
<4100 grams	25	55		
CT pelvimetry (Colcher-Sussman)			7	100
Contracted	2	0		
Adequate	28	61		
CT pelvimetry (Mengert)			10	98
Contracted	3	1		
Adequate	27	60		
Fetal-pelvic index			27	84
Positive	8	10		
Negative	22	51		

CT = computed radiography/tomography, U/S = ultrasound.
From Ferguson JE 2nd, Newberry YG, DeAngelis GA, et al: Am J Obstet Gynecol 1998; 179:1186–1192. Used by permission.

Source ▪

Colcher and Sussman based their criteria on extensive experience gained in developing their method of x-ray pelvimetry.[1] Mengert's cut-off levels were based on data from 592 patients who had x-ray pelvimetry.[2] Thurnau and Morgan's studies detail experiences with 406 patients in developing and using the FPI derived from x-ray pelvimetry.[4-9] Ferguson's subjects initially included 176 patients in the last trimester of pregnancy, with prior history and/or findings in the current pregnancy suspicious for fetal-pelvic disproportion, who had ultrasound and CT pelvimetry within 2 weeks of delivery. Of the 91 patients who fulfilled all inclusion criteria, 30 underwent cesarean section, and 61 had vaginal delivery.[10]

Comments ▪

Standard x-ray pelvimetry has been in use for over 50 years and, when combined with fetal size measurements at ultrasound (FPI), has yielded promising results, as shown by Thurnau and Morgan.[4-9] Because of concern for fetal radiation exposure, CT pelvimetry has been developed to obtain the same measurements with less than 10% to 50% of the fetal dose. However, Ferguson and associates found little clinical utility in applying the FPI and Colcher-Sussman criteria to CT-derived pelvimetry measurements. One possible explanation is that the definition of the AP-IN was slightly different between x-ray and CT pelvimetry (see separate sections on the Colcher-Sussman and CT methods). Obviously, the other potential explanation for the disparity of results involves differences in populations studied, experimental design, and obstetric practice patterns in different centers.

REFERENCES

1. Colcher AE, Sussman WA: A practical technique for roentgen pelvimetry with a new positioning. AJR Am J Roentgenol 1944; 51:207–214.
2. Mengert WF: Estimation of pelvic capacity. JAMA 1948; 138:169–174.
3. Cunningham FG, MacDonald PC, Gant NF, et al (eds): Williams Obstetrics, 29th ed. Stamford, CT, Appleton and Lange, 1997, pp 461–472.
4. Morgan MA, Thurnau GR, Fishburne JI: The fetal-pelvic index as an indicator of fetal-pelvic disproportion: A preliminary report. Am J Obstet Gynecol 1986; 155:608–613.
5. Morgan MA, Thurnau GR: Efficacy of the fetal-pelvic index for delivery of neonates weighing 4000 grams or greater. Am J Obstet Gynecol 1988; 158:1133–1137.
6. Morgan MA, Thurnau GR: Efficacy of the fetal-pelvic index in patients requiring labor induction. Am J Obstet Gynecol 1988; 159:621–625.
7. Thurnau GR, Morgan MA: Efficacy of the fetal-pelvic index as a predictor of fetal-pelvic disproportion in patients with abnormal labor patterns requiring labor augmentations. Am J Obstet Gynecol 1988; 159:1168–1672.
8. Thurnau GR, Scates DH, Morgan MA: The fetal-pelvic index: A method of identifying fetal-pelvic disproportion in women attempting vaginal birth after previous Cesarean delivery. Am J Obstet Gynecol 1991; 165:353–358.
9. Morgan MA, Thurnau GR: Efficacy of the fetal-pelvic index in nulliparous women at high risk for fetal-pelvic disproportion. Am J Obstet Gynecol 1992; 166:810–814.
10. Ferguson JE 2nd, Newberry YG, DeAngelis GA, et al: The fetal-pelvic index has minimal utility in predicting fetal-pelvic disproportion. Am J Obstet Gynecol 1998; 179:1186–1192.

CHAPTER 14

Vascular and Lymphatic Systems

∵

∵ FLOW IN NORMAL NECK VEINS
- ACR Code: 907 (Veins of the Neck)

Technique ▪

Pucheu and colleagues performed ultrasound of the internal jugular, innominate, and subclavian veins with an Ultramark 8 machine (ATL, Bellevue, WA) or a KONTRON Sigma 44 machine (Montigny-le-Bretonneux, France).[1] Muller used a model 1000 scanner (Diasonics) and 4.5-MHz pulsed-wave Doppler transducer to examine the internal jugular veins.[2] Examination was done with subjects supine and relaxed. The transducer was positioned so as to image the vein in question in longitudinal profile, and the duplex gate was placed in the lumen for Doppler measurements, which were angle corrected (<60 degrees). Gain, pulse repetition frequency, and wall filter settings were optimized to obtain the best possible tracing. Pucheu and colleagues performed continuous electrocardiogram monitoring, which was simultaneously displayed with Doppler tracings.[1]

Measurements ▪

Pucheu and colleagues measured the velocity in each vessel from frozen Doppler tracings at positions shown in Figure 1 during the mid-end systolic and diastolic portions (cardiopetal). Figure 2 shows three flow morphologies, along with their relative frequencies. Table 1 lists average measured flow velocities in each vessel (both left and right) and percentage respiratory variation as reported.[1] Muller and colleagues measured time-averaged mean velocities from the internal jugular veins over 7 to 8 seconds and multiplied the average velocity by the cross-sectional area of the vessel at the same site to obtain volume flow. Table 2 lists the flow volumes for both sides (summed) by age groups and by right and left sides.[2]

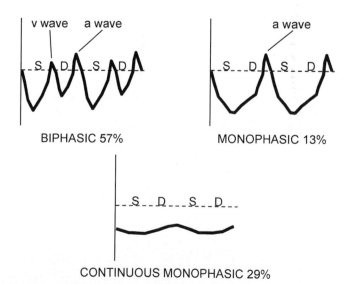

Figure 2 ▪ Different venous velocity profiles with relative frequencies found by Pucheu. Systole (S), diastole (D), the v wave, and a waves are shown. Generally, the profile morphologies were identical in all vessels examined in any one individual.[1]

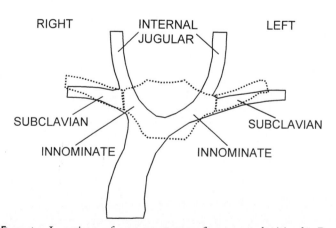

Figure 1 ▪ Locations of measurements of venous velocities by Pucheu. Muller measured volumetric flow from the internal jugular veins. The overlying sternum and medial clavicles (dotted lines) are shown.

Table 1 ▪ Flow Velocities in Neck Veins

MEASUREMENT LOCATION	MID END SYSTOLIC VELOCITY (cm/sec)		DIASTOLIC VELOCITY (cm/sec)		RESPIRATORY VARIATION (%)
	Mean ± SD	Range	Mean ± SD	Range	
R internal jugular	28 ± 15	5–77	21 ± 14	0–70	27
R innominate	33 ± 16	0–100	19 ± 10	0–62	31
R subclavian	16 ± 10	5–50	10 ± 7	0–35	38
L internal jugular	22 ± 16	0–67	18 ± 14	0–59	31
L innominate	22 ± 11	0–55	15 ± 8	0–40	40
L subclavian	11 ± 7	0–35	9 ± 6	0–28	42

cm/sec = centimeters per second, R = right, L = left, SD = standard deviation.
From Pucheu A, Evans J, Thomas D, et al: J Clin Ultrasound 1994; 22:367–373. Used by permission.

Table 2 ▪ Volume Flow in the Internal Jugular Veins

AGE (yr)	FLOW MEAN ± SD (ml/min)	
	Men	Women
21–30	766 ± 216	695 ± 162
31–40	816 ± 157	728 ± 212
41–50	726 ± 202	679 ± 242
51–60	787 ± 243	702 ± 199
All	773 ± 218	706 ± 195
	Both Sexes	
All	740 ± 209	
	Right	Left
All	770 ± 287	702 ± 193

ml/min = milliliters per minute, SD = standard deviation. All measurements except the bottom row are summed right and left flows.
From Muller HR, Hinn G, Buser MW: J Ultrasound Med 1990; 9:261–265. Used by permission.

Source ▪

Pucheu's group examined 198 neck vein systems (67 right, 131 left) in 148 patients (41 men, 107 women, mean age, 58.6 years, age range, 17 to 78 years). Any side previously catheterized, surgically damaged, or irradiated was excluded.[1] Muller's subjects were 84 volunteers and 16 patients having neurovascular checkups (normal findings) whose ages ranged from 21 to 70 years. They were evenly distributed by decade and gender (10 each).[2]

Comments ▪

There were no significant differences in velocities from side to side,[1] although the volumetric flow was greater on the right than on the left, with p <.001.[2] Pucheu and colleagues found diameters of the internal jugular and subclavian veins to average 9 mm, with a range of 5 to 15 mm, with increased diameters during deep expiration and Valsalva maneuvers and decreased size during rapid inspiration (sniffing). They also noted symmetry in Doppler flow patterns from side to side in individuals and stated that patients may serve as their own "control" when unilateral abnormality is suspected.[1]

REFERENCES

1. Pucheu A, Evans J, Thomas D, et al: Doppler ultrasonography of normal neck veins. J Clin Ultrasound 1994; 22:367–373.
2. Muller HR, Hinn G, Buser MW: Internal jugular venous flow measurement by means of a duplex scanner. J Ultrasound Med 1990; 9:261–265.

⠿ DIAMETER AND FLOW IN ARTERIES OF THE ARM AND HAND
- ACR Code: 91 (Arteries, Veins of Upper Limb)

Table 1 • Diameters and Flow Characteristics of Normal Upper Extremity Arteries

ARTERY	DIAMETER (mm)	FLOW VELOCITY (cm/sec)	FLOW VOLUME (ml/min)
Brachial	3.5 ± 0.9	75 ± 18	33.9 ± 28.4
Radial (wrist)	2.8 ± 0.6	57 ± 16	6.7 ± 4.1
Ulnar (wrist)	2.8 ± 0.6	66 ± 27	20.0 ± 23.8
Superficial arch (ulnar)	2.8 ± 0.6	48 ± 25	16.0 ± 18.9
Deep arch (radial)	2.6 ± 0.8	46 ± 15	14.6 ± 12.4
Ulnar digital			
thumb	1.3 ± 0.3	38.5 ± 11.6	—
index	1.3 ± 0.4	35.8 ± 15.8	—
long	1.2 ± 0.4	30.4 ± 14.9	—
ring	1.0 ± 0.3	24.5 ± 11.1	—
small	0.9 ± 0.4	20.5 ± 10.2	—
Radial digital			
thumb	1.1 ± 0.5	29.8 ± 16.4	—
index	1.0 ± 0.4	20.7 ± 9.2	—
long	1.1 ± 0.4	24.1 ± 11.7	—
ring	1.4 ± 0.3	29.4 ± 15.0	—
small	1.0 ± 0.4	23.5 ± 13.1	—

All measurements are given as mean ± standard deviation. mm = millimeters, cm/sec = centimeters per second, ml/min = millimeters per minute.
From Trager S, Pignataro M, Anderson J, Kleinert JM: J Hand Surgery [Am] 1993; 18:621–625. Used by permission.

Technique ▪

Ultrasound of the arm and hand was done with an Angio-Dynograph QAD 1 color flow system (Quantum Medical Systems, Issaquah, WA) with a 7.5-MHz transducer. Subjects sat for 30 minutes prior to the examination, and the room was kept at 20 degrees Centigrade or more.[1]

Measurements ▪

Measurements were made during longitudinal scanning through the vessel under study. The diameter (D), mean flow velocity over the cardiac cycle, and calculated flow volume were recorded for each vessel. For vessels larger than 1.5 mm, these three parameters could all be dynamically calculated by software in the machine. For smaller vessels, diameters and velocities were measured from frozen images and Doppler tracings. Table 1 lists the results.[1]

Source ▪

Subjects were 20 healthy volunteers (both male and female, age range, 20 to 45 years).[1]

Comments ▪

The arterial dominance at the wrist level was determined by comparing ulnar and radial flow volumes, with differences of greater than or equal to 25% considered significant. The radial artery was dominant in 35%, the ulnar in 55%, and there was balanced flow in 10%.[1]

REFERENCE

1. Trager S, Pignataro M, Anderson J, Kleinert JM: Color flow Doppler: Imaging the upper extremity. J Hand Surgery [Am] 1993; 18:621–625.

⠿ VELOCITIES IN PELVIC AND LOWER EXTREMITY ARTERIES
- ACR Code: 92 (Arteries of Lower Limb)

Technique ▪

Ultrasound of the pelvis, inguinal regions, and legs, with attention to the major arteries, was done with a QAD-1 Angiodynograph machine (Quantum, Issaquah, WA), with 3.0 to 5.0-MHz transducers. A wedged stand-off was used below the inguinal ligament. Duplex scanning guided by gray scale and color Doppler imaging was done from the midlumen of the artery in question, with the Doppler angle as close to 60 degrees as possible.[1]

Measurements ▪

From duplex tracings with a small sample volume made in the longitudinal plane, the peak systolic velocity (PSV) was

measured. Also, the quality of visualization of each vessel was noted and graded as good, poor, and not examinable.[1] Table 1 lists the results.

Source ▪

Subjects were 10 healthy volunteers (5 men, 5 women, age range, 22 to 46 years, mean age, 33 years).[1]

Comments ▪

The investigators state that an important qualitative finding in normal lower extremity arteries is that of reversed early diastolic flow. This is seen as a brief change in color after

Table 1 ▪ Visualization and Velocities from the Distal Aorta Through Calf Arteries in Normal Adults

| ARTERIAL SEGMENT | QUALITY OF EXAMINATION | | | NUMBER MEASURED | PSV (cm/sec) (Mean ± SD) |
	Good (%)	Poor (%)	Not Ex (%)		
Proximal aorta	90	—	10	9	95 ± 22
Distal aorta	80	10	10	9	92 ± 12
Proximal common iliac	85	—	15	17	86 ± 20
Distal common iliac	95	—	5	19	90 ± 21
Internal iliac	100	—	—	20	93 ± 18
Proximal external iliac	95	5	—	20	99 ± 22
Distal external iliac	100	—	—	20	96 ± 13
Proximal common femoral	95	—	5	19	89 ± 16
Distal common femoral	100	—	—	20	71 ± 15
Profunda femoris	100	—	—	20	64 ± 15
Proximal superficial femoral	100	—	—	20	73 ± 10
Midsuperficial femoral	95	—	5	19	74 ± 13
Distal superficial femoral	100	—	—	20	56 ± 12
Proximal popliteal	100	—	—	20	53 ± 9
Distal popliteal	100	—	—	20	53 ± 24
Tibioperoneal trunk	90	—	10	18	57 ± 14
Proximal anterior tibial	100	—	—	20	40 ± 7
Distal anterior tibial	100	—	—	20	56 ± 20
Proximal posterior tibial	95	—	5	16	42 ± 14
Distal posterior tibial	95	—	5	19	48 ± 23
Proximal peroneal	85	—	15	17	46 ± 14
Distal peroneal	75	5	20	16	44 ± 12

Not Ex = not examinable, PSV = peak systolic velocity, cm/sec = centimeters per second, SD = standard deviation.
From Hatsukami TS, Primozich J, Zierler RE, Strandness DE Jr: Ultrasound Med Biol 1992; 18:167–171. Used by permission.

peak systole and with duplex as a second wave (below the baseline) after the systolic. If reversal is present and there is a clear systolic window (no spectral broadening) in an artery, it is unlikely that there is significant stenosis or occlusion proximally.[1]

REFERENCE

1. Hatsukami TS, Primozich J, Zierler RE, Strandness DE Jr: Color Doppler characteristics in normal lower extremity arteries. Ultrasound Med Biol 1992; 18:167–171.

▪: DOPPLER CRITERIA FOR LOWER EXTREMITY ARTERIAL STENOSES
▪ ACR Code: 92 (Arteries of Lower Limb)

Technique ▪

Ultrasound studies of the distal aorta, pelvic arteries, and lower extremity arteries down to the knee were made with a 128 machine (Acuson, Mountain View, CA). A 3.0-MHz sector transducer was used to examine the aorta and iliac segments, and a 5.0-MHz linear transducer was used below the inguinal ligament. Duplex scanning through the midlumen in the longitudinal plane was done with the Doppler angle maintained at or near 60 degrees and the Doppler gate at 2 to 3 mm. Single-plane cut-film arteriograms, supplemented with additional views as needed, were made between 0 and 56 days (mean, 2.5 days) after the ultrasound.

Measurements ▪

Peak systolic velocity (PSV) was measured in a normal (Vn)-appearing portion of each defined arterial segment (Table 1). The maximum PSV in any suspected stenotic segment (Vs) was also recorded. A velocity ratio (Vr) was formed between these two measurements for each suspected stenosis (Vr = Vp/Vn). From arteriographic source films, stenosis was measured in terms of percent diameter

reduction by means of a ruler laid on the films. A total of 558 arterial segments in 86 legs was analyzed, and 70 of 86 legs (81%) had one or more significant stenoses (>50% diameter reduction). First-order stenoses (n = 58) were defined as the first or only lesion in any leg, and subsequent

Table 1 ▪ Arterial Velocities in Nondiseased Segments

| ARTERIAL SEGMENT | PSV (cm/sec) MEAN ± SD | |
	Normal Legs	All Legs
Aorta	76 ± 17	92 ± 46
Common iliac	111 ± 17	97 ± 40
External iliac	112 ± 49	106 ± 45
Common femoral	90 ± 41	93 ± 38
Proximal superficial femoral	89 ± 23	73 ± 44
Midsuperficial femoral	83 ± 25	65 ± 43
Distal superficial femoral	74 ± 21	60 ± 41
Popliteal	59 ± 12	47 ± 30

PSV = peak systolic velocity, cm/sec = centimeters per second, SD = standard deviation.
From Sacks D, Robinson ML, Marinelli DL, Perlmutter GS: J Ultrasound Med 1992; 11(3):95–103. Used by permission.

Table 2 ▪ Performance of Duplex Doppler Criteria for Lower Extremity Arterial Stenoses

% STENOSIS	PSV (cm/sec)	SENS/SPEC	PSV RATIO	SENS/SPEC
All Stenoses				
>50%	120	70/81	1.4	71/97
>70%	160	77/90	2.0	80/93
>90%	180	85/90	2.9	85/93
First-Order Stenoses				
>50%	120	87/82	1.4	82/98
>70%	160	94/93	2.0	94/96
>90%	180	83/93	2.9	83/96
Second-Order Stenoses				
>50%	120	56/82	1.4	62/98
>70%	160	63/92	2.0	68/95
>90%	180	86/94	2.9	86/96

PSV = peak systolic velocity in the stenosis (maximal), cm/sec = centimeters per second, PSV ratio = ratio between velocity in stenosis and in the normal artery, Sens/Spec = sensitivity and specificity.

From Sacks D, Robinson ML, Marinelli DL, Perlmutter GS: J Ultrasound Med 1992; 11(3):95–103. Used by permission.

stenoses or occlusions (n = 94) were termed second-order. Receiver operating characteristic (ROC) analysis was done using angiographic stenosis grades (>50%, >70%, or >90%) as cut-offs for disease positive/negative, with Vp or Vr as the tested variable. From this analysis, three cut-off levels of Vp and Vr were established. Table 1 lists PSV values in angiographically normal legs (n = 16) and in nonstenotic segments of the rest (n = 70). Table 2 lists test performance at various cut-off levels of Vp and Vr for the three angiographic stenosis grades.[1]

Source ▪

Subjects included 51 patients scheduled for lower extremity arteriogram who consented to have ultrasound evaluation prior to the angiogram.[1]

Comments ▪

The ultrasound evaluation was technically inadequate in 12 (23%) of the patients. This was due mostly to gas obscuring iliac arteries (n = 17). One distal superficial femoral artery was partly obscured by calcification. Examination of the infrainguinal was adequate in 50 of 51 patients (98%).[1]

REFERENCE

1. Sacks D, Robinson ML, Marinelli DL, Perlmutter GS: Peripheral arterial Doppler ultrasonography: Diagnostic criteria. J Ultrasound Med 1992; 11(3):95–103.

▪▪ INFRAINGUINAL ARTERIAL BYPASS GRAFT SURVEILLANCE WITH ULTRASOUND
▪ ACR Code: 92 (Arteries of Lower Limb)

Technique ▪

Ultrasound of the graft is done with machines that have real-time gray scale, color Doppler, and duplex Doppler capability and 5.0- to 7.5-MHz transducers. The patients are usually examined supine, and the leg to be examined is slightly flexed. The entire graft is examined (mostly in the longitudinal plane) with color Doppler to visualize the lumen and any stenotic segments. Careful attention must be paid to the anastomotic sites. Duplex Doppler is done with a sample gate of about 1.5 mm and an angle of <60 degrees. Angle correction of measured velocities is required.[1–5] A wedge-shaped stand-off pad may be useful in obtaining optimal Doppler angles.

Measurements ▪

The peak systolic velocity (PSV) is measured in the proximal, middle, and distal portions of the graft (Vbody) away from the anastomoses and any stenoses or tortuosities. PSV is also recorded from each anastomosis, as well as the native inflow and outflow arteries of the graft. If areas of stenosis or flow disturbance are detected at gray scale or color Doppler imaging, additional paired PSV measurements are done within the stenosis (Vs) and in an adjacent normal graft/artery segment (Vn). This allows calculation of a velocity ratio (Vr) to aid in grading the stenosis. Buth and colleagues calculated the inverse of VR (Vn/Vs) and used the term velocity index (VI). They also measured the end-diastolic velocity (EDV) in the narrowest part of the graft.[5] The relative positions of these measurements are shown in Figure 1 for different portions of the graft. Table 1 lists criteria from the technical bulletin by the American Institute of Ultrasound in Medicine (AIUM),[1] from two studies[3,4] abstracted in Beidle's review article,[2] and by Buth and colleagues.[5]

Source ▪

The Education Committee of the AIUM has produced an excellent technical bulletin on infrainguinal vein graft surveillance, and Beidle and colleagues reviewed the sub-

Table 1 ▪ Criteria for Abnormality During Infrainguinal Graft Surveillance

REFERENCE	CONDITION	CRITERIA (cm/sec)	SENS/SPEC (%)	PPV/NPV (%)
AIUM Tech Bull[1]	Low-flow graft	Vbody < 45	—	—
	Minimal criteria for flow-reducing lesion	Vs > 150 with spectral broadening and VR > 1.5	—	—
	≥50% stenosis	Vs > 200 and VR > 2.0	—	—
	≥75% stenosis	Vs > 400 and VR > 4.0	—	—
Taylor[3]	≥50% stenosis	VR ≥ 2.0 or Vbody < 45	100 / 98	96 / 100
Sladen[4]	≥50% stenosis	VR > 3.0 or Vs > 300 or Vbody < 45	98 / 87	80 / 90
Buth[5]	≥50% stenosis	VI < 0.65 (VR > 1.54)	89 / 92	85 / 95
		Vbody < 45	13 / 99	83 / 71
		EDV > 20	59 / 100	100 / 77
	≥70% stenosis	VI < 0.55 (VR > 1.82)	92 / 87	66 / 97
		Vbody < 45	16 / 98	67 / 81
		EDV > 20	91 / 100	100 / 97

cm/sec = centimeters per second, Sens/Spec = sensitivity/specificity, PPV = positive predictive value, NPV = negative predictive value. Criteria abbreviations as in Figure 1 and text.[1-6]

Vs=PSV IN STENOSIS, ALSO EDV (Buth)

Vn=PSV IN NORMAL SEGMENT

$$VR = \frac{Vs}{Vn} \quad VI = \frac{Vn}{Vs}$$

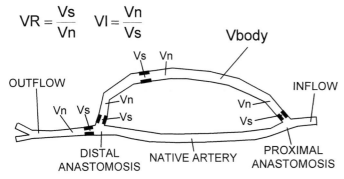

Figure 1 ▪ Doppler measurements from infrainguinal vein grafts for surveillance. The peak systolic velocity *(PSV)* is measured in the graft body *(Vbody)* in a nonstenotic straight segment. The maximum PSV in any identified stenoses *(Vs)* and in an adjacent normal graft/arterial segment *(Vn)* is measured as shown, depending on the position of the stenosis. The ratio of the two *(VR)* or an index *(VI)* may be calculated as shown.

ject.[1,2] Buth and associates studied 116 grafts in 112 patients with duplex and color Doppler ultrasound as well as digital subtraction angiography.[5]

Comments ▪

About one third of grafts develop significant stenoses, and most of these occur within 1 year of surgery, with a small percentage developing from 1 to 2 years. After 2 years, lesions develop at a rate of 2% to 3% per year.[1] Beidle and associates describe a typical ultrasound surveillance protocol with the first examination at 6 weeks and follow-up at 3, 6, 9, 12, and 18 months.[2] Some workers advocate using ankle-brachial pressure index (ABI) as a screening tool, with a decrease in ABI of 0.15 to 0.2 (compared with baseline postoperative values) signaling the need for ultrasound examination.[6-9] However, significant stenoses have been found in grafts that show a decrease in resting ABI of less than 0.1.[7,10] Idu and associates found that the assisted patency rate of infrainguinal grafts was 91% when regular ultrasound surveillance was undertaken, compared with 72% in those followed clinically.[7]

In addition to stenoses, arteriovenous fistulas involving the graft may be problematic. These can be detected with color Doppler by virtue of persistent diastolic flow above and through the fistula, as well as loss of diastolic flow reversal proximally on duplex tracings.[2]

REFERENCES

1. Education Committee, American Institute of Ultrasound in Medicine: Color duplex imaging for graft surveillance of the autologous vein graft. J Ultrasound Med 1998; 17:789–795.
2. Beidle TR, Brom-Ferral R, Letourneau JG: Surveillance of infrainguinal vein grafts with duplex sonography. AJR Am J Roentgenol 1994; 162:443–448.
3. Taylor PR, Tyrell MR, Crofton M, et al: Colour flow imaging in the detection of femoro-distal graft and native artery stenosis: Improved criteria. Eur J Vasc Surg 1992; 6:232–236.
4. Sladen JG, Reid JD, Cooperberg PL, et al: Color-flow duplex screening of infrainguinal grafts combining low- and high-velocity criteria. Am J Surg 1989; 158:107–112.
5. Buth J, Disselhoff B, Sommeling C, Stam L: Color-flow duplex criteria for grading stenosis in infrainguinal vein grafts. J Vasc Surg 1991; 14:716–728.
6. Mattos MA, van Bemmelen PS, Hodgson KJ, et al: Does correction of stenoses identified with color duplex scanning improve infrainguinal graft patency? J Vasc Surg 1993; 17:54–66.
7. Idu MM, Blankenstein JD, Gier P, et al: Impact of a color-flow duplex surveillance program on infrainguinal vein graft patency: A five-year experience. J Vasc Surg 1993; 17:42–53.
8. Grigg MJ, Nicolaides AN, Wolfe JH: Femorodistal vein bypass graft stenoses. Br J Surg 1988; 75:737–740.
9. Stierli P, Aeberhard P, Livers M: The role of colour flow duplex screening in infrainguinal vein grafts. Eur J Vasc Surg 1992; 6:293–298.
10. Brennan JA, Walsh AKM, Beard JD, et al: The role of simple non-invasive testing in infrainguinal vein graft surveillance. Eur J Vasc Surg 1991; 5:13–17.

▪: SIZE OF LEG VEINS AT ULTRASOUND
▪ ACR Code: 93 (Veins of Lower Limb)

Technique ▪

Ultrasound of the lower extremity vessels was done with HDI (ATL, Bothel, WA) and 128 or XP (Acuson, Mountain View, CA) machines and linear or curved array transducers from 3.5 to 7.0 MHz. Standard techniques were used, including gray scale graded compression, duplex Doppler, and color Doppler sonography.[1]

Measurements ▪

Anteroposterior (AP) vein and artery diameters were measured from frozen transverse images obtained at five levels: common femoral vein (CFV) in the groin, high superficial vein (High SFV) 1 to 2 cm below its origin, middle superficial vein (Mid SFV), low superficial vein (Low SFV) about 1 to 2 cm above the adductor canal, and popliteal vein (Pop Vein). The vein-to-artery ratio was calculated from each pair of measurements by dividing AP diameter of the vein by the adjacent artery.[1] Table 1 lists the vein diameters and vein/artery ratios at each level in patients with no evidence of deep venous thrombosis (DVT), those with acute DVT, and those with chronic DVT. Table 2 lists the differences in average values of vein diameters and vein/artery ratio between normal subjects and those with acute DVT, as well as between normal subjects and those with chronic DVT.

Source ▪

Sonograms were obtained from 975 legs of 721 symptomatic individuals referred for possible DVT. By standard ultrasound criteria, 768 legs were negative, 127 had acute DVT, 66 had chronic DVT, and 14 were indeterminate.

Table 1 ▪ Vein Diameters and Vein/Artery Ratios in Normal Subjects, Acute DVT, and Chronic DVT

VESSEL	VEIN DIAMETER (mm)		VEIN/ARTERY RATIO	
	Mean ± SD	Range	Mean ± SD	Range
	Normal			
CFV	10.57 ± 2.88	3.80–23.60	1.34 ± 0.37	0.52–2.93
High SFV	7.10 ± 1.96	2.60–14.80	1.24 ± 0.36	0.53–2.90
Mid SFV	6.41 ± 1.72	2.00–13.20	1.21 ± 0.33	0.42–2.76
Low SFV	6.52 ± 1.74	2.00–14.20	1.19 ± 0.32	0.45–2.74
Pop Vein	6.80 ± 2.11	1.50–15.70	1.22 ± 0.36	0.39–3.64
	Acute Deep Venous Thrombosis			
CFV	12.46	5.00–21.70	1.52	0.46–3.15
High SFV	9.14	3.40–19.50	1.58	0.55–3.43
Mid SFV	7.73	3.00–12.40	1.44	0.65–2.41
Low SFV	8.21	2.70–15.30	1.45	0.51–2.32
Pop Vein	8.82	3.80–14.40	1.49	0.80–2.55
	Chronic Deep Venous Thrombosis			
CFV	9.50 ± 2.74	5.00–13.90	1.25 ± 0.37	0.67–2.19
High SFV	6.79 ± 2.01	2.00–11.60	1.16 ± 0.42	0.23–2.77
Mid SFV	5.47 ± 2.48	2.00–16.00	1.00 ± 0.37	0.43–1.69
Low SFV	6.44 ± 2.04	3.00–10.80	1.13 ± 0.29	0.57–1.68
Pop Vein	5.90 ± 2.11	1.00–9.60	1.25 ± 0.37	0.64–1.91

Vessel abbreviations are given in text.
From Hertzberg BS, Kliewer MA, Delong DM, et al: AJR Am J Roentgenol 1997; 168:1253–1257. Used by permission.

Table 2 ▪ Differences in Vein Diameters and Vein/Artery Ratios Between Normal Subjects, Acute DVT, and Chronic DVT

VESSEL	DIFFERENCE (mm) ACUTE DVT–NORMAL		DIFFERENCE (mm) CHRONIC DVT–NORMAL	
	Vein Diameter	Vein/Artery Ratio	Vein Diameter	Vein/Artery Ratio
CFV	1.89	0.18	−1.07	−0.09
High SFV	2.04	0.34	−0.31	−0.08
Mid SFV	1.32	0.23	−0.94	−0.21
Low SFV	1.69	0.26	−0.08	−0.06
Pop Vein	2.02	0.27	−0.90	+0.03

Vessel abbreviations are given in text.
From Hertzberg BS, Kliewer MA, Delong DM, et al: AJR Am J Roentgenol 1997; 168:1253–1257. Used by permission.

Comments ▪

There were no significant differences between right and left sides. Veins with acute DVT were larger and veins with chronic DVT were smaller than negative veins, and the vein/artery ratio showed corresponding changes. However, the researchers found that there was considerable overlap in values between populations and recommend that vein diameters be interpreted in concert with other findings.[1] In a subsequent article, Hertzberg and associates compared diameter measurements with subjective impressions (small, normal, enlarged) of vein size. They felt that vein size can be reliably characterized by subjective impres-sions, obviating the need for routine measurement. In general, vein segments subjectively classified as small had measured diameters that were 60% to 80% less than normal, and those considered to be enlarged had measured diameters 140% to 160% larger than normal.[2]

REFERENCES

1. Hertzberg BS, Kliewer MA, DeLong DM, et al: Sonographic assessment of lower limb vein diameters: Implications for the diagnosis and characterization of deep venous thrombosis. AJR Am J Roentgenol 1997; 168:1253–1257.
2. Hertzberg BS, Kliewer MA, DeLong DM, et al: Sonographic estimates of vein size in the lower extremities: Subjective assessment compared with direct measurement. J Clin Ultrasound 1998; 26:113–117.

▪▪ DOPPLER PARAMETERS OF ABDOMINAL ARTERIES AND VEINS
▪ ACR Code: 95 (Arteries, Veins of Gastrointestinal System, Diaphragm, and Abdominal Wall)

Technique ▪

Abdominal ultrasound for evaluation of vascular structures is done with appropriate transducers, depending on the vessel to be interrogated and body habitus. Color Doppler is helpful to locate vessels and to guide Doppler gate placement in some cases.

Measurements ▪

Measurements are typically done in the longitudinal plane (with respect to the vessel being examined). For peak systolic velocity (PSV), end-diastolic velocity (EDV), and time-averaged velocity (Vmean), angle correction is required for accurate results, and the Doppler angle should

Table 1 ▪ Normal Ranges for Duplex-Sonographic Measurements in Various Abdominal Arteries

ARTERY	PSV (cm/sec)	EDV (cm/sec)	VMEAN (cm/sec)	RI	DIAMETER (mm)
Abdominal aorta	50–120	—	—	—	15–25
Celiac trunk	100–237	23–58	45–55	0.66–0.82	6–10
Splenic artery	70–110	—	15–40	—	4–8
Common hepatic artery	70–120	—	20–40	—	4–10
Left gastric artery	45–80	10–20	20–40	—	—
Gastroduodenal artery	13–29	—	—	—	2–5
Superior mesenteric artery	124–218	5–30	15–35	0.75–0.9	5–8
Renal artery	60–180	20–65	—	0.6–0.8	5–8
Inferior mesenteric artery	108–155	5–20	—	0.8–0.9	3–7
Ovarian artery	56–148	—	—	—	—
Uterine artery	—	—	—	0.8–0.9	—

PSV = peak systolic velocity, EDV = end-diastolic velocity, Vmean = time-averaged velocity, RI = resistive index.
From Hennerici M, Neuerburg-Heusler D: Thieme Medical Publishers, New York, 1998, pp 238–251. Used by permission.

Table 2 ▪ Normal Values for Duplex-Sonographic Measurements in Various Abdominal Veins

VEIN	PSV (cm/sec)	VMEAN (cm/sec)	FLOW RATE (ml/min/kg)	DIAMETER (mm)
Inferior vena cava	44–118	5–25	—	15–30
Hepatic veins	16–40	—	—	—
Portal vein	15–30	12–18	10–21	7–15
Splenic vein	9–30	5–12	2–5	5–10
Renal vein	18–33	10–20	—	4–9
Segmental veins	10–30	—	—	1–4
Superior mesenteric vein	8–40	9–18	3–9	4–13
Inferior mesenteric vein	—	—	—	3–7

PSV = peak systolic velocity, Vmean = time-averaged velocity, cm/sec = centimeters per second, ml/min/kg = milliliters per minute per kilogram of body weight, mm = millimeters.
From Hennerici M, Neuerburg-Heusler D: Thieme Medical Publishers, New York, 1998, pp 282–290. Used by permission.

be less than 60 degrees. For resistive index (RI), angle correction is not needed. Diameter (D) may be measured from frozen longitudinal or perpendicular transverse (with respect to the vessel) gray scale images with electronic calipers. The volume flow rate is calculated by multiplying Vmean by the area (pi/4 × D squared). Table 1 lists Doppler parameters and diameters of abdominal arteries, and Table 2 lists Doppler measurements and diameters of abdominal veins.[1, 2]

Source ▪

These tables are from an excellent text of vascular ultrasound and are derived from extensive review of the literature and the investigators' own clinical experience.[1, 2]

REFERENCES

1. Hennerici M, Neuerburg-Heusler D: Abdominal arteries; Normal findings. In Vascular Diagnosis with Ultrasound. Thieme Medical Publishers, New York, 1998, pp 238–251.
2. Hennerici M, Neuerburg-Heusler D: Abdominal veins; Normal findings. In Vascular Diagnosis with Ultrasound. Thieme Medical Publishers, New York, 1998, pp 282–290.

▪: MEASUREMENT OF SIZE OF MESENTERIC VESSELS[1]
▪ ACR Code: 95 (Mesenteric Arteries)

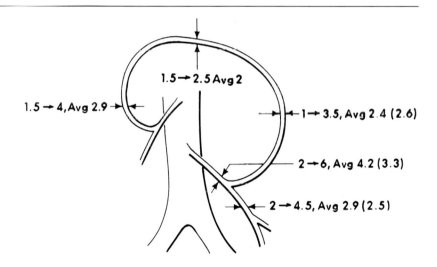

Figure 1 ▪ Measurement of mesenteric vessels to the colon beyond the mid-transverse colon. (From Wittenberg J, et al: AJR Am J Roentgenol 1975; 123:287. Used by permission.)

Technique ▪

Central ray: Perpendicular to plane of film.
Position: Anteroposterior.
Target-film distance: 40 inches.

Measurements ▪ (Figure 1)

The numbers represent the width of the vessels in millimeters as measured at points designated by the *arrows*. Both range and averages are given. The numbers in parentheses represent the average in millimeters for the same vessel as determined by Kahn and Abrams.[2]

Source ▪

Data are based on a study of 19 patients, 11 women and 8 men. The ages ranged from 56 to 89 years; the average age was 73 years.

REFERENCES

1. Wittenberg J, Athanasoalis CA, Williams LF Jr, et al: Ischemic colitis; Radiology and pathology. AJR Am J Roentgenol 1975; 123:287–300.
2. Kahn and Abrams: Radiology 1964; 82:429.

▪: DIAMETER AND FLOW IN SUPERIOR MESENTERIC AND CELIAC BRANCH ARTERIES

▪ ACR Code: 95 (Celiac and Superior Mesenteric Arteries)

Technique ▪

Ultrasound of the abdomen was performed with various machines and duplex Doppler-capable transducers ranging from 2 to 5 MHz. Examinations were done after fasting, supine, and during quiet breathing that was suspended during Doppler measurements.[1–4]

Measurements ▪

Gray scale scanning located the vessel in question, based on anatomic criteria. Doppler signals were obtained with the sample volume centrally placed within the lumen of the artery, within a few centimeters of the origin, guided by gray scale imaging through the long axis. Doppler insonation angles were maintained at less than 60 degrees for the most part. A Doppler tracing encompassing several cardiac cycles was obtained. The angle-corrected time-averaged velocity was then calculated on the ultrasound unit,[1, 3] by planimetry from paper recordings,[4] or after transfer of the spectrum to an off-line processor.[2] The diameter of the artery was also measured at the same point where Doppler signals were obtained. Volume flow rate was calculated by multiplying the time-averaged velocity by the vessel area ([pi × D squared]/4). Patient weights were used to calculate volume flow per kilogram.[1, 3, 4]

Figure 1 shows the vessels measured. Table 1 lists the results, including artery diameters, volume flow rate, and volume flow per kilogram. The sum of the splenic artery (SA) and the superior mesenteric artery (SMA) (SA + SMA) is shown as reported by Sato and Zwiebel and their colleagues.[1, 2] Table 2 gives results from Nakamura's study, including the pulsatility index (PI) in each vessel studied.[4]

Source ▪

Sato and colleagues studied 28 healthy adult volunteers, 27 adults with chronic hepatitis, and 32 adults with cirrhosis.[1] Zwiebel and associates evaluated 20 healthy adults and 20 patients with hepatic cirrhosis and portal hypertension.[2] Uzawa's subjects were 41 healthy adults.[3] The number column in Figure 1 lists the number of vessels successfully measured in each group. Nakamura and group evaluated healthy adult volunteers, and the numbers of subjects are given in Table 2.[4]

Comments ▪

Zwiebel and associates also measured the length of the spleen and found it to be greater than 13 cm in eight of the patients with cirrhosis. Within the cirrhosis group, volume flow rates in the SA, SMA, and SA + SMA were

---

Table 1 ▪ Diameters and Volume Flow Rates in Celiac Branches and Superior Mesentric Artery

REFERENCE/VESSEL	NO.	DIAMETER (mm)	FLOW (ml/min)	FLOW (ml/min/kg)
Sato (normal)				
SA	24	4.5 ± 0.5	179 ± 37	3.3 ± 0.7
SMA	21	6.4 ± 0.7	383 ± 90	7.0 ± 1.9
SA + SMA	18		578 ± 114	10.7 ± 2.3
Sato (chronic hepatitis)				
SA	25	5.0 ± 0.5	236 ± 89	4.1 ± 1.4
SMA	20	6.5 ± 0.8	399 ± 107	6.8 ± 1.5
SA + SMA	18		649 ± 162	11.4 ± 2.1
Sato (cirrhosis)				
SA	25	5.8 ± 0.9	432 ± 144	7.6 ± 2.4
SMA	26	6.4 ± 0.7	547 ± 111	9.6 ± 2.1
SA + SMA	19		989 ± 218	17.5 ± 4.0
Zwiebel (normal)				
SA	17		413 ± 110	
SMA	20		445 ± 63	
SA + SMA	17		853 ± 108	
Zwiebel (cirrhosis, PH)				
SA	17		599 ± 340	
SMA	20		574 ± 220	
SA + SMA	17		1130 ± 551	
Uzawa (normal)				
GDA	12	2.62 ± 1.4	67 ± 20	1.41 ± 0.50
PHA	12	2.74 ± 2.0	80 ± 65	1.57 ± 1.22
CHA	6	3.93 ± 2.5	195 ± 128	3.79 ± 2.10
CA	9	5.85 ± 3.6	516 ± 292	9.95 ± 6.72
SA	12	4.02 ± 3.3	247 ± 179	4.59 ± 3.19
SMA	11	6.13 ± 4.8	374 ± 210	7.01 ± 3.78

All measurements given as mean ± standard deviation. mm = millimeters, ml/min = milliliters per minute, ml/min/kg = milliliters per minute per kilogram body weight. PH = portal hypertension. Vessel abbreviations are given in Figure 1 legend.[1–3]

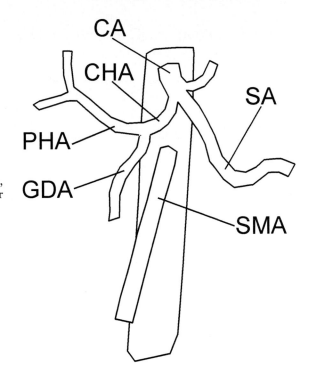

Figure 1 ▪ Arteries measured include: celiac *(CA)*, common hepatic *(CHA)*, proper hepatic *(PHA)*, gastroduodenal *(GDA)*, splenic *(SA)*, and superior mesenteric *(SMA)*.

Table 2 ▪ Doppler Flow Measurements in Normal Superior Mesentric, Splenic, and Common Hepatic Arteries

VESSEL	GENDER	NO.	DIAMETER (mm)	VELOCITY (cm/sec)	FLOW (ml/min)	FLOW (ml/min/kg)	PULSATILITY INDEX
SMA	Male	25	6.6±3.7	26.2±7.8	516+183	8.9±2.8	0.85±0.07
	Female	22	5.8±3.1	28.5±6.8	434±136	8.7±2.8	0.85±0.04
	TOTAL	47	6.2±3.6	27.3±7.4	478±166	8.8±2.8	0.85±0.06
SA	Male	15	4.8±2.7	36.1±10.1	398±202	6.8±2.0	0.74±0.10
	Female	6	4.6±2.5	31.0±7.2	301±96	5.9±1.9	0.76±0.08
	TOTAL	21	4.8±2.6	34.6±9.5	370±181	6.5±2.7	0.75±0.09
CHA	Male	12	4.3±2.4	30.3±10.0	267±154	4.7±3.0	0.80±0.05
	Female	6	4.1±2.5	33.7±19.3	226±70	4.6±1.5	0.77±0.07
	TOTAL	18	4.2±2.4	31.3±13.3	254±131	4.7±2.6	0.79±0.05

All measurements given as mean ± standard deviation. mm = millimeters, ml/min = milliliters per minute, ml/min/kg = milliliters per minute per kilogram body weight, cm/sec = centimeters per second. Vessel abbreviations given in Figure 1 legend.
From Nakamura T, Moriyasu F, Ban N, et al: J Clin Ultrasound 1989; 17:261–268. Used by permission.

all greater in those with enlarged spleens compared with those with normal spleen size (e.g., SA + SMA = 1463 ± 574 ml/min versus 1130 ± 551).[2] Zwiebel and group tested the measurement system with a flow phantom and found that it underestimated actual flow by 2% to 10%.[2] Sato and colleagues compared ultrasound (U/S) flow measurements with those obtained with an electromagnetic transducer (EMT) mounted directly on the same artery in dogs.[1] The following correlations were obtained:

EMT flow in SMA =
$$0.59 \times \text{U/S flow} + 23 \ (n = 14, r = 0.93).$$

EMT flow in SA =
$$0.62 \times \text{U/S flow} + 24 \ (n = 12, r = 0.93).$$

REFERENCES

1. Sato S, Ohnishi K, Sugita S, Okuda K: Splenic artery and superior mesenteric artery blood flow: Non-surgical Doppler US measurement in healthy subjects and patients with chronic liver disease. Radiology 1987; 164:347–352.
2. Zwiebel WJ, Mountford RA, Halliwell MJ, Wells PNT: Splanchnic blood flow in patients with cirrhosis and portal hypertension: Investigation with duplex Doppler US. Radiology 1995; 194:807–812.
3. Uzawa M, Karasawa E, Sugiura N, et al: Doppler color flow imaging in the detection and quantitative measurement of the gastroduodenal artery blood flow. J Clin Ultrasound 1993; 21:9–17.
4. Nakamura T, Moriyasu F, Ban N, et al: Quantitative measurement of abdominal arterial blood flow using image-directed Doppler ultrasonography: Superior mesenteric, splenic, and common hepatic arterial blood flow in normal adults. J Clin Ultrasound 1989; 17:261–268.

⁛ WAVEFORMS AND FLOW IN THE INFERIOR MESENTERIC ARTERY
▪ ACR Code: 956 (Inferior Mesenteric Artery)

Table 1 ▪ Doppler Flow Parameters and Diameter in the Inferior Mesenteric Artery

PARAMETER	UNITS	CONTROL GROUP	CA OR SMA OCCLUSION	ILIAC ARTERY OCCLUSION	AORTIC OCCLUSION
Number in group	—	24	5	9	19
Volume flow	(ml/min)	116 ± 76	1244 ± 963	550 ± 467	378 ± 275
Peak systolic velocity	(m/sec)	0.98 ± 0.30	1.89 ± 0.58	1.90 ± 0.88	1.26 ± 0.60
End-diastolic velocity	(m/sec)	0.11 ± 0.05	0.35 ± 0.22	0.18 ± 0.08	0.24 ± 0.15
Mean flow velocity	(m/sec)	0.25 ± 0.08	0.91 ± 0.51	0.61 ± 0.31	0.54 ± 0.28
Resistive index	—	0.89 ± 0.06	0.81 ± 0.11	0.89 ± 0.05	0.81 ± 0.09
Pulsatility index	—	4.50 ± 1.53	1.94 ± 0.62	3.07 ± 0.80	2.08 ± 0.97
Diameter	(mm)	3.08 ± 0.68	5.18 ± 1.10	4.13 ± 0.89	4.15 ± 0.87

CA = celiac artery, SMA = superior mesenteric artery, ml/min = milliliters per minute, m/sec = meters per second, mm = millimeters.
From Erden A, Yurdakul M, Cumhar T: AJR Am J Roentgenol 1998; 171:619–627. Used by permission.

Technique ▪

Ultrasound of the lower abdomen was done with an SSA-270A machine (Toshiba, Japan), with 3.75-MHz curved array or 7.5-MHz linear array transducers. Subjects were scanned in the supine position after an overnight fast.[1]

Measurements ▪

The proximal inferior mesenteric artery (IMA) was identified arising from the aorta anteriorly and to the left (usually around the L–3 level). Duplex scanning aided by color flow mapping in the longitudinal plane was done to obtain Doppler signals from the lumen of the IMA in the proximal 3 to 4 cm. If the proximal IMA was occluded, the distal main truncus was interrogated between the lower margin of the occlusion and the level of the aortic bifurcation.[1] Direct measurements were made from Doppler tracings using built-in software on the ultrasound machine. These included peak systolic velocity (PSV), end-diastolic velocity (EDV), and time-averaged mean flow velocity (Vmean). The diameter (D) of the vessel at the site of Doppler interrogation was also measured. From these the resistive index (RI), pulsatility index (PI), and blood flow volume (BFV) were calculated as follows:

$$RI = (PSV - EDV) / PSV$$
$$PI = (PSV - EDV) / Vmean$$
$$BFV = Vmean \times \pi D^2/4$$

Table 1 lists the results in normal controls and in three groups of patients with splanchnic, iliac, or aortic occlusion.

Source ▪

Subjects included 24 healthy adult volunteers (12 men, 12 women, age range, 23 to 75 years); 5 patients with celiac or superior mesenteric artery occlusion (3 men, 2 women, age range, 29 to 75 years); 9 men (age range, 46 to 73 years) with iliac occlusion; and 19 patients (18 men, 1 woman, range, 38 to 80 years). The vascular findings were confirmed at intra-arterial digital subtraction arteriography done within 48 hours of the ultrasound examinations.[1]

Comments ▪

One patient had occlusion of the origins of the IMA and the SMA, with retrograde filling of the IMA via the superior rectal artery from the right internal iliac. The ultrasound flow parameters were listed separately as follows: BFV = 250.8 ml/min, PSV = 0.5 m/sec, EDV = 0.29 m/sec, Vmean = 0.38 m/sec, RI = 0.43, PI = 0.58, and D = 3.8 mm. Previously reported success rates for detecting the IMA at ultrasound range from 77% to 92%.[2–4] The investigators were able to obtain measurements from 91% of their patients.[1] When examination of the IMA shows it to be unduly enlarged and Doppler study yields a monophasic, low-resistance, high-flow pattern, occlusive disease elsewhere in the abdomen may be inferred.

References

1. Erden A, Yurdakul M, Cumhar T: Doppler waveforms of the normal and collateralized inferior mesenteric artery. AJR Am J Roentgenol 1998; 171:619–627.
2. Sturm W, Judmaier G, Moriggi B, Kathrein H: Visualization of the inferior mesenteric artery in the ultrasound B image. Ultraschall Med 1995; 16:167–171.
3. Mirk P: Sonographic and Doppler assessment of the inferior mesenteric artery [letter]. J Ultrasound Med 1996; 15:78–79.
4. Denys AL, Lafortune M, Aubin B, et al: Doppler sonography of the inferior mesenteric artery: A preliminary study. J Ultrasound Med 1995; 14:435–439.

∴ HEPATIC DOPPLER PERFUSION INDEX FOR DETECTING METASTASES
▪ ACR Code: 958 DPI (Hepatic Perfusion)

Technique ▪

Ultrasound of the upper abdomen was done with a Spectra machine (Diasonics, Bedford, England) and a 3.5-MHz transducer, with pulsed Doppler at 3.0 MHz and a pulse repetition frequency of 3.7 MHz. Patients were examined after a 12-hour fast and were supine; measurements were made during suspended respiration (expiratory phase). Doppler angles were maintained in the range of 50% to 68% during duplex examinations.[1]

Measurements ▪

The method of measuring the Doppler perfusion index (DPI) is detailed in Figure 1 and Table 1. Normal values for each measured and calculated parameter from an earlier study are given in Table 1.[2] Figure 2 is a scatterplot of DPI with patients divided into three groups. From prior experience, the investigators established that DPI values of greater than 0.3 were abnormal and suspicious for metastases.[2] Table 2 lists performance of laparotomy, standard ultrasound (U/S), CT, and DPI in predicting the presence of metastases on presentation, and development of metastases within 1 year.[1]

Source ▪

Subjects were 161 patients with colorectal cancer scanned prior to laparotomy, at which time the liver was palpated and any suspicious lesions biopsied. The patients also had standard U/S and dynamic contrast-enhanced CT scanning done for staging purposes. After surgery, patients with apparently disease-free livers were followed up every 3 months with clinical examination, biochemical studies, and U/S of the liver. CT scans were repeated at 1 year (or sooner if clinically indicated). A combination of clinical, laparotomy, biopsy, U/S, and CT findings were used as the "gold standard" for the presence or absence of liver metastases on presentation and at 1-year follow-up. Initially, 56 patients had overt liver metastases. After 1 year, 70 of the 105 patients with initially disease-free livers had adequate follow-up: 23 had documented liver metastases, 4 died (no autopsy but 2 had local recurrence), 9 had local recurrence, and the rest were disease free.

Comments ▪

Leen and colleagues have published several other papers supporting the hypothesis that DPI is accurate in detecting/predicting hepatic metastases from colorectal cancer.[3-7] One study by Leen and colleagues of patients with gastric cancer reports good results with DPI in this setting as well.[8] Pennisi and associates have replicated Leen's results in patients with colorectal cancer and concluded that DPI may be superior to other modalities in detecting occult metastases at time of presentation. They also noted that a number of patients with a DPI greater than 0.30 also had smaller superior mesenteric arteries with slower flow, which supports the idea that a neoplastic humoral factor may be responsible for the hemodynamic changes.[9]

Walsh and associates[10] found a modestly elevated DPI in patients with hepatitis C compared with normal subjects (0.27 ± 0.14 versus 0.17 ± 0.06), and Leen and group[5] found that in cirrhosis the DPI is elevated into the same

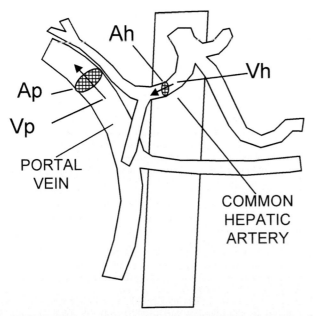

Figure 1 ▪ Depiction of measurements required to determine hepatic Doppler perfusion index. The area and time-averaged velocity are measured in the common hepatic (*Ah, Vh*) and portal vein (*Ap, Vp*) as shown.

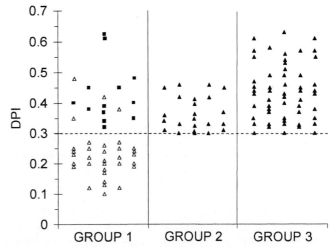

Figure 2 ▪ Scatterplot of Doppler perfusion index (*DPI*) values in three groups of patients with colorectal cancer. Group 1 = no overt metastases; 2 = initially free of metastases and developed overt metastases by 1 year; 3 = overt liver metastases at presentation. Disease-free (*open triangles*), overt liver metastases (*filled triangles*), and local recurrence (*filled squares*) conditions are shown. (From Leen E, Angerson WJ, Wotherspoon H, et al: Radiology 1995; 195:113–116. Used by permission.)

Table 1 ▪ Measurements and Calculations Required to Determine Hepatic Doppler Perfusion Index (DPI)

PARAMETER	NORMAL VALUE	DESCRIPTION
Hepatic artery velocity (Vh)	19.0 ± 10.0 cm/sec	Time-averaged velocity over four cardiac cycles from scans through the long axis of the common hepatic artery near the origin
Portal vein velocity (Vp)	15.0 ± 6.0 cm/sec	Time-averaged velocity over four cardiac cycles from scans through the long axis of the portal vein in its midportion
Hepatic artery area (Ah)	17.0 ± 5.0 mm^2	Average of four measurements of hepatic artery area made by perimeter mapping from perpendicular transverse images
Portal vein area (Ap)	15.0 ± 6.0 mm^2	Average of four measurements of portal vein area made by perimeter mapping from perpendicular transverse images
Hepatic artery flow (Qh)	194 ± 125 ml/min	Calculated by Vh $\times$ Ah
Portal vein flow (Qp)	1200 ± 640 ml/min	Calculated by Vp $\times$ Ap
DPI	0.14 ± 0.06	Calculated by Qh/(Qh + Qp)

cm/sec = centimeters per second, mm = millimeters, ml/min = milliliters per minute.

Table 2 ▪ Performance of Laparotomy, Ultrasound (U/S), Computed Tomography (CT), and Doppler Perfusion Index (DPI) in Detecting/Predicting Metastases

PROCEDURE	TRUE-POSITIVE	FALSE-POSITIVE	TRUE-NEGATIVE	FALSE-NEGATIVE
Laparotomy	36 / 36	0 / 0	105 / 82	20 / 43
U/S	27 / 27	5 / 5	100 / 77	29 / 52
CT	45 / 45	6 / 6	99 / 76	11 / 34
DPI	56 / 79	45 / 22	60 / 60	0 / 0

	SENSITIVITY (%)	SPECIFICITY (%)	PPV (%)	NPV (%)	ACCURACY (%)
Laparotomy	46 / 64	100 / 100	100 / 100	66 / 84	73 / 88
U/S	34 / 48	94 / 95	84 / 84	60 / 78	64 / 79
CT	57 / 80	93 / 94	88 / 88	69 / 90	75 / 89
DPI	100 / 100	73 / 57	78 / 55	100 / 100	86 / 72

Each data entry lists numbers as follows: presentation / 1-year follow-up. PPV = positive predictive value, NPV = negative predictive value.
From Leen E, Angerson WJ, Wotherspoon H, et al: Radiology 1995; 195:113–116. Used by permission.

range as that of patients with liver metastases (0.48 ± 0.19). The DPI also can be measured by scintigraphy, though the normal range seems to have a higher numeric value (up to 0.36).[11, 12]

Leen's group performed a reproducibility study of the DPI and found inter- and intraobserver coefficients of variation (20% and 16%, respectively) that were deemed clinically acceptable.[13] However, Fowler and two others independently measured the DPI in 9 healthy volunteers and demonstrated wide intraobserver variability with less marked interobserver variability. Of 270 separate measurements, 92 (34%) exceeded 0.3, and the overall mean value was 0.25.[14] Shuman cautioned that in addition to potential problems of reproducibility of this somewhat complex measurement, a 40% incidence of replaced/accessory hepatic arteries might cause problems.[15]

REFERENCES

1. Leen E, Angerson WJ, Wotherspoon H, et al: Detection of colorectal liver metastases: Comparison of laparotomy, CT, US, and Doppler perfusion index and evaluation of postoperative follow-up results. Radiology 1995; 195:113–116.

2. Leen E, Goldberg JA, Robertson J, et al: Early detection of occult colorectal hepatic metastases using duplex colour Doppler sonography. Br J Surg 1993; 80:1249–1251.
3. Leen E, Goldberg JA, Robertson J, et al: Detection of hepatic metastases using duplex/color Doppler sonography. Ann Surg 1991; 214:599–604.
4. Leen E, Goldberg JA, Robertson J, et al: Image-directed Doppler ultrasonography: A novel technique for the diagnosis of colorectal liver metastases. J Clin Ultrasound 1993; 21:221–230.
5. Leen E, Angerson WJ, Goldberg JA, et al: Hepatic arterial haemodynamics following intra-arterial angiotensin II infusion: Duplex colour Doppler sonography. Clin Radiol 1993; 47:321–324.
6. Leen E, Angerson WJ, Wotherspoon H, et al: Comparison of Doppler perfusion index and intraoperative ultrasonography in diagnosing colorectal liver metastases. Ann Surg 1994; 220:663–667.
7. Leen E, Angerson WG WG, Cooke TG, McArdle CS: Prognostic power of Doppler perfusion index in colorectal cancer. Correlation with survival. Ann Surg 1996; 223:199–203.
8. Leen E, Anderson JR, Robertson J, et al: Doppler index perfusion in the detection of hepatic metastases secondary to gastric carcinoma. Am J Surg 1997; 173:99–102.
9. Pennisi F, Ascanio B, Farina R: [Hemodynamic changes in patients with colorectal adenocarcinoma: The role of color Doppler US] Alterazioni emodinamiche nei pazienti affetti da adenocarcinoma colon-rettale: Ruolo dell'eco color Doppler. Radiol Med (Torino) 1998; 95:583–587.
10. Walsh KM, Leen E, MacSween RN, Morris AJ: Hepatic blood flow

changes in chronic hepatitis C measured by duplex Doppler color sonography: Relationship to histological features. Dig Dis Sci 1998; 43:2584–2590.

11. Warren HW, Gallagher H, Hemingway DM, et al: Prospective assessment of the hepatic perfusion index in patients with colorectal cancer. Br J Surg 1998; 85:1708–1712.

12. Gupta R, Sawant P, Parameshwar RV, et al: Gastric mucosal blood flow and hepatic perfusion index in patients with portal hypertensive gastrophy. J Gastroenterol Hepatol 1998; 13:921–926.

13. Oppo K, Leen E, Angerson WJ, et al: Doppler perfusion index: An interobserver and intraobserver reproducibility study. Radiology 1998; 208:453–457.

14. Fowler RC, Harris KM, Swift SE, et al: Hepatic Doppler perfusion index: Measurement in nine healthy volunteers. Radiology 1998; 209:867–871.

15. Shuman WP: Liver metastases from colorectal carcinoma: Detection with Doppler US-guided measurements of liver blood flow—past, present, future [editorial]. Radiology 1995; 195:9–10.

▪: NORMAL PORTAL VEIN DIAMETER IN CHILDREN
▪ ACR Code: 957 (Portal Vein, Splenic Vein)

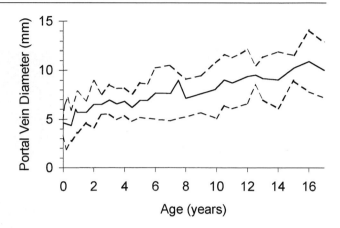

Figure 1 ▪ Portal vein diameter versus age. Mean *(solid line)* and limits of error *(dashed lines)* are shown. (From Patriquin HB, Perreault G, Grignon A, et al: Pediatr Radiol 1990; 20:451–453. Used by permission.)

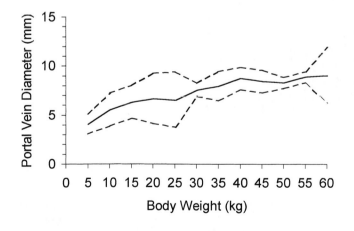

Figure 2 ▪ Portal vein diameter versus body weight. Mean *(solid line)* and limits of error *(dashed lines)* are shown. (From Patriquin HB, Perreault G, Grignon A, et al: Pediatr Radiol 1990; 20:451–453. Used by permission.)

Technique ▪

Ultrasound of the abdomen was done with various scanners and 5.0- to 7.5-MHz real-time sector transducers. Scanning was done with the subjects supine, 1 to 3 hours after the most recent meal, and during quiet breathing.[1]

Measurements ▪

The maximum diameter of the portal vein was measured with electronic calipers from frozen images through its long axis at the site of the hepatic artery crossing.[1] Figure 1 shows portal vein diameter versus age, and Figure 2 shows portal vein diameter versus body weight.

Source ▪

Subjects included 156 children (age range, birth to 16 years) undergoing abdominal ultrasound for conditions unrelated to the liver, spleen, or portal system. These were usually done to evaluate the genitourinary system or to diagnose pyloric stenosis in infants.[1]

Comments ▪

The portal vein diameter increased with advancing age (p = .0001) and with weight (p = .005).

REFERENCE

1. Patriquin HB, Perreault G, Grignon A, et al: Normal portal venous diameter in children. Pediatr Radiol 1990; 20:451–453.

▪▪ MEASUREMENT OF THE PORTAL VEIN BY REAL-TIME ULSTRASOUND[1]

▪ ACR Code: 957 (Portal Vein)

Technique ▪

1. All studies were made with a real-time mechanical sector scanner, using a 3.5-MHz transducer.
2. Patients were examined in the supine, right anterior oblique, and left lateral decubitus positions during suspended inspiration.

Measurements ▪ (Figures 1 and 2)

The measurements were obtained at the broadest point of the portal vein, just distal to the union of the splenic and superior mesenteric veins. There was no difference between measurements of male and female patients.

The overall mean diameter in patients aged 21 to 40

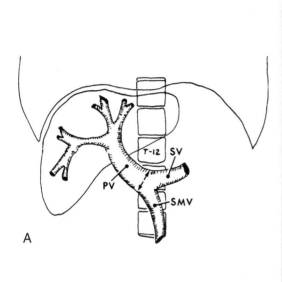

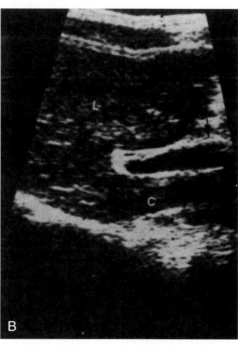

Figure 1 ▪ *A*, main portal vein *(PV)* formed by confluence of splenic vein *(SV)* and superior mesenteric vein *(SMV)*. *Arrows* indicate site of portal vein measurement. *B*, Real-time sagittal sonogram in right anterior oblique plane. *Arrows* indicate site of portal vein measurement. *L* = liver; *C* = inferior vena cava. (From Weinreb J, et al: AJR Am J Roentgenol 1982; 139:497. Used by permission.)

Figure 2 ▪ Portal vein measurements in 40 patients. (From Weinreb J, et al: AJR Am J Roentgenol 1982; 139:497. Used by permission.)

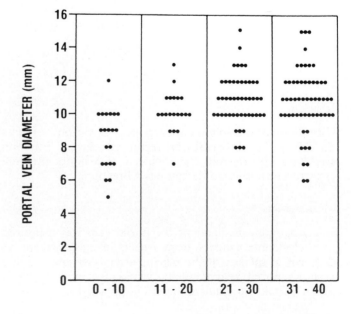

years was 11 ± 2 mm. Note that the Valsalva maneuver is reported to make the portal vein dilate.

Source ▪

One hundred forty-eight patients (83 females and 65 males) were studied, aged 0 to 40 years. The sonogram was performed for indications other than to evaluate portal vein

size. The only other criterion was that the extrahepatic portal vein be adequately visualized.

Reference

1. Weinreb J, Kumari S, Phillips G, Pochaczevsky R: Portal vein measurements by real-time sonography. AJR Am J Roentgenol 1982; 139:497–499.

▪: PORTAL, SUPERIOR MESENTERIC, AND SPLENIC VEIN DIAMETERS IN ADULTS
- ▪ ACR Code: 957 (Portal Vein, Splenic Vein)

Technique ▪

Abdominal ultrasound was performed with various machines and 3.5- to 5.0-MHz transducers. Baseline measurements were made with patients fasting, supine, and during suspended respiration (usually the inspiratory phase). Other measurements were made: in suspended expiration, left lateral (LL) decubitus position, and after a meal.[1–3]

Measurements ▪

The diameters of the extrahepatic portal vein and the superior mesenteric vein (SMV) were measured at the widest point from longitudinal or transverse images perpendic-

ular to the long axis.[1–3] The splenic vein diameter was also measured in two of the studies.[1, 3] Table 1 lists the normal vein diameters from all three studies in fasting patients, while supine, and during suspended inspiration; in expiration; and at various times after a meal. Also listed are diameter differences between inspiration/expiration, fasting/postprandial, and decubitus/supine. Diameters of the three veins from patients with portal hypertension (PH) are also included in the bottom row of Table 1, as reported by Goyal and colleagues.[3]

Source ▪

All three studies included groups of healthy adult volunteers, and their numbers are listed in Table 1. Goyal and colleagues also studied 50 patients (39 males, 11 females, mean age, 36 years, age range, 13 to 63 years) with PH mostly caused by cirrhosis. The diagnosis of PH was based on clinical features and documentation of varices by endoscopy.[3]

Comments ▪

Goyal and colleagues listed the upper limits of normal vein diameters (fasting, supine, inspiration) as follows: portal, 16 mm, splenic, 12 mm, and SMV, 11 mm. The normal portal vein, SMV, and splenic veins are all larger during inspiration compared with expiration, as well as after a meal, compared with the fasting state. They are smaller in the left lateral decubitus position compared with supine measurements. In patients with PH, the vein diameters are very often larger than normal, and the amount of respiratory variation is decreased.

Table 1 ▪ Diameters of the Portal, Superior Mesenteric, and Splenic Veins

REF/PATIENT GROUP	NO.	PORTAL (mm)	SMV (mm)	SPLENIC (mm)
Kurol (fasting)				
Inspiration	67	11.5 ± 1.8	9.0 ± 1.9	$7.2 + 1.7$
Expiration	67	8.5 ± 1.7	5.3 ± 2.0	2.8 ± 1.6
Insp–exp*	67	3.0 ± 1.8	3.7 ± 1.6	4.2 ± 1.7
Kurol (postmeal)				
Inspiration	15	12.8	9.4	7.3
Expiration	15	9.4	5.6	3.6
Insp–exp*	15	3.4	3.8	3.8
Bellamy (supine, insp)				
Fasting	13	7.2 ± 2.03	6.3 ± 2.5	—
30 min postmeal	13	10.4 ± 0.93	9.8 ± 2.04	—
1 hr postmeal	13	10.5 ± 2.05	10.3 ± 2.45	—
2 hr postmeal	13	7.8 ± 2.15	7.1 ± 2.53	—
3 hr postmeal	13	7.2 ± 1.96	6.2 ± 2.14	—
Goyal (normal)				
Fasting, supine, insp	96	10.4 ± 1.6	8.4 ± 1.3	8.1 ± 1.2
Insp–exp*	96	2.8 ± 0.7	3.4 ± 0.8	3.1 ± 0.8
Postmeal—fasting*	86	2.7 ± 1.4	3.2 ± 1.5	2.9 ± 1.4
LL decub—supine*	72	2.9 ± 1.0	3.9 ± 1.1	3.6 ± 1.1
Goyal (portal htn)				
Fasting, supine, insp	50	19.4 ± 2.4	14.3 ± 2.3	14.9 ± 3.0

*Indicates diameter difference between two measurement conditions. All measurements are given as mean ± standard deviation. mm = millimeters, insp = inspiration, exp = expiration, htn = hypertension, LL decub = left lateral decubitus.[1–3]

References

1. Kurol M, Forsberg L: Ultrasonographic investigation of respiratory influence on diameters of portal vessels in normal subjects. Acta Radiol 1986; 27:675–680.
2. Bellamy EA, Bossi MC, Cosgrove DO: Ultrasound demonstration of changes in the normal portal venous system following a meal. Br J Radiol 1984; 57:147–149.
3. Goyal AK, Pokhama DS, Sharma SK: Ultrasonic measurements of portal vasculature in diagnosis of portal hypertension: A controversial subject reviewed. J Ultrasound Med 1990; 9:45–48.

▪: DIAMETERS AND RESPIRATORY CHANGE IN THE PORTAL SYSTEM
▪ ACR Code: 957 (Portal Vein, Splenic Vein)

Technique ▪

Ultrasound of the upper abdomen with attention to the portal, splenic, and superior mesenteric veins was performed with an SSD-250 machine (Aloka, Tokyo, Japan) and a 2.5-MHz linear array transducer. Measurements of vein diameters were done: after a fast, with patients supine, during suspended expiration, and during a Valsalva maneuver (deep inspiration).[1]

Measurements ▪

The largest luminal diameter of each vessel was measured in the anteroposterior (AP) dimension from transverse and longitudinal scans. The portal vein was measured directly in front of the vena cava. The splenic vein was measured in front of the superior mesenteric artery and at the hilus of the spleen. The superior mesenteric vein was measured 2.0 cm before the confluence into the portal vein.[1] Table 1

Table 1 ▪ Diameters and Respiratory Change in Portal System in Normal Subjects and Patients with Cirrhosis

VESSEL/PARAMETER	NORMAL	CIRRHOSIS
Portal vein		
Expiration (mm)	10.9 ± 0.2	14.4 ± 0.3
Inspiration (mm)	12.6 ± 0.2	14.9 ± 0.2
Variation %	0–67 (17)	0–30 (0)
Variation (mm)	0–4 (2)	0–3 (0)
Superior mesenteric vein		
Expiration (mm)	5.3 ± 0.2	11.3 ± 0.3
Inspiration (mm)	10.0 ± 0.2	12.2 ± 0.2
Variation %	15–350 (83)	0–150 (7)
Variation (mm)	1–11 (4)	0–6 (1)
Splenic vein (near portal)		
Expiration (mm)	4.6 ± 0.2	10.9 ± 0.3
Inspiration (mm)	9.0 ± 0.2	12.0 ± 0.3
Variation %	15–300 (100)	0–300 (8)
Variation (mm)	1–11 (4)	0–9 (1)
Splenic vein (hilus)		
Expiration (mm)	5.2 ± 0.2	9.8 ± 0.3
Inspiration (mm)	7.1 ± 0.2	10.1 ± 0.3
Variation %	0–150 (33)	0–25 (0)
Variation (mm)	0–6 (2)	0–3 (0)

Diameters given as mean ± standard error. Respiratory variations given as range and (median). mm = millimeters.
From Zoli M, Dondi C, Marchesini G: J Ultrasound Med 1985; 4:641–646. Used by permission.

Table 2 ▪ Performance of Diameters and Respiratory Change in Diagnosing Cirrhosis

VESSEL(S)/PARAMETER	CUT-OFF	SENSITIVITY (%)	NPV (%)
Superior mesenteric vein			
Diameter (expiration)	>10 mm	60	72
Diameter (expiration)/BSA	>5.5 mm/m²	71	78
% Respiratory variation	<14	81	85
Respiratory variation	<1 mm	44	64
Splenic vein			
Diameter (expiration)	>10 mm	56	69
Diameter (expiration)/BSA	>5.3 mm/m²	69	76
% Respiratory variation	<14	72	78
Respiratory variation	<1 mm	43	64
Superior mesenteric + splenic vein			
Diameter (expiration)	>18 mm	73	79
Diameter (expiration)/BSA	>9.2 mm/m²	91	92
Superior mesenteric + splenic + portal vein			
Diameter (expiration)	>31 mm	75	81
Diameter (expiration)/BSA	>17.5 mm/m²	78	83

Cut-off points were chosen to give specificity of 100%. NPV = negative predictive value, BSA = body surface area, mm = millimeters, m = meters.
From Zoli M, Dondi C, Marchesini G: J Ultrasound Med 1985; 4:641–646. Used by permission.

Table 3 • Diameters of Portal System Vessels Grouped by Severity of Varices

VARICEAL GRADE	NONE	SMALL	MEDIUM	LARGE	ALL CASES
Number	33	24	24	19	67
Portal vein	13.3 ± 0.4	14.4 ± 0.4	14.8 ± 0.5	16.0 ± 0.7	14.9 ± 0.3
Superior mesenteric vein	10.0 ± 0.3	10.9 ± 0.5	12.8 ± 0.6	12.2 ± 0.6	11.9 ± 0.3
Splenic vein (near portal)	8.9 ± 0.6	10.4 ± 0.6	12.4 ± 0.6	12.7 ± 0.8	11.8 ± 0.4
Splenic vein (hilus)	8.7 ± 0.5	9.3 ± 0.5	10.5 ± 0.4	11.7 ± 0.9	10.4 ± 0.4

All measurements are in millimeters (mean ± standard error).
From Zoli M, Dondi C, Marchesini G: J Ultrasound Med 1985; 4:641–646. Used by permission.

lists the diameters of each vein (two locations of splenic) in inspiration, in expiration, and the variation between phases. Table 2 gives test performance (sensitivity and negative predictive value) of various parameters and cut-off values in detecting cirrhosis. Table 3 lists vein diameters in expiration from cirrhotic patients, grouped by presence and size of esophageal varices.

Source •

The study was carried out in 100 patients with liver cirrhosis (56 men, 44 women, age range, 19 to 77 years, median age, 57 years). Body weight and height were recorded to allow calculation of body surface area.[1] All patients underwent endoscopy, in which the presence and size/number of varices were graded according to Beppu and colleagues.[2] Control patients (n = 100) were carefully matched according to gender, age, height, and weight.[1]

Comments •

The diameter of the superior mesenteric vein in expiration is probably the single most useful measurement, with greater than 17 mm being 100% sensitive in predicting large varices. However, Zoli and coworkers found that using a cut-off of less than 8 mm would have avoided endoscopy in only 2 of 100 patients. These measurements may be useful in follow-up of patients undergoing drug therapy.[1]

REFERENCES

1. Zoli M, Dondi C, Marchesini G: Splanchnic vein measurements in patients with liver cirrhosis: A case-control study. J Ultrasound Med 1985; 4:641–646.
2. Beppu K, Inokuchi K, Koyanagi N, et al: Prediction of variceal hemorrhage by esophageal endoscopy. Gastrointest Endosc 1981; 27:213–218.

": THE CONGESTION INDEX OF THE PORTAL VEIN
■ ACR Code: 957 (Portal Vein, Splenic Vein)

Technique •

Ultrasound of the upper abdomen with attention to the portal vein was performed with an SAL 50A/SDL-01A machine (Toshiba, Japan), with a 5.0-MHz transducer that had Doppler capabilities. In the Doppler mode, ultrasound waves were emitted at 2.75 MHz with a repetition frequency of 4 to 6 KHz. Patients were all examined after fasting, at rest in semireclining posture (about 30 degrees), and during suspended quiet respiration. In a subset of patients, direct transhepatic portal pressure and transfemoral hepatic vein pressure were recorded.[1]

Measurements •

Doppler signals obtained from longitudinal scanning through the middle of the portal vein lumen were recorded onto paper. Orthogonal diameters (A and B) of the vessel were measured at the same site as velocity measurements after turning the transducer to be transverse to the vessel. The portal vein area was calculated from the formula for the area of an ellipse as follows:

$$\text{Vein area} = A \times B \times \pi/4.$$

The mean flow velocity was calculated by multiplying angle-corrected maximum portal velocity (Vmax) by 0.57 as follows:

$$\text{Flow velocity} = 0.57 \times V_{max}/\cos (\text{insonation angle}).$$

Volume flow rate was calculated by multiplying flow velocity by vessel area as follows:

$$\text{Flow volume} = \text{vein area} \times \text{flow velocity}.$$

The congestion index (CI) was calculated by dividing portal vein area by flow velocity as follows:

$$\text{Congestion index} = \text{vein area/flow velocity}.$$

Table 1 lists these Doppler portal vein parameters by disease class and includes direct portal and hepatic vein pressure measurements from the subset so examined.[1]

Source •

Normal adults as well as patients with acute hepatitis, chronic active hepatitis, liver cirrhosis, and idiopathic portal hypertension (IPH) were studied. The numbers of pa-

Table 1 ▪ Doppler and Direct Pressure Measurements in Normal Subjects and Liver Disease

	HEALTHY CONTROLS	ACUTE HEPATITIS	CHRONIC ACTIVE HEPATITIS	CIRRHOSIS	IDIOPATHIC PORTAL HTN
Number (Doppler, portal vein)	85	11	42	72	11
Diameter (mm)*	11.2 ± 6.0	11.6 ± 5.3	12.5 ± 7.2	13.8 ± 7.9	14.1 ± 7.6
Cross-sectional area (cm²)	0.99 ± 0.28	1.05 ± 0.22	1.22 ± 0.41	1.49 ± 0.49	1.56 ± 0.45
Blood flow velocity (cm/sec)	15.3 ± 4.0	15.0 ± 2.7	12.0 ± 3.5	9.7 ± 2.6	10.8 ± 3.8
Blood flow volume (ml/min)	899 ± 284	967 ± 356	851 ± 237	870 ± 289	1047 ± 381
Congestion index (cm/sec)	0.070 ± 0.029	0.071 ± 0.014	0.119 ± 0.084	0.171 ± 0.075	0.180 ± 0.107
Number (catheterization)	—	—	17	30	11
Portal vein pressure (mm Hg)	—	—	15.3 ± 4.1	20.9 ± 3.9	22.0 ± 4.4
Hepatic vein pressure (mm Hg)	—	—	5.6 ± 1.8	6.5 ± 2.1	7.2 ± 2.4
Portal-hepatic vein pressure (mm Hg)	—	—	9.7 ± 3.5	14.4 ± 3.6	14.8 ± 4.9
Portal vein pressure versus congestion index (r value)	—	—	−0.4	0.29	0.50

*Vein diameters calculated from areas assuming circular profile.
Measurements are given as mean ± standard deviation. HTN = hypertension. Measurement unit abbreviations are standard.
From Moriyasu F, Nishida O, Ban N, et al: AJR Am J Roentgenol 1986; 146:735–739. Used by permission.

tients in each group evaluated with Doppler ultrasound and direct pressure measurements are given in Table 1.

Comments ▪

Moriyasu and colleagues found that CI was 67% sensitive in detecting cirrhosis and IPH, with the cut-off set to mean ± 2 SD (0.128), whereas blood flow velocity and vein area were 55% and 6% sensitive, respectively.[1] Other investigators have validated the use of CI in detecting and following portal hypertension.[2-4] Rivolta and colleagues found that CI correlated with the severity of ascites and was a reliable measure of the severity of portal hypertension in those with ascites.[5] Ludwig found that the CI decreased after feeding in patients without a history of variceal bleeding (CI pre/CI post = 1.3 +/− 0.23) and increased in those with bleeding (CI pre/CI post = 0.86 +/− 0.29).[6]

REFERENCES

1. Moriyasu F, Nishida O, Ban N, et al: "Congestion index" of the portal vein. AJR Am J Roentgenol 1986; 146:735–739.
2. Siringo S, Bolondi L, Gaiani S, et al: The relationship of endoscopy, portal Doppler ultrasound flowmetry, and clinical and biochemical tests in cirrhosis. J Hepatol 1994; 20:11–18.
3. Siringo S, Bolondi L, Gaiani S, et al: Timing of the first variceal hemorrhage in cirrhotic patients: Prospective evaluation of Doppler flowmetry, endoscopy and clinical parameters. Hepatology 1994; 20:66–73.
4. Iwao T, Toyonaga A, Ikegami M, et al: Portal vein hemodynamics in cirrhotic patients with portal hypertensive gastropathy: An echo-Doppler study. Hepatogastroenterology 1994; 41:230–234.
5. Rivolta R, Maggi A, Cazzaniga M, et al: Reduction of renal cortical blood flow assessed by Doppler in cirrhotic patients with refractory ascites. Hepatology 1998; 28:1235–1240.
6. Ludwig D, Schwarting K, Korbel CM, et al: The postprandial portal flow is related to the severity of portal hypertension and liver cirrhosis. J Hepatol 1998; 28:631–638.

▪: PORTAL AND SPLENIC VEIN DUPLEX SONOGRAPHY IN PORTAL HYPERTENSION
▪ ACR Code: 957 (Portal Vein, Splenic Vein)

Technique ▪

Sonography of the upper abdomen was performed with an Ultramark 9 machine (Advanced Technology Laboratories, Solingen, Germany), with a 3.5-MHz phased-array transducer. Patients were fasting, and supine, and measurements were obtained during breathholding.[1] Transjugular catheterization of the portal vein (at the start of a transjugular intrahepatic portosystemic shunt = TIPS procedure) was accomplished, and pressures were measured in the main portal vein and inferior vena cava prior to tract dilation.[1]

Measurements ▪

Ultrasound measurements of the main portal vein were made halfway between the portal confluence and the bifurcation and of the splenic vein to the left of the aorta. Measurements included time-averaged maximum flow ve-

locity (MFV) and luminal diameter (D). Calculated parameters included cross-sectional area (A = π/4 × D squared) and volume flow (VolF = MFV/2 × A). The congestion index (CI = A / [MFV/2]) was calculated for the portal vein.[1] Table 1 lists the results.

Source ▪

The study group included 375 patients with symptomatic portal hypertension (247 male, 128 female, mean age, 53 years, age range, 10 to 84 years), admitted for elective treatment with TIPS. Of these, 296 had been treated for variceal bleeding and 79 for refractory ascites. There were 95 with Child-Pugh class A, 168 class B, and 112 class C. Eighteen patients with portal thrombosis at ultrasound were excluded from further analysis. Additionally, 100 age- and gender-matched normal control subjects were examined with ultrasound.[1]

Table 1 • Sonographic Findings, Portal Pressure, and Portosystemic Pressure Gradient

PARAMETER UNITS	PORTAL VEIN				SPLENIC VEIN			PORTAL VEIN PRESSURE (cm H₂O)	PORTAL-IVC GRADIENT (cm H₂O)
	Diameter (cm)	Velocity (cm/sec)	Flow (ml/min)	CONG INDEX (cm × sec)	Diameter (cm)	Velocity (cm/sec)	Flow (ml/min)		
Control	1.10 ± 0.20	26.5 ± 5.5	810 ± 180	0.07 ± 0.015	0.7 ± 0.1	25.1 ± 5.0	280 ± 75	<10	<5
All	1.44 ± 0.23	14.9 ± 9.5	759 ± 499	0.20	1.08 ± 0.28	15.0 ± 11.9	456 ± 436	39 ± 8	31 ± 7
Child-Pugh A	1.43 ± 0.24	18.2 ± 5.8	889 ± 414	0.17	1.10 ± 0.34	17.6 ± 8.1	556 ± 498	37 ± 7	29 ± 7
Child-Pugh B	1.44 ± 0.22	15.9 ± 9.0	817 ± 465	0.20	1.08 ± 0.26	15.6 ± 11.5	447 ± 409	39 ± 7	31 ± 7
Child-Pugh C	1.44 ± 0.22	10.8 ± 11.2	561 ± 556	0.25	1.07 ± 0.24	11.7 ± 14.6	372 ± 396	40 ± 8	32 ± 8

Measurements are given as mean ± standard deviation, except the congestion index (median). Cong Index = congestion index, IVC = inferior vena cava. Measurement unit abbreviations are standard.

From Haag K, Rossle M, Ochs A, et al: AJR Am J Roentgenol 1999; 172:631–635. Used by permission.

Comments •

Cumulative frequency analysis showed that portal vein diameter greater than 1.25 cm or a portal vein flow velocity of less than 21 cm/sec indicated portal hypertension, with sensitivity and specificity of 80%. If the congestion index exceeded 0.1, portal hypertension was diagnosed with sensitivity and specificity of 95%. Correlations between ultrasound parameters and portal pressure were found but not felt to be sufficiently strong to allow grading. There were no significant differences in ultrasound parameters between the variceal bleeding and ascites subgroups.[1]

REFERENCE

1. Haag K, Rossle M, Ochs A, et al: Correlation of duplex sonography findings and portal hypertension in 375 patients with portal hypertension. AJR Am J Roentgenol 1999; 172:631–635.

•: PORTAL MORPHOLOGY AND SPLEEN SIZE TO PREDICT VARICES
■ ACR Code: 957 (Portal Vein, Splenic Vein)

Technique •

Abdominal ultrasound with attention to the spleen, liver, portal system, and hepatic artery was done with an RA 1-2 (Diasonics, Milpital, CA) or an UltraMark U (ATL, Bothel, WA) machine. A 3.5-MHz real-time sector transducer was used.[1]

Measurements •

The diameter of the portal vein was measured anterior to the superior mesenteric artery and considered enlarged if greater than 13 mm.[2] The spleen was measured in three dimensions (transverse, TRV; anteroposterior, AP; and craniocaudal, CC). The upper limits of spleen size (TRV 8 cm, AP 12 cm, and CC 14 cm), given by Weill, were used.[3] Note was made of cut-off of intrahepatic portal vein branches, as well as any collateral vessels near the lower esophagus, around the spleen, around the umbilicus, and along the splenic vein. A scoring system was developed using these findings and is detailed in Table 1, which also shows sensitivity and specificity for varices on endoscopy. Table 2 lists the portal vein size, spleen length, and average sonographic score by patient group. Figure 1 is a scatterplot of sonographic score versus grade of varices for the cirrhotic patients.[4] When one or more of the findings described in Table 1 are seen, there is a high likelihood of significant varices on endoscopy; when two or more are present, the patient is very likely to have hematemesis.

Source •

The study subjects consisted of 42 adults with documented cirrhosis of the liver (31 by biopsy) and 20 normal adult

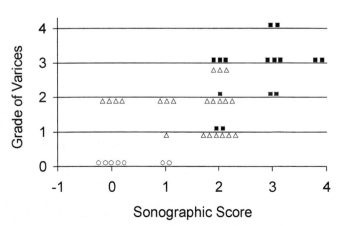

Figure 1 • Scatterplot of sonographic score from abdominal ultrasound versus severity of varices at endoscopy. Patients with no varices (circles), varices without hematemesis (triangles), and varices with hematemesis within 3 months (squares) are shown. (From Medhat A, Iber FL, Dunn M, et al: Am J Gastroenterol 1988; 83:58–63. Used by permission.)

Table 1 ▪ Scoring System for Abdominal Ultrasound to Predict Varices and Hematemesis

CRITERION	SCORE	NUMBER PRESENT/NUMBER IN GROUP			Sensitivity (%)	Specificity (%)
		+ Varices	− Varices	Controls		
						For Varices
Portal vein diameter >13 mm	+1	30/42	2/7	0/20	71	92
Spleen enlarged >1 dimension	+1	32/42	2/7	0/20	76	92
Cut-off of > 1 intrahepatic portal vein branch	+1	12/42	0/7	0/20	29	100
Collaterals: 1 or more bed	+1	16/42	0/7	0/20	38	100
TOTAL SCORE	>0				90	92
TOTAL SCORE	>1				84	100
						For Hematemesis
TOTAL SCORE	>1				100	88

The bottom row gives sensitivity/specificity for predicting hematemesis within 3 months of ultrasound. −Varices = no varices on endoscopy, +Varices = significant varices on endoscopy.[1]

Table 2 ▪ Portal Vein Diameter, Spleen Length, and Sonographic Scores

GROUP	NO.	PORTAL VEIN DIAMETER (mm)	SPLEEN LENGTH (cm)	SONOGRAPHIC SCORE	GRADE OF VARICES
Controls	20	11.2 ± 0.3	10.4 ± 0.3	0	—
Cirrhosis, − varices	7	12.3 ± 0.2	11.6 ± 0.6	0.55 ± 0.1	0
Cirrhosis, + varices	42	15.2 ± 0.4	13.8 ± 0.5	2.14 ± 0.2	2.30 ± 0.1
Cirrhosis, + varices, − hemat.	24	14.2 ± 0.6	12.6 ± 0.7	1.58 ± 0.2	2.00 ± 0.2
Cirrhosis, + varices, + hemat.	18	16.1 ± 0.6	15.3 ± 0.7	2.89 ± 0.2	2.75 ± 0.2

All measurements given as mean ± standard error. ± varices = with or without varices, ± hemat = with or without history of hematemesis.[1]

controls. All the cirrhotic patients underwent endoscopy within 10 days of ultrasound. Esophageal varices were graded from 0 to 4+, with 0 being none and 4+ representing the most severe.[4] Of the patients with documented varices, 18 had hematemesis within 3 months of the ultrasound.[1]

Comments ▪

Medhat and colleagues also measured hepatic artery as well as splenic vein diameter in most of the subjects and found no significant correlation with varices or hematemesis.[1]

REFERENCES

1. Medhat A, Iber FL, Dunn M, et al: Ultrasonographic findings with bleeding and nonbleeding esophageal varices. Am J Gastroenterol 1988; 83:58–63.
2. Weinreb J, Kamuri S, Phillips G, et al: Portal vein measurements by real-time sonography. AJR Am J Roentgenol 1982; 139:497.
3. Weill FS: The spleen: Examination techniques and echoanatomy. In Ultrasonography of Digestive Diseases. CV Mosby, St. Louis, 1982, 473–485.
4. Paquet J: Prophylactic endoscopic sclerosing treatment of the esophageal wall in varices: A prospective randomized trial. Endoscopy 1982; 14:4–5.

▪: ULTRASOUND SCORE TO PREDICT VARICEAL BLEEDING
▪ ACR Code: 957 (Portal Vein, Splenic Vein)

Technique ▪

Ultrasound of the upper abdomen was done with an SSH-160 machine (Toshiba, Japan) and a 3.75-MHz sector transducer with gray scale, color Doppler, and duplex Doppler analysis. Patients fasted overnight and were examined while supine and breathing quietly. Evaluation of respiratory variability in superior mesenteric vein (SMV) size was done between expiration and deep inspiration.[1]

Measurements ▪

The maximum diameters of the portal vein, splenic vein, SMV, and coronary (left gastric) vein were measured from frozen gray scale images perpendicular to the long axis.

The length of the spleen was measured. Maximum angle-corrected (<60 degrees) velocity of flow in the portal and splenic veins was measured with duplex scanning. Color Doppler and duplex scanning was used to determine flow direction in the coronary vein and to identify collateral channels at the gastroesophageal junction. The presence of any intraluminal thrombus was noted in the intra- and extrahepatic portal and splenic veins.[1] Respiratory variation in the SMV was defined as follows:

(Diameter at inspiration ×

100/diameter at expiration) − 100.

Table 1 lists the components of an ultrasound score based on results of the examination just described. The

Table 1 • Ultrasound Scoring System of Portal Hypertension

FIGURE 1	PARAMETER	SCORE
1	Portal/splenic vein flow	
	Velocity 5–10 cm/sec in portal vein or velocity < 5 cm/sec in splenic vein	1
	Velocity 1–4.9 cm/sec in portal vein	2
	Reversed (hepatofugal) flow in portal vein	0
2	Portal vein	
	Maximum diameter ≥ 13 mm	1
	Maximum diameter ≥ 17 mm	2
3	Superior mesenteric vein	
	Diameter ≥ 6 mm and respiratory variation < 40%	1
4	Spleen	
	Maximal longitudinal diameter ≥ 15 cm	1
5	Coronary (left gastric) vein	
	Maximum diameter ≥ 5 mm and hepatofugal flow	1
6	Gastroesophageal collaterals	
	Low velocity flow present at gastroesophageal junction	1
7	Vein thrombosis	
	Partial, intrahepatic portal vein thrombosis	1
	Extrahepatic portal or splenic vein thrombosis	2

Numbers in first column relate to Figure 1.
From Schmassmann A, Zuber M, Livers M, et al: AJR Am J Roentgenol 1993; 160:41–47. Used by permission.

assigned score was the sum of individual components and could range from 0 to 11. Figure 1 depicts the measurements/observations for the scoring system with numbers corresponding to components in Table 1. Table 2 lists results of various parameters in the three groups of subjects. Table 3 lists a subset of these parameters, as well as endoscopic score[2] and a modified (A = 5–6, B = 7–9, C = 10 15) Child's classification[3] in 12 patients who had recurrent bleeding and 18 who did not.[1]

Source •

Subjects included patients with biopsy-proved hepatic cirrhosis without history of variceal hemorrhage (21 men, 9 women, mean age, 58 years) and cirrhotic patients being treated for their first episode of gastrointestinal hemorrhage (20 men, 10 women, mean age, 62 years) requiring transfusion. A third group of 30 age- and gender-matched health control subjects was evaluated. Clinical follow-up of the patient groups was for 2 years and included subsequent episodes of bleeding.[1]

Comments •

Note that in Table 3 the only predictor of recurrent variceal hemorrhage within 2 years was the initial sonographic score. When the score was 4 or more, the prevalence of recurrent hemorrhage was 67%, whereas it was 22% when the score was less than 4. Based on their observations in the present study, literature review, and clinical experience, Schmassmann and colleagues stated that increased portal vein diameter, decreased response to respiration in the SMV, intrahepatic thrombosis (portal vein cut-off), and large spleen are associated with portal hypertension but not with an increased risk of variceal bleeding. Decreased velocity in the portal vein, enlargement of the coronary vein with hepatofugal flow, and detection of gastroesophageal collaterals are associated with esophageal hemorrhage.[1]

Figure 1 • Measurements/observations for the ultrasound scoring system listed in Table 1, numbered to correspond to table entries. *SMV* = superior mesenteric vein.

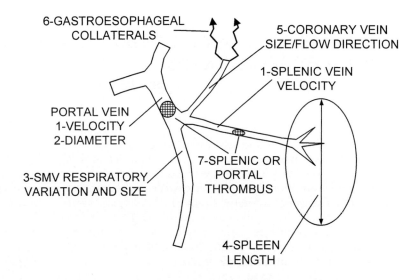

Table 2 ▪ Measurements/Observations in Controls, Cirrhosis, and Variceal Hemorrhage Groups

PARAMETER	CONTROL SUBJECTS	CIRRHOSIS GROUP	HEMORRHAGE GROUP	CIRRHOSIS VS. HEMORRHAGE
Number in group	30	30	30	
Portal vein				
Velocity (cm/sec)	27.2 ± 6	18.1 ± 5	14.2 ± 7	p <.05
Diameter (mm)	9.2 ± 1.5	12.7 ± 1.7	14.6 ± 5.0	NS
Splenic vein				
Velocity (cm/sec)	19.9 ± 4.6	14.6 ± 6.5	13.9 ± 5.5	NS
Diameter (mm)	4.6 ± 1.7	7.5 ± 1.6	10.1 ± 2.8	p <.01
SMV respiration change	89 ± 34	18 ± 12	13 ± 7	NS
Spleen length (cm)	10.3 ± 1.1	13.0 ± 2.4	14.9 ± 3.2	NS
Portosystemic collaterals				
To inferior vena cava (%)	0	30	50	NS
Gastroesophageal (%)	0	33	90	p <.001
Coronary vein ≥5 mm and hepatofugal flow (%)	0	15	43	p <.05
Intrahepatic portal vein thrombosis (%)	0	3	10	NS
Main portal or splenic vein thrombosis (%)	0	3	7	NS
Mean score	0	1.8 ± 0.8	3.8 ± 1.6	p <.0001
Score ≥4 (%)	0	7	40	p <.01

Measurements given as mean ± standard deviation. Observations given as percentage. NS = not significant, SMV = superior mesenteric vein.
From Schmassmann A, Zuber M, Livers M, et al: AJR Am J Roentgenol 1993; 160:41–47. Used by permission.

Table 3 ▪ Ultrasound, Endoscopic, and Clinical Findings in Patients With and Without Recurrent Bleeding

PARAMETER	NO REBLEEDING	REBLEEDING	NO VS. REBLEEDING
Number in group	18	12	—
Portal vein velocity (cm/sec)	17.2 ± 11	9.5 ± 9	NS
Portal vein diameter (mm)	13.2 ± 3.9	16.3 ± 6.2	NS
Portosystemic collaterals	83	100	NS
Coronary vein ≥ 5 mm (%)	22	50	NS
Ultrasound score	3.3 ± 1.5	5.0 ± 1.6	<0.05
Endoscopic score	− 0.2 ± 0.4	− 0.3 ± 0.2	NS
Pugh/Child classification	8.1 ± 2.3	8.9 ± 1.6	NS

Measurements given as mean ± standard deviation. Observations given as percentage. NS = not significant.
From Schmassmann A, Zuber M, Livers M, et al: AJR Am J Roentgenol 1993; 160:41–47. Used by permission.

REFERENCES

1. Schmassmann A, Zuber M, Livers M, et al: Recurrent bleeding after variceal hemorrhage: Predictive value of portal venous duplex sonography. AJR Am J Roentgenol 1993; 160:41–47.

2. Beppu K, Inokuchi K, Koyanagi N, et al: Prediction of variceal hemorrhage by esophageal endoscopy. Gastrointest Endosc 1981; 27:213–218.

3. Pugh RNH, Murray-Lyon IM, Dawson JL, et al: Transection of the esophagus for bleeding esophageal varices. Br J Surg 1973; 60:646–649.

▪: DOPPLER FINDINGS IN TRANSJUGULAR INTRAHEPATIC PORTOSYSTEMIC SHUNTS

▪ ACR Code: 959 (Transjugular Intrahepatic Portosystemic Shunt)

Technique ▪

Ultrasound of the liver and associated vasculature was done with a 128-XP machine (Acuson, Mountain View, CA) and 2- to 3.5-MHz phased-array transducers. Gray scale, duplex, and color Doppler scans were made of the transjugular intrahepatic portosystemic shunt (TIPS), hepatic arteries, and portal veins. Angle-corrected (60 degrees or less) velocities were measured with a duplex Doppler gate of 2 to 5 mm, maximal power output, low frequency wall filter, and gain set to maximum (free of noise).[1, 2]

Measurements ▪

Velocities in the TIPS were measured from scans through the long axis of the stent. From frozen duplex images the highest velocity in the displayed time interval was measured with electronic calipers. This was typically repeated three times and the highest velocity recorded. Foshager and colleagues did this in the proximal, middle, and distal portions of the shunt, and Feldstein and colleagues made measurements from the midportion (within hepatic parenchyma).[1, 2] Figure 1 depicts a duplex scan of a TIPS. Flow direction

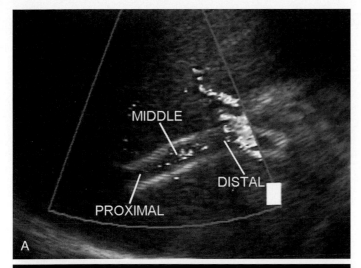

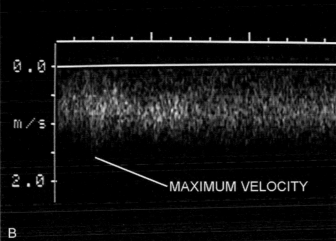

Figure 1 ▪ Duplex ultrasound of a transjugular intrahepatic portosystemic shunt (TIPS). *A*, Gray scale image with the transducer oriented along the long axis of the shunt through the midlumen. Velocities were measured in various portions of the shunt, as shown. *B*, Doppler tracing taken in the middle of the shunt. Typical turbulent flow is seen, and the maximum velocity is measured at the edge of the envelope (in this case 150 cm/sec).

in left and right intrahepatic portal branches was determined from color Doppler images. Foshager and group also measured peak systolic velocity in the hepatic artery.[1] Direct transjugular portal venography was performed through the stent, including measurement of the portosystemic pressure gradient.[1, 2]

Table 1 lists velocities in the TIPS and hepatic artery at various intervals following placement from Foshager and coworkers.[1] Table 2 lists performance of maximum velocity in the body of the shunt for predicting significant stenosis on venography, as defined by 50% or greater stenosis or a portosystemic gradient of 15 mm Hg or more.[2] Foshager and coworkers used a threshold of 60 cm/sec or less and found Doppler ultrasound to be 98% sensitive and 100% specific in detecting significant (50% or more) TIPS stenosis.[1]

Source ▪

Foshager and colleagues studied 40 patients who had undergone TIPS (22 males, 18 females, age range, 4 to 81

years, mean age, 51 years). A total of 200 duplex Doppler sonograms and 73 portal venograms was obtained from 1 day to 18 months after placement, resulting in 82 sonographic-venographic correlations, with time intervals ranging from less than 24 hours to 3 weeks.[1] Feldstein and groups evaluated 79 patients after TIPS who had 251 duplex Doppler sonograms and 116 portal venograms. The follow-up interval ranged from 1 day to 2.3 years (mean, 5.2 months).[2]

Table 1 ▪ Flow Velocities in TIPS and Hepatic Artery From 1 Day to 1 Year After the Procedure

| INTERVAL | NO. | SHUNT VELOCITY (cm/sec) | | |
		Peak ± SD	Minimum	Maximum
24 hr	40	198 ± 69	60	300
1–2 mon	25	178 ± 61	60	300
3–4 mon	7	171 ± 63	100	275
6 mon	9	150 ± 42	100	200
9 mon	7	156 ± 54	100	250
12 mon	4	135 ± 65	90	200

| INTERVAL | NO. | MEAN SHUNT VELOCITY (cm/sec) | | |
		Proximal	Middle	Distal
24 hr	36	174	163	118
1–2 mon	24	140	161	140
3–4 mon	7	135	168	76
6 mon	9	121	128	123
9 mon	6	131	146	86
12 mon	5	126	164	81

| INTERVAL | NO. | HEPATIC ARTERY VELOCITY (cm/sec) | | |
		Peak ± SD	Minimum	Maximum
Pre-TIPS	35	79 ± 43	20	175
24 hr	38	131 ± 67	35	375
1–2 mon	24	106 ± 48	50	230
3–4 mon	8	102 ± 35	50	160
6 mon	10	130 ± 65	35	230
9 mon	6	105 ± 46	65	180
12 mon	5	92 ± 16	70	110

SD = standard deviation, TIPS = transjugular intrahepatic portosystemic shunt.
From Foshager MC, Ferral H, Nazarian GK, et al: AJR Am J Roentgenol 1995; 165(1):1–7. Used by permission.

Table 2 ▪ Performance of Various Velocity Thresholds for Detecting Stenosis in TIPS

VMAX (cm/sec)	SENSITIVITY (%)	SPECIFICITY (%)
≤50	78	99
≤60	84	89
≤70	89	83
≤80	92	60
≤90	93	55
≤100	98	44

Vmax = maximum velocity in midportion of the shunt, cm/sec = centimeters per second.
From Feldstein VA, Patel MD, LaBerge JM: Radiology 1996; 201:141–147. Used by permission.

Table 3 ▪ Criteria Developed by Various Workers to Detect TIPS Malfunction[3-6]

REFERENCE	NO. TIPS EVALUATED	CRITERIA FOR SHUNT MALFUNCTION
Lafortune[3]	44	Decrease in flow > 20%
		Reversal of flow in portal vein branches or collaterals
Dodd[4]	45	Increase or decrease in peak shunt velocity > 50 cm/sec
Haskal[5]	64	Midshunt peak velocity < 60 cm/sec
		Main portal vein velocity < 40 cm/sec
Kanterman[6]	43	Peak shunt velocity < 90 or ≥ 190 cm/sec
		Increase in peak shunt velocity ≥ 60 cm/sec
		Decrease in peak shunt velocity > 40 cm/sec
		Distal shunt velocity < 90 or ≥ 220 cm/sec
		Main portal vein velocity < 30 cm/sec
		Antegrade flow in left or right portal vein

Comments ▪

The main portal vein velocity increased from 21.8 ± 11.9 cm/sec to 41.5 ± 18.5 cm/sec after TIPS. Flow in right portal branches became hepatofugal in 53%, remained hepatopetal in 41%, and was to and fro in 6%. Flow in left portal vein branches became hepatofugal in 55% and remained hepatopetal in 45%.[1] Feldstein and colleagues found that after TIPS, return of hepatopetal flow in portal vein branches beyond the stent was 100% sensitive and 92% specific for significant (50% or more) TIPS stenosis at portography.[2]

Several workers have conducted studies of groups of patients having TIPS placement and correlated various Doppler parameters with findings at angiographic evaluation of the same shunts, mostly including measurement of portosystemic gradients.[3-6] The criteria for shunt malfunction determined to be the most reliable in each series are presented in Table 3. Lin and coworkers evaluated 38 patients with 10-mm stents and 42 with 12-mm stents used to form the TIPS to determine whether there were significant Doppler velocities between the 10- and 12-mm stent groups.[7] They found no significant differences in baseline intrashunt flow velocity (10 mm = 132.4 ± 28.9 cm/sec, 12 mm = 126.7 ± 28.3 cm/sec). However, there were significant differences in flow velocity through the main portal vein (10 mm = 45.1 ± 13.8, 12 mm = 53.6 ± 18.4, p <.03).

Furst and Uggowitzer and their colleagues have experimented with intravenously administered galactose particle ultrasound contrast in evaluating TIPS patency. Contrast enhancement significantly improved visualization and measurement of flow in the TIPS.[8] Maximal peak velocities in the shunt were generally higher (mean ± SD = 12.6 ± 18.7 cm/sec) after contrast.[8] Contrast-enhanced scans showed better performance in detecting TIPS stenoses (similar criteria as described earlier, with the addition of focal peak velocity greater than 150 cm/sec) when compared with unenhanced scans. Sensitivity and specificity of enhanced scans were 78% and 100% compared with 47% and 50% without contrast.[9]

REFERENCES

1. Foshager MC, Ferral H, Nazarian GK, et al: Duplex sonography after transjugular intrahepatic portosystemic shunts (TIPS): Normal hemodynamic findings and efficacy in predicting shunt patency and stenosis. AJR Am J Roentgenol 1995; 165(1):1–7.
2. Feldstein VA, Patel MD, LaBerge JM: Transjugular intrahepatic portosystemic shunts: Accuracy of Doppler US in determination of patency and detection of stenoses. Radiology 1996; 201:141–147.
3. Lafortune M, Martinet J, Denys A, et al: Short and long-term hemodynamic effects of transjugular portosystemic intrahepatic shunts: A Doppler manometric correlative study. AJR Am J Roentgenol 1995; 164:997–1002.
4. Dodd GD III, Zajko AB, Orons PD, et al: Detection of transjugular portosystemic intrahepatic shunt dysfunction: Value of duplex Doppler sonography. AJR Am J Roentgenol 1995; 164:1119–1124.
5. Haskal ZJ, Carrol JW, Jacobs JE, et al: Sonography of transjugular portosystemic intrahepatic shunts: Detection of elevated portosystemic gradients and loss of shunt function. J Vasc Interv Radiol 1997; 8:549–556.
6. Kanterman RY, Darcy MD, Middleton WD, et al: Doppler sonography findings associated with transjugular intrahepatic portosystemic shunt malfunction. AJR Am J Roentgenol 1997; 168:467–472.
7. Lin EC, Middleton WD, Darcy MD, Teefey SA: Hemodynamics revealed by Doppler sonography in patients who have undergone creation of transjugular portosystemic intrahepatic shunts: Comparison of 10- and 12-mm metallic stents. AJR Am J Roentgenol 1999; 172:1245–1248.
8. Furst G, Malms J, Heyer T, et al: Transjugular intrahepatic portosystemic shunts: Improved evaluation with echo-enhanced color Doppler sonography, power Doppler sonography, and spectral duplex sonography. AJR Am J Roentgenol 1998; 170:1047–1054.
9. Uggowitzer MM, Kugler C, Machan L, et al: Value of echo-enhanced Doppler sonography in evaluation of transjugular intrahepatic portosystemic shunts. AJR Am J Roentgenol 1998; 170:1041–1046.

∷ HEPATIC VEIN WAVEFORM MORPHOLOGY AND VELOCITY
• ACR Code: 959 (Hepatic Veins)

Technique •

Ultrasound of the liver with attention to the hepatic veins (HV) was done using various machines and transducers with duplex Doppler capability. Subjects were typically supine, and observations/measurements were made in quiet respiration or during suspended respiration in various phases.[1-6]

Measurements •

Teichgraber and colleagues measured angle-corrected duplex Doppler flow velocities in the middle hepatic vein of subjects during different phases of respiration as well as before and after exercise.[1] Figure 1 shows a normal HV waveform with different components labeled. Table 1 lists velocities as well as the systolic to diastolic (S:D) ratio from

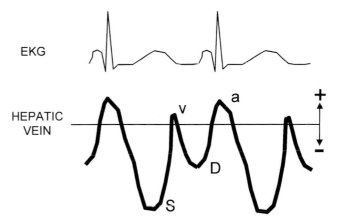

Figure 1 • Normal triphasic hepatic vein Doppler waveform (2 cycles), with electrocardiogram *(EKG)* tracing superimposed. Forward flow during systole *(S)* from movement of the tricuspid annulus toward the apex, retrograde wave *(v)* from right atrial overfilling, antegrade diastolic flow *(D)* after the tricuspid valve opens, retrograde wave *(a)* from atrial contraction. Doppler flow toward the heart *(S, D)* has a negative sign in most scanning configurations.

Table 1 • **Normal Velocities of Hepatic Vein Waveform Components**

CONDITION	S (cm/sec)	D (cm/sec)	a (cm/sec)	S:D RATIO
Full inspiration	− 17 ± 2.4	− 14 ± 1.3	7 ± 1.0	1.21 ± 0.009
Midinspiration	− 21 ± 1.9	− 16 ± 1.6	8 ± 1.1	1.31 ± 0.014
Expiration	− 29 ± 2.0	− 18 ± 1.6	− 10 ± 1.0	1.61 ± 0.011
Resting	− 23 ± 9.4	− 15 ± 4.0	8 ± 1.6	—
After exercise	− 58 ± 14.6	− 35 ± 35.7	35 ± 28.7	—
Rest-exercise change (%)	148	139	372	—

All measurements given as mean ± standard deviation. cm/sec = centimeters per second, S:D Ratio = systolic to diastolic ratio. Waveform abbreviations are listed in the text and Figure 1.
From Teichgraber UKM, Gebel M, Benter T, Manns MP: J Ultrasound Med 1997; 16:549–554. Used by permission.

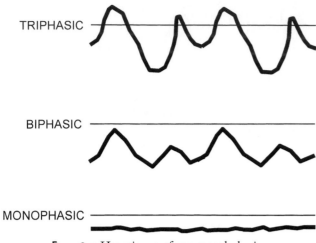

TRIPHASIC

BIPHASIC

MONOPHASIC

Figure 2 ▪ Hepatic waveform morphologies.

REFERENCE/GROUP	NO.	TRIPHASIC (%)	BIPHASIC (%)	MONOPHASIC (%)
Shapiro[2]				
Normal	75	68 (91)	(mono or biphasic) 7 (9)	
Roobottom[3]				
Pregnant women				
10–20 wk	25	16 (64)	5 (20)	4 (16)
20–30 wk	25	3 (12)	5 (20)	17 (68)
30–40 wk	25	2 (8)	3 (12)	20 (80)
Bolondi[4]				
Normal controls	65	65 (100)	0	0
Cirrhosis	60	30 (50)	19 (32)	11 (18)
Dietrich[5]				
Normal controls	75	56 (75)	7 (9)	12 (16)
Chronic hepatitis C	135	64 (47)	23 (17)	48 (36)
Gorka[6]				
Cirrhosis − varices	7	7 (100)	0	0
Cirrhosis + varices	43	18 (42)	13 (30)	12 (28)

Table 2 ▪ Hepatic Vein Waveform Morphologies Observed in Different Populations

Teichgraber and colleagues.[1] The other studies included observations of HV waveform morphology.[2–6] Figure 2 shows the different identified morphologies, and Table 2 lists percentages of these morphologies observed in various groups of patients.[2–6]

Source ▪

Teichgraber and coworkers evaluated 25 healthy adults at different respiratory phases and 8 volunteers before and after performing 50 to 100 sit-ups.[1] Subjects included in the other studies included normal controls, pregnant women, patients with chronic hepatitis C, and patients with cirrhosis with or without varices.[2–6] Numbers of patients in each group are given in Table 2.

Comments ▪

Teichgraber and coworkers also measured HV velocities in 20 fasting adults and after carbohydrates or protein-lipid meals and found no significant changes in HV velocities.[1] Gorka and group found progressive dampening of the HV waveform (biphasic to monophasic) to be associated with worsening hepatic fibrosis and portal hypertension. In fact, simple recognition of HV morphology was superior to portal vein velocimetry in predicting varices, with sensitiv-

ity of 92% for monophasic, 62% for biphasic, and 76% monophasic or biphasic.[6] However, biphasic and monophasic morphologies have been observed in some normal subjects[2, 5] and are common in late pregnancy.[3]

REFERENCES

1. Teichgraber UKM, Gebel M, Benter T, Manns MP: Effect of respiration, exercise, and food intake on hepatic vein circulation. J Ultrasound Med 1997; 16:549–554.
2. Shapiro RS, Winsberg F, Maldjian C, et al: Variability of hepatic vein Doppler tracings in normal subjects. J Ultrasound Med 1993; 12:701–703.
3. Roobottom CA, Hunter JD, Wesszton MJ, Dubbins PA: Hepatic venous Doppler waveforms: Changes in pregnancy. J Clin Ultrasound 1995; 23:477–482.
4. Bolondi L, Bassi SL, Gaiani S, et al: Liver cirrhosis: Changes of Doppler waveform of the hepatic veins. Radiology 1991; 178:513–516.
5. Dietrich CF, Lee JH, Gottschalk R, et al: Hepatic and portal vein flow pattern in correlation with intrahepatic fat deposition and liver histology in patients with chronic hepatitis C. AJR Am J Roentgenol 1998; 171:436–443.
6. Gorka W, Mulla AA, Sebayel MA, et al: Qualitative hepatic venous Doppler sonography versus portal flowmetry in predicting the severity of esophageal varices in hepatitis C cirrhosis. AJR Am J Roentgenol 1997; 169:511–515.

▪▪ HEPATIC VEIN DOPPLER IN HEART FAILURE AND TRICUSPID REGURGITATION
▪ ACR Code: 959 (Hepatic Veins)

Technique ▪

Ultrasound of the liver with attention to the hepatic veins (HV) was done with 3.5-MHz real-time transducers and machines capable of duplex Doppler imaging. Patients were fasting and supine, and measurements were made during suspended breathing.[1, 2]

Measurements ▪

Abu-Yousef measured velocities of middle HV waveforms from duplex tracings and simultaneous electrocardiographic tracings to aid in cardiac cycle timing. The maximum systolic velocity (S), maximum diastolic velocity (D), their ratio (S:D), the a wave velocity (a), and the diameter

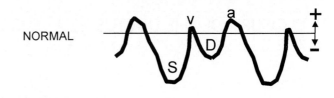

Figure 1 • Hepatic vein waveforms in normal subjects and tricuspid regurgitation that may be associated with congestive heart failure (*CHF*). Standard nomenclature for the components (*S, D, a, v*) is shown. In typical scanning orientation, antegrade flow is positive (above the baseline) on duplex tracings.

Table 1 • Hepatic Vein Velocities and Diameters in Normal Subjects, Congestive Heart Failure, and Tricuspid Regurgitation

REFERENCE/GROUP	MIDDLE HEPATIC VEIN DIAMETER (mm) AND FLOW (cm/sec)				
	Diameter	S	D	a	S:D Ratio
Abu Yousef					
Normal (n = 24)	7	−29	−23	10	1.5
Mean (range)	(3, 10)	(−22, −47)	(−12, −42)	(0, 18)	(0.8, 2.4)
CHF, TR (n = 15)	10	12	−52	22	−0.2
Mean (range)	(8, 18)	(55, −32)	(−18, −82)	(10, 43)	(−0.9, 0.9)

	RIGHT HEPATIC VEIN DIAMETER (mm)			
	Mean ± SD	(Range)	Mean − 2 SD	Mean + 2 SD
Henriksson				
Normal men (n = 20)	6.2 ± 1.43	(4, 9)		9.1
Normal women (n = 20)	5.6 ± 1.66	(3, 9)		8.9
CHF, − effusion (n = 12)	8.8 ± 1.26	(7, 11)	6.3	
CHF, + effusion (n = 17)	13.3 ± 1.74	(10, 18)	9.8	

TR = tricuspid regurgitation, S:D ratio = systolic to diastolic ratio, SD = standard deviation, CHF = congestive heart failure, S, D, a, v = standard nomenclature for hepatic vein waveforms as shown in Figure 1.[1, 2]

of the HV were all measured and recorded.[1] Henriksson and colleagues measured the diameter of the right HV near the confluence from frozen gray scale images.[2] Figure 1 shows typical waveforms obtained in normal subjects and patients with congestive heart failure (CHF) and tricuspid regurgitation (TR). Table 1 lists velocities and diameter of the middle HV from Abu-Yousef, as well as diameter of the right HV in normal subjects and patients with CHF and/or TR.

Source •

Abu-Yousef evaluated 24 normal volunteers (9 men, 15 women, mean age, 29 years, age range, 14 to 74 years) and 15 patients (6 men, 9 women, mean age, 53 years, age range, 38 to 77 years), of whom 13 had TR and 1 had aortic–right atrial fistula from a ruptured sinus of Valsalva aneurysm.[1] Henriksson and colleagues studied 40 normal controls (20 men, 20 women, mean age, 62 years, age range, 52 to 76 years), 12 of whom had CHF without pleural effusion (mean age, 70 years, age range, 54 to 84

years), and 17 of whom had CHF and pleural effusion (mean age, 72 years, age range, 52 to 84 years).[2]

Comments •

A cut-off of 10 mm appears to be useful for HV diameter in diagnosing CHF. The hepatic veins and inferior vena cava are often visually distended and lack normal pulsations at gray scale sonography. Analysis of HV waveforms (Figure 1) in TR reveals a decrease in systolic antegrade velocity (S:D <0.6), no systolic flow or reversal of the S component, as well as an increased tendency for the v wave to be retrograde.[2]

REFERENCES

1. Abu-Yousef MM: Duplex Doppler sonography of the hepatic vein in tricuspid regurgitation. AJR Am J Roentgenol 1991; 156(1):79–83.
2. Henriksson L, Hedman A, Johansson R, Lindstrom K: Ultrasound assessment of liver veins in congestive heart failure. Acta Radiol 1982; 23:361–363.

⁛ CLOSURE OF THE DUCTUS VENOSUS IN NEONATES

■ ACR Code: 959 (Other Veins of Abdomen)

EXAM TIME (days)	PREMATURE (28–32 weeks)		PREMATURE (33–36 weeks)		TERM	
	Open/Total	Cum. Percent	Open/Total	Cum. Percent	Open/Total	Cum. Percent
1–2	27/27	100	101/103	98	73/73	100
6–7	22/26	85	54/95	56	41/60	68
9–10	18/22	69	26/47	31	14/32	30
13–14	11/18	42	11/24	14	7/13	16
17–18	8/11	31	5/9	8	2/3	11
21	7/8	27	0/4	0		
28	4/6	18				

Table 1 ■ Closure of the Ductus Venosus in Neonates

Cum. Percent = cumulative patency rate expressed as percentage of initially scanned subjects.
From Loberant N, Herskovits M, Barak M, et al: AJR Am J Roentgenol 1992; 172:227–229. Used by permission.

Technique ■

Ultrasound of the upper abdomen was done with an SSD-870 machine (Aloka Company, Tokyo, Japan) and a 5.0-MHz sector transducer.[1, 2]

Measurements ■

The ductus venosus was identified within the liver, lying between the portal vein and the hepatic venous confluence in a sagittal orientation. It was mostly visible at gray scale imaging, but in smaller neonates could be identified only with color Doppler. The length and width were measured. Duplex Doppler was done in the midlumen and the angle-corrected (<60 degrees) velocity recorded. The ductus was considered to be closed when the channel was obliterated and there was no demonstrable Doppler flow within it.[1, 2] Table 1 lists numbers of neonates scanned, the number with patent ductus venosus, and the cumulative percentage remaining open during the follow-up intervals. Table 2 lists length, width, and flow velocities of the ductus venosus on the initial (1 to 2 days) scan. In each neonate, the flow velocity gradually decreased from the initial scan until closure.[1, 2]

Source ■

In the first report, 73 healthy term neonates were evaluated at 1 to 2 days after birth and in follow-up (four times) over 18 days after birth.[1] The second study included two groups: 27 premature infants (gestational age range, 28 to 32 weeks, birth weight range, 865 to 1950 grams) and 103 premature infants (gestational age range, 33 to 36 weeks, birth weight range, 1258 to 2825 grams). The premature babies were otherwise healthy, and none underwent umbilical vein catheterization. Initial scans were done 1 to 2 days after delivery in both groups. Follow-up in the first cohort consisted of six additional scans over 28 days and in the second group five more scans over 21 days.[2] In both studies, follow-up was discontinued for that individual once the ductus had closed. As the studies progressed, some infants were lost to follow-up before their ductus had closed, and the investigators corrected for these in the cumulative patency percentage calculations.[1, 2]

PARAMETER	PREMATURE (28–32 weeks) Mean	PREMATURE (33–36 weeks) Mean	TERM Range
Length (mm)	10.5	11.3	11–19
Width (mm)	—	—	1–2
Velocity (cm/sec)	40	40	15–70

Table 2 ■ Size and Flow Velocity in the Ductus Venosus[1, 2]

REFERENCES

1. Loberant N, Barak M, Gaitini D, et al: Closure of the ductus venosus in neonates: Findings on real-time gray-scale, color-flow Doppler, and duplex Doppler sonography. AJR Am J Roentgenol 1992; 159:1083–1085.
2. Loberant N, Herskovits M, Barak M, et al: Closure of the ductus venosus in premature infants: Findings on real-time gray-scale, color-flow Doppler, and duplex Doppler sonography. AJR Am J Roentgenol 1992; 172:227–229.

˙: MEASUREMENT OF RENAL ARTERY SIZE[1]
▪ ACR Code: 961 (Renal Artery)

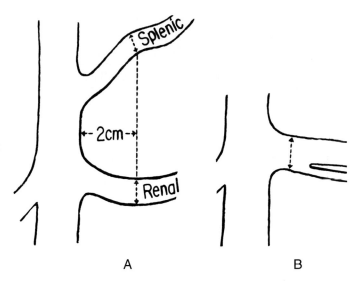

Figure 1 ▪ Measurement of renal and splenic artery diameters (see text for details). (Adapted from Maluf NSR: Surg Gynecol Obstet 1958; 107:415.)

A   B

Table 1 ▪ Internal Diameter of Renal Artery		
	DIAMETER (mm)	SD
Two normal kidneys	6.5–6.7	0.75–0.88
One healthy hypertrophied kidney	8.4–8.6	0.71–0.83

Technique ▪

Central ray: Perpendicular to plane of film centered over the interspace between the first and second lumbar vertebral bodies.
Position: Anteroposterior.
Target-film distance: 32 inches. Measurements are reduced by 10% for distortion.

Measurements ▪ (Figure 1 and Table 1)

1. The renal and splenic arteries are measured where they intersect a line 2 cm from and parallel to the lateral border of the aorta. The measurements are made at right angles to the longitudinal axis of the vessel at the 2-cm intersection.
2. When the renal artery bifurcates at a point closer than 2 cm from the aorta, it is measured proximal to this bifurcation. When a kidney receives more than one artery from the aorta, the equivalent diameter (D) is obtained from the equation:

$$D = 4\sqrt{D_1^4 + D_2^4 + \dots D_n^4}$$

in which D_1 and D_2 are the diameters of two such arteries and D_n the diameter of the nth such artery.

Of greater value is the ratio (see below) of internal diameter of the renal artery to the splenic artery. This is typically greater than unity when the kidney is normal. The ratio rises in renal hypertrophy and falls in renal hypoplasia or reduced renal function. A narrow renal artery always indicates reduced renal function, but an artery of normal caliber does not necessarily imply normal renal function. Normal ratio:

$$\frac{\text{Diameter of renal artery}}{\text{Splenic artery}} = \,>1$$

Source ▪

The data are based on measurements of 18 young patients with normal kidneys, 9 young patients with only one healthy hypertrophied kidney, and 32 patients with unilateral or bilateral renal abnormality.

REFERENCE

1. Maluf NSR: Surg Gynecol Obstet 1958; 107:415.

•: POSITION OF RENAL ARTERY ORIGINS

- ACR Code: 961 (Renal Artery)

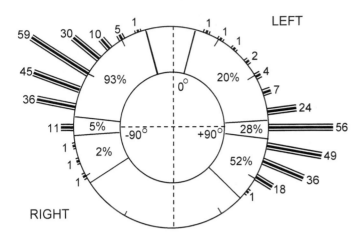

Figure 1 • Location and distribution of the right and left renal arteries in the transverse plane in 200 patients. Numbers of arteries are outside the circle and percentages inside. The radial reference frame is described in the text. (From Verschuyl EJ, Kaatee R, Beek FJ, et al: Radiology 1997; 203:71–75. Used by permission.)

Technique •

Contrast-enhanced spiral CT of the abdomen was performed with a Tomoscan SR 7000 machine (Philips Medical Systems, Eindhoven, Netherlands).[1, 2]

Measurements •

From axial slices through the renal artery origins, the position and profile angle (perpendicular to the orifice) of the right and left renal artery origins were determined. The profile angles were assigned positive or negative values corresponding to angiographic projection with the image intensifier above a supine patient. Thus, a truly lateral vessel would be best imaged with a profile angle of 0 degrees (posteroanterior view), and an anterior vessel such as the celiac artery would be best imaged with a profile angle of 90 degrees (lateral view). Figure 1 shows the location and distribution of the right and left renal arteries in the transverse plane.[1] Table 1 lists various angiographic projections and the percent of origins that would be seen in profile on an angiogram done in that projection.[2]

The profile angle of the right renal artery origin was 24 ± 15 (mean ± SD) degrees, with a range of −26 to −70 degrees, the profile angle of the left renal artery origin was 5 ± 16 degrees, with a range of −75 to −38 degrees.[1]

Source •

CT scans were studied of 200 patients (89 male, 111 female, mean age, 54 years, age range, 12 to 91 years), many of whom had significant atherosclerosis.[1] A second study included 70 patients all having significant atherosclerosis and suspected renal artery stenosis. Many of these were also included in the first study,[1] and they also underwent digital subtraction angiography.[2]

Comments •

Regardless of gender, the 20-degree left anterior oblique (LAO) projection tends to depict the largest number of renal artery origins bilaterally. The right renal origin was best depicted on a 20-degree LAO view, and the next best projection was a 40-degree LAO view. The left renal artery origin was best seen on an AP view, with the next best being a 20-degree LAO. The angle between right and left renal artery origins is greater in females than in males, so a single view is more likely to be successful in females.[2]

Table 1 • Angiographic Projections That Provide the Best Profiles of Renal Artery Origins

PROJECTION	LEFT (%)	RIGHT (%)	LEFT AND/ OR RIGHT (%)
All patients (n = 200)			
20° RAO	16 (8)		8 (4)
AP	94 (47)	32 (16)	62 (31)
20° LAO	78 (39)	100 (50)	90 (45)
40° LAO	8 (4)	58 (29)	32 (16)
60° LAO		10 (5)	
Male patients (n = 89)			
40° RAO	3 (3)		
20° RAO	10 (11)		
AP	47 (53)	8 (9)	28 (31)
20° LAO	25 (28)	50 (56)	38 (43)
40° LAO		27 (30)	13 (15)
60° LAO		5 (6)	
Female patients (n = 111)			
20° RAO	6 (5)		3 (3)
AP	47 (42)	23 (21)	36 (32)
20° LAO	51 (46)	50 (45)	50 (45)
40° LAO	6 (5)	32 (29)	19 (17)
60° LAO		4 (4)	

Percentages in parentheses. RAO = right anterior oblique, LAO = left anterior oblique, AP = anteroposterior.
From Verschuyl EJ, Kaatee R, Beek FJA, et al: Radiology 1997; 205:115–120. Used by permission.

REFERENCES

1. Verschuyl EJ, Kaatee R, Beek FJ, et al: Renal artery origins: Location and distribution in the transverse plane at CT. Radiology 1997; 203:71–75.
2. Verschuyl EJ, Kaatee R, Beek FJ, et al: Renal artery origins: Best angiographic projection angles. Radiology 1997; 205:115–120.

⬝: DETECTION OF NATIVE RENAL ARTERY STENOSIS BY ULTRASOUND
▪ ACR Code: 961 (Renal Artery)

Technique ▪

Ultrasound of the kidneys is performed with real-time sector or curved-array transducers, usually 3.5 MHz. Lower-frequency transducers may be helpful for larger patients, and children and asthenic adults might benefit from higher-frequency probes. Having the patient fast before the examination helps reduce gas. Scanning is done from the lateral and posterolateral aspects of the flanks to minimize the distance to the kidneys. Oblique or decubitus positioning with the side of interest up can help.

The main renal artery (RA) is visualized as best as possible from the aorta to the renal hilum (sometimes scanning from the anterior abdomen may provide the best window). For duplex Doppler analysis, the gate is swept along the course of the artery to find the highest velocity flow. Color Doppler may be helpful to distinguish this area. Angle-corrected duplex sweeps are obtained with the Doppler frequency set to ensure that the peak velocity is within the display and not subject to aliasing.

For intrarenal analysis, smaller arteries (segmental or sometimes interlobar) at the junction of the renal sinus and parenchyma are interrogated. Color Doppler can help find them, though discriminatory features are obtained mainly from duplex velocimetry. Doppler parameters are optimized with small gate, lower-frequency, moderate to high gain, and low wall filter settings to obtain a tracing that fills the display as much as possible. Angle correction is harder to perform in these small arteries and is needed only for calculation of acceleration. A fast sweep speed (2 seconds) helps in measuring acceleration. Usually, three or more regions of each kidney are sampled, and results may be averaged or the most abnormal recorded to enhance sensitivity. Figure 1 depicts the relevant renal arterial anatomy.

To enhance accuracy of the intrarenal arterial features, the examination may be done 1 hour after administration of 25 to 50 mg of captopril (crushed and diluted in a glass of water). Patients with increased creatinine, decreased creatinine clearance, hyperkalemia, or sensitivity to angiotensin-converting enzyme (ACE) inhibitors may not be candidates for captopril. Suggested precautions include intravenous hydration (normal saline, 100 ml/min, for at least 2 hours prior to the study), and frequent blood pressure checks for at least 2 hours after captopril administration.[1, 2]

Measurements ▪

Early investigations of ultrasound to detect renal artery stenosis (RAS) concentrated on the main RA and used the highest (associated with the stenosis itself) peak systolic velocity (PSV) and the ratio of PSV between the RA and aorta. Test performance was disappointing, examination times were long, and technically adequate studies were obtained only in 30% to 40%.[3, 4]

Most recent work has focused on intrarenal segmental arterial analysis, which is technically successful in 98% to 100%.[5, 6] Figure 2 shows typical normal intrarenal waveforms with various intervals and velocities identified. Resistive index (RI) is often reduced in arteries downstream from a stenosis, and Figure 3 depicts measurements needed to calculate it.[6, 7] Probably the most useful intrarenal parameters reflect the phenomenon of pulsus tardus et parvus (delayed and decreased) waveforms downstream from the

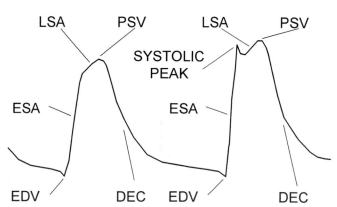

Figure 1 ▪ Renal artery anatomy. Direct measurements (*) relating to the stenosis itself are made from the main renal artery and compared with aortic velocities. Intrarenal measurements are made in segmental (occasionally interlobar) branches at the periphery of the renal sinus.

Figure 2 ▪ Normal intrarenal Doppler signals. The waveform to the right has an early systolic peak (ESP) and the one to the left does not. The general consensus is that both types may be seen in normal subjects. The early systolic acceleration *(ESA)* is between end-diastole *(EDV)* and either the ESP or the inflection point at the beginning of the late systolic acceleration *(LSA)*. The deceleration *(DEC)* and peak systolic velocity *(PSV)* are also shown.

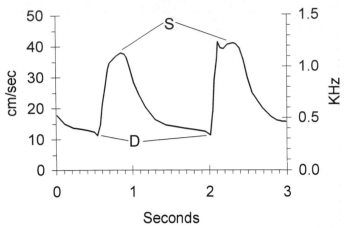

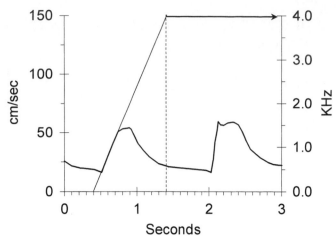

Figure 3 ▪ Measurements for an intrarenal resistive index include peak systolic velocity *(S)* and end-diastolic velocity *(D)*. Peak systolic velocity in the aorta and at the stenosis (Saorta and Smax in Table 1) in the main renal artery have been used as well.

Figure 5 ▪ Measurement of the acceleration index (AI). A line is drawn tangential to the early rapid upstroke and extended for 1 second along the X-axis. The frequency shift *(arrow,* in KHz*)* is divided by transducer frequency (in MHz). The resulting numbers are similar to systolic acceleration (Figure 6). Angle correction is helpful, if possible, to obtain accurate results.

stenosis. This can be characterized qualitatively (Figure 4) or with quantitative parameters relating to the early systolic acceleration (Figures 5 and 6). Numerous studies have dealt with these morphologic and quantitative features of the waveform, with test performances ranging from excellent to poor.[6-11] Table 1 lists the various parameters that have been described, and Table 2 gives cut-off values and test performance (sensitivity/specificity). The lower limits of sensitivity and specificity in the bottom three rows of Table 2 are strongly influenced by Kliewer's[11] data and are otherwise at least above 75%.

Captopril administration causes an increase in vascular

compliance and decreases systemic blood pressure, which leads to exaggeration of the parvus/tardus phenomenon in vessels distal to stenoses.[1, 2, 12] Both Rene and Oliva and their coworkers found significant improvement in sensitivity and specificity of qualitative and quantitative features (less with RI) to diagnose RAS after captopril compared with identical evaluations done without captopril. Both workers concluded that studies done without captopril are adequate for detecting greater than 70% stenoses, whereas the addition of captopril allows more confident diagnosis (or exclusion) of greater than 50% stenoses.[1, 2]

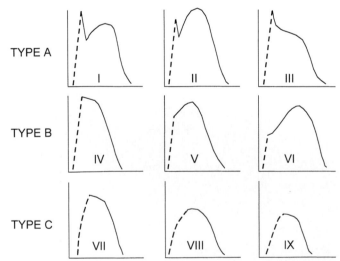

Figure 4 ▪ Morphologic grades of intrarenal arterial Doppler signals. Many systems have fewer grades. The early systolic acceleration is shown with a *dashed line.* Type A exhibits an early systolic peak, Type B does not but still has a rapid acceleration, and Type C is abnormal, showing slowing of the upstroke and varying amounts of decrease in velocity. (From Oliva VL, Soulez G, Lesage D, et al: AJR Am J Roentgenol 1998; 170:169–175. Used by permission.)

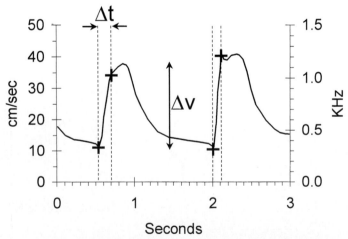

Figure 6 ▪ Early systolic acceleration can be calculated automatically from the operator's console of most newer machines. Cursors (+) are placed at the beginning and end of the early rapid upstroke. The change in velocity *(delta v)* is divided by the time interval *(delta t).* The acceleration time is simply delta t. Angle correction is helpful to obtain accurate results for acceleration and is not needed for acceleration time.

Table 1 ▪ Doppler Parameters for Detecting Renal Artery Stenosis

PARAMETER (Abbreviation)	LOCATION (Fig. 1)	FIGURE	ANGLE CORRECTED	UNITS	FORMULAS
Maximum velocity (PSVmax)	Main (at stenosis)	1, 2	yes	meters/sec	S_{MAX}
Renal aorta ratio (RAR)	Main (at stenosis) and aorta	1, 2	yes	none	$\dfrac{S_{MAX}}{S_{AORTA}}$
Resistive index (RI)	Segmental	3	no	none	$\dfrac{S - D}{S}$
RI difference (ΔRI)	Interlobar	3	no	none	$RI_{HIGH} - RI_{LOW}$
Acceleration index (AI)	Segmental	5	yes	none or sec^{-1}	$\dfrac{\text{freq after 1 sec (KHz)}}{\text{xducer freq (MHz)}}$
Early systolic acceleration (ESA, SA, or A)	Segmental	6	yes	meters/sec^2	$\dfrac{\Delta v}{\Delta t}$
Acceleration time (AT)	Segmental	6	no	seconds	Δt
Waveform analysis	Segmental	4	no	Rating scale score or normal/abnormal	None

Abbreviations in the formulas are as in Figures 1 through 6.

Table 2 ▪ Cut-off Values and Performance of Doppler Parameters in Detecting Renal Artery Stenosis

PARAMETER	CUT-OFF	SENSITIVITY	SPECIFICITY	COMMENTS
Maximum velocity	>1.0	0–70%	37–80%	Technically difficult, may miss stenosis in one of multiple arteries
Renal aorta ratio	>3–3.5	0–70%	37–90%	As above
Resistive index	<0.6–0.7	50–65%	43–72%	Better discrimination after captopril
RI difference	>5–7	77–100%	92–100%	The side with the low RI is abnormal % stenosis = 0.6 × ΔRI + 57.0
Acceleration index	<4	—	—	Excellent discrimination of >75% stenosis in children
Early systolic acceleration	<3–4.7	70–90%	35–83%	<3–3.5 most commonly cited
Acceleration time	>0.07–0.12	57–78%	20–91%	>0.07 most commonly cited
Waveform analysis	Only type C = positive; types B&C positive	46–95%	67–100%	Mostly only type C positive

"Positive" in waveform analysis is diagnostic of stenosis.

REFERENCES

1. Rene PC, Oliva VL, Bui BT, et al: Renal artery stenosis: Evaluation of Doppler US after inhibition of angiotensin-converting enzyme with captopril. Radiology 1995; 196:675–679.
2. Oliva VL, Soulez G, Lesage D, et al: Detection of renal artery stenosis with Doppler sonography before and after administration of captopril: Value of early systolic rise. AJR Am J Roentgenol 1998; 170:169–175.
3. Berland LL, Koslin DB, Routh WD, Keller FS: Renal artery stenosis: Prospective evaluation of diagnosis with color duplex US compared with angiography. Radiology 1990; 174:421–423.
4. Desberg AL, Paushter DM, Lammert GK, et al: Renal artery stenosis: Evaluation with color Doppler flow imaging. Radiology 1990; 177:749–753.
5. Schoenberg SO, Knopp MV, Bock M, et al: Renal artery stenosis: Grading of hemodynamic changes with cine phase-contrast MR blood flow measurements. Radiology 1997; 203:45–53.
6. Handa N, Fukanaga R, Etani H, et al: Efficacy of echo-Doppler examination for the evaluation of renovascular disease. Ultrasound Med Biol 1988; 14:1–5.
7. Patriquin HB, Lafortune M, Jequier J, et al: Stenosis of the renal artery: Assessment of slowed systole in the downstream circulation with Doppler sonography. Radiology 1992; 184:479–485.
8. Lafortune M, Patriquin H, Demeule E, et al: Renal arterial stenosis; Slowed systole in the downstream circulation: Experimental study in dogs. Radiology 1992; 184:475–487.
9. Halpern EJ, Needleman L, Nack TL, East SA: Renal artery stenosis: Should we study the main renal artery or segmental vessels? Radiology 1995; 195:799–804.
10. Stavros AT, Parker SH, Yakes WF, et al: Segmental stenosis of the renal artery: Pattern recognition of tardus and parvus abnormalities with duplex sonography. Radiology 1992; 184:487–492.
11. Kliewer MA, Tupler RH, Carrol BA, et al: Renal artery stenosis: Analysis of Doppler waveform parameters and tardus-parvus pattern. Radiology 1993; 189:779–787.
12. Bude RO, Rubin JM: Detection of renal artery stenosis with Doppler sonography: It is more complicated than originally thought. Radiology 1995; 196:612–613.

▪: DIMENSIONS OF THE INFRARENAL INFERIOR VENA CAVA
▪ ACR Code: 982 (Inferior Vena Cava)

Technique ▪

Ultrasound of the inferior vena cava was done with several machines and 3.5- to 5.0-MHz mechanical and phased-array sector transducers. Patients were examined supine in quiet respiration, during breathholding after deep inspiration, and during leg raising to produce Valsalva physiology.[1]

Measurements ▪

The long and short axis diameters of the inferior vena cava (IVC) were measured about 1 cm below the level of the left renal vein from transverse images.[1] A single diameter was calculated by arithmetic mean, geometric mean, or a formula based on the Ramanujan method for estimating the perimeter of an ellipse.[2] Using the results of all three equations (which gave similar results), the mean IVC diameters were 17.2 mm (range, 5.1 to 28.9 mm) during quiet breathing, 17.6 mm (range, 9.7 to 31 mm) during leg lifting, and 18.8 mm (range, 7.7 to 31.3 mm) during breathholding. In the whole population there was an average 9.3% increase of the diameter during breathholding compared with quiet respiration (p <.001) and leg lifting (p <.005). In one of four of the patients, there was a larger change with breathholding (mean increase, 3.5 mm, range, 0.5 to 7.4 mm). The calculated diameter was greater than 28 mm in 2% during quiet breathing, 5% during breathholding, and 5.6% during quiet breathing or breathholding. There was a modest tendency toward increasing IVC diameter with advancing age (r = 0.20, p =.0027 in quiet respiration and r = 0.31, p =.0012 with breathholding) and no significant correlation with gender, height, or weight.[1]

The midinfrarenal IVC diameter at cavography had an average value of 21.3 mm (range, 10 to 31 mm), and the mean length (confluence to renal veins) was 9.6 cm (range, 8 to 14.2 cm).[3] Grant and colleagues studied qualitative changes in IVC size during various respiratory maneuvers and found that it got larger during breathholding and smaller during inspiration and Valsalva.[4]

Source ▪

A total of 156 patients with no history of cardiac disease, compressing abdominopelvic masses, or lower extremity deep venous thrombosis was initially evaluated. In 48 (31%) the IVC was not seen well enough to measure. Measurements for the remaining 108 (32 men, 76 women, mean age, 45.2 years, age range, 19 to 87 years) were reported.[1]

Comments ▪

These findings may have application in assessment of patients needing vena cava filter placement. However, the IVC was obscured and unmeasurable by ultrasound in one third of the patients examined by Sykes and colleagues.[1] The simple arithmetic mean ([long axis + short axis]/2) of diameters is probably sufficient for most purposes as it gives values that are at most 6% lower than the other two equations.

REFERENCES

1. Sykes AM, McLoughlin RF, So CB, et al: Sonographic assessment of infrarenal inferior vena caval dimensions. J Ultrasound Med 1995; 14(9):665–668.
2. Birnholz JC: On calculating the perimeter of an ellipse. J Clin Ultrasound 1984; 12:55–56.
3. Bonnichon P, Guardard F, Ouakil E, et al: Biometry of infrarenal inferior vena cava measured by cavography: Clinical applications. Surg Radiol Anat 1989; 11:149–154.
4. Grant E, Rendano F, Levine E, et al: Normal inferior vena cava: Caliber changes observed by dynamic ultrasound. AJR Am J Roentgenol 1990; 135:335–338.

⁘ MEASUREMENT OF THE ABDOMINAL AORTA
- ACR Code: 981 (Abdominal Aorta)

In Children[1] •

Technique

Central ray: Perpendicular to plane of film.
Position: Anteroposterior.
Target-film distance: 40 inches.

Measurements (Figure 1)

Aortic diameter was measured in three sites. Site A is at the level of the pedicles of the 11th thoracic vertebra, Site B just above the renal arteries, and Site C at the aortic bifurcation. The renal arteries were measured between 1 and 2 cm from their aortic origin. Renal lengths were measured from the nephrographic phase of the arteriograms. The measurements were correlated with body surface areas from the known height and weight of the patients. Results are shown in Figures 2 and 3.

Source

Data are derived from aortograms of 45 patients, ranging in age from 1 day to 15 years.

In Adults[2] •

Technique

Central ray: Perpendicular to plane of film centered over midabdomen.
Position: Anteroposterior.
Target-film distance: 48 inches.

Measurements (Figure 4)

Measurements were made at the following sites:

1. The 11th rib, the level where the aorta pierces the diaphragm.

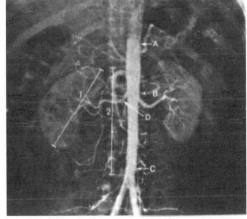

Figure 1 ▪ Measurements obtained from abdominal aortograms. *A* = aortic diameter at the level of the pedicles of the eleventh thoracic vertebra; *B* = aortic diameter at the level of renal arteries; *C* = aortic diameter at bifurcation; *D* = diameter of renal artery; *1* = renal length at greatest longitudinal axis; *2* = distance between the first and fourth lumbar vertebrae. (From Taber P, et al: Radiology 1972; 102:129. Used by permission.)

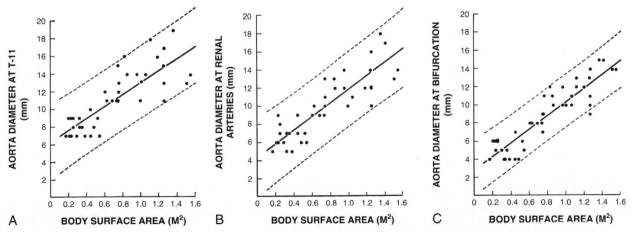

Figure 2 ▪ Aortic diameter related to body surface area. *A*, At eleventh thoracic vertebra. *B*, At renal arteries. *C*, At aortic bifurcation. The *dotted lines* represent the 95% confidence limits of the regression curve. (From Taber P, et al: Radiology 1972; 102:129. Used by permission.)

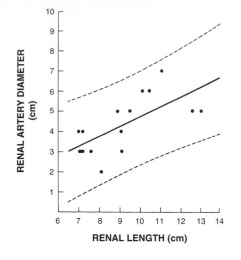

Figure 3 ▪ Diameter of the renal artery related to ipsilateral kidney length. (From Taber P, et al: Radiology 1972; 102:129. Used by permission.)

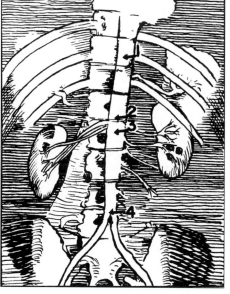

Figure 4 ▪ Measurement of the abdominal aorta in adults (see text for details). (From Steinberg CR, et al: AJR 1965; 95:703. Used by permission.)

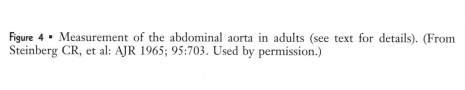

Table 1 ▪ Average Age and Diameter (in mm) of the Abdominal Aorta at Sites Measured

GENDER AND DIAGNOSIS	NO. OF CASES	AGE	AT 11TH RIB	ABOVE RENAL ARTERIES	BELOW RENAL ARTERIES	AT BIFURCATION OF AORTA	DIFFERENCE BETWEEN 11TH RIB AND BIFURCATION OF AORTA
Male							
Normal	29	53.9±13.7	26.9±3.96	23.9±3.92	21.4±3.65	18.7±3.34	8.14±2.14
Hypertensive	49	48.6±15.1	27.7±4.62	24.5±4.43	21.3±4.37	19.5±3.08	8.16±3.70
Occlusive	109	56.8±9.9	27.2±3.42	23.6±3.29	20.5±3.30	18.2±3.68	9.08±3.72
Abdominal aneurysm	90	63.6±7.1	33.5±6.05	31.2±8.36	34.3±12.56	31.8±10.53	1.76±10.23
Female							
Normal	44	56.9±14.3	24.4±3.45	21.6±3.16	18.7±3.36	17.5±2.52	6.80±4.54
Hypertensive	45	53.8±13.0	25.6±2.85	21.7±3.02	19.5±3.29	17.5±2.92	8.09±2.22
Occlusive	48	57.0±8.5	24.7±2.96	20.7±2.71	17.6±2.74	15.7±3.02	8.92±3.48
Abdominal aneurysm	18	67.2±7.3	30.5±6.05	28.5±6.94	32.2±14.00	25.4±6.21	5.05±6.40

From Steinberg CR, et al: AJR Am J Roentgenol 1965; 95:703. Used by permission.

2. Above the renal arteries, at a site that is almost at one half the length of the abdominal aorta and is below the celiac axis.
3. Below the renal arteries.
4. At the bifurcation of the abdominal aorta.

The values for male and female normal subjects, hypertensive patients, and patients with occlusive arterial disease and abdominal aneurysms are given in Table 1. Hypertension and thrombotic occlusive disease do not alter the mean diameter. In arteriosclerotic aneurysmal disease, there is enlargement of the aorta at each site, suggesting that aortic dilatation is a significant accompaniment of the aneurysm.

Source

Measurements are based on a study of 500 consecutive patients referred for intravenous abdominal aortography.

REFERENCES

1. Taber P, Korobkin MT, Gooding CA, et al: Growth of the abdominal aorta and renal arteries in childhood. Radiology 1972; 102:129–134.
2. Steinberg CR, Archer M, Steinberg I: Measurement of the abdominal aorta after intravenous aortography in health and arteriosclerotic peripheral vascular disease. AJR Am J Roentgenol 1965; 95:703–708.

▪: MEASUREMENT OF THE ABDOMINAL AORTA BY CT (ALSO APPLICABLE TO ULTRASONOGRAPHY)[1]

▪ ACR Code: 981 (Abdominal Aorta)

Technique ▪

1. Studies were performed on a Siemens Somatom 2 CT system.
2. Images were obtained:
   a. Immediately caudal to the origin of the superior mesenteric artery.
   b. Approximately midway between the superior mesenteric artery and the bifurcation.
   c. Immediately cranial to the bifurcation.

Measurements ▪ (Figure 1)

An average aortic diameter is calculated by taking the mean of the three measurements.

The mean "aortic diameters" are shown in Figure 2.

The aortic diameter increases with advancing age. In women, the diameter varies from 12.3 mm in the second decade to 16.9 mm in the sixth decade. In men, the diameter increases from 12.2 mm in the second decade to 22.8 mm in the sixth decade. An aortic diameter greater than 30 mm on ultrasound is considered abnormal.[2]

Note: Studies correlating measurements obtained on cross-table lateral radiographs, made at a 40-inch tube-to-

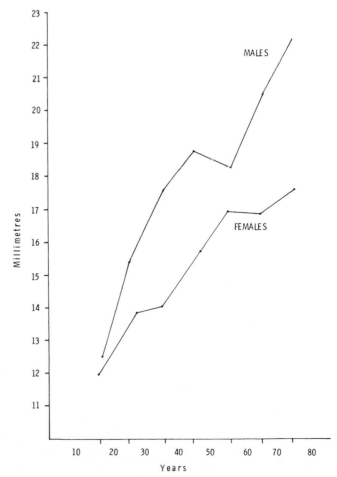

Figure 1 ▪ Normal aorta shown by CT: no calcification. Electronic calipers traverse the aorta to give measurement of diameter of 20 mm *(L + 41)*. (From Dixon AK, et al: Clin Radiol 1984; 35:33–37. Used by permission.)

Figure 2 ▪ Graph of mean "aortic diameter" in males and females of each group plotted against age. (From Dixon AK, et al: Clin Radiol 1984; 35:33–37. Used by permission.)

film distance, are larger than sonographic measurements by a factor of 1.3.[3]

Source ▪

Data are based on CT examinations of 257 patients with a variety of clinical problems but without suspected aortic disease. Patient ages ranged from the second to eighth decade.

References

1. Dixon AK, Lawrence JP, Mitchell RA: Age-related changes in the abdominal aorta shown by computed tomography. Clin Radiol 1984; 35:33–37.
2. Sarti DA: Diagnostic Ultrasound: Text and Cases, 2nd ed. Year Book Medical Publishers, Chicago, 1987, p 284.
3. Hardy DC, Lu JK, Weyman PJ, Nelson GL: Measurement of the abdominal aortic aneurysm. Plain radiographic and ultrasonographic correlation. Radiology 1981; 141:821–823.

▪: DIAMETER OF AORTA AND ILIAC AND FEMORAL ARTERIES AT CT
▪ ACR Code: 981 (Abdominal Aorta)

Technique ▪

Computed tomography of the abdomen and pelvis were done with a 9800 scanner (General Electric, Milwaukee, WI) with 10-mm-slice thickness, mostly during intravenous iodinated contrast administration.[1]

Measurements ▪

Maximal vessel diameter of the aorta (three levels), each common iliac artery, and each common femoral artery were measured from hard copy images with calipers calibrated to the distance scale on the films. Figure 1 shows measure-

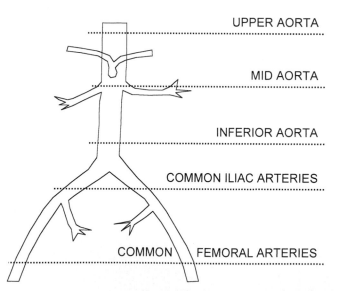

Figure 1 ▪ Locations of slices from which measurements of the aorta, iliac, and femoral arterial diameters were made.

DECADE (n = 26 each) MEAN AGE (yr)	4th 34	5th 45	6th 55	7th 66	8th 75
Upper aorta	2.07 ± 0.21	2.15 ± 0.24	2.41 ± 0.32	2.50 ± 0.24	2.72 ± 0.35
Midaorta	1.75 ± 0.02	1.80 ± 0.25	1.99 ± 0.30	2.00 ± 0.21	2.10 ± 0.20
Lower aorta	1.60 ± 0.17	1.69 ± 0.23	1.77 ± 0.33	1.84 ± 0.23	1.96 ± 0.21
R common iliac	1.04 ± 0.17	1.06 ± 0.19	1.17 ± 0.20	1.23 ± 0.20	1.30 ± 0.19
L common iliac	1.04 ± 0.17	1.06 ± 0.19	1.17 ± 0.20	1.22 ± 0.20	1.30 ± 0.19
R common femoral	0.96 ± 0.13	0.96 ± 0.16	1.05 ± 0.17	1.12 ± 0.20	1.20 ± 0.18
L common femoral	0.97 ± 0.14	0.95 ± 0.16	1.04 ± 0.17	1.11 ± 0.20	1.20 ± 0.18

Table 1 ▪ Diameters of Aorta and Iliac, and Femoral Arteries with CT in Men

Measurements are in centimeters (mean ± standard deviation). R = right, L = left.
From Horejs D, Gilbert PM, Burstein S, Vogelzang RL: J Comput Assist Tomogr 1988; 12:602–603. Used by permission.

Table 2 ▪ Diameter of Aorta and Iliac, and Femoral Arteries with CT in Women

DECADE (n = 26 Each) MEAN AGE (yr)	4th 35	5th 45	6th 55	7th 65	8th 74
Upper aorta	1.91 ± 0.22	1.96 ± 0.25	2.10 ± 0.27	2.31 ± 0.27	2.18 ± 0.26
Midaorta	1.53 ± 0.22	1.58 ± 0.22	1.66 ± 0.22	1.78 ± 0.23	1.75 ± 0.29
Lower aorta	1.43 ± 0.15	1.50 ± 0.18	1.47 ± 0.21	1.59 ± 0.23	1.62 ± 0.26
R common iliac	0.95 ± 0.14	0.98 ± 0.18	0.97 ± 0.19	1.03 ± 0.15	1.10 ± 0.21
L common iliac	0.95 ± 0.14	0.98 ± 0.18	0.97 ± 0.19	1.02 ± 0.15	1.10 ± 0.21
R common femoral	0.81 ± 0.11	0.83 ± 0.13	0.78 ± 0.11	0.85 ± 0.07	0.92 ± 0.12
L common femoral	0.97 ± 0.14	0.82 ± 0.13	0.78 ± 0.11	0.85 ± 0.07	0.92 ± 0.12

Measurements are in centimeters (mean ± standard deviation). R = right, L = left.
From Horejs D, Gilbert PM, Burstein S, Vogelzang RL: J Comput Assist Tomogr 1988; 12:602–603. Used by permission.

ment locations, Table 1 lists measurements for men, and Table 2 lists measurements for women.[1]

Source ▪

Measurements were made from CT scans of 260 patients (180 men, 180 women, n = 26 in each decade from 30 to 80 years) who were examined for nonvascular complaints or history.[1]

REFERENCE

1. Horejs D, Gilbert PM, Burstein S, Vogelzang RL: Normal aortoiliac diameters by CT. J Comput Assist Tomogr 1988; 12:602–603.

▪: CHANGE IN AORTIC DIAMETER AT ULTRASOUND WITH AGE
▪ ACR Code: 981 (Abdominal Aorta)

Technique ▪

Ultrasound of the aorta was done with a 150S portable unit (Pie Data Ltd., United Kingdom), with a 3.5-MHz mechanical annular array sector transducer.[1]

Measurements ▪

The abdominal aorta was examined in longitudinal and transverse planes. Measurements of the anteroposterior (AP) diameter of the vessel were taken from frozen transverse images perpendicular to the long axis made from the renal artery origins to the bifurcation. The largest measurement was recorded.[1] Data analysis included calculation of median and 8 percentile values (including 75%, 87.5%, 93.75%, 96.875% above the median) for each age from 60 to 75 years. Robust regression of the 93.75 percentile against age was used to produce suggested cut-off values. Figure 1 shows cumulative percentage of subjects versus diameter at 60, 65, 70, and 75 years. Table 1 lists the median, the upper two percentiles (labeled 94th and 97th), percentage measuring 40 mm or more, and suggested cut-off values by age.[1]

Source ▪

A total of 13,000 men in general medical practices in the United Kingdom were invited to participate in the study, of whom 10,061 (76%) accepted. The aorta was adequately visualized and measured in 9771 cases, which form the basis for the data.[1]

Comments ▪

In the whole study population, 7.2% had measurements of 30 mm or more, and 2.3% measured 40 mm or more. The

Figure 1 ▪ Cumulative percentiles of anteroposterior diameter of the infrarenal aorta in men aged 60, 65, 70, and 75 years. Note how the curves below the median remain the same, whereas there is greater skewing in the upper percentiles with advancing age.[1]

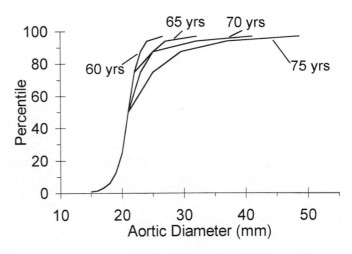

Table 1 ▪ Infrarenal Aorta Anteroposterior Diameters in Men Aged 60 to 75 Years

AGE (yr)	MEDIAN & PERCENTILE VALUES (mm)			% ABOVE 40 mm	SUGGESTED CUT-OFF (mm)
	Median	94th	97th		
60	21.0	24.0	26.5	0.6	>25.0
61	21.0	26.0	29.0	1.4	>25.5
62	21.0	27.0	30.0	0.8	>26.0
63	21.0	27.5	33.0	1.7	>27.0
64	21.0	28.0	31.0	2.0	>27.5
65	21.0	27.0	32.0	1.1	>28.0
66	21.0	27.0	33.5	1.4	>29.0
67	21.0	30.0	35.0	2.8	>30.0
68	21.0	35.0	41.0	3.4	>30.5
69	21.0	30.0	39.5	3.1	>31.0
70	21.0	32.0	41.0	3.5	>32.0
71	21.0	33.5	41.0	3.2	>32.5
72	21.0	32.0	40.0	3.4	>33.0
73	21.0	32.0	40.0	3.6	>34.0
74	21.0	35.0	47.0	4.6	>35.0
75	21.0	37.0	48.5	5.7	>35.5

From Grimshaw G, Thompson J: J Clin Ultrasound 1997; 25:7–13. Used by permission.

median value (21 mm) and the distribution of measurements below the median remained stable with increasing age, whereas the distribution of measurements above the median became increasingly skewed with advancing age. Grimshaw and Thompson were unable to determine whether younger subjects with wider aortic diameters went on to develop aneurysms in this cross-sectional study. They suggest that upper limits of normal may need to be adjusted upward in older men to avoid the expense of serial follow-up in too many otherwise healthy patients.[1]

REFERENCE

1. Grimshaw G, Thompson J: Changes in diameter of the abdominal aorta with age: An epidemiological study. J Clin Ultrasound 1997; 25:7–13.

▪: SIZE OF THE TERMINAL THORACIC DUCT
▪ ACR Code: 995 (Thoracic Duct, Cisterna Chyli)

Technique ▪

Real-time ultrasound of the left side of the neck was done with 3.5- to 5.0-MHz curved-array transducers. Patients were fasting and supine and had the neck slightly hyperextended.[1]

Measurements ▪

Scanning was done to locate a vessel draining into the left internal jugular or subclavian vein near the confluence that had no detectable flow at color Doppler interrogation. From frozen images depicting the terminus of this vessel (the thoracic duct) into the vein, its maximum internal diameter was measured with electronic calipers at 3 to 10 mm from the vein. The duct was seen well enough to measure in 78% to 79% of subjects. Figure 1 shows the scanning and measurement technique. The duct measured 1.9 ± 0.5 mm in healthy subjects and 3.1 ± 1.2 mm in those with portal hypertension. There was a positive correlation between duct diameter and age in the healthy subjects (r squared = 0.388, p <.05), ranging from just over 1.0 mm at 20 years to about 2.5 mm at 80 years (estimated from a graph). There was no significant change in duct diameter with age in the cirrhotic patients nor was there any relationship between duct size and Child class. Table 1 lists sensitivity and specificity for different duct sizes in detecting portal hypertension.[1]

Source ▪

Subjects included 23 healthy volunteers and 24 patients with history, clinical evidence (including liver biopsy in 20), and imaging findings of cirrhosis of the liver complicated

Table 1 ▪ Performance of Thoracic Duct Diameter in Predicting Portal Hypertension

THORACIC DUCT DIAMETER (mm)	SENSITIVITY (%)	SPECIFICITY (%)
1.5	95	22
2.0	79	55
2.5	68	88
3.0	38	94
3.5	26	100

From Zironi G, Cavalli G, Casali A, et al: AJR Am J Roentgenol 1995; 165:863–866. Used by permission.

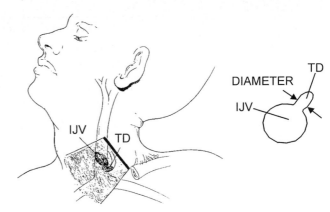

Figure 1 ▪ Technique of measuring the terminal thoracic duct *(TD)* diameter. Scanning of the lower left neck to locate the confluence of the thoracic duct at or near the confluence of the left internal jugular *(IJV)* and subclavian veins is depicted on the right. Measurement of the terminal duct diameter is shown on the left. (From Zironi G, Cavalli G, Casali A, et al: AJR Am J Roentgenol 1995; 165:863–866. Used by permission.)

by portal hypertension. Correlation of thoracic duct diameter was done with age, as well as Child classification[2] and Beppu's endoscopic scores[3] when available.[1]

Comments ▪

The flow rate in the thoracic duct has been shown to be between 14 and 110 ml/hr in normal subjects[4] and can be as high as 720 ml/hr in patients with cirrhosis.[5] The velocity of flow in the normal thoracic duct may be estimated (assuming a diameter range of 2 to 7 mm) to be 0.4 to 6.0 cm/sec.[6] This slow rate is not expected to be detectable with current Doppler ultrasound equipment.[1]

REFERENCES

1. Zironi G, Cavalli G, Casali A, et al: Sonographic assessment of the distal end of the thoracic duct in healthy volunteers and in patients with portal hypertension. AJR Am J Roentgenol 1995; 165:863–866.
2. Pugh RNH, Murray-Lyon IM, Dawson JL, et al: Transection of the esophagus for bleeding esophageal varices. Br J Surg 1973; 60:646–649.
3. Japanese Research Society for Portal Hypertension: The general rules for recording endoscopic findings on esophageal varices. Jpn J Surg 1980; 10:84–93.
4. Ross KJ: A review of surgery of the thoracic duct. Thorax 1961; 16:12–21.
5. Dumont AE, Mulholand JH: Alterations in thoracic duct lymph flow in hepatic cirrhosis: Significance in portal hypertension. Ann Surg 1962; 156:668–677.
6. Rosenberger A, Abrams HL: Radiology of the thoracic duct. AJR Am J Roentgenol 1971; 111:807–820.

▪▪ NONFATTY AXILLARY NODES ON MAMMOGRAMS
▪ ACR Code: 997 (Supraclavicular, Cervical, and Axillary Nodes)

Technique ▪

Film-screen mammography was done in routine clinical practice for screening or diagnostic purposes on several machines.[1]

Measurements ▪

The largest diameter of the largest nonfatty node was measured from the source mammograms. The anatomic distribution (unilateral versus bilateral), nodal border characteristics, and presence of intranodal calcifications were noted. Table 1 lists the findings grouped by nodal pathology. Table 2 gives odds ratios for malignancy at various nodal size cut-offs (1).

Source ▪

From a database of 33,031 mammograms, 174 (0.53%) with reported axillary findings were selected for review.

Table 1 ▪ Clinical, Pathologic, and Mammographic Findings in Patients with Axillary Adenopathy

NODAL DIAGNOSIS	AGE RANGE	NO.	PROOF PATH/CLIN	DISTRIBUTION UNILAT/BILAT	SIZE (mm) MEAN (Range)
Nonspecific benign lymphadenopathy	31–75	22	6/16	17/5	18.7 (12–32)
Metastatic breast cancer	35–90	20	15/5	20/0	28.3 (12–65)
Chronic lymphocytic leukemia, small (well-differentiated) (lymphocytic lymphoma)	51–79	13	13/0	1/12	38.5 (16–85)
Collagen vascular disease	29–71	6	1/5	2/4	24.3 (20–33)
Miscellaneous lymphadenopathy	38–61	6	2/4	4/2	26.3 (17–40)
Lymphoma (other than well-differentiated) (lymphocytic lymphoma)	46–78	3	3/0	1/2	19.3 (14–24)
Metastases, nonbreast primary site	42–66	3	2/1	3/0	40.0 (18–63)
Metastases, unknown primary site	59–72	3	3/0	3/0	27.3 (18–32)

Path = pathologic, Clin = clinical, Unilat = unilateral, Bilat = bilateral.
From Walsh R, Kornguth PJ, Soo MS, et al: AJR Am J Roentgenol 1997; 168:33–38. Used by permission.

Table 2 ▪ Odds Ratios for Malignancy for Size of
Nonfatty Axillary Nodes

LENGTH OF NODE (mm)	ODDS RATIO FOR MALIGNANCY	95% CI OF ODDS RATIO
20	1.00	1.00–1.00
30	2.44	1.31–4.53
40	5.93	1.72–20.50
50	14.44	2.25–92.80
60	35.16	2.94–419.89
70	85.63	3.86–1900.74
80	208.51	5.05–8604.15

CI = confidence interval.
From Walsh R, Kornguth PJ, Soo MS, et al: AJR Am J Roentgenol 1997;
168:33–38. Used by permission.

From these, 94 (0.28%) with nonfatty axillary lymph nodes that had adequate pathologic correlation (n = 52) or clinical follow-up (n = 42) were included in the subsequent analysis. The clinical follow-up interval ranged from 5 to 48 months.[1]

Comments ▪

Using nodal size greater than 33 mm as test-positive yielded a sensitivity of 31% and specificity of 97% for malignancy. With size greater than 15 mm as test-positive, sensitivity was 95% and specificity was 26% for malignancy. Ill-defined or spiculated margins were found in 9 of 42 cases with nodal malignancy and 2 of 34 cases with benign nodes. Intranodal calcifications were seen only twice, and both were in metastatic nodes from breast cancer. Walsh and colleagues state that normal axillary lymph nodes on mammograms are typically less than 15 mm in size, though when fat-infiltrated they may measure up to several centimeters in length. In general, homogeneously dense (nonfatty) axillary lymph nodes were strongly associated with malignancy when they were longer than 33 mm, had ill-defined or spiculated margins, or contained microcalcifications.[1]

REFERENCE

1. Walsh R, Kornguth PJ, Soo MS, et al: Axillary lymph nodes: Mammographic, pathologic, and clinical correlation. AJR Am J Roentgenol 1997; 168:33–38.

▪: SIZE OF NORMAL ABDOMINAL AND PELVIC LYMPH NODES
▪ ACR Code: 998 (Abdominal and Pelvic Nodes)

Technique ▪

Dorfman and colleagues performed dynamic contrast-enhanced computed tomography with GE 9800 (General Electric, Milwaukee, WI) or 1200 SX (Picker, Highland Heights, OH) machines. Contrast (150 ml, 182 mg/ml) was given as a bolus, and 10-mm contiguous slices were made through the abdomen.[1] Vinnicombe and colleagues performed abdominopelvic CT (scanner model and technique not given). CT scans were performed both before and after bipedal lymphangiography.[2]

Measurements ▪

In both studies the maximal short axis diameter (MSAD) of individual lymph nodes in each identified node-bearing area was measured from appropriate CT slices windowed at soft tissue settings. The number of patients having visible nodes in each area was noted and reported as well.[1, 2] Dorfman and colleagues used a nonparametric tolerance interval method on node size and histogram analysis to determine upper limits of normal nodal size.[1, 3, 4] Mean and standard deviation MSAD were also reported. Vinnicombe and colleagues also used nonparametric methods to determine median and percentile values for MSAD.[2] Table 1 lists the number of normal nodes seen in each area, observed MSAD (mean ± SD or median), and upper limits of normal or upper percentiles of MSAD.[1, 2]

Source ▪

Dorfman and group studied 130 patients scanned for blunt abdominal trauma with no other pertinent medical history (85 men, 45 women, age range, 16 to 90 years).[1] Vinnicombe and group evaluated 40 men with stage I germ cell tumors of the testes for staging. No patients had stage II or higher disease, and none had pelvic adenopathy during 5- to 7-year follow-up after the initial scans. Other exclusion criteria included chemo- or radiation therapy and incidental pelvic disease.[2]

Comments ▪

CT scans done after lymphangiography revealed more nodes (total number in 40 patients was 1801 after lymphangiography versus 187 before) with larger MSAD (99th percentile range = 9.4 to 12 mm after lymphangiography versus 7.4 to 8 mm before).

Table 1 ▪ Number and Maximal Short Axis Diameters of Normal Abdominal and Pelvic Lymph Nodes

REFERENCE/ ANATOMIC SITE	PATIENTS WITH NODES/TOTAL (%)	DIAMETER (mean ± SD)	UPPER LIMIT BY TOL. INT.	UPPER LIMIT BY HISTOGRAM
Dorfman				
Paracardiac	33/130 (25)	3.9±0.2	6.8	8.0
Retrocrural space	64/130 (49)	3.0±0.1	5.0	6.0
Gastrohepatic ligament	25/130 (19)	4.1±0.3	6.8	8.0
Upper para-aortic (celiac to renal)	58/130 (45)	3.7±0.2	7.0	9.0
Lower para-aortic (renal to bifurcation)	130/130 (100)	3.4±0.1	10.0	11.0
Porta hepatis	13/130 (10)	3.2±0.4	6.0	7.0
Portacaval space	30/130 (23)	5.3±0.4	8.0	10.0

		DIAMETER (Median)	95th PERCENTILE	99th PERCENTILE
Vinnicombe				
Common iliac	18/40 (45)	3	6.5	8
External iliac	13/40 (33)	3	6	7.4
Obturator	10/40 (25)	3	5.1	6
Internal iliac	6/40 (15)	3	4	4

All measurements are in millimeters. SD = standard deviation, Tol. Int. = tolerance interval.[1, 2]

REFERENCES

1. Dorfman RE, Alpern MB, Gross BH, Sandler MA: Upper abdominal lymph nodes: Criteria for normal size determined with CT [see comments]. Radiology 1991; 180(2):319–322.
2. Vinnicombe SJ, Norman AR, Nicolson V, Husband JE.: Normal pelvic lymph nodes: Evaluation with CT after bipedal lymphangiography. Radiology 1995; 194:349–355.
3. Glazer GM, Gross BH, Quint LE, et al: Normal mediastinal lymph nodes: Number and size according to American Thoracic Society mapping. AJR Am J Roentgenol 1985; 144:261–265.
4. Reed AH, Henry RJ, Mason WB: Influence of statistical method used on the resulting estimate of normal range. Clin Chem 1971; 17:275–284.

Index

■

Note: Page numbers in *italics* refer to illustrations; page numbers followed by t refer to tables.

ISBN 0-323-00161-0